MOLECULAR IMAGING
OF THE LUNGS

LUNG BIOLOGY IN HEALTH AND DISEASE

Executive Editor

Claude Lenfant

Former Director, National Heart, Lung, and Blood Institute
National Institutes of Health
Bethesda, Maryland

1. Immunologic and Infectious Reactions in the Lung, *edited by C. H. Kirkpatrick and H. Y. Reynolds*
2. The Biochemical Basis of Pulmonary Function, *edited by R. G. Crystal*
3. Bioengineering Aspects of the Lung, *edited by J. B. West*
4. Metabolic Functions of the Lung, *edited by Y. S. Bakhle and J. R. Vane*
5. Respiratory Defense Mechanisms (in two parts), *edited by J. D. Brain, D. F. Proctor, and L. M. Reid*
6. Development of the Lung, *edited by W. A. Hodson*
7. Lung Water and Solute Exchange, *edited by N. C. Staub*
8. Extrapulmonary Manifestations of Respiratory Disease, *edited by E. D. Robin*
9. Chronic Obstructive Pulmonary Disease, *edited by T. L. Petty*
10. Pathogenesis and Therapy of Lung Cancer, *edited by C. C. Harris*
11. Genetic Determinants of Pulmonary Disease, *edited by S. D. Litwin*
12. The Lung in the Transition Between Health and Disease, *edited by P. T. Macklem and S. Permutt*
13. Evolution of Respiratory Processes: A Comparative Approach, *edited by S. C. Wood and C. Lenfant*
14. Pulmonary Vascular Diseases, *edited by K. M. Moser*
15. Physiology and Pharmacology of the Airways, *edited by J. A. Nadel*
16. Diagnostic Techniques in Pulmonary Disease (in two parts), *edited by M. A. Sackner*
17. Regulation of Breathing (in two parts), *edited by T. F. Hornbein*
18. Occupational Lung Diseases: Research Approaches and Methods, *edited by H. Weill and M. Turner-Warwick*
19. Immunopharmacology of the Lung, *edited by H. H. Newball*
20. Sarcoidosis and Other Granulomatous Diseases of the Lung, *edited by B. L. Fanburg*

The opinions expressed in these volumes do not necessarily represent the views of the National Institutes of Health.

MOLECULAR IMAGING OF THE LUNGS

Edited by

Daniel P. Schuster
Washington University
St. Louis, Missouri, U.S.A.

Timothy S. Blackwell
Vanderbilt University
Nashville, Tennessee, U.S.A.

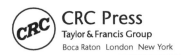

CRC Press
Taylor & Francis Group
Boca Raton London New York

CRC Press is an imprint of the
Taylor & Francis Group, an **informa** business

CRC Press
Taylor & Francis Group
6000 Broken Sound Parkway NW, Suite 300
Boca Raton, FL 33487-2742

First issued in paperback 2019

© 2010 by Taylor & Francis Group, LLC
CRC Press is an imprint of Taylor & Francis Group, an Informa business

No claim to original U.S. Government works

ISBN-13: 978-1-57444-854-2 (hbk)
ISBN-13: 978-0-367-39281-9 (pbk)

A CIP record for this book is available from the British Library.

Library of Congress Cataloging-in-Publication Data available on application

**Visit the Taylor & Francis Web site at
http://www.taylorandfrancis.com**

**and the CRC Press Web site at
http://www.crcpress.com**

Introduction

Since the middle of the past century, we have witnessed an explosion of knowledge in many fields that has served medicine exceptionally well. All the same, prospects for further advances and progress are virtually infinite. The development and completion of the Human Genome Project has led forward-looking scientists and physicians to conceptualize and operationalize molecular therapies. For these therapies to be fully effective, however, it will be necessary to identify (and observe) the molecular disorders that need to be corrected and treated.

The opportunity for physicians to see organs *in vivo* began 120 years ago with Wilhelm Roentgen's discovery and development of radiography. Since then, and especially during the past few decades, researchers have devised new and ever more precise methods of radiology—such as positron emission tomography, computed tomography, magnetic resonance imaging—which, along with optical imaging, have considerably improved diagnostic capability.

Understanding the molecular and genetic process of disease is contingent on the ability to "see" at the molecular level in order to establish a diagnosis and evaluate possible molecular therapies. Talk of "individualized therapy" is heard everywhere today, but to exploit this concept fully, the visualization of gene expression will be necessary. And, in addition to enabling customized therapies, we can hope that our ability to uncover disorders at the molecular level will enable us to correct a problem before patients become aware of their symptoms. The public health potential of this approach is enormous, especially in the case of chronic conditions with slow progression. Chronic obstructive pulmonary disease, for example, would be a perfect candidate for such investigation.

The series of monographs Lung Biology in Health and Disease would fail its purpose if it were not a tool and conduit to bring new research advances to clinicians. After all, the ultimate goal of the series is to assist basic and clinical scientists in arriving and remaining at the forefront of what is known. *Molecular Imaging of the Lungs*, edited by Drs. Daniel P. Schuster and Timothy S. Blackwell, sets a new standard for the series by bringing an area of basic science to a practical level with very significant applications from which patients will benefit tremendously.

I am very grateful to the editors and authors for giving the series the opportunity to present this volume to the readership. I have no doubt that physicians who read it will recognize how richly and extensively research will ultimately serve their practice and their patients.

Claude Lenfant, M.D.
Gaithersburg, Maryland

Preface

A suite of emerging techniques, known collectively as "molecular imaging," now offer scientists an unprecedented opportunity to identify, follow, and quantify biologic processes at the cellular level with molecular specificity in intact organisms. For instance, it is now possible to evaluate, with imaging, the distribution, magnitude, and timing of gene expression in genetically altered animals (1–3). Even though nonimaging methods are also available to monitor gene expression, such methods—usually based on tissue sampling—are invasive and unattractive as routine procedures for clinical investigations. In contrast, molecular imaging can provide a seamless translation from studies in animals to later studies in humans.

While most studies that employ molecular imaging have so far focused on non-organ specific applications (such as cancer detection or treatment monitoring, and gene therapeutics), the ability to image fundamental processes (such as gene expression, inflammation, cell trafficking, apoptosis), provides ample reason to employ these methods in studies of lung biology. This rapidly developing, multidisciplinary field capitalizes on recent advances in the techniques of molecular and cell biology, on new highly specific probes that serve as sources for the imaging signal, and on dramatic improvements in imaging instrumentation (especially for small animals).

The number of options already available is dazzling. For instance, noninvasive real-time analysis of gene expression is possible using reporter genes with optical signatures [e.g., green fluorescent protein (*gfp*), firefly luciferase (3,4), and bacterial luciferase]. Key advances in detector technology for imaging low levels of light now enable imaging of these probes in living animals with charge coupled device (CCD) cameras. Alternatively, gene expression imaging can be accomplished with radionuclide-based techniques such as positron emission tomography (PET) or single photon emission computed tomography (SPECT) (5). In these cases, gene expression is monitored by measuring the accumulation of highly specific radiotracers in tissues expressing the target gene. Gene expression can also be followed by magnetic resonance imaging (MRI) using probes that, again, only accumulate in tissues expressing a target gene capable of activating a specific nanomagnetic probe (5).

Even within one type of imaging modality, choices are rapidly increasing in number. For instance, three general strategies have already evolved for optical molecular imaging *in vivo*: use of endogenous fluorochromes; use of reporter genes that generate internal light from specific biochemical reactions or external illumination (bioluminescence and fluorescent proteins); and use of injected optical contrast agents incorporating visible light fluorophores, near-infrared fluorophores, or activatable fluorophores (1,4,6).

Added to this array of new techniques for molecular imaging is a growing capability to perform anatomic or structural imaging in small animals. So-called "micro" computed tomography (CT), MRI, and ultrasound scanners and instruments now allow one to measure morphologic properties such as airway caliber or right ventricular dimensions, even in mice or other rodents. In many cases, these structural measurements can be coupled with various physiologic measurements relevant to lung physiology and pathophysiology, such as ventilation, perfusion, lung water, and pulmonary arterial pressure, among others. Furthermore, since each of the modern molecular imaging technologies like PET, MRI, and optical imaging has specific advantages and weaknesses, it makes sense to identify ways to benefit from each through so-called "fusion imaging," allowing detailed mapping of structure to function (e.g., with X-ray CT and PET). The use of multifunctional reporter genes that link two or more modalities is another approach that should be highly informative (4). Fusion genes that encode bioluminescent and fluorescent reporter proteins effectively couple the powerful *in vivo* capabilities of bioluminescence with the subset-discriminating capabilities of fluorescence-activated cell sorting (4,7). Similarly, dual reporters that combine nuclear imaging techniques (e.g., PET) with fluorescence and/or bioluminescence for gene expression studies have also been developed (8–11).

These exciting developments will allow pulmonary scientists to study *in vivo* lung biology at an unprecedented cellular and molecular level. New and established basic scientists, as well as physician-scientists interested in emerging techniques for noninvasive imaging of molecular events in the lungs of intact animals and in humans, need to become aware of these approaches to studying lung biology, both for their promise and limitations. Thus, this volume is divided into two main sections. In the first, "Methodologies," topics are presented and reviewed relevant to the underlying techniques themselves, including instrumentation, radionuclide-based methods, optical imaging approaches, magnetic resonance methods, and ultrasonography. In the second, "Applications," the focus turns to how these methods have already been—and will be in the future—applied to studies involving the lungs, including such diverse topics as gene expression imaging, inflammation imaging, imaging pulmonary cytokine regulation, molecular imaging of lung cancer, and imaging cell death, among others.

Taking advantage of these new capabilities should allow pulmonary scientists a "view" on lung biology that could not be imaged—or even imagined—a few years ago.

References

1. Weissleder R, Mahmood U. Molecular imaging. Radiology 2001; 219(2):316–333.
2. Massoud T, Gambhir S. Molecular imaging in living subjects: seeing fundamental biological processes in a new light. Gene Dev 2003; 17:545–580.
3. Contag PR, Olomu IN, Stevenson DK, Contag CH. Bioluminescence indicators in living mammals. Nat Med 1998; 4:245–247.
4. Contag C, Ross B. It's not just about anatomy: in vivo bioluminescence imaging as an eyepiece into biology. J Magn Reson Imag 2002; 16:378–387.
5. Wu J, Inubushi M, Sundaresan G, Schelbert H, Gambhir S. Positron emission tomography imaging of cardiac reporter gene expression in living rats. Circulation 2002; 106:180–183.
6. Weissleder R. Scaling down imaging: molecular mapping of cancer in mice. Nat Rev Cancer 2002; 2:11–18.
7. Day R, Kawecki M, Berry D. Dual-function reporter protein for analysis of gene expression in living cells. Biotechniques 1998; 25:848–856.
8. Doubrovin M, Ponomarev V, Beresten T. Imaging transcriptional regulation of p53-dependent genes with positron emission tomography in vivo. Proc Natl Acad Sci USA 2001; 98:9300–9305.
9. Luker G, Sharma V, Pica C, Dahlheimer J, Li W, Ochesky J, Ryan C, Piwnica-Worms H, Piwnica-Worms D. Noninvasive imaging of protein–protein interactions in living animals. Proc Natl Acad Sci USA 2002; 99:6961–6966.
10. Luker GD, Sharma V, Piwnica-Worms D. Visualizing protein–protein interactions in living animals. Methods 2003; 29:110–122.
11. Gelovani Tjuvajev J, Blasberg R. In vivo imaging of molecular-genetic targets for cancer therapy. Cancer Cell 2003; 3:327–332.

Contributors

Tomohiro Asai, Ph.D. *Department of Medical Biochemistry, University of Shizuoka, School of Pharmaceutical Sciences, Shizuoka, Japan*

Timothy S. Blackwell, M.D. *Departments of Medicine and Cell and Developmental Biology, Vanderbilt University School of Medicince, Nashville, Tennessee, USA*

Ronald G. Blasberg, M.D. *Department of Neurology, Memorial Sloan-Kettering Cancer Center, New York, New York, USA*

Delphine L. Chen, M.D. *Departments of Radiology and Surgery, Washington University School of Medicine, St. Louis, Missouri, USA*

Ann V. Clough, Ph.D. *Department of Mathematics, Statistics and Computer Science, Marquette University, Milwaukee, Wisconsin, USA*

Christopher H. Contag, Ph.D. *Department of Pediatrics, Microbiology & Immunology, and Radiology, Stanford University School of Medicine, Stanford, California, USA*

Johannes Czernin, M.D.   *Department of Molecular and Medical Pharmacology, David Geffen School of Medicine at UCLA, Los Angeles, California, USA*

Michael Doubrovin, M.D., Ph.D.   *Department of Neurology, Memorial Sloan-Kettering Cancer Center, New York, New York, USA*

Armin Ernst, M.D.   *Division of Pulmonary and Critical Care Medicine, Beth Israel Deaconess Medical Center, Boston, Massachusetts, USA*

Sanjiv S. Gambhir, M.D., Ph.D.   *The Crump Institute for Molecular Imaging, Los Angeles, California, USA; Department of Molecular & Medical Pharmacology, David Geffen School of Medicine at UCLA; Department of Diagnostic Radiology, Stanford University School of Medicine, Stanford, California, USA*

Joel R. Garbow, Ph.D.   *Departments of Chemistry and Radiology, Washington University, St. Louis, Missouri, USA*

Steven T. Haworth, Ph.D.   *Division of Pulmonary and Critical Care Medicine, Medical College of Wisconsin, Milwaukee, Wisconsin, USA*

Eric A. Hoffman, Ph.D.   *Department of Radiology, University of Iowa, Iowa City, Iowa, USA*

Meera Iyer, Ph.D.   *The Crump Institute for Molecular Imaging, Los Angeles, California, USA; Department of Molecular & Medical Pharmacology, David Geffen School of Medicine at UCLA*

E. Duco Jansen, Ph.D.   *Departments of Biomedical Engineering and Nerosurgery, Vanderbilt University School of Medicine, Nashville, Tennessee, USA*

Hazel A. Jones, Ph.D.   *Section on Experimental Medicine and Toxicology, Imperial College, London, UK*

Richard LaForest, Ph.D.   *Department of Radiology Radiation-Sciences, Washington University School of Medicine, St. Louis, Missouri, USA*

Kathryn E. Luker, Ph.D.   *Department of Radiology, Washington University School of Medicine, St. Louis, Missouri, USA*

William Lunn, M.D.   *Department of Interventional Pulmonology, Harvard Medical School, Boston, Massachusetts, USA*

Robert H. Mach, Ph.D.   *Department of Radiology Radiation-Sciences, Washington University School of Medicine, St. Louis, Missouri, USA*

Philipp Mayer-Kuckuk, M.D., Ph.D.   *Department of Neurology, Memorial Sloan-Kettering Cancer Center, New York, New York, USA*

Geoffrey McLennan, M.D., Ph.D.   *Department of Medicine, University of Iowa, Iowa City, Iowa, USA*

Wayne Mitzner, Ph.D. *Department of Environmental Health Sciences, Johns Hopkins University, Baltimore, Maryland, USA*

Jeffrey J. Neil, M.D., Ph.D. *Department of Neurology, Washington University, St. Louis, Missouri, USA*

Naoto Oku, M.D. *Department of Medical Biochemistry, University of Shizuoka, School of Pharmaceutical Sciences, Shizuoka, Japan*

Cassandra B. Orellana, M.D. *Department of Newborn Medicine, Washington University, St. Louis, Missouri, USA*

David R. Piwnica-Worms, M.D., Ph.D. *Departments of Radiology and Molecular Biology and Pharmacology, Washington University School of Medicine, St. Louis, Missouri, USA*

Wolfgang Recheis, Ph.D. *Department of Radiology, University of Iowa, Iowa City, Iowa, USA*

Buck E. Rogers, Ph.D. *Department of Radiation Oncology, Washington University School of Medicine, St. Louis, Missouri, USA*

Alan F. Ross, M.D. *Department of Anesthesia, University of Iowa, Iowa City, Iowa, USA*

Raffaella Rossin, Ph.D. *Mallinckrodt Institute of Radiology, Washington University School of Medicine, St. Louis, Missouri, USA*

Daniel P. Schuster, M.D. *Departments of Radiology Radiation-Sciences and Internal Medicine, Washington University School of Medicine, St. Louis, Missouri, USA*

Inna Serganova, Ph.D. *Department of Neurology, Memorial Sloan-Kettering Cancer Center, New York, New York, USA*

Victor M. Villalobos, Ph.D. *Department of Radiology, Washington University School of Medicine, St. Louis, Missouri, USA*

Elizabeth Wagner, Ph.D. *Division of Pulmonary and Critical Care Medicine, Johns Hopkins Asthma and Allergy Center, Baltimore, Maryland, USA*

Wolfgang Weber, M.D. *Department of Nuclear Medicine, Technische Universitaet Muenchen, Muenchen, Germany*

Michael J. Welch, Ph.D. *Department of Radiology Radiation-Sciences, Washington University School of Medicine, St. Louis, Missouri, USA*

Contents

SECTION 2: APPLICATION TO THE LUNGS

Section 1: Methodologies

1

Molecular Imaging Probes for PET and SPECT

RAFFAELLA ROSSIN and MICHAEL J. WELCH

Washington University School of Medicine,
St. Louis, Missouri, USA

I. Introduction

The term "molecular imaging" can be broadly defined as the *in vivo* characterization and measurement of biological processes at the cellular and subcellular (molecular) levels (1). The traditional approach for diagnosing disease is largely based on assessing anatomical and physiological changes that are late manifestations of molecular changes. However, advances in molecular and cellular biology techniques (manipulation of nucleic acids, DNA sequencing,

3

reverse transcription, polymerase chain reaction, etc.) allow development of novel tools, reagents, and methods to image-specific pathways *in vivo*, particularly those involved in disease processes (2–8). The completion of the first draft of the human genome (9) and the subsequent developments in proteomics are expected to lead to new understanding of the disease processes and to new medical therapies and diagnostics previously not imagined.

Molecular imaging monitors gene expression *in vivo* by targeting DNA, mRNA transcripts, products of gene expression (receptors, enzymes, proteins), or specific functions of these products (2). Successful use of these targets depends on the development of high-affinity ligands and/or efficient signal amplification strategies. Appropriate target selection is critical. Although high-affinity antisense tracers have been synthesized, the number and density of targets for antisense imaging are low (just two DNA strands per cell and up to 10^5 mRNA molecules per cell for some highly expressed genes). Therefore, imaging of DNA and mRNA transcripts requires extreme signal amplification for adequate image visualization. Accordingly, attention has been focused on the products of gene expression. In fact, receptors, enzymes, and proteins can be both overexpressed (up to 10^6 molecules per cell) and available to ligands (cell membrane-bound receptors and antigens); the use of molecular imaging and reporter gene strategies to study gene expression is rapidly progressing (2,4,10).

Once the molecular target is chosen, the next step is administration of an exogenous contrast agent to visualize target location by means of an imaging system. Molecular imaging probes are typically composed of a signaling component and an affinity component. The signaling component can be a radionuclide (nuclear imaging), a paramagnetic atom (magnetic resonance imaging), a fluorochrome (optical imaging), or an echoing microbubble (ultrasonography). The affinity component can be a small molecule (receptor ligand, enzyme substrate, peptide, antisense oligonucleotide) or a higher molecular weight ligand (monoclonal antibody, recombinant protein). The mechanisms exploited for targeting are receptor–ligand, antigen–antibody, enzyme–substrate, and transporter–substrate specific interactions.

For a tracer to be successful as a molecular imaging probe, it must be distributable throughout the body, accumulate at the target, remain at the target long enough to be detectable *in vivo*, and clear from nontarget tissues. In short, successful *in vivo* screening of potential molecular imaging agents must overcome significant hurdles.

Stability of the imaging probe in the blood after intravenous administration is of paramount importance. The signaling moiety must be anchored to the circulating affinity moiety (or to its active metabolite) long enough for the collected images to show biodistribution of the drug and not the label. A stable bond between signaling and affinity components also reduces nonspecific binding to plasma proteins and nontarget tissues, improving the signal-to-noise ratio at the target. At the same time, the biological properties of the parent molecule (transport mechanism, affinity for the target, etc.) must be maintained. Molecular modeling and high-throughput combinatorial chemistry techniques are currently used by the pharmaceutical industry to build libraries of new high-affinity tracers, and sophisticated organic synthesis approaches are commonly used to obtain stable labeled compounds with improved plasma stability to proteolytic enzymes (11).

Delivery to the target is another key consideration. The labeled molecule must be able to leave the blood stream (either by a transport mechanism or by a passive diffusion) to interact with extracellular targets. In some instances, the imaging probe must go farther, crossing the membrane to enter the intracellular compartment. Delivery barriers are typically the most challenging to deal with, particularly for large probes, but even low-molecular weight molecules may not be taken into cells. To circumvent existing delivery barriers, strategies developed include the use of small, neutrally charged, lipophilic probes to cross the blood–brain barrier (12) and the use of internalizing peptides and small proteins (the human immunodeficiency virus type 1 TAT peptide and the third helix of the homeodomain of Antennapedia) (13) to shuttle the imaging probe across the cellular membrane. To improve blood circulation and reduce immunogenicity, probes may be conjugated to (polyethylene)glycol, a nontoxic polymer which shelters the circulating drugs by hampering recognition by the reticuloendothelial system (14).

As no imaging probe is 100% specific, minimizing the background created by nonspecifically bound (or nonexcreted) contrast agent is a key goal in imaging probe development. To reduce background noise, the imaging probe must clear rapidly from the nontarget tissues and from the blood after specific interaction with the target. Blood clearance can be improved by tuning the chemical structure or reducing the size of the administered probe (e.g., by using peptides or antibody fragments derivatives instead of intact antibodies) to increase kidney excretion. "Clearing agents" have also been administered before the imaging procedure to eliminate the probe from the blood (e.g., injection of streptavidin derivatives to eliminate radiolabeled-biotinylated antibodies) (15).

Another strategy to reduce background noise and improve tracer uptake at the target site is the pre-targeting approach. In a pre-targeting approach, a bulky targeting species with poor clearance (e.g., an antibody), a contrast agent with optimal pharmacokinetic properties, and a high affinity for the targeting moiety are used. The signaling moiety is administered after the targeting species has accumulated at the target site and cleared from the blood, enhancing the signal-to-noise ratio (16).

In addition, background noise has been reduced by using activatable "smart probes" (also referred to as sensors or beacons) that carry a signaling moiety that "lights up" only when interacting with the target (e.g., near-infrared fluorescent probes for optical imaging) (4,17). This feature is not available with radiolabeled probes, which produce signal constantly through decay of the radioisotope. With radiotracers, images are collected after nonspecifically distributed surplus probe has cleared and the signal comes primarily from those probe molecules that are specifically bound to the target.

Another approach to improve the differentiation of target and background is to use imaging probes that can be converted by an intracellular enzyme substrate into a "trapped" product, amplifying the imageable signal [e.g., 2-deoxy-2-[^{18}F]fluoro-D-glucose (^{18}FDG)].

II. Radionuclides for PET and SPECT Molecular Imaging Probes

A radionuclide is an unstable nucleus, which spontaneously reaches a more stable state by emitting some sort of radiation. Radionuclides decay by one or more of six processes: fission, α-decay, β^- (beta)-decay, β^+ (positron)-decay, electron capture, and isomeric transition. The radionuclides used to synthesize imaging probes for positron emission tomography (PET) and single photon emission tomography (SPECT) are β^+-emitters and γ-emitters, respectively. Positron (β^+) emission from a proton-rich nucleus occurs after the conversion of a proton into a neutron, with simultaneous emission of a neutrino (ν). The positron is the antiparticle to the electron and the energy of emission can take a continuum of values up to a maximum, which depends on the difference between the energetic states of the parent–daughter nuclei. After emission from the nucleus, the positron loses kinetic energy by collisions and scattering with surrounding atoms. The positron eventually combines with an electron and annihilates, which releases two 0.511 MeV photons in opposite directions (ca. 180° to each other) to conserve momentum. The distance traveled by the positron before annihilation depends on its initial energy.

Gamma (γ) rays are photons deriving from isomeric transitions. Isomeric transitions occur when a nucleus remains in an excited state after a particle emission or a decay by electron capture. These intermediate levels are referred to as *isomeric states* (or *metastable states*), and each decays to a lower state (either the ground state or another intermediate state) with lifetimes from picoseconds to years. Gamma ray emissions are characteristic of the radionuclide, and the energies of the emitted photons depend on the energy differences between the initial excited state and the next one.

Radionuclides are primarily produced in cyclotrons or reactors, depending on the nuclear reaction required. Very short-lived radionuclides such as ^{11}C, ^{15}O, and ^{13}N are available only in institutions that have a cyclotron facility, and this limits their widespread use. Remote facilities rely on commercially available long- and medium-lived radionuclides (^{123}I, ^{111}In, ^{67}Ga, etc.) and radionuclides produced by generators (e.g., ^{99m}Tc). The most commonly used radionuclides in PET and SPECT imaging are listed in Table 1.1. A complete discussion about radionuclide production, labeling conditions, and recent progresses in radiochemistry can be found elsewhere (18–20).

Table 1.1 Radionuclides for PET and SPECT

$T_{1/2}$		Decay modes (%)	Main γ keV (%)	β_{max} MeV (β_{ave})	Production (18)
SPECT radionuclides					
^{99m}Tc	6.01 h	IT	140 (89.1)		^{99}Mo/^{99m}Tc generator
^{123}I	13.27 h	EC	159 (83.3)		^{124}Te(p,2n)^{123}I
^{67}Ga	78.27 h	EC	93 (39.2); 185 (21.2); 300 (16.8)		^{68}Zn(p,2n)^{67}Ga
^{111}In	67.31 h	EC	171 (90.7); 245 (94.1)		^{111}Cd(p,n)^{111}In ^{112}Cd(p,2n)^{111}In
^{201}Tl	72.91 h	EC	167 (10.0)		^{203}Tl(p,3n)^{201}Pb:^{201}Tl
^{133}Xe	5.24 days	β^-	81 (38.0)	0.346 (0.100)	^{235}U fission
PET radionuclides					
^{11}C	20.39 min	β^+ (99.8) EC (0.2)	511 (199.5)	0.960 (0.386)	^{14}N(p,α)^{11}C
^{13}N	9.96 min	β^+ (99.8) EC (0.2)	511 (199.6)	1.198 (0.492)	^{16}O(p,α)^{13}N
^{15}O-	122.24 s	β^+ (99.9) EC (0.1)	511 (199.8)	1.732 (0.735)	^{14}N(d,n)^{15}O ^{15}N(p,n)^{15}O
^{18}F	109.8 min	β^+ (97) EC (3)	511 (193.5)	0.633 (0.250)	^{18}O(p,n)^{18}F ^{20}Ne(d,α)^{18}F
^{124}I	4.18 days	β^+ (23) EC (77)	511 (46); 603 (62.9); 723 (10.3)	2.138 (0.820)	^{124}Te(p,n)^{124}I ^{124}Te(d,2n)^{124}I
^{75}Br	96.7 min	β^+ (73) EC (27)	287 (90); 511 (146)	2.008 (0.719)	^{76}Se(p,2n)^{75}Br ^{76}Se(d,3n)^{75}Br

(continued)

Table 1 *Continued*

$T_{1/2}$		Decay modes (%)	Main γ keV (%)	β_{max} MeV (β_{ave})	Production (18)
^{76}Br	16.2 h	β^+ (55)	511 (109); 559 (74.0)	3.941	^{76}Se(p,n)^{76}Br
		EC (45)	657 (15.9); 1854 (14.7)	(1.180)	^{76}Se(d,2n)^{76}Br
^{66}Ga	9.49 h	β^+ (56)	511 (112); 1039 (36.0)	4.153	^{63}Cu(α,n)^{66}Ga
		EC (44)	2752 (23.3)	(1.740)	
^{68}Ga	67.71 min	β^+ (89)	511 (178.3)	1.899	^{68}Ge/^{68}Ga generator
		EC (11)		(0.829)	
^{60}Cu	23.7 min	β^+ (93)	511 (185); 826 (21.7)	3.772	^{60}Ni(p,n)^{60}Cu
		EC (7)	1332 (88.0); 1792 (45.4)	(0.970)	
^{61}Cu	3.33 h	β^+ (61)	511 (123); 656 (10.8)	1.215	^{61}Ni(p,n)^{61}Cu
		EC (39)		(0.500)	
^{62}Cu	9.7 min	β^+ (97)	511 (194.9)	2.926	^{62}Zn/^{62}Cu generator
		EC (3)		(1.314)	
^{64}Cu	12.7 h	β^+ (17)	511 (34.8)	0.653	^{64}Ni(p,n)^{64}Cu
		EC (44)		(0.278)	
		β^- (39)			
^{94m}Tc	52.0 min	β^+ (70)	511 (140.4); 871 (94.2)	2.438	^{94}Mo(p,n)^{94m}Tc
		EC (30)		(1.072)	

Source: Available on http://www.nndc.bnl.gov.

The most commonly used PET radionuclides are ^{11}C, ^{13}N, ^{15}O, and [18]F. [11]C, ^{15}O, and ^{13}N have stable isotopes in most of the chemical entities existing in life and can substitute atoms belonging to biomolecules without changing the biomolecule itself. [18]F is often substituted for a hydroxyl group or a hydrogen atom. As the van der Waals radius of fluorine is similar to that of hydrogen, ^{18}F-labeling causes very little steric alteration of the biomolecule. However, the electronegative nature of fluorine can alter the binding properties or reactivity of the labeled molecule.

[11]C is a positron-emitting radionuclide (99.8%) with a 20.4 min half-life. The half-life of this radionuclide allows both multi-step syntheses of radiotracers and repeated studies in patients and animals in a short time frame. For these reasons, ^{11}C has been used to synthesize a multitude of diagnostic agents (e.g., [^{11}C]choline, ^{11}C-labeled amino acids, [^{11}C]flumazenil, and many others) and is widely used in both clinical practice and research.

[13]N and [15]O are positron-emitters with a 10 min half-life and a 122 s half-life, respectively. Similar to ^{11}C, both ^{13}N and [15]O allow *in vivo* evaluation of a wide range of important biological processes. However, their very short half-life precludes the use of time-consuming synthetic and purification steps. At the same time, both ^{13}N and [15]O can be used repeatedly during the same imaging procedure.

[18]F is probably the most important PET radionuclide, as it is used to produce [18]FDG and other tracers including [18]FDOPA, fluoromisonidazole ([18]FMISO), and so on. [18]F decays 97% by positron emission and 3% by electron capture. The maximum energy of the emitted positrons (0.635 MeV) is ideal for imaging with PET cameras, because these positrons have a short mean range before annihilation (2.4 mm in water), providing the highest resolution of all PET radionuclides. The relatively long half-life of [18]F (109.8 min) allows for a variety of synthetic strategies to be accomplished and extended imaging protocols to be carried out. Furthermore, ^{18}F-labeled radiotracers can be transported within a few hours drive from commercial sources.

Other attractive radiohalogens for the synthesis of PET tracers are [76]Br and [124]I (21,22). Both of these radiohalogens have a longer half-life compared with [18]F (16.1 h and 4.2 days, respectively) allowing more protracted imaging studies to be carried out. Unfortunately, complex decay schemes and high end-point energies of the emitted positrons result in a lower image quality for both [76]Br and [124]I when compared with [18]F (23). However, as PET techniques are gaining importance over traditional SPECT, new radiotracers labeled with less-than-ideal PET radionuclides may find clinical application. Some new candidate PET radiotracers labeled with [124]I and [76]Br will be considered in the following sections.

Iodine isotopes are also widely used in SPECT imaging procedures. For over four decades, the γ- and β^--emitting, reactor-produced ^{131}I was used for both radiotherapy of thyroid pathologies and diagnostic imaging. Now, ^{123}I is replacing this "classic" iodine isotope in SPECT imaging, because it gives a much lower radiation dose. Furthermore, ^{123}I emits 159 keV gamma radiation, ideal for imaging with gamma cameras. The cyclotron-produced radionuclide ^{123}I decays by electron capture with a half-life of 13.3 h.

The chemistry of iodine radionuclides used in nuclear medicine has been extensively explored. Isotopic exchange procedures, direct iodination approaches (those using chloramine-T and iodogen), and indirect approaches (the Bolton–Hunter method) are but a few of the well-known synthetic strategies to label biomolecules with iodine (24). Some of the most important ^{123}I-labeled imaging tracers [I-labeled iodoazomycin arabinoside (^{123}IAZA), I-labeled vasoactive intestinal peptide (^{123}I-VIP), etc.] will be discussed in the following sections.

Copper radionuclides are promising candidates for both PET imaging (^{60}Cu, ^{61}Cu, ^{62}Cu, ^{64}Cu) and radiotherapy (^{64}Cu and ^{67}Cu) (25). Copper radionuclides decay by β^+- and/or β^--emission, and γ-emission, with half-lives ranging from 10 min (^{62}Cu) to 62 h (^{67}Cu). ^{60}Cu, ^{61}Cu, and ^{64}Cu can be produced on a medical cyclotron, whereas the long-lived β^--emitter ^{67}Cu is produced on high-energy accelerators. ^{62}Cu is obtained from the decay of cyclotron-produced ^{62}Zn, and the development of a ^{62}Zn/^{62}Cu generator may allow for its more widespread use. However, the relatively short half-life of ^{62}Zn (9.2 h) limits the life span of the ^{62}Zn/^{62}Cu parent–daughter generator to 1–2 days.

As the other radiometals used in nuclear medicine, copper radionuclides cannot be covalently bound to biomolecules. Instead, a bifunctional chelating agent (BFCA), containing coordinating sites for the metal, must be conjugated to the targeting molecule. Until recently, ligands of choice are the tetraazamacro-cyclics DOTA and TETA. However, preliminary clinical trials with ^{64}Cu-tracers revealed the instability of Cu–TETA complexes *in vivo*. Therefore, a series of a new chelators (TE2A, tachpyr, SarAr, etc.) with improved *in vivo* stability have been developed and are under evaluation for Cu-labeling of antibodies, proteins, peptides, and so on (26).

Gallium is one of the most important radiometals in nuclear medicine, largely because of the widespread use of ^{67}Ga-citrate in SPECT imaging studies. In addition, positron-emitting ^{66}Ga and ^{68}Ga are gaining importance in the development of unconventional PET tracers (25). Both ^{67}Ga and ^{66}Ga are cyclotron-produced radionuclides. The widespread use of ^{67}Ga for SPECT imaging is due to its emission of 184.6 keV gamma rays, excellent for SPECT detectors. Furthermore, its relatively long half-life (78 h) allows ^{67}Ga-radiopharmaceuticals to be marketed. In contrast, ^{66}Ga has a less-than-ideal decay (23). However, it emits high-energy positrons and gamma rays, and is therefore a potential radiodiagnostic/radiotherapic tracer.

^{68}Ga is a better PET imaging tracer than ^{66}Ga, as it decays 90% by positron emission with an end-point positron energy of 1.90 MeV. Of these three gallium radionuclides, ^{68}Ga has the shortest half-life (68.3 min). However, marketing of the available ^{68}Ge/^{68}Ga-generator may be a keystone for PET expansion. In fact, the parent radionuclide (^{68}Ge) decays to ^{68}Ga by electron capture with a half-life of 275 days, and this allows for long-term use (over 2 years) of the ^{68}Ge/^{68}Ga-generator in institutions with no in-house cyclotron.

Like copper, gallium must also be stabilized in a coordination complex conjugated to a biomolecule. The BFCAs of choice to label biomolecules with gallium are the versatile DTPA and DOTA ligands. Some of the target-specific tracers obtained by conjugating these ligands to biomolecules will be considered in the following sections.

The establishment and evolution of diagnostic nuclear medicine can probably be attributed to the existence of ^{99m}Tc (27). Since the introduction of gamma cameras in hospitals, ^{99m}Tc has been the most used γ-emitter. Even now, 80% of the diagnostic imaging procedures are carried out using ^{99m}Tc-labeled radiopharmaceuticals. The prominent role of ^{99m}Tc is due to its optimal nuclear properties. ^{99m}Tc decays >99% by isomeric transition and emits a 140 keV gamma photon, ideal for imaging with gamma cameras. Furthermore, the ^{99m}Tc half-life (6.01 h) is optimal for preparing and administering the radiopharmaceutical to the patient, and yet it is short enough to minimize the adsorbed radiation dose. Finally, ^{99m}Tc is widely available in health and research institutions because of the existence of a user friendly and inexpensive generator.

The ^{99}Mo/^{99m}Tc generator consists of an alumina column in which ^{99}Mo (a fission- or reactor-produced radionuclide) is adsorbed as ^{99}Mo-molybdate. ^{99}Mo decays 87% to ^{99m}Tc, and a ^{99m}Tc-pertechnetate solution is easily obtained by eluting the column with sterile saline solution. ^{99m}Tc-radiopharmaceuticals are then synthesized by adding the generator eluate to one of the many commercially available radiopharmaceutical kits. Because the parent radionuclide decays to ^{99m}Tc with a half-life of 66 h, the ^{99}Mo/^{99m}Tc generator can be used daily for up to 1 week.

Much effort has been devoted to development of BFCAs for this versatile radiometal. The most common Tc(V) complexes are usually obtained by conjugating the biomolecules with BFCAs containing nitrogen and sulfur atoms [$N_xS_{(4-x)}$ coordination set], but stable complexes can also be obtained with phosphino-, carboxylate-containing ligands, and so on. The coordination approach may vary as well [tetradentate complexes, mixed $(3 + 1)$ approach, Tc(I)(CO)$_3$ approach, direct labeling, etc.], depending on the biomolecule to be labeled (27,28).

Another technetium isotope with potential application in nuclear medicine is ^{94m}Tc. ^{94m}Tc is a cyclotron-produced radionuclide with a 53 min half-life. It decays 72% by emission of 2.47 MeV positrons, and is a candidate PET tracer. Recent studies have shown that ^{94m}Tc-pertechnetate can replace ^{99m}Tc-pertechnetate in commercially available kits (29). ^{94m}Tc-labeled tracers and PET imaging could provide image resolution superior to that of the corresponding SPECT ^{99m}Tc-labeled agents. Furthermore, in pre-clinical and clinical trials, imaging studies using ^{94m}Tc-tracers could provide quantitative information for analogous ^{99m}Tc-compounds and shorten the time necessary to evaluate new radiopharmaceuticals (25).

Like ^{99m}Tc and ^{67}Ga, ^{111}In is another widely used radiometal in SPECT imaging procedures. ^{111}In is a cyclotron-produced radionuclide with a half-life of 2.83 days, which allows commercial distribution. ^{111}In decays by electron capture and emits two major gamma radiations including one at 171 keV, which is useful for detection by gamma cameras.

Like the congener gallium, ^{111}In forms stable complexes with DTPA and DOTA. To date, ^{111}In-labeled white blood cells and somatostatin (SST) analogs are commonly used to detect inflammation foci and SST receptor-positive tumors in patients, respectively (30).

III. Radiotracers for Molecular Imaging

The premise of molecular imaging is that "sick" cells are different from their "normal" neighbors, that is, they have a distinctive phenotype because of altered expression or processing of gene products. Molecular imaging takes advantage of a variety of specific markers induced by pathological cell alterations to detect disease much earlier and to predict or assess therapeutic response, putting a version of Ehrlich's "magic bullet" into practice.

Among all molecular imaging techniques, nuclear imaging has a position of prominence resulting from the high sensitivity, which allow *in vivo* evaluation of high affinity, low abundance molecular targets such as receptors, enzymes, antigens, neurotransmitters, and so on. Several PET and SPECT radiotracers have been developed to probe molecular events. These agents have been translated from concept to human studies largely because a radiotracer is administered in nanomolar quantities so pharmacological effect is likely to be negligible.

In the following sections, we will discuss some examples of PET and SPECT radiotracers developed to image tumor metabolism, proliferation, hypoxia, receptor, and gene expression. Although few studies are focused on lung-specific applications, the underlying principles should still be relevant to many lung diseases (e.g., lung cancer). More examples of molecular probes to detect inflammation, angiogenesis, cell apoptosis, and so on will be discussed in other chapters of this book.

A. Tumor Metabolism

About 70 years ago, Warburg demonstrated that tumor cells have a great capacity for aerobic glycolysis, which causes an increase in lactate production (31). This important discovery led to the development of ^{18}FDG (32) to measure glucose metabolism *in vivo*. ^{18}FDG, as an analog of glucose, is transported into tumor cells by a number of specific membrane transporter proteins. In the cell, ^{18}FDG is converted to ^{18}FDG-6-phosphate by hexokinase. However, unlike glucose, ^{18}FDG-6-phosphate does not undergo further enzymatic reaction and is trapped in the cell. The high glycolytic phenotype of most human tumors depends on upregulation of both glucose transporters (33) and hexokinase (34).

In vivo measurement of glucose metabolism with ^{18}FDG PET is used to better differentiate between benign and malignant lesions and to pre-operatively delineate tumors from normal tissues. Furthermore, ^{18}FDG standard uptake is used for tumor grading, as a marker of response to antitumor therapy, to determine disease relapse, and as a prognostic indicator (35). However, ^{18}FDG uptake is not tumor specific, and false positive findings can occur in inflammatory lesions (36). Furthermore, high radioactivity background in certain tissues, including brain and bladder, can obscure subtle increases in tumor uptake and makes it difficult to assess small changes in tumor size in or near these tissues (37).

In clinical practice, ^{18}FDG PET is currently used with a variety of human cancers such as nonsmall cell lung cancers, colorectal, esophageal, breast, and thyroid carcinomas, melanomas, lymphomas, head and neck cancers, and other tumors (38).

Another interesting target for metabolic tumor imaging is increased protein metabolism. Cells use amino acids for protein synthesis, as metabolic fuel or as building blocks for secretory products. The process of malignant transformation requires cells to acquire and use nutrients efficiently. For this reason, malignant cells generally upregulate expression of amino acid transporters (39). Nearly all the existing amino acids have been radiolabeled, mostly with ^{11}C, and evaluated as potential radiotracers to measure tumor metabolism (40).

Because inflammatory cells exhibit low protein metabolism when compared with their glucose metabolism, inflammatory tissues obscure radiolabeled amino acid uptake less than they do ^{18}FDG uptake (41). Similarly, labeled amino acids may be useful tools to evaluate brain lesions, or lesions that show hypo- or isometabolic uptake of ^{18}FDG (42).

The majority of PET studies in oncology have been performed with ^{11}C-labeled methionine, which is relatively easy to synthesize (41–43). Because of its low uptake in the brain, [^{11}C]methionine has been proven to be a sensitive and specific tool for brain tumors, able to differentiate nonneoplastic from malignant lesions (42,44). Methionine uptake reflects the amino acid transport, whereas [^{11}C]tyrosine has been used to quantify protein synthesis rate in brain tumors (45,46). An ^{123}I-iodinated tyrosine analog (IMT) also has been proposed to assess tumor cells proliferation by means of SPECT imaging. ^{123}IMT uptake in glioma cells *in vitro* (47) and in soft-tissue sarcomas *in vivo* (48) was shown to be induced by rapid proliferation.

1-[^{11}C]Acetate is a well-known PET imaging agent. In the myocardium, 1-[^{11}C]acetate is rapidly converted to ^{11}CO$_2$ via the TCA cycle, and therefore is used to evaluate changes in oxidative metabolism in patients with recent infarction (49). Recently, 1-[^{11}C]acetate has been reported to be a promising alternative to ^{18}FDG for tumor detection, especially in brain, renal, and prostatic malignancies (50). Acetate metabolism is different in tumor cells than in myocardium. In tumor cells, 1-[^{11}C]acetate is incorporated into lipids, which are then used for cell membrane synthesis (51). Consequently, high uptake of

1-[^{11}C]acetate in tumors may be due to enhanced lipid synthesis compared with normal tissues.

Choline is another essential substrate for cell membrane synthesis, as it is a precursor for the biosynthesis of phosphatidylcholine (52). In preliminary clinical studies, [^{11}C]choline has shown potential for detection of tumors in areas where ^{18}FDG lacks sensitivity (53–55). High tumor to background ratios were found for many malignant brain tumors. However, in these tumors, [^{11}C]choline PET did not allow for malignancy grade estimation (Table 1.2) (55).

B. Tumor Proliferation

Tumor lesions are characterized by uncontrolled cellular proliferation, and high histological indices of mitotic activity are typically associated with increased cellular anaplasia and increased tumor aggressiveness. The growth fraction of a tumor is defined as the number of clonogenic cells in S-phase. In most human tumors, this fraction constitutes $\sim$3–15% of the total cell mass, and high percentages reflect a high malignancy. These rapidly duplicating cells are the best candidates for DNA damage, for example, with radiotherapy, which decreases cells capacity to proliferate. Thus, a proliferation-targeted imaging tracer could be useful to predict the overall chance of survival and response to specific cancer therapies or to identify patients likely to benefit from more aggressive treatment strategies (56).

Because cell growth requires an adequate energy supply, ^{18}FDG uptake has often been used as an indirect measure of tumor proliferation (57). Correlation between ^{18}FDG uptake and tumor cells proliferation was confirmed in glioma (58), meningioma (59), lymphoma (60), ovarian epithelial carcinoma (57), lung cancer (61–63), and squamous-cell carcinoma of the head and neck (64). 1-[^{11}C]Acetate, [^{11}C]choline, and radiolabeled amino acids are other PET tracers used to indirectly measure tumor proliferation, because cell growth and proliferation inevitably necessitate membrane constituents and proteins (65).

Table 1.2 Examples of Tumor Metabolism Imaging Tracers

Tracer	Target	Application	References
^{18}FDG	Glucose metabolism	PET	32, 35, 38
[^{11}C]Methionine	Protein metabolism	PET	40–44
[^{11}C]Tyrosine		PET	40, 45, 46
^{18}FET		PET	40
^{123}I-IMT		SPECT	40, 47, 48
1-[^{11}C]Acetate	Lipid metabolism	PET	49–51
[^{11}C]Choline		PET	53–55

More direct indicators of proliferation have also been evaluated. As cell replication entails DNA synthesis, most of the published work to date has focused on nucleosides analogs (66). DNA is synthesized from nucleotides containing four different bases; whereas adenosine, cytosine, and guanosine are also incorporated into RNA, only thymidine is uniquely incorporated into DNA (56). Thymidine is transported into cells from the bloodstream (salvage pathway) or is derived from local production (*de novo* pathway) (67). It is then phosphorylated by the cytosolic form of the mammalian thymidine kinase (TK1) and incorporated into DNA. Thymidine has been labeled with ^{11}C either in the methyl-5-position (5-[methyl-^{11}C]thymidine) or in the ring-2-position (2-[^{11}C]thymidine), and it has been evaluated in a panel of human tumors (68–72). Following IV injection, ^{11}C-labeled thymidine is rapidly metabolized, and so time–activity curves obtained from blood samples, and related kinetic models, must be used to correctly evaluate tumor uptake. This complicated quantification, together with the short half-life of ^{11}C (20 min), has led to the development and evaluation of a series of thymidine analogs with improved plasma stability and labeled with longer half-life isotopes (e.g., $^{123/124/131}$I-, ^{76}Br-, ^{18}F-labeled deoxyuridine, etc.) (73–81).

To date, the most promising new marker for imaging tumor cells proliferation is a thymidine analog labeled with ^{18}F (^{18}FLT) (82,83). Like other thymidine analogs, ^{18}FLT enters cells depending on their duplication rate, utilizing the salvage pathway for DNA synthesis. It is then trapped in the cell after phosphorylation by the human TK1, and the 3′ substitution prevents further incorporation into DNA (84). A number of pre-clinical and clinical studies are being carried out by research groups to validate the use of ^{18}FLT in assessing tumor proliferation (85–88). The tumor uptake values obtained clearly contrast with background activity in nonproliferating tissues. However, high physiological ^{18}FLT uptake in highly proliferating organs (e.g., liver and bone marrow) hampers detection of metastases in these tissues. On the other hand, ^{18}FLT may be more suitable than ^{18}FDG for imaging of brain metastases, because of its low uptake in the brain (Table 1.3) (87).

Table 1.3 Tumor Proliferation Imaging Tracers

Tracer	Target	Application	References
2-[^{11}C]Thymidine	Thymidine kinase 1 activity	PET	68–71
5-[^{11}C-Methyl]thymidine		PET	72
^{18}FLT		PET	82–88
Labeled deoxyuridine		PET/SPECT	73–78
^{18}FDG	Glucose metabolism	PET	57–64
Labeled amino acids	Protein synthesis	PET/SPECT	40, 65
1-[^{11}C]Acetate	Cell membranes synthesis	PET	51, 65
[^{11}C]Choline		PET	65

C. Tumor Hypoxia

In recent years, the detection of hypoxic cells within human tissues has become the subject of intense research, as hypoxia occurs in several kinds of tumors and also is a consequence of ischemic strokes. Distribution of oxygen within a tumor is heterogeneous. Oxygen concentration usually shows a gradient, and is lowest in the less vascularized center of the tumor. Hypoxia induces an aggressive phenotype in tumors, increasing metastatic potential and promoting progression (89). It is suggested that low oxygen tension in the primary tumor provides a physiological signal that forces the tumor to select a cell subpopulation with the highest potential to survive in adverse conditions (90). Furthermore, tumor hypoxia promotes angiogenesis through the induction of pro-angiogenic factors such as the vascular endothelial growth factor (91). Tumor hypoxia also induces resistance to both radiotherapy and chemotherapy, due to lack of reactive oxygen radicals, slower tumor cell proliferation, and vascular insufficiency (91).

Significant hypoxia has been detected in nearly 40% of head and neck cancers, in soft-tissue sarcomas, breast cancers, and glioblastoma multiforme. However, hypoxia levels cannot be predicted by tumor size, grade, extent of necrosis, or blood hemoglobin status (89). Much effort has been dedicated to develop clinically relevant techniques to assess the presence of hypoxia in tissues and tumors (92). Despite their usefulness, these techniques are usually invasive (needle electrodes, analysis of biopsy samples) and limited when trying to detect dynamic changes in hypoxic tissues. On the other hand, *in vivo* imaging offers a noninvasive method for real-time evaluation of hypoxia in whole organs and tumors, and when time-dependent changes in oxygen distribution occur over time.

When tissues become hypoxic, there is a tendency to switch from Krebs cycle metabolism to glycolysis, resulting in a 2-fold increase in glycolysis (93). For this reason, [18]FDG has been evaluated for hypoxia imaging in pre-clinical and clinical studies (89,94,95). However, multiple reports provide clear evidence that hypoxia and accelerated glycolysis are common but independent manifestations, because hypoxia is not the only trigger for increased glucose metabolism in cancer cells (93). As a result, other molecular imaging probes have been developed for identification and quantification of hypoxia. Some of these tracers are summarized in Table 1.4.

For imaging hypoxia by PET and SPECT, both nitroimidazole- and nonnitroimidazole-containing imaging agents have been developed.

Inside cells, 2-nitroimidazole acts as a bioreductive molecule. It undergoes a single electron reduction in hypoxic environments, forming reactive radicals that bind to intracellular protein thiols and become trapped (96). Because nitroimidazole uptake requires intact nitroreductase enzymes, 2-nitroimidazole, in principle, could be exploited to distinguish between normoxic, hypoxic (but viable), and necrotic tissues (90).

Table 1.4 Examples of Hypoxia Imaging Tracers

Tracer		Application	References
[18]FMISO	Nitroimidazole-containing tracers	PET	89, 90, 97, 99
[18]FETA		PET	100
[18]FETNIM		PET	101
^{18}F-EF5		PET	102
[123]IAZA		SPECT	98, 103
[18]FAZA		PET	90
[124]IAZG		PET	104
^{99m}Tc-BMS-181321		SPECT	105
^{99m}Tc-BRU59-21		SPECT	106
[99m]Tc N2IPA		SPECT	107
^{99m}Tc-HL91	Non nitroimidazole-containing tracers	SPECT	108, 109
[60/61/62/64]Cu-ATSM		PET	110–113

The initial imaging studies of tumor hypoxia with 2-nitroimidazole were performed with the ^{18}F-labeled PET tracer [18]FMISO (97) and the ^{123}I-labeled SPECT tracer [123]IAZA (98).

Among potential PET hypoxia tracers, [18]FMISO is the most widely studied, but its high lipophilicity results in high background that reduces the quality of the images (90). Furthermore, it has been reported that fluoromisonidazole undergoes extensive metabolism, with only 3% of injected radioactivity excreted in urine as unchanged drug (99). Some more polar compounds, such as [18]FETA (100), [18]FETNIM (101), and ^{18}F-EF5 (102), have been evaluated to overcome the slow clearance and some of the nonoxygen-dependent metabolism seen with [18]FMISO.

Although originally developed for SPECT imaging of tumor hypoxia, [123]IAZA was also used clinically to image hypoxia induced by diabetes, blunt brain trauma, and rheumatoid arthritis (103). The favorable *in vivo* behavior of the azomycin arabinoside moiety also has been exploited in the development of two new potential PET tracers, [18]FAZA (90), and [124]IAZG (104). These two new PET tracers may overcome the major limitation of [18]FMISO. In fact, [18]FMISO takes several hours to clear from normoxic tissues, jeopardizing image quality, given the half-life of [18]F (90).

2-Nitroimidazole derivatives also have been labeled with ^{99m}Tc by using different chelator systems for SPECT imaging of hypoxia. In BMS-181321 (105) and BRU59-21 (106), the nitroimidazole moiety is coupled to a propylene amine oxime-type chelator. These two tracers show affinity for hypoxic cells, but their *in vivo* use is limited by high blood levels and extended hepatobiliary excretion due to high lipophilicity. Recently, N2IPA has been obtained by conjugating 2-nitroimidazole with a hydroxyiminoamide chelator. Preliminary results indicate N2IPA as a promising ^{99m}Tc-labeled tracer for tumor hypoxia (107).

The nonimidazole-containing hypoxia tracers most widely studied so far are ^{99m}Tc-butylene amine oxime (^{99m}Tc–BnAO, HL91) and Cu–diacetyl-*bis*(N^4-methylthiosemicarbazone) (Cu–ATSM).

HL91 was evaluated as a potential hypoxia imaging agent because the metal core of certain ^{99m}Tc 2-nitroimidazole derivatives showed even greater hypoxia selectivity than the nitro-containing complex (108). ^{99m}Tc HL91 has shown similar tumor-to-muscle and tumor-to-blood ratios as ^{18}FMISO and ^{123}IAZA, and has the advantage of being easily prepared from a kit at low cost. Furthermore, HL91 showed rapid blood clearance and kidney excretion (109). Despite these promising features, this compound is no longer in commercial development.

Copper complexes of a methylthiosemicarbazone moiety were recently developed for imaging hypoxic tissues with PET. The Cu–ATSM system showed high cell membrane permeability and a low redox potential (110). In pre-clinical experiments, Cu–ATSM imaging was compared to needle electrode oxygen readings and a correlation between high ^{64}Cu–ATSM uptake and low tissue pO_2 was observed (111). Studies with ^{60}Cu–ATSM have been performed in patients with lung cancer (112) and cervical cancer (113) with promising results.

D. Tumor Receptors

Cells functions depend on the interactions between receptors and specific ligands such as neurotransmitters and hormones. In recent years, it has been shown that human cancers can upregulate a variety of receptors, and that these receptors can be targeted for diagnostic or therapeutic purposes. The success of ^{111}In-labeled octreotide (114) and ^{123}I-labeled VIP (115) in highlighting tumors because of interaction with tumor cell receptors has intensified research into other receptors that could be tumor markers for diagnosis and therapy. Besides SST and VIP receptors, a variety of receptors have been investigated in the last two decades, and many targeting ligands have been synthesized and evaluated for *in vivo* imaging of tumors with PET and SPECT. Some of these receptors and tracers are listed in the following sections (Table 1.5).

SST Receptors

SST is a family of 14-amino acid (SST-14) and 28-amino acid (SST-28) cyclic disulfide-containing peptides. SST is widely distributed in the human body, in particular in the central and peripheral nervous system, endocrine glands, immune system, and gastrointestinal tract, where it acts as neurotransmitter, neurohormone, or local hormone. Moreover, SST and SST analogs have been shown to inhibit tumor growth in many animal tumor models (116–118).

Table 1.5 Examples of Tumor Receptor Targeting Imaging Tracers

Tracer	Target	Application	References
[111]In-Pentretreotide	SST receptors	SPECT	114, 117, 118, 120, 121
[99m]Tc-Depreotide		SPECT	122, 123
^{123}I-VIP	VIP receptors	SPECT	115, 140
^{99m}Tc-TP 3659		SPECT	141–143
^{111}In-DTPA-Glu-minigastrine	CCK-B/Gastrin	SPECT	145, 146
^{111}In-DTPA-Glu-CCK8	Receptors	SPECT	145, 147
^{99m}Tc-RP257	GRP receptors	SPECT	151
[99m]Tc-Leu-13-BN1		SPECT	160–163
^{111}In-DTPA-BN		SPECT	148, 149, 159
[99m]Tc-Demobesin 1		SPECT	154
^{111}In-DTPA-Folate	Folate receptors	SPECT	168, 175
^{99m}Tc-EC20		SPECT	173
P-^{123}I-MBA	Sigma receptors	SPECT	181, 187

SST receptors have been identified *in vitro* on the membrane of a variety of tumor cells, especially in neuroendocrine tumors, tumors of the nervous system, lymphomas, breast cancers, prostate cancers, gastric cancers, and so on (116,117). In addition, some human tumors (such as colorectal cancers) that exhibit no detectable SST receptor still have a high receptor density in vascular systems surrounding the tumor tissues (119).

In vivo imaging and therapy of SST receptors overexpressing tumors are usually performed with SST analogs such as octreotide and other small cyclic peptides with high receptor affinity, improved plasma stability, and fast clearance. These small peptides have excellent tissue permeability and lack of undesired side effects when administered at tracer concentrations (116).

Initially, *in vivo* imaging of SST positive tumors in humans was performed with the SPECT tracer [^{123}I,Tyr[3]]octreotide (120). However, this tracer's limitations include a difficult radiosynthesis and consistent abdominal uptake *in vivo*. These drawbacks were solved with DTPA conjugation of octreotide, followed by ^{111}In-labeling.

[^{111}In-DTPA[0]]octreotide (^{111}In-pentetreotide, Octreoscan) (121) is now commercially available and is the most widely used radiotracer for *in vivo* imaging of tumors expressing high levels of SST receptor, such as neuroendocrine tumors (carcinoids), meningiomas, and medulloblastomas (116).

Another commercially available SPECT tracer for imaging receptor-positive tumors is ^{99m}Tc-depreotide (^{99m}Tc-P829, Neotect) (122). P829 is a synthetic peptide containing the conformationally constrained pharmacophore with affinity for the receptor, but lacking the disulfide bridge of octreotide. For this reason, P829 can be directly labeled with ^{99m}Tc by using generator-produced pertechnetate solution and a reducing agent, without loss of affinity for the SST receptors (122). Despite its lower sensitivity in detecting endocrine tumors compared with ^{111}In-pentetreotide (123), ^{99m}Tc-depreotide recently has been approved by the Food and Drug Administration for detection of solitary pulmonary nodules in humans.

Owing to the paramount interest in diagnosis and therapy of SST receptor-positive human tumors, octreotide and other SST analogs have been conjugated with a variety of ligands including deferoxamine (124) for [67/68]Ga-labeling and a series of azamacrocycles [DOTA (125–129), NOTA (130), and TETA (131,132) for [67/68]Ga-, [111]In-, [86/90]Y-, [177]Lu-, and ^{64}Cu-labeling]. Furthermore, SST derivatives have been coupled to a N_4-type BFCA (133) and to a HYNIC (134) for ^{99m}Tc-labeling. More recently, SST analogs have been labeled with [124]I (126), [76]Br (135), [110m]In (136), and [18]F (137), yielding promising new tracers to detect SST receptor-positive tumors with PET *in vivo* imaging.

VIP Receptors

The VIP is a 28-amino acid neuropeptide belonging to the family of secretin-like peptides (138). VIP plays an important role in the gut as neurotransmitter and has a neuromodulatory role in the central nervous system (139). VIP receptors are expressed in many healthy tissues such as gastrointestinal mucosa, lobules and duct of the breast, prostatic glands, bladder urothelium, and smooth muscles of the stomach. Interest in using VIP for *in vivo* early tumor diagnosis builds on the finding that VIP receptors are expressed by most primary human tumors (cancers of the lung, colon, rectum, breast, prostate, liver, etc.); in many cases, VIP receptor density is much higher than SST receptors (116). Unfortunately, this broad expression of VIP receptors hampers the use of labeled VIP derivatives for cancer imaging, and VIP tumor scintigraphy is limited to those sites expressing a low physiological receptor density (e.g., colorectal cancer).

As VIP has two Tyr residues in its sequence, it has been successfully labeled with the SPECT radionuclide [123]I (115). Although ^{123}I-VIP has been reported to be a poor candidate to detect neuroendocrine malignancies compared with ^{111}In-pentetreotide, as well as small pulmonary lesions (140), it has been successfully used in clinical practice to detect a variety of cancers including colorectal cancer, pancreatic carcinoma, and gastric cancer (115).

A newer candidate for SPECT imaging of VIP receptor-positive tumors is ^{99m}Tc-TP 3659 (141). TP 3659 is a synthetic VIP analog containing a C-terminal Gly–Gly–Ala–Gly tetrapeptide suitable for stabilizing [99m]Tc (N_4 chelating set). ^{99m}Tc-TP 3659 has been successfully tested in a small number of patients with different tumors (142) and it was proven to be a promising candidate for detection of colon cancer, despite some hepatobiliary excretion (143).

For PET imaging purposes, ^{18}F-labeled VIP has been evaluated in a preliminary study with a breast cancer model, where it demonstrated low tumor uptake compared with [18]FDG (144).

Other Receptors

Cholecystokinin (CCK) and gastrin are gastrointestinal peptides acting as neurotransmitters in the brain and as regulators of various functions in the gastrointestinal tract (116,145). The CCK/gastrin receptor CCK-2 is overexpressed in medullary thyroid cancers (MTCs) and in several other tumors, such as small cell lung cancers, stromal ovarian cancers, and astrocytomas (116,145). The interest in developing CCK/gastrin-based radiotracers, as well as therapeutic agents, arises mainly from the lack of SST receptors in MTCs, which prevent octreotide imaging and radioiodine therapy (145). For imaging purposes, several synthetic peptides containing the receptor-active C-terminal tetrapeptide Trp-Met-Asp-Phe-NH_2 and either a sulfated Tyr (as in CCK) or a Glu_5 sequence (as in gastrin) have been evaluated (146,147). In patients with known and occult metastatic MTCs, the derivative ^{111}In-DTPA-D-Glu-minigastrin visualized tumor lesions as early as 1 h post-injection. Due to these encouraging results, labeled minigastrin derivatives are now under evaluation for radiotherapy of patients with advanced metastatic MTC.

High density of gastrin-releasing peptide (GRP) receptors has been identified in all the prostatic carcinomas and in many breast cancers, as well as in the metastases of these tumors (116). A series of potential diagnostic tracers for GRP receptor-expressing tumors have been developed by labeling bombesin (BN), the amphibian counterpart of GRP. BN and BN(7–14), a truncated BN derivative, have been labeled with [111]In (148,149), [99m]Tc (150–157), and [64]Cu (158).

Following pre-clinical evaluation, ^{111}In-DTPA-BN biodistribution was found suitable for *in vivo* imaging of GRP receptor-expressing tumors (159). The results from a phase I clinical trial in patients with invasive prostate carcinoma are awaited. The promising BN analogs ^{99m}Tc-RP257 (151) and ^{99m}Tc-Leu-13-BN1 (160) have been proven useful in detecting primary prostate cancers as well as metastases in pilot clinical studies. In other small-scale clinical studies, ^{99m}Tc-Leu-13-BN1 clearly visualized tumor lesions in colon cancer patients (161) and breast cancer patients (162), and has been used successfully for scintigraphic-driven breast biopsies (163). Recently, the GRP receptor-targeting SPECT tracer ^{99m}Tc-Demobesin 1 exhibited good clearance from target and nontarget tissues and considerable tumor uptake in prostate tumor-bearing mice (154). Clinical studies with ^{99m}Tc-Demobesin 1 in prostate cancer patients are in progress.

The folate receptor α-isoform is another attractive target for tumor diagnosis and therapy, because it is physiologically expressed in only limited regions of the body and is overexpressed by a number of human tumors and, notably, by all ovarian and endometrial carcinomas (164,165). For imaging purposes, several folate conjugates have been labeled with gallium isotopes (166,167), [111]In (168), [99m]Tc (169–173), and [64]Cu (174). In a recent preliminary clinical study, ^{111}In-DTPA-folate SPECT was able to identify both newly diagnosed and recurrent ovarian cancers with high sensitivity (175). ^{99m}Tc-EC20 (173), a new promising radiolabeled folate conjugate, is currently undergoing clinical evaluation.

Sigma receptors (σ_1 and σ_2) are membrane-bound proteins, originally classified as subtypes of the opiate receptors (176). The observed overexpression of σ-receptors in a variety of human tumors (177) suggests the use of σ-specific imaging agents for tumor diagnosis (178–181). Recently, as σ_2 receptors were identified as markers of tumor proliferation (182) and administration of σ_2-specific targeting compounds was suggested to result in high contrast images (183), high affinity and selective σ_2-receptor targeting ligands have been synthesized as candidate breast cancer imaging tracers (184–186). To our knowledge, the only clinical trial with σ-specific tracers in breast cancer patients was performed with a radioiodinated benzamide (P-^{123}I-MBA) expressing affinity for both σ_1 and σ_2 receptors (181). In this pilot SPECT study, focal uptake of P-^{123}I-MBA was observed in patients with confirmed breast cancer and no uptake was found in fibrocystic disease or local inflammation (187).

E. Reporter Genes

The tracers discussed so far are useful for directly imaging cell phenotypes which are consequences of disease. However, there is a growing interest in indirect monitoring of disease status by imaging the expression of genes encoding for these phenotypes. *In vivo* targeting of DNA and RNA with radiolabeled antisense oligonucleotides has been largely unsuccessful so far due to fast tracer metabolism and difficult delivery to the target (188). To date, the most successful strategy for *in vivo* imaging of gene expression exploits the use of reporter genes coupled to reporter probes (Table 1.6). An example of a reporter

Table 1.6 Examples of Reporter Probes for Reporter Gene Imaging

Tracer	Target	Application	References
[$^{123/124/131}$I]FIAU	HSV1-*tk* and HSV1-*sr39tk*	PET/SPECT	189, 196, 197, 199
[^{11}C]FMAU		PET	192
[^{18}F]PCV		PET	193
[^{18}F]GCV		PET	193
^{18}FHBG		PET	194
^{18}FHPG		PET	195
[^{18}F]Fluoroethylspiperone	h*D2R*	PET	203
^{111}In-Pentretreotide	h*SSTR2*	SPECT	121
[$^{123/124/131}$I]Iodide	h*NIS*	PET/SPECT	202
^{99m}Tc-Pertechnetate		SPECT	204
^{99m}Tc-Glucoheptonate	PEP-MT	SPECT	205, 206

gene is a transgene placed under the control of the same promoter that activates the expression of the target gene. Therefore, expression of the target gene leads to expression of the reporter, and the product of the reporter gene expression (e.g., an enzyme, a receptor, etc.) can be monitored by means of a reporter probe (2–5). The main advantage of the reporter gene imaging strategy is that a small number of well-characterized reporter gene–reporter probe pairs can be used in many different reporter constructs, that is, to monitor many different molecular events. Conversely, direct targeting of receptors, enzymes, and so on requires *de novo* synthesis, characterization, and biological evaluation of unique molecular imaging probes for each target, and this is a time-consuming, costly effort.

However, a reporter gene needs to be introduced into the cells to be imaged. Viral gene vectors (retrovirus, adenovirus, *Herpes simplex* virus, etc.) have a high transfection efficiency, but may lead to immunogenic response, whereas nonviral systems (naked DNA, liposomes, etc.) are less immunogenic and easier to manufacture, but lead to a less efficient transfection (3).

To date, the reporter gene imaging approach is used to evaluate gene delivery systems or to track transgenic cancer cells and xenografts in animal models. In the future, this approach may be useful to monitor the effectiveness of gene therapy in humans.

The wild-type *Herpes simplex* virus-1 thymidine kinase gene (HSV1-*tk*) (189) and a mutant HSV1-*tk* gene (HSV1-*sr39tk*) (190) are the most studied genes for therapeutic and imaging applications. Viral thymidine kinase, product of HSV1-*tk* expression, enables higher phosphorylation of nucleoside analogs (such as ganciclovir) when compared with endogenous thymidine. The resulting mono-phosphorylated nucleoside is trapped within the cell and subsequently converted to nucleoside triphosphate, which terminates DNA synthesis resulting in cell death (191). The HSV1-*tk* gene is not present in nontransfected mammalian cells, and cells that do not express the HSV1-*tk* gene do not accumulate ganciclovir.

For nuclear imaging purposes, nucleoside analogs are labeled with positron- or gamma-emitting radionuclides. These tracers freely cross the plasma membrane by means of active transports and are trapped in cells expressing the HSV1-*tk* reporter gene, thus producing an imageable signal. Because the reporter probes are administered in tracer amount, they do not cause toxicity. Candidate PET reporter probes for HSV1-*tk* are pyrimidine nucleosides derivatives, such as 2'-fluoro-2'-deoxy-1-β-D-arabinofuranosyl-5-[[124]I]iodouracyl ([124]I]FIAU) (189), and [11C]-2'-fluoro-5-methyl-1-β-D-arabinofuranosyluracil ([11C]FMAU) (192), 18F-labeled acycloguanosine analogs, such as penciclovir ([18F]PCV), and ganciclovir ([18F]GCV) (193), and their side chain substituted 18F-derivatives 9-(4-fluoro-3-hydroxy-methylbutyl)guanine (18FHBG) (194), and 9-[(3-fluoro-1-hydroxy-2-propoxy)methyl]guanine (18FHPG) (195). A SPECT tracer candidate to image the reporter gene HSV1-*tk* is [[123/131]I]FIAU (196,197). Several studies have compared these different radiolabeled reporter probes for imaging HSV1-*tk* expression *in vitro* and *in vivo*. Most of these studies have used stably transfected cell lines in cell culture and/or in xenograft models, whereas some have used adenoviral-mediated gene delivery (transient transfection). As the mechanism of reporter gene introduction is an important variable for determining the optimal reporter gene/reporter probe combination (198), a rigorous comparison of the performances of these reporter constructs is difficult.

In a preliminary clinical trial, [124I]FIAU PET imaging was useful in monitoring experimental HSV-1-*tk* suicide-gene treatment of glioblastomas. [124I]FIAU imaging revealed the location, magnitude, and extent of vector-mediated HSV-1-*tk* gene expression delivered by direct intratumoral infusion of cationic liposomes in a phase I/II clinical trial for recurrent glioblastoma in patients (199). Although still in validation, it appears that the PET reporter-gene imaging will be able to provide supplementary gene delivery information in gene therapy trials.

Reporter genes can also encode for extracellular receptors such as dopamine D2 (200) and SST type-2 receptors (201), or membrane transporters such as the sodium/iodide symporter (202). These human genes have been suggested as candidate reporter genes because they exhibit limited expression in the body. At the same time, radiolabeled tracers with high affinity for these extracellular gene-products have been extensively studied and are approved for human use [e.g., [18F]fluoroethylspiperone for D2 receptors (203), 111In-pentetreotide for SST receptors (121), and 123/124/131I or 99mTc-pertechnetate for the sodium/iodide symporter (202,204)]. Furthermore, as these are human genes, the products of gene expression are less likely to be immunogenic.

More recently, new reporter genes encoding for "artificial" membrane receptors have been developed (205,206). These genes encode for metallothionein-based proteins and other proteins exhibiting oxotechnetate-binding properties upon expression on the cell surface. Therefore, noninvasive mapping of gene expression can be achieved by administering commercially available 99mTc-radiopharmaceuticals such as 99mTc-glucoheptonate, 99mTc-DTPA and so on. This strategy overcomes the drawback of natural background expression of receptors, such as dopamine and serotonin receptors, in nontransfected tissues. Furthermore, it does not require mutagenesis to decouple receptors from signal transduction cascades.

IV. Summary

In this chapter, we have described some classes of radiopharmaceuticals developed for molecular imaging. Although only a limited number of these have been used to date for pulmonary imaging, many are suitable for studies of lung cancer, lung inflammation, or gene transfer to the lungs. The chapter describes the broad variety of agents that can be utilized. Similar agents can be developed for new molecular targets in the lungs as they are identified.

References

1. Wagenaar DJ, Weissleder R, Hengerer A. Glossary of molecular imaging terminology. Acad Radiol 2001; 8:409–420.
2. Sharma V, Luker GD, Piwnica-Worms D. Molecular imaging of gene expression and protein function *in vivo* with PET and SPECT. J Magn Res Imaging 2002; 16:336–351.
3. Weissleder R, Mahmood U. Molecular imaging. Radiology 2001; 219:316–333.
4. Massoud TF, Gambhir SS. Molecular imaging in living subjects: seeing fundamental biological processes in a new light. Gene Dev 2003; 17:545–580.
5. Mountz JD, Hsu HC, Wu Q, Liu HG, Zhang HG, Mountz JM. Molecular imaging: new applications for biochemistry. J Cell Biochem Suppl 2002; S39:162–171.
6. Hnatowich DJ. Observations on the role of nuclear medicine in molecular imaging. J Cell Biol Suppl 2002; S39:18–24.
7. Gambhir SS. Molecular imaging of cancer with positron emission tomography. Nat Rev Cancer 2002; 2:683–693.
8. Britz-Cunningham SH, Adelstein SJ. Molecular targeting with radionuclides: state of the science. J Nucl Med 2003; 44:1945–1961.
9. Pennisi E. Human genome: finally, the book of life and instructions for navigating it. Science 2000; 288:2304–2307.
10. Budinger TF, Benaron DA, Koretsky AP. Imaging transgenic animals. Annu Rev Biomed Eng 1999; 1:611–648.
11. Okarvi SM. Peptide-based radiopharmaceuticals: future tools for diagnostic imaging of cancer and other diseases. Med Res Rev 2004; 24:357–397.
12. Lever SZ. Evolution of radiopharmaceuticals for diagnosis and therapy. J Cell Biol Suppl 2002; S39;60–64.
13. Green I, Christison R, Voyce CJ, Bundell KR, Lindsay MA. Protein transduction domains: are they delivering? Trends Pharmacol Sci 2003; 24:213–215.
14. Harris JM, Chess RB. Effect of pegylation on pharmaceuticals. Nat Rev Drug Discov 2003; 2:214–221.
15. Govindan SV, Griffiths GL, Michel RB, Adrews PM, Goldenberg DM, Mattes MJ. Use of galactosylated-streptavidin as a clearing agent with ^{111}In-labeled biotinylated antibodies to enhance tumor/non-tumor localization ratios. Cancer Biother Radiopharm 2002; 17:307–316.
16. Lewis MR, Wang M, Axworthy DB, Theodore LJ, Mallet RW, Fritzberg AR, Welch MJ, Anderson CJ. *In vivo* evaluation of pretargeted ^{64}Cu for tumor imaging and therapy. J Nucl Med 2003; 44:1284–1292.
17. Cherry SR. *In vivo* molecular and genomic imaging: new challenges for imaging physics. Phys Med Biol 2004; 49:R13–R48.
18. Welch MJ, Redvanly CS. Handbook of Radiopharmaceuticals: Radiochemistry and Applications. Chichester: Wiley, 2003.
19. Valk PE, Bailey DL, Townsend DW, Maisey MN. Positron Emission Tomography: Basic Science and Clinical Practice. London: Springer, 2003.
20. Nicolini M, Mazzi U. Technetium, Rhenium and Other Metals in Chemistry and Nuclear Medicine. Vol. 6. Padova: SG Editoriali, 2002.
21. Mason NS, Mathis CA. Radiohalogens for PET imaging. In: Valk PE, Bailey DL, Townsend DW, Maisey MN, eds. Positron Emission Tomography: Basic Science and Clinical Practice. London: Springer, 2003:217–250.

22. Rowland DJ, McCarthy TJ, Welch MJ. Radiobromine for imaging and therapy. In: Welch MJ, Redvanly CS, eds. Handbook of Radiopharmaceuticals: Radiochemistry and Applications. Chichester: Wiley, 2003:441–465.

23. Laforest R, Rowland DJ, Welch MJ. MicroPET imaging with nonconventional isotopes. IEEE Trans Nucl Sci 2002; 49:2119–2126.

24. Finn R. Chemistry applied to iodine radionuclides. In: Welch MJ, Redvanly CS, eds. Handbook of Radiopharmaceuticals: Radiochemistry and Applications. Chichester: Wiley, 2003:423–440.

25. McQuade P, McCarthy DW, Welch MJ. Metal radionuclides for PET imaging. In: Valk PE, Bailey DL, Townsend DW, Maisey MN, eds. Positron Emission Tomography: Basic Science and Clinical Practice. London: Springer, 2003:251–264.

26. Sun X, Anderson CJ. Production and application of copper-64 radiopharmaceuticals. Methods Enzymol 2004; 386:237–261.

27. Banerjee S, Pillai MRA, Ramamoorthy N. Evolution of Tc-99m in diagnostic radiopharmaceuticals. Semin Nucl Med 2001; 31:260–277.

28. Mahmood A, Jones AG. Technetium radiopharmaceuticals. In: Welch MJ, Redvanly CS, eds. Handbook of Radiopharmaceuticals: Radiochemistry and Applications. Chichester: Wiley, 2003:323–362.

29. Bigott HM, Welch MJ. Technetium-94m-sestamibi. Preparation and quality control for human use. In: Nicolini M, Mazzi U, eds. Technetium, Rhenium and Other Metals in Chemistry and Nuclear Medicine. Vol. 6. Padova: SG Editoriali, 2002:559–561.

30. Weiner RE, Thakur ML. Chemistry of gallium and indium radiopharmaceuticals. In: Welch MJ, Redvanly CS, eds. Handbook of Radiopharmaceuticals: Radiochemistry and Applications. Chichester: Wiley, 2003:363–399.

31. Warburg O. The Metabolism of Tumors. New York: Richard Smith, 1931.

32. Ido T, Wan CN, Casella V, Fowler JS, Wolf AP, Reivich M, Kuhl DE. Labeled 2-deoxy-D-glucose analogs, ^{18}F-labeled 2-deoxy-2-fluoro-D-glucose, 2-deoxy-2-fluoro-D-mannose and ^{14}C-2-deoxy-2-fluoro-glucose. J Labelled Compd Radiopharm 1978; 14:171–183.

33. Flier JS, Mueckler MM, Usher P, Lodish HF. Elevated levels of glucose transport and transporter messenger RNA are induced by ras or src oncogenes. Science 1987; 235:1492–1495.

34. Bustamante E, Morris HP, Pedersen PL. Energy metabolism of tumor cells. Requirement for a form of hexokinase with a propensity for mitochondrial binding. J Biol Chem 1981; 256:8699–8704.

35. Brock CS, Meikle SR, Price P. Does fluorine-18 fluorodeoxyglucose metabolic imaging of tumours benefit oncology? Eur J Nucl Med 1997; 24:691–705.

36. Shreve PD, Anzai Y, Wahl RL. Pitfalls in oncologic diagnosis with FDG PET imaging: physiologic and benign variants. Radiographics 1999; 19:61–77.

37. Eary JF, Mankoff DA, Spence AM, Berger MS, Olshen A, Link JN, O'Sullivan F, Krohn KA. 2-[C-11]Thymidine imaging of malignant brain tumors. Cancer Res 1999; 59:615–621.

38. Rohren EM, Turkington TG, Coleman RE. Clinical applications of PET in oncology. Radiology 2004; 231:305–332.

39. Isselbacher KJ. Sugar and amino acid transport by cells in culture—differences between normal and malignant cells. N Engl J Med 1972; 286:929–933.

40. Jager PL, Vaalburg W, Pruim J, de Vries EG, Langen KJ, Piers DA. Radiolabeled amino acids: basic aspects and clinical applications in oncology. J Nucl Med 2001; 42:432–445.

41. Kubota K, Matsuzawa T, Fujiwara T, Sato T, Tada M, Ido T, Ishiwata K. Differential diagnosis of AH109A tumor and inflammation by radioscintigraphy with L-[methyl-^{11}C]-methionine. Jpn J Cancer Res 1989; 80:778–782.

42. Chung JK, Kim YK, Kim S, Lee YJ, Paek S, Yeo JS, Jeong JM, Lee DS, Jung HW, Lee MC. Usefulness of ^{11}C-methionine PET evaluation of brain lesions that are hypo- or isometabolic on ^{18}F-FDG PET. Eur J Nucl Med Mol Imaging 2003; 29:176–182.

43. Inoue T, Kim EE, Wrong FC, Yang DJ, Bassa P, Wong WH, Korkmaz M, Tansey W, Hicks K, Podoloff DA. Comparison of fluorine-18-fluorodeoxyglucose and carbon-11-methionine PET in detection of malignant tumors. J Nucl Med 1996; 37:1472–1476.

44. Herholz K, Holzer T, Bauer B, Schroder R, Voges J, Ernestus RI, Mendoza G, Weber-Luxenburger G, Lottgen J, Thiel A, Wienhard K, Heiss WD. ^{11}C-methionine PET for differential diagnosis of low-grade gliomas. Neurology 1998; 50:1316–1322.

45. Pruim J, Willemsen AT, Molenaar WM, van Waarde A, Paans AM, Heesters MA, Go KG, Visser GM, Franssen EJ, Vaalburg W. Brain tumors: L-[1-C-11]tyrosine for visualization and quantification of protein synthesis rate. Radiology 1995; 197:221–226.

46. Kole AC, Plaat BEC, Hoekstra HJ, Vaalburg W, Molenaar WM. FDG and L-[1-^{11}C]-tyrosine imaging of soft-tissue tumors before and after therapy. J Nucl Med 1999; 40:381–386.

47. Langen KJ, Muhlensiepen H, Holschbach M, Hautzel H, Jansen P, Coenen HH. Transport mechanism of 3-[^{123}I]iodo-α-methyl-L-tyrosine in a human glioma cell line: comparison with [^{3}H-methyl]-L-methionine. J Nucl Med 2000; 41:1250–1255.

48. Jager PL, Plaat BE, de Vries EG, Molenaar WM, Vaalburg W, Piers DA, Hoekstra HJ. Imaging of soft-tissue tumors using L-3-[iodine-123]iodo-alpha-methyl-tyrosine single photon emission tomography: comparison with proliferative and mitotic activity, cellularity and vascularity. Clin Cancer Res 2000; 6:2252–2259.

49. Walsh MN, Geltman EM, Brown MA, Henes CG, Weinheimer CJ, Sobel BE, Bergmann SR. Noninvasive estimation of regional myocardial oxygen consumption by positron emission tomography with carbon-11 acetate in patients with myocardial infarction. J Nucl Med 1989; 30:1798–1808.

50. Liu RS. Clinical application of [C-11]acetate in oncology. Clin Positron Imaging 2000; 3:185.

51. Yoshimoto M, Waki A, Yonekura Y, Sadato N, Murata T, Omata N, Takahashi N, Welch MJ, Fujibayashi Y. Characterization of acetate metabolism in tumor cells in relation to cell proliferation: acetate metabolism in tumor cells. Nucl Med Biol 2001; 28:117–122.

52. Zeisel SH. Dietary choline: biochemistry, physiology, and pharmacology. Annu Rev Nutr 1981; 1:95–121.

53. Hara T, Kosaka N, Shinoura N, Kondo T. PET imaging of brain tumor with [methyl-^{11}C]choline. J Nucl Med 1997; 38:842–847.

54. de Jong IJ, Pruim J, Elsinga PH, Jongen MM, Mensink HJ, Vaalburg W. Visualisation of bladder cancer using [^{11}C]-choline PET: first clinical experience. Eur J Nucl Med Mol Imaging 2002; 29:1283–1288.

55. Utriainen M, Komu M, Vuorinen V, Lehikoinen P, Sonninen P, Kurki T, Utriainen T, Roivainen A, Kalimo H, Minn H. Evaluation of brain tumor metabolism with [^{11}C]choline PET and ^{1}H-MRS. J Neurooncol 2003; 62:329–338.

56. Van de Wiele C, Lahorte C, Oyen W, Boerman O, Goethals I, Slegers G, Dierckx RA. Nuclear medicine imaging to predict response to radiotherapy: a review. Int J Rad Oncol Biol Phys 2003; 55:5–15.

57. Kurokawa T, Yoshida Y, Kawahara K, Tsuchida T, Okazawa H, Fujibayashi Y, Yonekura Y, Kotsuji F. Expression of Glut-1 glucose transfer, cellular proliferation activity and grade of tumor correlate with [F-18]-fluorodeoxyglucose uptake by positron emission tomography in epithelial tumors of the ovary. Int J Cancer 2004; 109:926–932.

58. Chung JK, Lee YJ, Kim SK, Jeong JM, Lee DS, Lee MC. Comparison of [^{18}F]fluorodeoxyglucose uptake with glucose transporter-1 expression and proliferation rate in human glioma and non-small-cell lung cancer. Nucl Med Commun 2004; 25:11–17.

59. Lippitz B, Cremerius U, Mayfrank L, Bertalanffy H, Raoofi R, Weis J, Bocking A, Bull U, Gilsbach JM. PET-study of intracranial meningiomas: correlation with histopathology, cellularity and proliferation rate. Acta Neurochir Suppl (Wien) 1996; 65:108–111.

60. Hoffmann M, Kletter K, Becherer A, Jager U, Chott A, Raderer M. ^{18}F-Fluorodeoxyglucose positron emission tomography (^{18}F-FDG-PET) for staging and follow-up of marginal zone B-cell lymphoma. Oncology 2003; 64: 336–340.

61. Sasaki M, Sugio K, Kuwabara Y, Koga H, Nakagawa M, Chen T, Kaneko K, Hayashi K, Shioyama Y, Sakai S, Honda H. Alteration of tumor suppressor genes (*Rb, p16, p27* and *p53*) and an increased FDG uptake in lung cancer. Ann Nucl Med 2003; 17:189–196.

62. Higashi K, Ueda Y, Yagishita M, Arikasa Y, Sakurai A, Oguchi M, Seki H, Nambu Y, Tonami H, Yamamoto I. FDG PET measurement of the proliferative potential of non-small cell lung cancer. J Nucl Med 2000; 41:85–92.

63. Vesselle H, Schmidt RA, Pugsley JM, Li M, Kohlmyer SG, Vallires E, Wood DE. Lung cancer proliferation correlates with [F-18]fluorodeoxyglucose uptake by positron emission tomography. Clin Cancer Res 2000; 6:3837–3844.

64. Jacob R, Welkoborsky HJ, Mann WJ, Jauch M, Amadee R. [Fluorine-18]fluorodeoxyglucose positron emission tomography, DNA ploid and growth fraction in squamous-cell carcinomas of the head and neck. ORL J Otorhinolaryngol Relat Spec 2001; 63:307–313.

65. Krohn KA. Evaluation of alternative approaches for imaging cellular growth. Q J Nucl Med 2001; 45:174–178.

66. Schwartz JL, Tamura Y, Jordan R, Grierson JR, Krohn KA. Monitoring tumor cell proliferation by targeting DNA synthetic processes with thymidine and thymidine analogs. J Nucl Med 2003; 44:2027–2032.

67. Cleaver JE. Thymidine Metabolism and Cell Kinetics. Amsterdam: North Holland Publishing Co., 1967.

68. Wells P, Gunn RN, Alison M, Steel C, Golding M, Ranicar AS, Brady F, Osman S, Jones T, Price P. Assessment of proliferation *in vivo* using 2-[^{11}C]thymidine

positron emission tomography in advanced intra-abdominal malignancies. Cancer Res 2002; 62:5698–5702.

69. Wells JM, Mankoff DA, Eary JF, Spence AM, Muzi M, O'Sullivan F, Vernon CB, Link JM, Krohn KA. Kinetic analysis of 2-[^{11}C]thymidine PET imaging studies of malignant brain tumors: preliminary patient results. Mol Imaging 2002; 1:145–150.

70. Shields AF, Mankoff DA, Link JM, Graham MM, Eary JF, Kozawa SM, Zheng M, Lewellen B, Lewellen TK, Grierson JR, Krohn KA. Carbon-11-thymidine and FDG to measure therapy response. J Nucl Med 1998; 39:1757–1762.

71. Martiat P, Ferrant A, Labar D, Cogneau M, Bol A, Michel C, Michaux JL, Sokal G. *In vivo* measurement of carbon-11 thymidine uptake in non Hodgkin's lymphoma using positron emission tomography. J Nucl Med 1988; 29:1633–1637.

72. Van Eijkeren ME, Thierens H, Seuntjens J, Goenthals P, Lemahieu I, Strijckmans K. Kinetics of [methyl-^{11}C]thymidine in patients with squamous cell carcinoma of the head and neck. Acta Oncol 1996; 35:737–741.

73. Tjuvajev JG, Macapinlac HA, Daghighian F, Scott AM, Ginos JZ, Finn RD, Kothari P, Desai R, Zhang J, Beattie B. Imaging of brain tumor proliferative activity with iodine-131-iododeoxyuridine. J Nucl Med 1994; 35:1407–1417.

74. Guenther I, Wyer L, Knust EJ, Finn RD, Koziorowski J, Weinreich R. Radiosynthesis and quality assurance of 5-[^{124}I]iodo-2'-deoxyuridine for functional PET imaging of cell proliferation. Nucl Med Biol 1998; 25:359–365.

75. Bergstrom M, Lu L, Fasth KJ, Wu F, Bergstrom-Pettermann E, Tolmachev V, Hedberg E, Cheng A, Langstrom B. *In vitro* and animal validation of bromine-76-bromodeoxyuridine as a proliferation marker. J Nucl Med 1998; 39:1273–1279.

76. Seitz U, Wagner M, Vogg AT, Glatting G, Neumaier B, Greten FR, Schmid RM, Reske SN. *In vivo* evaluation of 5-[^{18}F]fluoro-2'-deoxyuridine as tracer for positron emission tomography in a murine pancreatic cancer model. Cancer Res 2001; 61:3853–3857.

77. Borbath I, Gregoire V, Bergstrom M, Laryea D, Langstrom B, Pauwels S. Use of 5-[^{76}Br]bromo-2'-fluoro-2'-deoxyuridine as a ligand for tumour proliferation: validation in an animal tumour model. Eur J Nucl Med Mol Imaging 2002; 29:19–27.

78. Toyohara J, Hayashi A, Sato M, Tanaka H, Haraguchi K, Yoshimura Y, Yonekura Y, Fujibayashi Y. Rationale of 5-^{125}I-iodo-4'-thio-2'-deoxyuridine as a potential iodinated proliferation marker. J Nucl Med 2002; 43:1218–1226.

79. Kim CG, Yang DJ, Kim EE, Cherif A, Kuang LR, Li C, Tansey W, Liu CW, Li SC, Wallace S, Podoloff DA. Assessment of tumor cell proliferation using [^{18}F]fluorodeoxyadenosine and [^{18}F]fluoroethyluracil. J Pharm Sci 1996; 85:339–344.

80. Conti PS, Alauddin MM, Fissekis JR, Schmall B, Watanabe KA. Synthesis of 2'-fluoro-5-[^{11}C]-methyl-1-beta-D-arabinofuranosyluracil ([^{11}C]-FMAU): a potential nucleoside analog for *in vivo* study of cellular proliferation with PET. Nucl Med Biol 1995; 22:783–789.

81. Mangner TJ, Klecker RW, Anderson L, Shields AF. Synthesis of 2'-deoxy-2'-[^{18}F]fluoro-beta-D-arabinofuranosyl nucleosides, [^{18}F]FAU, [^{18}F]FMAU, [^{18}F]FBAU and [^{18}F]FIAU, as potential PET agents for imaging cellular proliferation. Nucl Med Biol 2003; 30:215–224.

82. Shields AF, Grierson JR, Dohmen BM, Machulla HJ, Stayanoff JC, Lawhorn-Crews JM, Obradovich JE, Muzik O, Mangner TJ. Imaging proliferation *in vivo* with [F-18]FLT and positron emission tomography. Nat Med 1998; 4:1334–1336.

83. Buck AK, Halter G, Schirrmeister H, Kotzerke J, Wurziger I, Glatting G, Mattfeldt T, Neumaier B, Reske SN. Imaging proliferation in lung tumors with PET: ^{18}F-FLT versus ^{18}F-FDG. J Nucl Med 2003; 44:1426–1431.

84. Mier W, Haberkorn U, Eisenhut M. [^{18}F]FLT: portrait of a proliferation marker. Eur J Nucl Med Mol Imaging 2002; 29:165–169.

85. Oyama N, Ponde DE, Dence C, Kim J, Tai YC, Welch MJ. Monitoring of therapy in androgen-dependent prostate tumor model by measuring tumor proliferation. J Nucl Med 2004; 45:519–525.

86. Barthel H, Cleij MC, Collingridge DR, Hutchinson OC, Osman S, He Q, Luthra SK, Brady F, Price PM, Aboagye EO. 3′-Deoxy-3′-[^{18}F]fluorothymidine as a new marker for monitoring antiproliferative therapy *in vivo* with positron emission tomography. Cancer Res 2003; 63:3791–3798.

87. Dittmann H, Dohmen BM, Paulsen F, Eichhorn K, Eschmann SM, Horgen M, Wehrmann M, Machulla HJ, Bares R. [^{18}F]FLT PET for diagnosis and staging of thoracic tumours. Eur J Nucl Med Mol Imaging 2003; 30:1407–1421.

88. Visvikis D, Francis D, Mulligan R, Costa DC, Croasdale I, Luthra SK, Taylor I, Ell PJ. Comparison of methodologies for the *in vivo* assessment of ^{18}FLT utilization in colorectal cancer. Eur J Nucl Med Mol Imaging 2004; 31:169–178.

89. Rajendran JG, Mankoff DA, O'Sullivan F, Peterson LM, Schwartz DL, Conrad EU, Spence AM, Muzi M, Farwell DG, Krohn KA. Hypoxia and glucose metabolism in malignant tumors: evaluation by [^{18}F]fluoromisonidazole and [^{18}F]fluoro-deoxyglucose positron emission tomography imaging. Clin Cancer Res 2004; 10:2245–2252.

90. Sorger D, Patt M, Kumar P, Wiebe LI, Barthel H, Seese A, Dannenberg C, Tannapfel A, Kluge R, Sabri O. [^{18}F]Fluoroazomycinarabinofuranoside (^{18}FAZA) and [^{18}F]fluoromisonidazole (^{18}FMISO): a comparative study of their selective uptake in hypoxic cells and PET imaging in experimental rat tumors. Nucl Med Biol 2003; 30:317–326.

91. Brown JM. The hypoxic cell: a target for selective cancer therapy—eighteenth Bruce F. Cain Memorial Award Lecture. Cancer Res 1999; 59:5863–5870.

92. Evans SM, Koch CJ. Prognostic significance of tumor oxygenation in humans. Cancer Lett 2003; 195:1–16.

93. Larson SM. Positron emission tomography-based molecular imaging in human cancer: exploring the link between hypoxia and accelerated glucose metabolism. Clin Cancer Res 2004; 10:2203–2204.

94. Burgman P, Odonoghue JA, Humm JL, Ling CC. Hypoxia-induced increase in FDG uptake in MCF-7 cells. J Nucl Med 2001; 42:170–175.

95. Bentzen L, Keiding S, Horsman MR, Falborg L, Hansen SB, Overgaard J. Feasibility of detecting hypoxia in experimental mouse tumours with ^{18}F-fluori-nated tracers and positron emission tomography—a study evaluating [^{18}F]fluoro-2-deoxy-D-glucose. Acta Oncol 2000; 39:629–637.

96. Nunn A, Linder K, Strauss HW. Nitroimidazoles and imaging hypoxia. Eur J Nucl Med 1995; 22:266–280.

97. Koh WJ, Rasey JS, Evans ML, Grierson JR, Lewellen TK, Graham MM, Krohn KA, Griffin TW. Imaging hypoxia in human tumors with [F-18]fluoromisonidazole. Int J Radiat Oncol Biol Phys 1992; 22:199–212.

98. Parliament MB, Chapman JD, Urtasun RC, McEwan AJ, Goldberg L, Mercer JR, Mannan RH, Wiebe LI. Non-invasive assessment of human tumor hypoxia with ^{123}I-iodoazomycin arabinoside: preliminary report of a clinical study. Br J Cancer 1992; 65:90–95.

99. Graham MM, Peterson LM, Link JM, Evans ML, Rasey JS, Koh WJ, Caldwell JH, Krohn KA. Fluorine-18-fluoromisonidazole radiation dosimetry in imaging studies. J Nucl Med 1997; 38:1631–1636.

100. Rasey JS, Hofstrand PD, Chin LK, Tewson TJ. Characterization of [^{18}F]fluoroetanidazole, a new radiopharmaceutical for detecting tumor hypoxia. J Nucl Med 1999; 40:1072–1079.

101. Lehtio K, Oikonen V, Nyman S, Gronroos T, Roivainen A, Eskola O, Minn H. Quantifying tumour hypoxia with fluorine-18 fluoroerythronitroimidazole ([^{18}F]FETNIM) and PET using the tumour to plasma ratio. Eur J Nucl Med Mol Imaging 2003; 30:101–108.

102. Ziemer LS, Evans SM, Kachur AV, Shuman AL, Cardi CA, Jenkins WT, Karp JS, Alavi A, Dolbier WR Jr, Koch CJ. Noninvasive imaging of tumor hypoxia in rats using the 2-nitroimidazole ^{18}F-EF5. Eur J Nucl Med Mol Imaging 2003; 30:259–266.

103. Stypinski D, McQuarrie SA, Wiebe LI, Tam YK, Mercer JR, McEwan AJB. Dosimetry estimations for ^{123}I-IAZA in healthy volunteers. J Nucl Med 2001; 42:1418–1423.

104. Zanzonico P, O'Donoghue J, Chapman JD, Schneider R, Cai S, Larson S, Wen B, Chen Y, Finn R, Ruan S, Gerweck L, Humm J, Ling C. Iodine-124-labeled iodo-azomycin-galactoside imaging of tumor hypoxia in mice with serial microPET scanning. Eur J Nucl Med Mol Imaging 2004; 31:117–128.

105. Ng CK, Sisanus AJ, Zaret BL, Soufer R. Kinetic analysis of technetium-99m-labeled nitroimidazole (BMS-181321) as a tracer of myocardial hypoxia. Circulation 1995; 92:1261–1268.

106. Melo T, Duncan J, Ballinger JR, Rauth M. BRU59–21, a second-generation ^{99m}Tc-labeled 2-nitroimidazole for imaging hypoxia in tumors. J Nucl Med 2000; 41:169–176.

107. Chu T, Li R, Hu S, Liu X, Wang X. Preparation and biodistribution of technetium-99m-labeled 1-(2-nitroimidazole-1-yl)-propanhydroxyiminoamide (N2IPA) as a tumor hypoxia marker. Nucl Med Biol 2004; 31:199–203.

108. Archer CM, Edwards B, Kelly JD, King AC, Burke JF, Riley ALM. Technetium labelled agents for imaging tissue hypoxia *in vivo*. In: Nicolini M, Bandoli G, Mazzi U, eds. Technetium, Rhenium and Other Metals in Chemistry and Nuclear Medicine. Vol. 4. Padova: SG Editoriali, 1995: 535–539.

109. Yutani K, Kusuoka H, Fukuchi K, Tatsumi M, Nishimura T. Applicability of ^{99m}Tc-HL91, a putative hypoxic tracer, to detection of tumor hypoxia. J Nucl Med 1999; 40:854–861.

110. Fujibayashi Y, Taniuchi H, Yonekura Y, Ohtani H, Konishi J, Yokoyama A. Copper-62-ATSM: a new hypoxia imaging agent with high membrane permeability and low redox potential. J Nucl Med 1997; 38:1155–1160.

111. Lewis JS, Sharp TL, Laforest R, Fujibayashi Y, Welch MJ. Tumor uptake of copper-diacetyl-*bis*[*N*(4)-methylthiosemicarbazone]: effect of changes in tissue oxygenation. J Nucl Med 2001; 42:655–661.

112. Dehdashti F, Mintun MA, Lewis JS, Bradley J, Govindan R, Laforest R, Welch MJ, Siegel BA. *In vivo* assessment of tumor hypoxia in lung cancer with ^{60}Cu–ATSM. Eur J Nucl Med Mol Imaging 2003; 30:844–850.

113. Dehdashti F, Grigsby PW, Mintun MA, Lewis JS, Siegel BA, Welch MJ. Assessing tumor hypoxia in cervical cancer by positron emission tomography with ^{60}Cu–ATSM: relationship to therapeutic response–a preliminary report. Int J Radiat Oncol Biol Phys 2003; 55:1233–1238.

114. Krenning EP, Kwekkeboom DJ, Bakker WH, Breeman WA, Kooij PP, Oei HY, van Hagen M, Postema PT, de Jong M, Reubi JC, Visser TJ, Reijs AEM, Hofland LJ, Koper JW, Lamberts SWJ. Somatostatin receptor scintigraphy with [^{111}In-DTPA-D-Phe^1]- and [^{123}I-Tyr^3]-octreotide: the Rotterdam experience with more than 1000 patients. Eur J Nucl Med 1993; 20:716–731.

115. Virgolini I, Raderer M, Kurtaran A, Angelberger P, Banyai S, Yang Q, Li S, Banyai M, Pidlich J, Niederle B, Scheithauer W, Valent P. Vasoactive intestinal peptide-receptor imaging for the localization of intestinal adenocarcinomas and endocrine tumors. N Engl J Med 1994; 331:1116–1121.

116. Reubi JC. Peptide receptors as molecular targets for cancer diagnosis and therapy. Endocr Rev 2003; 24:389–427.

117. van der Lely AJ, de Herder WW, Krenning EP, Kwekkeboom DJ. Octreoscan radioreceptor imaging. Endocrine 2003; 20:307–311.

118. Breeman WA, de Jong M, Kwekkeboom DJ, Valkema R, Bakker WH, Kooij PP, Visser TJ, Krenning EP. Somatostatin receptor-mediated imaging and therapy: basic science, current knowledge, limitations and future perspectives. Eur J Nucl Med 2001; 28:1421–1429.

119. Reubi JC, Mazzucchelli L, Hennig I, Laissue JA. Local up-regulation of neuropeptide receptors in host blood vessels around human colorectal cancers. Gastroenterology 1996; 110:1719–1726.

120. Becker W, Marienhagen J, Scheubel R, Saptogino A, Bakker WH, Breeman WA, Wolf F. Octreotide scintigraphy localizes somatostatin receptor-positive islet cell carcinomas. Eur J Nucl Med 1991; 18:924–927.

121. Bakker WH, Albert R, Bruns C, Breeman WA, Hofland LJ, Marbach P, Pless J, Pralet D, Stolz B, Koper JW, Lamberts SWJ, Visser TJ, Krenning EP. [^{111}In-DTPA-D-Phe^1]-octreotide, a potential radiopharmaceutical for imaging of somatostatin receptor-positive tumors: synthesis, radiolabeling and *in vitro* validation. Life Sci 1991; 49:1583–1591.

122. Vallabhajosula S, Moyer BR, Lister-James J, McBride BJ, Lipszyc H, Lee H, Bastidas D, Dean RT. Preclinical evaluation of technetium-99m-labeled somatostatin receptor-binding peptides. J Nucl Med 1996; 37:1016–1022.

123. Lebtahi R, Le Cloirec J, Houzard C, Daou D, Sobhani I, Sassolas G, Mignon M, Bourguet P, Le Guludec D. Detection of neuroendocrine tumors: ^{99m}Tc-P829 scintigraphy compared with ^{111}In-pentetreotide scintigraphy. J Nucl Med 2002; 43:889–895.

124. Smith-Jones PM, Stolz B, Bruns C, Albert R, Reist HW, Fridrich R, Macke HR. Gallium-67/gallium-68-[DFO]-octreotide—a potential radiopharmaceutical for

PET imaging of somatostatin receptor-positive tumors: synthesis and radiolabeling *in vitro* and preliminary *in vivo* studies. J Nucl Med 1994; 35:317–325.

125. Heppeler A, Froidevaux S, Maecke HR, Jermann E, Behe M, Powell P, Hennig M. Radiometal-labelled macrocyclic chelator-derivatised somatostatin analogue with superb tumor-targeting properties and potential for receptor-mediated internal radiotherapy. Chem Eur J 1999; 5:1974–1981.

126. Li WP, Lewis JS, Kim J, Bugaj JE, Johnson MA, Erion JL, Anderson CJ. DOTA-D-Tyr^1-octreotate: a somatostatin analogue for labeling with metal and halogen radionuclides for cancer imaging and therapy. Bioconjug Chem 2002; 13:721–728.

127. Virgolini I, Britton K, Buscombe J, Moncayo R, Paganelli G, Riva P. In- and Y-DOTA-lanreotide: results and implications of the MAURITIUS trial. Semin Nucl Med 2002; 32:148–155.

128. Jamar F, Barone R, Mathieu I, Walrand S, Labar D, Carlier P, de Camps J, Schran H, Chen T, Smith MC, Bouterfa H, Valkema R, Krenning EP, Kvols LK, Pauwels S. ^{86}Y-DOTA-D-Phe^1-Tyr^3-octreotide (SMT487)—a phase 1 clinical study: pharmacokinetics, biodistribution and renal protective effect of different regimens of amino acid co-infusion. Eur J Nucl Med Mol Imaging 2003; 30:510–518.

129. Kwekkeboom DJ, Bakker WH, Kooij PP, Konijnenberg MW, Srinivasan A, Erion JL, Schmidt MA, Bugaj JL, de Jong M, Krenning EP. [^{177}Lu-DOTA^0,Tyr^3]octreotate: comparison with [^{111}In-DTPA^0]octreotide in patients. Eur J Nucl Med 2001; 28:1319–1325.

130. Eisenwiener KP, Prata MI, Buschmann I, Zhang HW, Santos AC, Wenger S, Reubi JC, Macke HR. NODAGATOC, a new chelator-coupled somatostatin analogue labeled with [$^{67/68}$Ga] and [^{111}In] for SPECT, PET, and targeted therapeutic applications of somatostatin receptor (hsst2) expressing tumors. Bioconjug Chem 2002; 13:530–541.

131. Lewis JS, Srinivasan A, Schmidt MA, Anderson CJ. *In vitro* and *in vivo* evaluation of ^{64}Cu-TETA-Tyr^3-octreotate. A new somatostatin analog with improved target tissue uptake. Nucl Med Biol 1999; 26:267–273.

132. Anderson CJ, Dehdashti F, Cutler PD, Schwarz SW, Laforest R, Bass LA, Lewis JS, McCarthy DW. ^{64}Cu-TETA-octreotide as a PET imaging agent for patients with neuroendocrine tumors. J Nucl Med 2001; 42:213–221.

133. Maina T, Nock B, Nikolopoulou A, Sotiriou P, Loudos G, Maintas D, Cordopatis P, Chiotellis E. [^{99m}Tc]demotate, a new ^{99m}Tc-based [Tyr^3]octreotate analogue for the detection of somatostatin receptor-positive tumours: synthesis and preclinical results. Eur J Nucl Med Mol Imaging 2002; 29:742–753.

134. Decristoforo C, Mather SJ, Cholewinski W, Donnemiller E, Riccabona G, Moncayo R. ^{99m}Tc-EDDA/HYNIC-TOC: a new ^{99m}Tc-labelled radiopharmaceutical for imaging somatostatin receptor-positive tumours; first clinical results and intra-patient comparison with ^{111}In-labelled octreotide derivatives. Eur J Nucl Med 2000; 27:1318–1325.

135. Yngve U, Khan TS, Bergstrom M, Langstrom B. Labeling of octreotide using Br-76 prosthetic groups. J Labelled Compd Radiopharm 2001; 44:561–573.

136. Lubberink M, Tolmachev V, Widstrom C, Bruskin A, Lundqvist H, Westlin JE. ^{110m}In-DTPA-D-Phe^1-octreotide for imaging of neuroendocrine tumors with PET. J Nucl Med 2002; 43:1391–1397.

137. Wester HJ, Schottelius M, Scheidhauer K, Meisetschlager G, Herz M, Rau FC, Reubi JC, Schwaiger M. PET imaging of somatostatin receptors: design, synthesis and preclinical evaluation of a novel ^{18}F-labelled, carbohydrated analogue of octreotide. Eur J Nucl Med Mol Imaging 2003; 30:117–122.

138. Ulrich CD II, Holtmann M, Miller LJ. Secretin and vasoactive intestinal peptide receptors: members of a unique family of G protein-coupled receptors. Gastroenterology 1998; 114:382–397.

139. Waschek JA. Vasoactive intestinal peptide: an important trophic factor and developmental regulator? Dev Neurosci 1995; 17:1–7.

140. Raderer M, Kurtaran A, Leimer M, Angelberger P, Niederle B, Vierhapper H, Vorbeck F, Hejna MH, Scheithauer W, Pidlich J, Virgolini I. Value of peptide receptor scintigraphy using ^{123}I-vasoactive intestinal peptide and (111)In-DTPA-D-Phe[1]-octreotide in 194 carcinoid patients: Vienna University Experience, 1993 to 1998. J Clin Oncol 2000; 18:1331–1336.

141. Pallela VR, Thakur ML, Chakder S, Rattan S. ^{99m}Tc-labeled vasoactive intestinal peptide receptor agonist: functional studies. J Nucl Med 1999; 40:352–360.

142. Thakur ML, Marcus CS, Saeed S, Pallela V, Minami C, Diggles L, Pham HL, Ahdoot R, Kalinowski EA, Moody T. Imaging tumors in humans with Tc-99m-VIP. Ann NY Acad Sci 2000; 921:37–44.

143. Rao PS, Thakur ML, Pallela V, Patti R, Reddy K, Li H, Sharma S, Pham HL, Diggles L, Minami C, Marcus CS. [99m]Tc labeled VIP analog: evaluation for imaging colorectal cancer. Nucl Med Biol 2001; 28:445–450.

144. Jagoda EM, Aloj L, Seidel J, Lang L, Moody TW, Green S, Caraco C, Daube-Witherspoon M, Green MV, Eckelman WC. Comparison of an ^{18}F labeled derivative of vasoactive intestinal peptide and 2-deoxy-2-[^{18}F]fluoro-D-glucose in nude mice bearing breast cancer xenografts. Mol Imaging Biol 2002; 4:369–379.

145. Behe M, Behr TM. Cholecystokinin-B (CCK-B)/gastrin receptor targeting peptides for staging and therapy of medullary thyroid cancer and other CCK-B receptor expressing malignancies. Biopolymers 2002; 66:399–418.

146. Behr TM, Jenner N, Behe M, Angerstein C, Gratz S, Raue F, Becker W. Radiolabeled peptides for targeting cholecystokinin-B/gastrin receptor-expressing tumors. J Nucl Med 1999; 40:1029–1044.

147. Aloj L, Panico M, Caraco C, Del Vecchio S, Arra C, Affuso A, Accardo A, Mansi R, Tesauro D, De Luca S, Pedone C, Visentin R, Mazzi U, Morelli G, Salvatore M. *In vitro* and *in vivo* characterization of indium-111 and technetium-99m labeled CCK-8 derivatives for CCK-B receptor imaging. Cancer Biother Radiopharm 2004; 19:93–98.

148. Breeman WA, De Jong M, Bernard BF, Kwekkeboom DJ, Srinivasan A, van der Pluijm ME, Hofland LJ, Visser TJ, Krenning EP. Pre-clinical evaluation of [^{111}In-DTPA-Pro[1], Tyr[4]]bombesin, a new radioligand for bombesin-receptor scintigraphy. Int J Cancer 1999; 83:657–663.

149. Hoffman TJ, Gali H, Smith CJ, Sieckman GL, Hayes DL, Owen NK, Volkert WA. Novel series of ^{111}In-labeled bombesin analogs as potential radiopharmaceuticals for specific targeting of gastrin-releasing peptide receptors expressed on human prostate cancer cells. J Nucl Med 2003; 44:823–831.

150. Baidoo KE, Lin KS, Zhan Y, Finley P, Scheffel U, Wagner HN Jr. Design, synthesis, and initial evaluation of high-affinity technetium bombesin analogues. Bioconjug Chem 1998; 9:218–225.

151. Van de Wiele C, Dumont F, Vanden Broecke R, Oosterlinck W, Cocquyt V, Serreyn R, Peers S, Thornback J, Slegers G, Dierckx RA. Technetium-99m RP527, a GRP analogue for visualisation of GRP receptor-expressing malignancies: a feasibility study. Eur J Nucl Med 2000; 27:1694–1699.

152. Okarvi SM, al-Jammaz I. Synthesis, radiolabelling and biological characteristics of a bombesin peptide analog as a tumor imaging agent. Anticancer Res 2003; 23:2745–2750.

153. Varvarigou AD, Scopinaro F, Leondiadis L, Corleto V, Schillaci O, De Vincentis G, Sourlingas TG, Sekeri-Pataryas KE, Evangelatos GP, Leonti A, Xanthopoulos S, Delle Fave G, Archimandritis SC. Synthesis, chemical, radiochemical and radiobiological evaluation of a new ^{99m}Tc-labelled bombesin-like peptide. Cancer Biother Radiopharm 2002; 17:317–326.

154. Nock B, Nikolopoulou A, Chiotellis E, Loudos G, Maintas D, Reubi JC, Maina T. [^{99m}Tc]demobesin 1, a novel potent bombesin analogue for GRP receptor-targeted tumour imaging. Eur J Nucl Med Mol Imaging 2003; 30:247–258.

155. Karra SR, Schibli R, Gali H, Katti KV, Hoffman TJ, Higginbotham C, Sieckman GL, Volkert WA. ^{99m}Tc-labeling and *in vivo* studies of a bombesin analogue with a novel water-soluble dithiadiphosphine-based bifunctional chelating agent. Bioconjug Chem 1999; 10:254–260.

156. La Bella R, Garcia-Garayoa E, Langer M, Blauenstein P, Beck-Sickinger AG, Schubiger PA. *In vitro* and *in vivo* evaluation of a ^{99m}Tc(I)-labeled bombesin analogue for imaging of gastrin releasing peptide receptor-positive tumors. Nucl Med Biol 2002; 29:553–560.

157. Smith CJ, Sieckman GL, Owen NK, Hayes DL, Mazuru DG, Kannan R, Volkert WA, Hoffman TJ. Radiochemical investigations of gastrin-releasing peptide receptor-specific [^{99m}Tc(X)(CO)$_3$-Dpr-Ser-Ser-Ser-Gln-Trp-Ala-Val-Gly-His-Leu-Met-(NH$_2$)] in PC-3, tumor-bearing, rodent models: syntheses, radiolabeling, and *in vitro/in vivo* studies where Dpr = 2,3-diaminopropionic acid and X = H$_2$O or P(CH$_2$OH)$_3$. Cancer Res 2003; 63:4082–4088.

158. Rogers BE, Bigott HM, McCarthy DW, Della Manna D, Kim J, Sharp TL, Welch MJ. MicroPET imaging of a gastrin-releasing peptide receptor-positive tumor in a mouse model of human prostate cancer using a ^{64}Cu-labeled bombesin analogue. Bioconjug Chem 2003; 14:756–763.

159. Breeman WA, de Jong M, Erion JL, Bugaj JE, Srinivasan A, Bernard BF, Kwekkeboom DJ, Visser TJ, Krenning EP. Preclinical comparison of ^{111}In-labeled DTPA- or DOTA-bombesin analogs for receptor-targeted scintigraphy and radionuclide therapy. J Nucl Med 2002; 43:1650–1656.

160. Scopinaro F, De Vincentis G, Varvarigou AD, Laurenti C, Iori F, Remediani S, Chiarini S, Stella S. ^{99m}Tc-bombesin detects prostate cancer and invasion of pelvic lymph nodes. Eur J Nucl Med Mol Imaging 2003; 30:1378–1382.

161. Scopinaro F, De Vincentis G, Corazzieri E, Massa R, Osti M, Pallotta N, Covotta A, Remediani S, Di Paolo M, Monteleone F, Varvarigou A. Detection of colon cancer

with ^{99m}Tc-labeled bombesin derivative (^{99m}Tc-leu-13-BN1). Cancer Biother Radiophar 2004; 19:245–252.

162. Scopinaro F, Varvarigou AD, Ussof W, De Vincentis G, Sourlingas TG, Evangelatos GP, Datsteris J, Archimandritis SC. Technetium labeled bombesin-like peptide: preliminary report on breast cancer uptake in patients. Cancer Biother Radiopharm 2002; 17:327–335.

163. Soluri A, Scopinaro F, De Vincentis G, Varvarigou A, Scafe R, Massa R, Schillaci O, Spanu A, David V. ^{99m}Tc [13Leu] bombesin and a new gamma camera, the imaging probe, are able to guide mammotome breast biopsy. Anticancer Res 2003; 23:2139–2142.

164. Antony AC. Folate receptors. Annu Rev Nutr 1996; 16:501–521.

165. Ke CY, Mathias CJ, Green MA. Folate-receptor-targeted radionuclide imaging agents. Adv Drug Deliv Rev 2004; 56:1143–1160.

166. Wang S, Lee RJ, Mathias CJ, Green MA, Low PS. Synthesis, purification, and tumor cell uptake of ^{67}Ga-deferoxamine-folate, a potential radiopharmaceutical for tumor imaging. Bioconjug Chem 1996; 7:56–62.

167. Mathias CJ, Lewis MR, Reichert DE, Laforest R, Sharp TL, Lewis JS, Yang ZF, Waters DJ, Snyder PW, Low PS, Welch MJ, Green MA. Preparation of ^{66}Ga- and ^{68}Ga-labeled ^{III}Ga-deferoxamine-folate as potential folate-receptor-targeted PET radiopharmaceuticals. Nucl Med Biol 2003; 30:725–731.

168. Wang S, Luo J, Lantrip DA, Waters DJ, Mathias CJ, Green MA, Fuchs PL, Low PS. Design and synthesis of [^{111}In]DTPA-folate for use as a tumor-targeted radiopharmaceutical. Bioconjug Chem 1997; 8:673–679.

169. Mathias CJ, Hubers D, Low PS, Green MA. Synthesis of [^{99m}Tc]DTPA-folate and its evaluation as a folate-receptor-targeted radiopharmaceutical. Bioconjug Chem 2000; 11:253–257.

170. Trump DP, Mathias CJ, Yang Z, Low PS, Marmion M, Green MA. Synthesis and evaluation of ^{99m}Tc(CO)$_3$-DTPA-folate as a folate-receptor-targeted radiopharmaceutical. Nucl Med Biol 2002; 29:569–573.

171. Guo W, Hinkle GH, Lee RJ. ^{99m}Tc-HYNIC-folate: a novel receptor-based targeted radiopharmaceutical for tumor imaging. J Nucl Med 1999; 40:1563–1569.

172. Wedeking PW, Wager RE, Arunachalam T, Ramalingam K, Linder KE, Ranghanatan RS, Nunn AD, Raju N, Tweedle M. Metal complexes derivatized with folate for use in diagnostic and therapeutic application. US Patent 6221334, 2002.

173. Leamon CP, Parker MA, Vlahov IR, Xu LC, Reddy JA, Vetzel M, Douglas N. Synthesis and biological evaluation of EC20: a new folate-derived, ^{99m}Tc-based radiopharmaceutical. Bioconjug Chem 2002; 13:1200–1210.

174. Ke CY, Mathias CJ, Yang ZF, Luo J, Low PS, Waters DJ, Green MA. Synthesis and evaluation of folate-*bis*(thiosemicarbazone) and folate–CYCLAM conjugates for possible use as folate-receptor-targeted copper radiopharmaceuticals. J Labelled Compd Radiopharm 1999; 42:S821–S823.

175. Siegel BA, Dehdashti F, Mutch DG, Podoloff DA, Wendt R, Sutton GP, Burt RW, Ellis PR, Mathias CJ, Green MA, Gershenson DM. Evaluation of ^{111}In-DTPA-folate as a receptor-targeted diagnostic agent for ovarian cancer: initial clinical results. J Nucl Med 2003; 44:700–707.

176. Ferris CD, Hirsch DJ, Brooks BP, Snyder SH. Sigma receptors: from molecule to man. J Neurochem 1991; 57:729–737.

177. Vilner BJ, John CS, Bowen WD. Sigma-1 and sigma-2 receptors are expressed in a wide variety of human and rodent tumor cell lines. Cancer Res 1995; 55:408–413.

178. John CS, Vilner BJ, Gulden ME, Efange SM, Langason RB, Moody TW, Bowen WD. Synthesis and pharmacological characterization of 4-[^{125}I]-N-(N-benzylpiperidin-4-yl)-4-iodobenzamide: a high affinity sigma receptor ligand for potential imaging of breast cancer. Cancer Res 1995; 55:3022–3027.

179. Waterhouse RN, Chapman J, Izard B, Donald A, Belbin K, O'Brien JC, Collier TL. Examination of four ^{123}I-labeled piperidine-based sigma receptor ligands as potential melanoma imaging agents: initial studies in mouse tumor models. Nucl Med Biol 1997; 24:587–593.

180. John CS, Vilner BJ, Geyer BC, Moody T, Bowen WD. Targeting sigma receptor-binding benzamides as *in vivo* diagnostic and therapeutic agents for human prostate tumors. Cancer Res 1999; 59:4578–4583.

181. John CS, Bowen WD, Fisher SJ, Lim BB, Geyer BC, Vilner BJ, Wahl RL. Synthesis, *in vitro* pharmacologic characterization, and preclinical evaluation of N-[2-(1'-piperidinyl)ethyl]-3-[^{125}I]iodo-4-methoxybenzamide (P[^{125}I]MBA) for imaging breast cancer. Nucl Med Biol 1999; 26:377–382.

182. Wheeler KT, Wang LM, Wallen CA, Childers SR, Cline JM, Keng PC, Mach RH. Sigma 2 receptors as a biomarker of proliferation in solid tumours. Br J Cancer 2000; 82:1223–1232.

183. Mach RH, Huang Y, Buchheimer N, Kuhner R, Wu L, Morton TE, Wang L, Ehrenkaufer RL, Wallen CA, Wheeler KT. [(18)F]N-(4'-fluorobenzyl)-4-(3-bromo-phenyl) acetamide for imaging the sigma receptor status of tumors: comparison with [^{18}F]FDG, and [^{125}I]IUDR. Nucl Med Biol 2001; 28:451–458.

184. Choi SR, Yang B, Plossl K, Chumpradit S, Wey SP, Acton PD, Wheeler K, Mach RH, Kung HF. Development of a Tc-99m labeled sigma-2 receptor-specific ligand as a potential breast tumor imaging agent. Nucl Med Biol 2001; 28:657–666.

185. Berardi F, Ferorelli S, Abate C, Colabufo NA, Contino M, Perrone R, Tortorella V. 4-(Tetralin-1-yl)- and 4 (naphthalen-1-yl)alkyl derivatives of 1-cyclohexylpipera-zine as sigma receptor ligands with agonist sigma2 activity. J Med Chem 2004; 47:2308–2317.

186. Rowland DJ, Tu Z, Mach RH, Welch MJ. Investigation of a new sigma 2 receptor ligand for detection of breast cancer. Labelled Compd Radiopharm 2003; 46:S6.

187. Caveliers V, Everaert H, John CS, Lahoutte T, Bossuyt A. Sigma receptor scintigraphy with N-[2-(1'-piperidinyl)ethyl]-3-^{123}I-iodo-4-methoxybenzamide of patients with suspected primary breast cancer: first clinical results. J Nucl Med 2002; 43:1647–1649.

188. Younes CK, Boisgard R, Tavitian B. Labelled oligonucleotides as radiopharmaceuticals: pitfalls, problems and perspectives. Curr Pharm Des 2002; 8:1451–1466.

189. Tjuvajev JG, Avril N, Oku T, Sasajima T, Miyagawa T, Joshi R, Safer M, Beattie B, DiResta G, Daghighian F, Augensen F, Koutcher J, Zweit J, Humm J, Larson SM, Finn R, Blasberg R. Imaging herpes virus thymidine kinase gene transfer and expression by positron emission tomography. Cancer Res 1998; 58:4333–4341.

190. Gambhir SS, Bauer E, Black ME, Liang Q, Kokoris MS, Barrio JR, Iyer M, Namavari M, Phelps ME, Herschman HR. A mutant herpes simplex virus type 1

thymidine kinase reporter gene shows improved sensitivity for imaging reporter gene expression with positron emission tomography. Proc Natl Acad Sci USA 2000; 97:2785–2790.

191. Ram Z, Culver KW, Walbridge S, Frank JA, Blaese RM, Oldfield EH. Toxicity studies of retroviral-mediated gene transfer for the treatment of brain tumors. J Neurosurg 1993; 79:400–407.

192. de Vries EF, van Waarde A, Harmsen MC, Mulder NH, Vaalburg W, Hospers GA. [^{11}C]FMAU and [^{18}F]FHPG as PET tracers for herpes simplex virus thymidine kinase enzyme activity and human cytomegalovirus infections. Nucl Med Biol 2000; 27:113–119.

193. Namavari M, Barrio JR, Toyokuni T, Gambhir SS, Cherry SR, Herschman HR, Phelps ME, Satyamurthy N. Synthesis of 8-[^{18}F]fluoroguanine derivatives: *in vivo* probes for imaging gene expression with positron emission tomography. Nucl Med Biol 2000; 27:157–162.

194. Alauddin MM, Conti PS. Synthesis and preliminary evaluation of 9-(4-[^{18}F]-fluoro-3-hydroxymethylbutyl)guanine ([^{18}F]FHBG): a new potential imaging agent for viral infection and gene therapy using PET. Nucl Med Biol 1998; 25:175–180.

195. Alauddin MM, Conti PS, Mazza SM, Hamzeh FM, Lever JR. 9-[(3-[^{18}F]-Fluoro-1-hydroxy-2-propoxy)methyl]guanine ([^{18}F]-FHPG): a potential imaging agent of viral infection and gene therapy using PET. Nucl Med Biol 1996; 23:787–792.

196. Tjuvajev JG, Finn R, Watanabe K, Joshi R, Oku T, Kennedy J, Beattie B, Koutcher J, Larson S, Blasberg RG. Noninvasive imaging of herpes virus thymidine kinase gene transfer and expression: a potential method for monitoring clinical gene therapy. Cancer Res 1996; 56:4087–4095.

197. Haubner R, Avril N, Hantzopoulos PA, Gansbacher B, Schwaiger M. *In vivo* imaging of herpes simplex virus type 1 thymidine kinase gene expression: early kinetics of radiolabelled FIAU. Eur J Nucl Med 2000; 27:283–291.

198. Min JJ, Iyer M, Gambhir SS. Comparison of [^{18}F]FHBG and [^{14}C]FIAU for imaging of HSV1-tk reporter gene expression: adenoviral infection vs stable transfection. Eur J Nucl Med Mol Imaging 2003; 30:1547–1560.

199. Jacobs A, Voges J, Reszka R, Lercher M, Gossmann A, Kracht L, Kaestle C, Wagner R, Wienhard K, Heiss WD. Positron-emission tomography of vector-mediated gene expression in gene therapy for gliomas. Lancet 2001; 358:727–729.

200. MacLaren DC, Gambhir SS, Satyamurthy N, Barrio JR, Sharfstein S, Toyokuni T, Wu L, Berk AJ, Cherry SR, Phelps ME, Herschman HR. Repetitive, non-invasive imaging of the dopamine D2 receptor as a reporter gene in living animals. Gene Ther 1999; 6:785–791.

201. Zinn KR, Buchsbaum DJ, Chaudhuri TR, Mountz JM, Grizzle WE, Rogers BE. Noninvasive monitoring of gene transfer using a reporter receptor imaged with a high-affinity peptide radiolabeled with ^{99m}Tc or ^{188}Re. J Nucl Med 2000; 41:887–895.

202. Mandell RB, Mandell LZ, Link CJ Jr. Radioisotope concentrator gene therapy using the sodium/iodide symporter gene. Cancer Res 1999; 59:661–668.

203. Barrio JR, Satyamurthy N, Huang SC, Keen RE, Nissenson CH, Hoffman JM, Ackermann RF, Bahn MM, Mazziotta JC, Phelps ME. 3-(2′-[^{18}F]Fluoroethyl)-spiperone: *in vivo* biochemical and kinetic characterization in rodents, nonhuman primates, and humans. J Cereb Blood Flow Metab 1989; 9:830–839.

204. Moon DH, Lee SJ, Park KY, Park KK, Ahn SH, Pai MS, Chang H, Lee HK, Ahn IM. Correlation between ^{99m}Tc-pertechnetate uptakes and expressions of human sodium iodide symporter gene in breast tumor tissues. Nucl Med Biol 2001; 28:829–834.
205. Simonova M, Shtanko O, Sergeyev N, Weissleder R, Bogdanov A Jr. Engineering of technetium-99m-binding artificial receptors for imaging gene expression. J Gene Med 2003; 5:1056–1066.
206. Bogdanov AA Jr, Simonova M, Weissleder R. Engineering membrane proteins for nuclear medicine: applications for gene therapy and cell tracking. Q J Nucl Med 2000; 44:224–235.

2

"Micro"-Instruments for Molecular Imaging with PET and SPECT

RICHARD LAFOREST

Washington University,
St. Louis, Missouri, USA

I. Introduction

The ever increasing popularity of small animal imaging with radio-tracers has been made possible by recent technological progress in image resolution and machine sensitivity (1). The ability to trace the spatial and temporal evolution and distribution of radio-labeled molecules in appropriate animal models offers researchers the opportunity to study disease progression, tumor growth, gene expression, and pharmacokinetics of new drugs in new and valuable ways.

Advancements in molecular biology have made genetically modified mice, the animal of choice, as models of human diseases. However, for *in vivo* imaging, the size of the mouse, $\sim$20 g, requires high spatial resolution and high sensitivity (the efficiency at which the instrument detects and records emitted radiation).

To be able to perform the same types of studies that are currently performed on humans (average adult weight of 70 kg), small animal imaging devices must have a spatial resolution scaled appropriately to the object of interest. Typical human clinical scanners have a spatial resolution of $\sim$5–10 mm. Because the typical human chest has a diameter of 30–50 cm, spatial resolution in the mouse, with a chest diameter of 2–3 cm, must improve by a factor of at least 10, that is <1 mm. Spatial resolution demands of this sort have required new and improved technologies of both detector and overall camera design.

Performance requirements are also dictated by a wide array of applications typically desired in a research imaging environment. For example, flow studies with ^{15}O-H$_2$O necessitate the injection of a large amount of activity into the subject. Due to the short half-life of ^{15}O, the camera is required to have both high sensitivity and high counting rate capabilities to collect as many decay events as possible which are needed to produce images with an acceptable signal-to-noise ratio. On the other hand, when receptor studies are performed with a long half-lived nuclide like ^{64}Cu, the concentration of radioactivity in an image region-of-interest is usually low (depending on the concentration of the receptor) but remains in place for a long period of time (depending on receptor affinity). In such cases, sensitivity (the fraction of decay events detected compared to the true total number during the period of counting) is of crucial importance.

The paradigm that is common to all imaging devices that operate by counting photons can be expressed as follows: when the dimensions of the image resolution element are reduced to provide higher spatial resolution, a decreased number of counts will be detected within each element, resulting in a degradation in the imaging signal-to-noise ratio. Small animal imaging devices push this paradigm to the limit. Typical human PET cameras exhibit sensitivities of $\sim$2–3%, while the resolution volume element is $\sim$125 μL (5 mm^3). To maintain similar performance in small animal imaging devices with a typical resolution volume element of $\sim$1 μL (1 mm^3), sensitivity would have to increase by two orders of magnitude—a level of performance not yet achievable.

Thus, all camera designs, both for SPECT and for PET, are subjected to a compromise between sensitivity and resolution. Some tracers with short-lived radio-nuclides, like glucose or radioactive water, can be injected in larger amounts, thus compensating for the lack in sensitivity. In this case, the limitations on signal-to-noise will mostly be determined by the ability of the camera to acquire data at high counting rates. However, dead-time in the detectors and processing electronics may limit the counting capability of the imaging device, thereby reducing the signal-to-noise ratio achievable in the reconstructed images despite the high amounts of radioactivity administered (see Section IV). In addition, in PET, the acquisition of random (false) coincidences increases with the square of the amount of activity administered, whereas the acquisition of valid events only increases proportionally. This leads to acquisition of more random than true events at high counting rates, which also lowers signal-to-noise in the reconstructed images.

In this chapter, we will review the latest major technological developments for *in vivo* radio-tracer imaging. The two modalities described in this section, namely single photon emission computed tomography (SPECT) and positron emission computed tomography (PET), employ radio-nuclides attached to biological molecules, such as genes, proteins, peptides, antibodies, or antibody fragments. The propagation of the tracer occurs in the living animal through the vascular system or through the airways in the lungs. In particular, the progress made recently in developing these techniques for the imaging of laboratory animal models, like the mouse and the rat, will be presented. Other imaging modalities like magnetic resonance imaging (MRI), optical imaging (OI) and ultrasound (US) will be discussed in other chapters.

II. Single Photon Emission Computed Tomography

Typically, gamma cameras employ a single large sheet of scintillating material, usually NaI(Tl), together with an array of light sensing devices, such as photomultiplier tubes (PMTs), to collect the scintillation light. A collimator then completes the detector assembly. The purpose of the latter is to project an image of the object onto the scintillation detector by limiting gamma rays recorded by the detector to those impinging at normal angles (as in the case of a parallel-hole collimator). The gamma rays emitted by the radio-isotope produce scintillation light at the point where the gamma rays interact with the detector crystal. The scintillation light is then collected by an array of light sensing devices and its location is determined by Anger logic. The precision of this localization is measured as the intrinsic spatial resolution. A typical intrinsic spatial resolution for a clinical gamma camera is $\sim 2-4$ mm. For small animal imaging, the requirement for spatial resolution needs to be higher.

For SPECT imaging, a gamma camera is rotated around the subject to acquire complete tomographic views and the projection images are collected in a step-shoot mode. While this method of image acquisition makes it possible to generate tomographic images, it also means that one must assume that the radio-pharmaceutical bio-distribution does not change during the period of scanning.

Gamma camera performance is determined primarily by collimator design and the characteristics of the scintillation material. In the case of a parallel collimator, the collimator design parameters are the hole diameter, their number, the distance between the holes (hole pitch), and the collimator thickness. The specific combination of these affects the sensitivity and the spatial resolution of the camera. Likewise, thick scintillating material limits spatial resolution, whereas a thin scintillation crystal yields lower sensitivities.

Both sensitivity and resolution are determined by collimator design. Parallel-hole collimator geometry, although having a lower sensitivity than a small pinhole collimator, has a sensitivity and a field-of-view (FOV) that is independent of subject-collimator distance. Thus, a parallel-hole collimator is recommended when a larger FOV is required (assuming that the requirement for spatial resolution is not less than ~2.5 mm).

Typical system spatial resolution and geometric sensitivity for pin-hole collimator apertures of 0.5 and 1 mm are plotted in Fig. 2.1(a). These calculations assumed an intrinsic spatial resolution of 1 mm and an aperture angle of 60°. As can be seen, the dependence of camera sensitivity decreases as the square of the subject to collimator aperture distance. Optimum configuration is thus achieved by placing the subject very close to the collimator aperture. Moreover, spatial resolution degrades approximately linearly with subject to collimator distance,

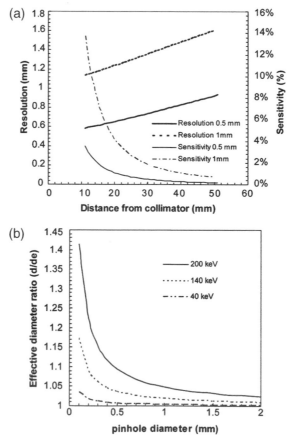

Figure 2.1 (a) Theoretical spatial resolution and geometric sensitivity along the central axis as a function of distance for a typical pin-hole collimator in a SPECT system. (b) Aperture penetration in typical pin-hole configuration for three gamma ray energies showing the inherent spatial limitation in SPECT when using high energy photons.

which is another incentive to place the subject close to the collimator. The drawback, however, is that the FOV is reduced, limiting applicability of this technique if only a part of the animal can be imaged at any one time. Aperture penetration shown in Fig. 2.1(b) is more important for high-energy photons and will reduce the ability of the scanner to achieve high resolution as the effective diameter will be larger.

A pinhole collimator design (unlike a parallel collimator design) is often adopted when imaging small animals with SPECT cameras (2–7) because it allows for a higher spatial resolution. Commercial small animal SPECT cameras are now available through a variety of vendors, including Gamma Medica (CA, USA) (8,9) (distributing through Siemens Medical Systems). Imtek Inc. (Knoxville, TN) has recently released a combined small animal SPECT-CT instrument using two opposed pinhole gamma cameras. Several research institutions have also developed dedicated small animal SPECT systems, including the University of Arizona (10) and the University of Amsterdam (which specifically developed a collimator for small animal studies using a clinical gamma camera) (3,11–13). The spatial resolution of these cameras can be as high as 0.5 mm; however, to achieve this spatial resolution, sensitivity is usually quite low (meaning that higher doses of radioactivity must be administered to achieve images of acceptable quality). Other collimator designs [like the multi-pinhole collimator (14–16)] are currently under investigation. A first commercial SPECT camera using this technology was now made available by BIOSCAN, which offers a product with a selection of collimators with various multiple holes configuration. In each case, the goal is to achieve improvements in spatial resolution (sub-millimeter), camera sensitivity (thereby lowering the radiation dose required), and overall FOV (optimally making it possible to image the entire animal with one bed position).

So far, most of these cameras have used scintillation techniques as the method for collecting and recording gamma rays emitted from the animal or subject. A replacement for the traditional scintillator and PMT combination has long being sought (17). New semiconductor detectors offer the possibility of detecting gamma rays with smaller detectors (allowing high spatial resolution). However, the intrinsic sensitivity must also be high to justify the associated increase in overall cost of building such machines. Recently, the University of Arizona has built a small animal imaging system with many of these features (18,19), and an even more recent upgrade includes X-ray computer tomography functionality (20).

A major advantage of using SPECT instruments for imaging is the large array of off-the-shelf tracers that are already available. A second advantage is the possibility of performing studies that employ multiple tracers in a single imaging session, each labeled with a different isotope. Especially in small animal imaging, Tc-99 and I-125 radio-labeled probes can be imaged simultaneously with very high resolution and with minimal attenuation of radioactivity within the animal.

III. Positron Emission Tomography

Imaging with PET requires the use of positron emitting nuclides that are generally produced with the use of a cyclotron. A radio-nuclide undergoing a β^+ (positron) decay results in the emission of both a positron and a neutrino. These two emitted particles will escape the nucleus with a total energy determined by the difference in nuclear masses between the mother and the daughter nuclei. While the neutrino will escape from the body of the subject (indeed, even the laboratory without being detected), the positron will rapidly collide with other charged particles, mostly atomic electrons in molecules of surrounding tissue, losing energy at every collision until it comes to a stop. When the positron has lost sufficient energy (typically when its kinetic energy is comparable to the energy of atomic electrons), the positron, being the anti-particle of the electron, will annihilate with an atomic electron. This annihilation event releases two gamma rays of equal energy (511 keV), emitted almost in opposite directions from one another. The detection of these two annihilation photons on either side of the subject forms the basis of PET [Fig. 2.2(a)]. The distance of travel of the positron before annihilation (also known as the positron range) and the fact that the positron–electron annihilation photons do not travel exactly opposite from one another are the fundamental limiting factors that determine the spatial resolution of PET cameras.

By far, the most widely used isotope for PET imaging is ^{18}F as it possesses many desirable decay characteristics: it has a half-life of 109.77 min, which is sufficiently long for production, separation, and processing of radio-labeling chemistry. Its decay characteristics also make it an almost ideal isotope for PET imaging: the energy of the emitted positron (maximum of 635 keV) is the lowest among all positron emitters. In addition, no other types of gamma rays are emitted during the decay of this isotope. Other popular isotopes in PET imaging are ^{11}C, ^{13}N, and ^{15}O. Several nonconventional beta-decaying nuclides are also being investigated for use (21,22) (see Chapter 1).

Most PET cameras use a cylindrical geometry design (unlike the planar design of most gamma cameras) in which the radiation detectors are arranged in a ring surrounding the subject [as in Fig. 2.2(a)]. This configuration maximizes the packing of the detectors, which in turn affects sensitivity and uniformity of radiation detection across the subject (crucial to create accurate maps of radioactivity concentrations within tissues).

The choice of scintillation material and thickness affects spatial resolution and camera efficiency in detecting the emitted photons. A scintillation material with a high photoelectric absorption fraction can stop 511 keV gamma rays very efficiently. Compton scattering causes energy depositions in two or more crystals (typically 1–2 cm apart), which makes measurement of the point of interaction between the photon and the detector array imprecise. Thus, the best spatial resolution in PET cameras is achieved by using small size scintillation crystals with high stopping efficiency (e.g., detectors made with

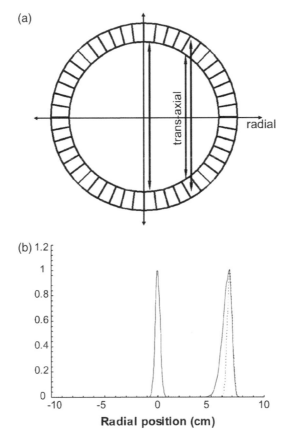

Figure 2.2 (a) Illustration of the basic construction of a PET camera with detector arranged in a cylindrical arrangement. In this ring geometry, the uncertainty due to the depth of interaction (b), in the accurate identification of the radial position of the line on response is illustrated. Typical radial profile through the image of a point source imaged by PET at two radial positions shows a broadening of the profile at large offsets.

LSO (Lu_2SiO_5:Ce) (23) or GSO (Gd_2SiO_5:Ce) (24). A summary of commonly used PET and SPECT scintillation material is presented in Table 2.1.

Until recently, PET cameras employed physical septa between the detectors to limit the acquisition of gamma rays to only those emitted in transverse planes relative to the subject (so-called "2-D imaging"), allowing accurate estimates of regional tissue radioactivity in transverse image sections. This practice obviously reduces the amount of overall radioactivity used in image reconstruction (i.e., reduces the overall sensitivity of the camera). PET imaging without the use of septa (referred to as "3-D imaging") greatly improves sensitivity and also increases the number of random (i.e., fortuitous) coincidences

Table 2.1 Physical and Optical Properties of Commonly Used Scintillation Material in PET and SPECT

Scintillation material	Density (g/cm^3)	Effective atomic number	Primary decay constant (ns)	Emission intensity (%NaI)	Emission wavelength (nm)	Attenuation coefficient at 511 keV (cm^{-1})
Lu_2SiO^5	7.40	65	40	75	420	0.86
Gd_2SiO_5	6.71	59	60	30	430	0.70
$Bi_4Ge_3O_{12}$	7.13	75	300	15	480	0.95
YAP	5.55	32	27	40	347	0.37
BaF_2	4.88	53	2	12	220, 310	0.45
YSO	4.45	36	70	45	550	0.36
LGSO	7.23	65	60	40	420	0.84
LuAP	8.34	64	17	30	365	0.87
NaI(Tl)	3.67	51	230	100	410	0.35

of unrelated decays as well as the fraction of scattered radiation (both sources of noise in reconstructing an accurate image map of regional tissue radioactivity). Scatter and randoms rejection are also important in small animal PET, though not as crucial as in human PET imaging. Septa are generally not present in order to maximize sensitivity of the imaging device.

As previously noted, positron range and photon nonacolinearity are the factors that ultimately limit the spatial resolution that can be achieved in PET, regardless of camera design. Positron range (i.e., the distance traveled by the positron in tissue before annihilation) will vary for each isotope being used for imaging. Photon nonacolinearity, on the other hand, refers to the fact that both annihilation photons are not always emitted at exactly 180° relative to each other. At the time of annihilation, the positron and electron may each have a small velocity relative to the laboratory frame of reference. To conserve energy and momentum, the photons travel at an angle from the annihilation event that is slightly different than 180° from one another. If this variance is not accounted for (which is generally the case), then the accuracy of the PET images as maps of the concentration of regional radioactivity will be affected. For small animal PET tomographs, due to their relatively small diameter, the effect of image "blurring" due to photon nonacolinearity is small when compared with the degradation in spatial resolution caused by positron range or by camera design.

On the basis of the fundamental physics of positron decay, the limit for spatial resolution of a PET image using fluorine-18 (again, a nearly ideal isotope for PET imaging purposes) should be in the range of 0.5–0.75 mm. However, it is possible that in the future, software solutions that make corrections in image reconstruction for the loss of resolution due to the physical process of

Table 2.2 Summary of Characteristics of a Several Complete Small Animal PET Cameras

System	FOV axial xTX (cm)	Crystal size (mm)	Scintillation material	Light sensing device	Number of detectors	Number of crystals	Resolution (mm)	Sensitivity (CFOV, %)
UCLA microPET-I (26)	1.8 × 11.25	2 × 2 × 10	LSO	PS-PMT	30	1,920	1.8	0.56
UCLA microPET-II (27)	4.9 × 8.0	0.975 × 0.975 × 12.5	LSO	PS-PMT	120	23,520	1.25	2.25
CMS microPET-R4 (28)	7.8 × 11	2.24 × 2.24 × 10	LSO	PS-PMT	96	6,144	2.4	3.4
CMS microPET-P4 (29)	7.8 × 19	2.24 × 2.24 × 10	LSO	PS-PMT	168	10,752	2.4	2.25
CMS microPET-F120	7.8 × 11	1.51 × 1.51 × 10	LSO	PS-PMT	96	13,824	1.8	6.5
CMS microPET-F220 (30)	7.8 × 19	1.51 × 1.51 × 10	LSO	PS-PMT	168	24,192	1.8	3.4
Phillips Medical MOSAIC (31)	12.8 × 21	2 × 2 × 10	GSO	PMT	288	14,456	2.3	1.8
General Electric SUINSA, ARGUS	4.6 × 6	1.8 × 1.8 × 15	LGSO + GSO	PS-PMT	36	2 × 6,084	2	4.4
NIH ATLAS (32)	2.3 × 6.9	2 × 2 × 15	LGSO + GSO	PS-PMT	18	2 × 1,458	2	1.8
Ferrara YAP-PET (33)	4 × 4	2 × 2 × 30	YAP	PS-PMT	4	1,600	2	1.7
Julich Tier-PET (36)	4 × 4	2 × 2 × 15	YAP	PS-PMT	4	1,600	2	0.32
Sherbrooke Animal PET (34)	1.05 × 18	3 × 5 × 20	BGO	APD	256	4,096	2.1	0.4
Oxford Positron Systems Quad HIDAC (35)	17 × 28	0.5 mm pitch	Lead converted plates	MWPC	32	14 millions	0.95	1.8
Indianapolis IndyPET-II (37)	15 × 23	3.75 × 6.75 × 30	BGO	PMT	120	6,720	2.5,4.1	7.05
Seattle MiCe2 (38)	9 × ~10	0.8 × 0.8 × 10	MLS	PS-PMT	72	34,848		
Massachusetts General Hospital MMP-II (39)	1.2 × 12	1.2 × 4.5 × 7	LSO	PMT	36	360	1.8	0.16
Brussels VUB-PET (40)	5.2 × 17	3 × 3 × 20	BaF$_2$	Photosensitive wire-chambers		3,000	2.6	3

nuclear decay, that is, positron range and photon nonacolinearity may become available.

Several PET cameras have been specifically designed for small animal PET imaging (25,40). A summary of their characteristics and performance is given in Table 2.2. Photos of actual commercially available instruments are shown in Figs. 2.3 and 2.4. An example of the quality and spatial resolution which can be achieved with current generation PET instruments is shown in a bone scan of a rat in Fig. 2.5. Figure 2.3(a) shows the detector block arrangement of the microPET-FOCUS from Concorde MicroSystem (30). The PET detectors in this camera were based on the original design from UCLA small animal PET system (41). These detectors are composed of an array of LSO scintillator crystals coupled to position sensitive PMT via a bundle of optical fibers. This detector design was developed for the UCLA prototype later commercialized by Concorde MicroSystems under the appellation microPET-R4 and -P4. Among many improvements brought to the commercial models, the most noticeable is on the sensitivity with the inclusion of four detector rings instead one as compared to the original prototype. Recently, this vendor released the microPET-FOCUS-220 (30) and -120 which employed similar block detectors made of smaller cut crystals and improved packing fraction which resulted in a combined increased spatial resolution and sensitivity. Figure 2.3(b), shows the unique cylindrical crystal array of GSO crystals from the MOSAIC (31) (distributed by Philips Medical Systems). The light sensing devices of this camera are composed of an array of single channel PMTs where position information for crystal identification is obtained from Anger logic. The Oxford Positron System Quad-HIDAC (35) uses four banks of high-density avalanche chamber. The intrinsic resolution of this type of detector can achieve sub-millimeter resolution. The Argus from SUINSA (Spain), distributed by General Electric Medical Systems, uses a block detector design developed for the NIH-ATLAS (32), which allows for depth of interaction (DOI) measurement with two layer scintillator detectors in "phoswich" mode. The depth of interaction uncertainty is another limiting factor for the spatial resolution, which affects more severely compact ring cameras [see Fig. 2.2(b)]. Cameras using detectors with DOI capability attempt to overcome this limitation.

The last commercial camera pictured in Fig. 2.4 is the YAP-PET developed at the University of Ferrara (33) and now commercialized by COMECER. This system uses the ultra fast YAP scintillator in four planar detector heads rotating around the animal. This camera can be configured to be operated in SPECT mode with the addition of parallel-hole collimator.

The ideal characteristics of a SPECT or PET camera are given in Table 2.3. Key factors include spatial resolution, sensitivity, image contrast, counting rate ability, and scatter fraction. Issues related to spatial resolution and instrument sensitivity have already been discussed, but resolution and sensitivity by themselves do not suffice to fully characterize these imaging systems or to fully compare the different models. In clinical SPECT and PET imaging, the National

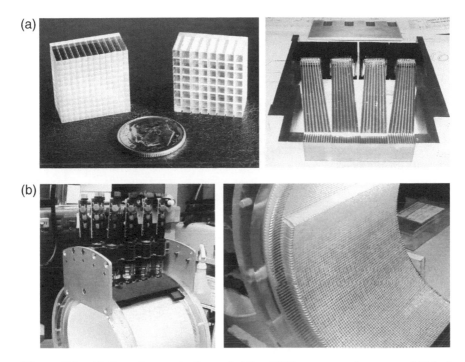

Figure 2.3 (a) Crystal arrays in Concorde MicroPET cameras and cassette of 4 block detector assembly showing the LSO arrays, optical fiber light guide, and position sensitive phototubes and (b) cylindrical array of GSO scintillation crystal (PIXELAR GSO technology) in the MOSAIC™ small animal PET, with phototube arrangement to the light-guide and exposed views of the crystal array. [Courtesy of Robert Nutt (CTI Concorde microSystems LLC) and Dr. Joel Karp (University of Pennsylvania).]

Electronic Manufacturer Association has published reports on standardized performance measurement procedures (42–44). Those techniques generally are not directly applicable to small animal PET imaging due to the smaller FOV.

Good image contrast is the result of a complex combination of resolution, radioactivity counting statistics, specificity of tracer uptake, ability of the camera to reject randoms, and the accuracy of scatter and random corrections during image reconstruction. Signal-to-noise characteristics depend on sensitivity, counting rate, and also the radio-pharmaceutical for a given applications. Insufficient counting statistics combined with poor image contrast due to low specific uptake will lead inexorably to images that are difficult to interpret.

Another very important parameter is the counting rate ability of the camera. As noted previously, to be comparable to currently available clinical scanners, high resolution imaging systems for imaging small animals would require an improvement in sensitivity of more than two orders of magnitude (which is yet to be achieved in existing small animal cameras). To overcome the loss of

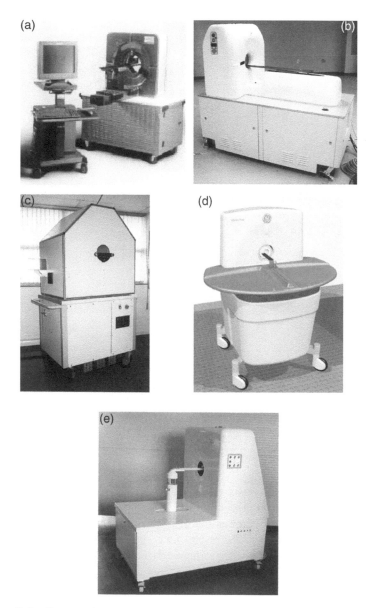

Figure 2.4 Commercially available small animal PET cameras: (a) microPET-P4 from Concorde microSystems, (b) MOSAIC from Phillips Medical System, (c) Quad-HIDAC from Oxford Positron Systems, (d) ARGUS by SUINSA, and (e) YAP-PET from the University of Ferrarra, sold by COMECER. (Courtesy of Robert Nutt, Concorde MicroSystems, Dr. Joel Karp, University of Pennsylvania, Dr. Alan Jeavons, Oxford Positron System, SUINSA, and COMECER.)

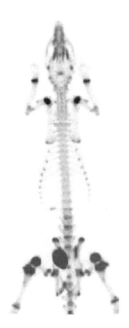

Figure 2.5 A rat bone scan acquired in a microPET-FOCUS camera. The animal was scanned in three bed positions, 1.5 h postinjection of 0.88 mCi of ^{18}F$^-$. Image reconstruction was performed using a FORE followed by 2D-filtered back projection.

sensitivity, one can inject more activity into the animal if the camera is capable of recording high count rates. Unfortunately, there are limits on count rate. The front-end electronic or coincidence processing electronic circuits can be busy processing the signals of a first decay when a second decay triggers the same detector. In such a case, the system is said to be "dead" and the latter event is lost. Event loss due to system dead-time is a very important parameter affecting the ability to detect activity and to quantify the amount of activity in the animal

Table 2.3 Ideal Characteristics of a PET or SPECT Camera

Fine granularity for improved spatial resolution
High efficiency detector material for high sensitivity
High photo-electric fraction for maximum stopping power
High energy resolution to allow for scatter rejection based on gamma energy
Large axial coverage to allow imaging of the whole animal
No loss of resolution due to DOI
High counting rate capability
Fast scintillation material to allow short timing coincidence window to reduce detection of fortuitous coincidences
Low cost.

being scanned. Scintillation materials with fast decay constants allow instruments to be produced with less system dead-time, thereby improving the counting rate performance of the camera. A standard way of reporting the counting rate performance of a PET camera is through the use of the noise equivalent count (45).

Another parameter of importance is the scatter fraction, that is, the fraction of events arising from scatter of one of the emitted photons within the animal. Again, no standard methods have yet been adopted for measuring scatter in small animal PET instruments. However, it is reasonable to expect that standards for performance measurements should be published soon. These will allow easier and more in-depth comparisons of the different camera models.

IV. Combined Systems

Several small animal systems have already been produced that combine X-ray-CT with gamma detectors (46,47). Adding anatomical maps generated by X-ray-CT helps in the interpretation of the functional (PET) data (e.g., where a region-of-interest on the PET image is positioned within the thorax). The CT data can also be used to correct the PET images for variable attenuation of radioactivity within the thorax (because tissue density is so variable within the chest). On the other hand, the radiation dose from X-ray-CT of small animals can be considerable (on the order of 5 cGy for relatively low-resolution images, ~ 100 μm), potentially limiting the possibility of serial studies (due to radiation-induced tissue injury).

Other dual modality imaging systems are being developed like MRI and PET, or OI and PET. The main problem in combining PET with an MR camera is that the intense magnetic field of the MR camera disturbs the PMTs, and they likewise disrupt the uniformity of the magnetic field. Nevertheless, a combined PET and MR system has been proposed with an array of LSO crystals with long optical fibers guiding the scintillation light to PMTs placed outside the MR field (48).

There is still an active debate whether combined systems should consist of two separate imaging cameras or one functional unit in which the two modalities co-exist. If separate, CT and SPECT or PET cameras could be used independently, allowing maximum usage of each camera. However, a combined system allows for immediate anatomic registration of anatomical to functional imaging, whereas with separate systems, registration has to be performed with software tools. This procedure is often tedious, needs trained personnel and is subject to errors if there is movement of the animal. For the present, cost considerations will make it likely that small animal CT and PET instruments will remain as two separate units, despite the obvious technical advantage of easy image co-registration in a combined unit. The technology for PET/CT exists and in the foreseeable future, a combined small animal PET/CT is likely to become available. Already, combined SPECT/CT systems are commercially produced. There is no doubts that future PET technology will include development of high resolution detector with depth of interaction capability to address both questions of resolution and sensitivity. The major limitation in SPECT is sensitivity and this point will be addressed in novel SPECT designs with multi-pinhole collimators.

V. Conclusions

It seems safe to say that we have seen only the tip of the iceberg with respect to advances in instrumentation for small animal imaging. Many laboratories throughout the world continue to develop instrumentation or new image reconstruction algorithms that undoubtedly will eventually find their way into new cameras. As the demand for small animal SPECT or PET imaging increases, new cameras with increased functionality will become available, opening the door to even more exciting biological research.

References

1. Chatziioannou AF. Molecular imaging of small animals with dedicated PET tomographs. Eur J Nucl Med 2002; 29:98–114.
2. Ishizu K, Mukai T, Fujita T, Yonekura Y, Nishizawa S, Tamaki N, Konishi J. Less than 2 mm high resolution SPECT with pinhole collimator for small animals. J Nucl Med 1993; 34:194P.
3. Jaszczak RJ, Li J, Wang H, Zalutsky R, Coleman RE. Pinhole collimation for ultra-high-resolution, small field-of-view SPECT. Phys Med Biol 1994; 39:425–437.
4. Erlandsson K, Ivanovic M, Strand SE, Sjogren K, Weber DA. High resolution pinhole SPECT for small animal imaging. J Nucl Med 1993; 34:9P.
5. Moore RY, Ohtani H, Khaw BA, Strauss HW. High resolution pinhole sequence imaging for small laboratory animals. J Nucl Med 1991; 32:987.
6. Olsson LE, Ahlgren L. Tomographic scintigraphy using pinhole collimator and a rotating gamma camera. Nucl Med 1990; 29:47–50.
7. Palmer J, Wollmer P. Pinhole emission computed tomography: method and experimental evaluation. Phys Med Biol 1990; 35:339–350.
8. McElroy DP, MacDonald LR, Beekman FJ, Wang Y, Patt BE, Iwanczyk JS, Tsui BMW, Hoffman EJ. Performance evaluation of A-SPECT: a high resolution desktop pinhole SPECT system for imaging small animals. IEEE Trans Nucl Sci 2002; 49:2139–2147.
9. Macdonal LR, Patt BE, Iwanczyk JS, Tsui BMW, Wang Y, Frey EC, Wessell DE, Acton PD. Pinhole SPECT of mice using the LumaGEM gamma camera. IEEE Trans Nucl Sci 2001; 48:830–836.
10. Furenlid LR, Wilson DW, Chen Y-C, Kim H, Pietraski PJ, Crawford MJ, Barrett HH. Fastspect-II: a second-generation high-resolution dynamic SPECT imager. IEEE Trans Nucl Sci 2004; 51:631–635.
11. Ogawa K, Kawade T, Nakamura K, Kubo A, Ichidara T. Ultra-high resolution pinhole SPECT for small animal study. IEEE Trans Nucl Sci 1998; 45:3122–3126.

12. Habraken JBA, de Bruin K, Shehata M, Booji J, Bennink R, van Eck Smit BLF, Busemann Sokole E. Evaluation of high-resolution pinhole SPECT using a small rotating animal. J Nucl Med 2001; 42:1863–1869.
13. Schramm NU, Wirrwar A, Sonnenberg F, Halling H. Compact high resolution detector for small animal SPECT. IEEE Trans Nucl Sci 2000; 47:1163–1167.
14. Meikle SR, Kench P, Weisenberger AG, Wojcik R, Smith MF, Majewski S, Eberl S, Fulton RR, Rosenfeld AB, Fulham MJ. A prototype coded aperture detector for small animal SPECT. IEEE Trans Nucl Sci 2002; 49:2167-2171.
15. Meikle SR, Kench P, Wojcik R, Smith MF, Weisenberger AG, Majewski S, Lerch M, Rosenfeld AB. Performance evaluation of a multipinhole small animal SPECT system. IEEE Med Imaging Conf 2003;
16. Schramm NU, Ebel G, Engeland U, Schurrat T, Behe M, Behr TM. High-resolution SPECT using miltipinhole collimation. IEEE Trans Nucl Sci 2003; 50:315–320.
17. Dilmanian FA, Weber DA, Coderre JA, Joel DD, Shi K-C, Meinken GE, Som P, Tang Y-N, Volkow ND, Yee C, Brill AB, Watanabe M, Inuzuka E, Oba K, Gerson R, Iida H, Hiruma A. A high-resolution SPECT system based on a micro-channel-plate imager. IEEE Trans Nucl Sci 1990; 37:687–695.
18. Kastis GA, Barber HB, Barrett HH, Gifford HC, Pang IW, Patton DD. High resolution SPECT imager for three-dimensional imaging of animals. J Nucl Med 1998; 39:9P.
19. Kastis GA, Wu MC, Balzer SJ, Wislon DW, Furenlid LR, Peterson TE, Barber HB, Barrett HH, Woolfenden JM, Kelly P, M A. Tomographic small-animal imaging using a high-resolution semicondustor camera. IEEE Trans Nucl Sci 2002; 49:172–175.
20. Kastis GA, Fruenlid LR, Wilson DW, Peterson TE, Barber HB, Barrett HH. Compact CT/SPECT small animal-imaging system. Trans Nucl Sci 2004; 51:63–67.
21. Nickles J. Production of a broad range of radionuclides with an 11 MeV proton cyclotron. J Labelled Compd Rad 1991; 30:120–122.
22. McCarthy TJ, McCarthy DW, Laforest R, Wüst F, Reichert D, Lewis MJ, Welch MJ. Non-standard Isotope production and applications at Washington University. CAARI 2000.
23. Melcher CL, Schweitzer JS. Cerium-doped lutetium oxyorthosilicate: a fast, efficient new scintillator. IEEE Trans Nucl Sci 1992; 39:502–505.
24. Takagi K, Fukazawa T. Cerium-activated Gd_2SiO_5 single crystal scintillator. Appl Phys Lett 1983; 42:43–45.
25. Cherry SR, Shao Y, Silverman RW, Meadors K, Siegel S, A C, Young JW, Jones W, Moyers JC, Newport D, Boutefnouchet A, Farquar TH, Andreaco M, Paulus MJ, Binkley DM, Nutt R, Phelps ME. MicroPET: a high resolution PET scanner for imaging small animals. IEEE Trans Nucl Sci 1997; 44.
26. Chatziioannou AF, Cherry SR, Shao Y, Silverman RW, Meadors K, Farquhar TH, Pedarsani M, Phelps ME. Performance evaluation of microPET: a high-resolution lutetium oxyorthosilicate PET scanner for animal imaging. J Nucl Med 1999; 40:1164–1175.
27. Tai Y-C, Chatziioannou AF, Yang Y, Silverman RW, Meadors K, Siegel S, Newport DF, Stickel JR, Cherry SR. MicroPET II: design, development and initial performance of an improved microPET scanner for small-animal imaging. Phys Med Biol 2003; 48:1519.

28. Knoess C, Siegel S, Smith A, Newport D, Richerzhagen N, Winkeler A, Jacobs A, Goble RN, Graf R, Wienhard K, Heiss WD. Performance evaluation of the micro-PET R4 PET scanner for rodents. Eur J Nucl Med 2003; 30.

29. Tai YC, Chatzioannou A, Cherry S. Performance evaluation of the microPET-P4: a PET system dedicated to animal imaging. Phys Med Biol 2001; 46:1845.

30. Tai YC, Ruangma A, Siegel S, Newport D, Laforest R. Performance evaluation of microPET focus: a third generation microPET scanner decicated to animal imaging. J Nucl Med 2004.

31. Surti S, Karp JS, Perkins AE, Freifelder R, Muehllehner G. Design evaluation of A-PET: a high sensitivity animal PET camera. IEEE Med Imaging Conf 2002.

32. Siedel J, Vaquero JJ, Green MV. Resolution uniformity and sensitivity of the NIH ATLAS small animal PET scanner: comparison to simulated LSO scanners without depth-of-interaction capability. IEEE Trans Nucl Sci 2003; 50:1347–1645.

33. Del Guerra A, Damiani C, Di Domenico G, Motta A, Giganti M, Marchesini R, Piffanelli A, Sabba N, Sartori L, Zavattini E. An integrated PET-SPECT small animal imager: preliminary results. IEEE Trans Nucl Sci 2000; 47:1537–1540.

34. Lecomte R, Cadorette J, Rodrigue S, Lapointe D, Rouleau D, Benrourkia M, Yao R, Msaki P. Initial results from the Sherbrooke avalanche photodiode positron tomograph. IEEE Trans Nucl Sci 1996; 43:1952-1957.

35. Jeavons AP, Chandler RA, Dettmar CAR. A 3D HIDAC-PET camera with sub-millimeter resolution for imaging small animals. IEEE Trans Nucl Sci 1999; 46:468–473.

36. Weber A, Herzog H, Cremer M, Engels R, Hmacher K, Kehren F, Muehlensiepen H, Ploux L, Reinartz R, Reinhart P, Rongen F, Sonnenberg F, Coenen HH, Halling H. Evaluation of TierPET system. IEEE Trans Nucl Sci 1999; 46:1177–1183.

37. Rouze NC, Hutchins GD. Design and characterization of IndyPET-II: a high-resolution, high-sensitivity dedicated research scanner. IEEE Trans Nucl Sci 2003; 50:1491–1497.

38. Lee K, Kinahan PE, Miyaoka RS, Kim JS, Lewellen TK. Impact of system design parameters on image figures of merit for a mouse PET scanner. IEEE Trans Nucl Sci 2004; 51:27–33.

39. Correia JA, Burnham CA, Kaufman D, Brownell AL, Fischman AJ. Performance evaluation of MMP-II: a second generation small animal PET. IEEE Trans Nucl Sci 2004; 51:26–27.

40. Tavernier S, Brurndonckx P, Debruyne J, Etienne L, Folger H, Hartmann W, Rajeswaran S, Smolik W, Van Lancker L, Zhang S. First results from a prototype PET scanner using BaF_2 scintillator and photosensitive wire chambers. IEEE NSS-MIC 1994.

41. Cherry SR, Shao Y, Silverman RE, Meadors K, Siegel S, Chatziioannou A, Young JW, Jones W, Moyers JC, Newport D, Boutefnouchet A, Farquar TH, Andreaco M, Paulus MJ, Binkley DM, Nutt R, Phelps ME. MicroPET: a high resolution PET scanner for imaging small animals. IEEE Trans Nucl Sci 1997; 44:1161–1166.

42. NEMA Standards Publication NU 2-1994. Performance Measurements of Positron Emission Tomographs. National Electrical Manufacturers Association, 1994.

43. NEMA Standards Publication NU 2-2001. Peformance Measurements of Positron Emission Tomographs. National Electrical Manufacturers Association, 2001.

44. NEMA Standards Publication NU 1-2001. Performance Measurements of Scintillation Cameras. National Electrical Manufacturers Asscociation, 2001.
45. Strother SC. Measuring PET scanner sensitivity: relating countrates to image signal-to-noise ratios using noise equivalent counts. IEEE Trans Nucl Sci 1990; 37:783–788.
46. Lang TF, Hasegawa BH, Soo Chin L, Keenan Brown J, Blankespoor SC, Reilly SM, Gingold EL, Cann CE. Description of a prototype emission-transmission computed tomography imaging system. J Nucl Med 1992; 33:1881–1887.
47. Kalki K, Blankespoor SC, Brown JK, Hasegawa BH, Dae MW, Chin M, Stillson C. Myocardial perfusion imaging with a combined X-ray CT and SPECT system. J Nucl Med 1997; 38:1535–1540.
48. Slates R, Cherry S, Boutefnouchet A, Shao Y, Dahlbom M, Frahani K. Design of a small animal MR compatible PET scanner. IEEE Trans Nucl Sci 1999; 46:565–570.

3

PET and SPECT as Platforms for Molecular Imaging

BUCK E. ROGERS

Washington University,
St. Louis, Missouri, USA

I. Introduction

With the development of new molecular imaging probes, sophisticated animal models, and small-animal imaging devices as well as advances in molecular biology techniques, molecular imaging has become increasingly important for understanding basic biological processes in living subjects. Molecular imaging can be defined as the characterization of biological processes at the cellular and molecular levels in living animals or humans using remote imaging detectors (1). This can differ from "classical" diagnostic imaging that focuses on imaging the end result of these biological processes (2). Molecular imaging modalities include nuclear imaging, optical imaging, magnetic resonance imaging (MRI), computed tomography (CT), and ultrasound. All of these modalities offer differ-ent advantages and limitations for molecular imaging. Most of these advanta-ges and limitations are centered on issues of spatial and temporal resolution, sensitivity, molecular probe availability, image acquisition and analysis time, and cost. The focus of this chapter will be on nuclear imaging, in particular single photon emission computed tomography (SPECT) and positron emission tomography (PET). These techniques have the advantages of having a high sensitivity, being extremely quantitative, and having a number of probes readily available. They are, however, relatively expensive, expose the subject to radiation, and have lower spatial resolution than some of the other imaging modalities. This chapter will describe the basics of SPECT and PET imaging, describe the advantages and disadvantages of each modality, and give examples of how each platform is used for molecular imaging applications.

II. SPECT Imaging

A. Principles of SPECT Imaging

SPECT imaging differs from CT in that the radiation source is located within the subject instead of outside the subject. Both SPECT and PET imaging rely upon the detection and quantification of molecular probes that have been tagged with radionuclides and injected into living subjects. SPECT imaging uses radio-nuclides that emit γ-ray photons, whereas PET imaging uses radionuclides that emit positrons (positively charged electrons emitted from the nucleus). A scinti-llation camera (gamma camera) consists of a lead collimator that only allows γ-rays traveling parallel to the collimator holes to pass through to scintillation crystals. The collimator essentially focuses the γ-rays as they are too energetic to be focused by a lens (3). In general, the sensitivity and resolution of collimators are inversely related with high-resolution collimators having low sensitivity and vice-versa. The scintillation crystals then convert the γ-ray energy into visible light that can then be processed for image reconstruction. The gamma camera provides a 2-dimensional image by "compressing" the region of interest into a single image, referred to as *planar imaging*. Planar gamma camera images are difficult to interpret because each point in the image represents all activity above and below that point and that objects perpendicular to the imaging plane appear shortened or are difficult to view (3). When the detectors are rotated around the subject, 3-dimensional tomographic images are produced (SPECT imaging). The 3-dimensional nature of SPECT produces volumetric images that can be analyzed for information in every slice through the image. These SPECT images do not have the overlap from radioactivity that has accumulated in structures above or below the site of interest as with planar gamma camera imaging. The SPECT images, however, generally require longer acquisition times and can generate very large data sets (4). A schematic of SPECT data acquisition for a single-headed camera is depicted in Fig. 3.1. The use of multiple detector SPECT systems with more than one scintillation camera can decrease these acquisition times or they can increase the sensitivity by acquiring more

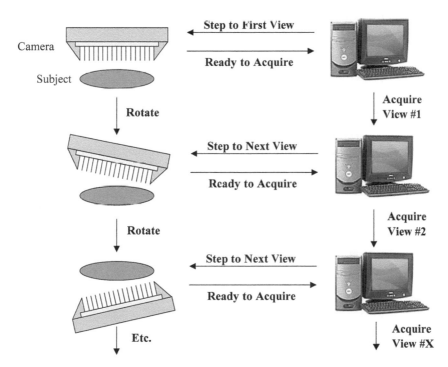

Figure 3.1 Schematic of SPECT data acquisition for a single-headed camera. The computer tells the camera to rotate to the next viewing angle and after the camera sends a message back to the computer that it is ready to acquire, the data are acquired for that angle for a certain period of time. The time for each view includes the data acquisition time and the camera step time. The total acquisition time is the time for each view multiplied by the number of views (X). Figure adapted from Ref. (7).

counts. This gain in sensitivity can be traded for greater resolution by the use of higher resolution collimators. These multiple SPECT systems consist of two or three detectors. Drawbacks to these multiple detector systems include an increase in quality control requirements to ensure there are no decreases in camera performance and a loss in flexibility of movement that may be necessary for some types of planar imaging because the multiple detectors do not need to be rotated 360°.

After acquisition of the data, the images must be reconstructed. This is accomplished through the use of image-reconstruction algorithms, the details of which are beyond the scope of this chapter. Finally, other factors that influence SPECT images include the attenuation of photons, Compton scattering of photons, and loss of resolution with increasing distance from the collimator. Non-uniform attenuation of separate photons emitted from a single point in the subject is the result of the photons passing through different density tissues. Compton scattering of photons results in data that do not accurately predict the origin of the photon. These concepts are illustrated in Fig. 3.2. A more detailed discussion of algorithms and the physical factors that influence SPECT images are described elsewhere (3,5–7).

B.   Radionuclides Used in SPECT Imaging

A list of radionuclides commonly used for SPECT imaging is presented in Table 3.1. Technetium-99m (^{99m}Tc) and thallium-201 (^{201}Tl) are generator produced, whereas gallium-67 (^{67}Ga), indium-111 (^{111}In), and iodine-123 (^{123}I) are cyclotron produced (8). ^{201}Tl is a monovalent cationic metal that is used for cardiac imaging as a chloride salt. ^{67}Ga is used in the form of ^{67}Ga-citrate for imaging tumors and sites of inflammation. Both of these are commercially available for clinical use. ^{111}In is used for imaging many different biological processes

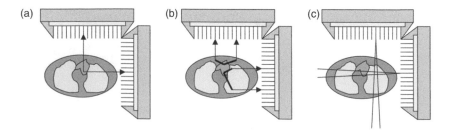

Figure 3.2 Physical factors that influence SPECT images. (a) Photon attenuation occurs when photons emitted from a single point pass through different density tissues, (b) Compton scattering results in photons that do not appear to originate from the original emission, and (c) for a single point, resolution is lost with increasing distance to the camera. Figure adapted from Ref. (3).

Table 3.1 Half-lives and Percent Abundance of Major γ-Emissions from Commonly Used SPECT Radionuclides

Radionuclide	$t_{1/2}$ (h)	γ keV (%)
^{99m}Tc	6.0	140.5 (89.1)
^{201}Tl	72.9	135.3 (2.6), 167.4 (10.0)
^{67}Ga	78.3	93.3 (39.2), 184.6 (21.2), 300.2 (16.8)
^{111}In	67.3	171.3 (90.7), 245.4 (94.1)
^{123}I	13.3	159.0 (83.3)

when conjugated to a variety of biomolecules. Because of the great stability of indium with transferrin, chelators are conjugated to the biomolecule that form strong complexes with indium. ^{123}I is generally attached to proteins and peptides directly through tyrosine residues for tumor imaging. Other ^{123}I compounds include: ^{123}I-sodium iodide for thyroid imaging, ^{123}I-iodoamphetamine for brain imaging, and ^{123}I-labeled fatty acids for myocardial imaging. ^{99m}Tc is the most widely used radionuclide for a variety of nuclear medicine procedures. For imaging studies, ^{99m}Tc must be reduced and attached to carriers. A number of ^{99m}Tc-labeled imaging agents exist, including blood pool, skeletal, lung, renal, cardiac, hepatobiliary, and brain. Similar to ^{111}In, ^{99m}Tc is generally conjugated to biomolecules through the use of chelators. A more detailed review of molecular imaging probes is found in Chapter 1 of this book.

The physical properties of these radionuclides contribute greatly to the quality of the images in SPECT. Some of the reasons for the widespread use of ^{99m}Tc are its physical properties that include a half-life ($t_{1/2}$) of 6 h, no beta decay, and a 140 keV photon (89% abundance). Another reason is the availability of the ^{99m}Tc generator system. The relatively short half-life of ^{99m}Tc allows for a greater number of photon emissions during SPECT imaging, which improves the imaging statistics (9). The fact that no beta radiation is emitted lowers the absorbed radiation dose to the patient that allows for the injection of a greater amount of radioactivity, thus also increasing the imaging statistics. SPECT imaging with radionuclides that have high photon energies ($>\sim$170 keV) results in lower quality images because of reduced localization of the photon absorption in the detector and increased penetration of the collimator that results in blurred images (6). The 140 keV photon of ^{99m}Tc fits these criteria and also provides good tissue penetration that reduces attenuation. ^{123}I is an attractive radionuclide due to the 13.2 h half-life and 159 keV photon emission. The longer half-lives of ^{201}Tl, ^{67}Ga, and ^{111}In make them less desirable as well as some of their higher energy photon emissions. It should be noted that multiple radionuclides with different γ-ray energies can be imaged simultaneously by SPECT because the detector can be set to discriminate between the different energies. Thus, there are a wide variety of radionuclides available for SPECT imaging of biological processes in living subjects.

III. PET Imaging

A. Principles of PET Imaging

As mentioned earlier, PET imaging uses radionuclides that emit positively charged particles from the nucleus. These particles have the same physical properties as electrons except for the positive charge emitted upon the decay of radionuclides that are proton-rich. The positron can travel up to several millimeters prior to interacting with an electron, this is called an annihilation event, which converts the energy into two photons of 511 keV each that are ~180° apart. This is illustrated in Fig. 3.3. These photons are detected with scintillation crystals that are placed in a ring around the subject. In general, dedicated PET scanners will have 18–30 consecutive rings of crystals (10). In commercial scanners, two alternative designs have been used that are less expensive but sacrifice sensitivity and resolution. One design uses less expensive crystals with only a few large detectors that are hexagonally arranged. Another system uses only two

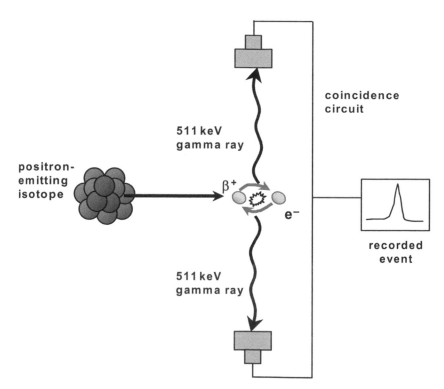

Figure 3.3 The concept of annihilation. A positron is emitted from a nucleus and can travel several millimeters before annihilating with an electron. The two 511 keV photons resulting from the annihilation travel in opposite directions and are recorded by rings of detectors.

opposing 60° arcs of detectors that are rotated as opposed to the full 360° of detectors. In addition to these human systems, small animal imaging systems have been a major development in recent years and are discussed in Chapter 2 of this book.

The two 511 keV photons emitted during positron annihilation are traveling along a common line, as they are ~180° apart, and should hit two opposite detectors about the same time. Therefore, if two crystals 180° apart register a photon event at the same time, the system then records the coincident event on a line of response (LOR) between the two detectors. To account for short time delays a coincidence window is set to record events within a certain time period (usually 6–20 ns) (10,11). Most dedicated PET scanners have septa that are positioned between the rings of detectors that limit events to those within the same detector ring and that reduce the scatter and random photons that are generated outside that ring of detectors. When the septa are in place, the scanner is said to be operating in 2-dimensional mode because a single slice of information is obtained from the plane of one ring of detectors. When the septa are removed, coincidences are allowed for detectors from different rings, thus allowing for 3-dimensional acquisition. This is illustrated in Fig. 3.4. More quantitative data is obtained in 2-dimensional mode, whereas the 3-dimensional mode is more sensitive but also more prone to distortion that is difficult to correct.

Similar to SPECT imaging, the PET images must be reconstructed after acquisition of the data using a variety of algorithms. In addition, photon

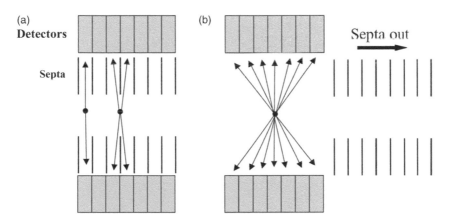

Figure 3.4 The two-dimensional mode of a PET scanner is shown in (a). This mode only allows for data to be collected that originates within a plane of detectors that limits sensitivity. Allowing for coincidences that originate between rings can increase sensitivity. The three-dimensional mode is shown in (b). When the septa are removed, coincidences are allowed from large axial angles that increase the sensitivity. Figure adapted from Ref. (10).

attenuation and scatter must be corrected. Additional corrections for PET scanning must be made to ensure that all arriving photons are accounted for. If two photons arrive so close in time that their energy registers >511 keV, the data will be discarded and both photons will be lost. Another situation for photon loss is when the second photon arrives while the detector is processing the information from the first photon such that the signal from the second photon is not recorded. This is referred to as the *system dead-time*. A more detailed description of the algorithms used for image reconstruction and the steps to correct for system limitations can be found elsewhere (10–12).

B. Radionuclides Used in PET Imaging

A list of common positron emitting radionuclides are listed in Table 3.2. Oxygen-15 (^{15}O), nitrogen-13 (^{13}N), carbon-11 (^{11}C), fluorine-18 (^{18}F), and copper-64 (^{64}Cu) are all cyclotron produced, whereas rubidium-82 (^{82}Rb), copper-62 (^{62}Cu), and gallium (^{68}Ga) are generator produced (8). The short half-lives of the cyclotron-produced radionuclides often require an onsite cyclotron although many centralized pharmacies now supply regional hospitals with ^{18}F-labeled radiopharmaceuticals. PET radiopharmaceuticals labeled with ^{15}O are limited to ^{15}O-labeled water, ^{15}O-labeled oxygen gas, ^{15}O-labeled carbon dioxide, and ^{15}O-labeled carbon monoxide. These agents are used to determine blood flow, blood volume, and oxygen extraction. ^{13}N is mostly used as ^{13}N-labeled ammonia for cerebral and myocardial blood flow studies. There is an extensive list of ^{11}C-labeled PET radiopharmaceuticals, with ^{11}C-labeled acetate, ^{11}C-labeled glucose, and ^{11}C-labeled butanol being some of the more common agents for blood flow and metabolism studies. The most frequently used ^{18}F-labeled radiopharmaceutical is ^{18}F-labeled glucose (FDG) that is Food and Drug administration (FDA) approved for indication of a variety of cancers. Other examples of ^{18}F-labeled radiopharmaceuticals are ^{18}F-labeled L-dopa for dopamine receptor binding and ^{18}F-labeled estradiol for estrogen receptor binding. ^{82}Rb is used for determining myocardial perfusion as the potassium salt, and

Table 3.2 Decay Properties of Commonly Used PET Radionuclides

Radionuclide	$t_{1/2}$ (min)	Positron yield (%)	$E_{\beta+}$ max (MeV)
^{15}O	2.0	99.9	1.73
^{13}N	10.0	99.8	1.20
^{11}C	20.4	99.8	0.96
^{18}F	110.0	96.7	0.63
^{64}Cu	762.0	17.4	0.65
^{82}Rb	1.3	81.8	3.38
^{62}Cu	9.8	97.2	2.93
^{68}Ga	68.1	87.9	1.90

[68]Ga-citrate is used to determine plasma volume. [62]Cu-PTSM is used for blood flow studies, while ^{64}Cu, with its longer half-life, can be attached to tumor-targeting biomolecules for tumor imaging. A more detailed discussion of molecular probes labeled with PET radionuclides is found in Chapter 1 of this book.

Physical factors of the radionuclides used for PET imaging that contribute to the quality of the PET images include the energy of the positron and whether the radionuclide has other radioactive emissions. The energy of the positron will affect the resolution of the resulting image. Positrons with higher energy will travel farther from their point of emission prior to annihilation that will result in a loss of resolution. If a radionuclide has emissions in addition to positrons, such as γ-rays, these emissions will compete in the detection process, allowing coincidence events to go undetected compared to a pure positron emitter that would not have the competition of detecting the coincidence events. If γ-rays are tying up the detector, this will increase dead time and decrease resolution. It should also be noted that, in general, the half-lives of PET radionuclides are shorter than the half-lives of SPECT radionuclides, requiring the use of facile chemistries to incorporate these radionuclides into the desired probes.

IV. SPECT Imaging vs. PET Imaging

There are several factors involved when deciding to use SPECT or PET for molecular imaging applications. Some of these factors include the resolution that is necessary to observe the biological process of interest, the availability of the appropriate radionuclides and molecular probes for a given biological process, the ability to observe multiple processes simultaneously, and the relative cost of the two modalities. These comparisons are summarized in Table 3.3. The need for a lead collimator in SPECT imaging (as opposed to electronic collimation in PET resulting from the coincidence photons) is the main difference from PET imaging that affects resolution. In SPECT, there is always a compromise between resolution and sensitivity due to the collimator. Improving the resolution

Table 3.3 Comparison of SPECT and PET Imaging. The Modality Marked with an X has an Advantage Over the Other

	SPECT	PET
Resolution/sensitivity		X
Quantitative degree		X
Probe availability[a]	X	X
Image multiple processes simultaneously	X	
Cost	X	

[a]Both modalities have many probes available, but in general, PET radionuclides are used to radiolabel small organic compounds and SPECT radionuclides are used to radiolabel larger peptides and proteins.

by using a collimator with smaller holes results in a loss of sensitivity because more photons are being prevented from reaching the detectors. Only $\sim 0.01\%$ of the emitted γ-rays are detected in SPECT because of the collimation that results in SPECT being about an order of magnitude less sensitive when PET (4). PET has a sensitivity of $\sim 1-10 \, \text{pmol/L}$ that is independent of the positron-labeled probe. Budinger (13) demonstrated that a three-detector SPECT system designed for human brain imaging is ~ 15 times less sensitive when compared with PET imaging if 1 cm resolution is required. Therefore, if a high degree of quantitation (sensitivity) is needed at a given resolution, then PET is the modality of choice. However, if the process being investigated does not require a high level of resolution, then sensitivity can be gained and SPECT may be satisfactory.

The standard PET radionuclides listed in Table 3.2 consist of atoms that are naturally occurring and can be substituted in organic-based molecular probes for the corresponding nonradioactive atom. In general, fluorine is not naturally occurring in organic molecules but labeling with ^{18}F only results in a minor change in the structure of the probe because its size is similar to that of a hydrogen atom that is being replaced. Substitution of these naturally occurring atoms allows for the native molecule to be evaluated without perturbation to the biological system, as long as a synthetic route is available for the production of the desired probe in a timely fashion. This differs from many of the metal radionuclides used in SPECT imaging. In general, these metal radionuclides must be attached to the probe of interest through the use of a bifunctional chelator that may have a dramatic effect on the biological action of the probe. Therefore, only selected probes that maintain their biological integrity after conjugation and radiolabeling with these radionuclides can be evaluated. A good example of this is steroid-based probes for imaging the estrogen receptor (14). There have been many derivatives radiolabeled with ^{18}F for PET imaging, however, it has proven more difficult to find probes that can be labeled with ^{99m}Tc for SPECT imaging (14). This is usually less of an issue when radiolabeling larger molecules, such as peptides or antibodies, in which the bifunctional chelating agent is a small percentage of the total size of the biomolecule. Overall, the molecular probe and target of interest will dictate whether PET or SPECT (or both) radionuclides can be used to image particular biological processes.

Another aspect when considering PET or SPECT imaging is whether there is a need for evaluating multiple biological processes simultaneously. As PET detects the two 511 keV γ-rays after annihilation for all positron-emitters, it cannot distinguish between two or more different radionuclides. Thus, when imaging multiple processes, the molecular probes must be injected in sequence such that the first radionuclide decays prior to administration of the second probe. This differs from what can be accomplished with SPECT, as different radionuclides can be detected simultaneously by discriminating between their γ-ray energies. The windows on the SPECT detectors can be set to register photons from one radionuclide during a first imaging session and then the windows can be reset to register photons from another radionuclide during a second imaging session. This allows for the probes radiolabeled with different radionuclides to be injected simultaneously, unlike the injection stagger that is necessary for PET imaging. Therefore, at least in theory, SPECT imaging should possess advantages over PET imaging with regard to imaging multiple events simultaneously.

Finally, the cost of the two modalities may be a factor when starting a molecular imaging program. PET imaging is more expensive due to the cost of the equipment and the cost per study. PET scanners are more expensive generally due to the large number of crystals that are needed for full-ring systems compared with the fewer number of crystals in a SPECT scanner that does not encompass the entire 360°. In addition, a cyclotron is required to produce the radionuclides for conducting many standard PET studies, although, centralized pharmacies are becoming more common for supplying ^{18}F-labeled radiopharmaceuticals (as the half-life of ^{18}F is long enough to allow for shipment) to regional hospitals and PET facilities. In addition to the hardware costs, the cost of a PET study is greater than the cost of a SPECT study (4). Overall, there are many factors that should be considered when choosing a modality for conducting a nuclear molecular imaging study.

V. Applications of PET and SPECT Molecular Imaging

There are several targets that can be chosen when conducting a molecular imaging study. In general, these can be DNA, messenger RNA (mRNA), expressed protein, and functional protein. Molecular imaging of DNA would be difficult as there are only two target molecules per cell and the signal from imaging one or both DNA strands will likely not be distinguishable from nonspecific probe accumulation. Imaging of mRNA with fifties to thousands of targets per cell is more realistic, although, there are still challenges regarding nonspecific uptake and binding of probes. The most prevalent targets for molecular imaging studies are proteins and the function of proteins. There are hundreds to millions of protein targets per cell and targeting to protein function can lead to exponential increases in reporter probe amplification. In this section, examples of attempts to image RNA will be discussed followed by an overview of molecular imaging of proteins and protein function. Another area that will be discussed in this section is the molecular imaging of exogenous marker genes. In recent years, marker genes have been used to evaluate gene transfer for potential gene therapy applications and to monitor protein–protein interactions to elucidate molecular pathways *in vivo* and for potential drug screening.

A. Imaging of RNA

Molecular imaging of mRNA can provide information on the expression pattern of genes at the cellular level and potentially determine early changes in disease states prior to phenotypic changes. However, molecular imaging of mRNA is difficult owing to the relatively low number of target molecules as mentioned earlier and difficulty in delivering antisense probes to intracellular sites. Despite these hurdles, various mRNA imaging strategies have been pursued and recent advances leave this target in the realm of possibility.

A number of oligonucleotide analogs have been synthesized and evaluated with their structures described elsewhere (15). Unmodified phosphodiester DNAs are rapidly degraded by nucleases *in vivo* which greatly limits their use for imaging mRNA (15). DNA phosphorothioates are limited as imaging agents due to the rapid degradation of the target RNA and their nonspecific binding to serum and tissue proteins (16). Methylphosphonates and 2′-O-methyl RNAs maintain the ribose backbone and do not result in degradation of the target RNA. However, the methylphosphonates have lower binding affinity to complementary RNA than DNA (17). Peptide nucleic acids (PNAs), morpholino (MORF), and *trans*-4-hydroxy-l-proline nucleic acid-phosphono nucleic acid (HypNA-pPNA) are other promising analogs that have an artificial backbone in place of the ribose backbone.

As there are only a limited number of target mRNA molecules, a high specific activity must be achieved. A variety of radionuclides have been used for radiolabeling oligonucleotide analogs for potential SPECT and PET imaging. Tavitian et al. (18) labeled antisense DNA with ^{18}F at specific activities >1000 Ci/mmol for potential PET imaging. Liu et al. have labeled MORF analogs with ^{111}In and ^{99m}Tc at ~500 and ~1500 Ci/mmol, respectively, whereas Lewis et al. have demonstrated labeling of a PNA conjugate with ^{111}In at >1000 Ci/mmol (19,20). Thus, radiolabeling of oligonucleotide analogs at high specific activities can be achieved for imaging of mRNA.

Delivery and penetration of oligonucleotides to target cells are issues that must be addressed for imaging mRNA. In this regard, several PNAs have been conjugated to cell membrane permeation peptides or cellular transmembrane receptors. Cell membrane permeant peptides that have been investigated include the homeodomain of Antennapedia (21) and the basic domain of human immunodeficiency virus 1 (HIV-1) Tat protein (22,23). Lewis et al. (19) conjugated a PNA to a synthetic transduction peptide (PTD-4) and demonstrated that the PTD-4 and chelate did not inhibit PNA binding to its target. One issue with using cell permeant peptides is that they are not targeted to a cell or tissue of interest. They will deliver the oligonucleotide of interest to all cells, where specific binding to mRNA will occur only in target cells, which will likely not lead to great target accumulation. In this regard, cell-specific targeting peptides have been investigated. Meir et al. (24) conjugated a PNA to an octreotide analog for targeting to tumor-associated somatostatin receptors. They demonstrated high selective uptake when the conjugate was radiolabeled with ^{125}I in a rat pancreatic tumor model. Rao et al. (25) conjugated a PNA to the type 1 insulin growth factor (IGF-1), radiolabeled it with ^{99m}Tc and demonstrated selective tumor uptake in MCF-7 breast tumor xenografts.

Despite these advances, only a small number of imaging studies using antisense agents for mRNA detection have been published. Dewanjee et al. (26) used an ^{111}In-labeled antisense phosphorthioate oligonucleotide to image D1 mouse mammary tumors 2 h after intravenous injection that was not observed when using the corresponding ^{111}In-labeled sense probe. Sato et al. (27) used an antisense oligodeoxynucleotide targeted to *c-erbB-2* conjugated with a dendrimer or avidin that was radiolabeled with ^{111}In to detect intraperitoneal SHIN3 human ovarian tumors 24 h after intraperitoneal administration of the radiolabeled conjugate. However, negative control experiments were not performed in this study. Tian et al. (28) evaluated ^{99m}Tc-labeled PNA conjugates conjugated to IGF-1. This study demonstrated that an IGF-1 labeled peptide without the PNA did not accumulate in IGF-1 receptor negative tumors and that a labeled PNA without the IGF-1 peptide did not accumulate in receptor positive tumors. However, the investigators have presented unpublished data that demonstrate that the ^{99m}Tc-PNA-IGF-1 conjugate accumulated in IGF-1 receptor positive tumors. These studies demonstrate the potential of using radiolabeled antisense agents for the noninvasive imaging of mRNA. It is anticipated that further advances in this field will allow for PET and SPECT molecular imaging of mRNA for the diagnosis and staging of disease.

B. Imaging of Endogenous Proteins and Protein Function

A comprehensive list of molecular imaging studies that utilize a variety of radiolabeled probes targeted to different proteins is given by Massoud and Gambhir (4). In general, the imaging of proteins and protein function can be divided between the imaging of intracellular proteins and the imaging of transmembrane proteins. A discussion, in this chapter, of intracellular proteins that are targets of molecular imaging studies will be limited to hexokinase, mammalian thymidine kinase, and estrogen/androgen receptors. Some of the transmembrane proteins that will be discussed in this chapter include neurotransmitters and neuroreceptors, tumor receptors, tumor antigens, and multidrug resistance (MDR) transporters.

Imaging of Intracellular Proteins

The imaging of hexokinase, which catalyzes the initial rate-limiting step in glycolysis, using FDG is one of the most widely studied targets in PET imaging. FDG enters cells via glucose transporters and is phosphorylated by hexokinase. As the phosphorlyated FDG is not further metabolized like glucose itself, it remains trapped within the cell, leading to accumulation of radioactivity at the target site for detection. FDG has been used widely for the detection of normal and pathologic function in the brain and heart and has been gaining significance in oncology for the diagnosis and staging of disease (29–32). Thus, molecular imaging of the enzymatic activity of hexokinase with FDG has been studied widely with PET and is used routinely in the clinic for a variety of malignancies.

It should be noted that radiolabeled glucose analogs for SPECT imaging have been investigated, but as of yet it is unclear if these agents will have widespread utility (33).

One of the issues with FDG PET imaging in oncology is that FDG uptake is not limited to tumor-specific glucose metabolism, but can occur in other glucose-utilizing cells (1). Thus, one approach toward tumor-selective uptake of radio-pharmaceuticals has been the development of tumor proliferation markers. Thymidine and thymidine analogs are rapidly incorporated into DNA and radiolabeled analogs have been used to determine cell proliferation in cell culture and in animal models for years. Endogenous thymidine kinase is upregulated just prior to S phase and then declines in G2 and is responsible for the phosphorylation of thymidine and thymidine analogs (34–37). For molecular imaging purposes, thymidine analogs have been radiolabeled with ^{18}F for PET imaging of cell proliferation. The most promising compound has been ^{18}F-labeled 3'-deoxy-3'-fluorothymidine (FLT) which is trapped intracellularly after phosphorylation (38). FLT has been used to demonstrate proliferation in both cell culture and animal models and a recent clinical trial shows a good correlation between immunostaining of cell proliferation in pulmonary nodules and FLT standard uptake values (39,40).

Imaging of nuclear steroid receptors has been of interest for tailoring therapeutic interventions based on the presence or absence of a receptor (41,42). Determination of estrogen receptor status is critical for treatment planning in the management of breast cancer. The most widely studied ligand for imaging the estrogen receptor has been an ^{18}F-labeled derivative of estradiol for PET imaging. This derivative has demonstrated good localization in estrogen receptor positive tissues and tumors both preclinically and clinically (43–45). It has also been shown to have clinical utility for predicting the "metabolic flare" response that occurs after tamoxifen therapy (46,47). In recent years, ^{99m}Tc-labeled steroid and nonsteroid ligands have been synthesized for potential SPECT imaging of the estrogen receptor, however, none of these derivatives have demonstrated good estrogen receptor-mediated uptake in animal models as of yet (14). Molecular imaging of the androgen receptor for monitoring the pathophysiology of metastatic prostate cancer has been evaluated using ^{18}F-labeled dihydrotestosterone analogs (48,49). One of these analogs (^{18}F-FDHT) has demonstrated potential in nonhuman primate imaging and in a clinical imaging study (48,50). An example of how ^{18}F-FDHT can be used to monitor the expression of the androgen receptor in response to therapy is shown in Fig. 3.5.

Imaging of Transmembrane Proteins

Neuroimaging is one of the most widely studied areas for PET and SPECT. In particular, imaging of neurotransmitters and neuroreceptors in Parkinson's disease, schizophrenia, and cocaine addiction have been areas of particular interest (51). It is imperative that the radiolabeled substrates readily cross the

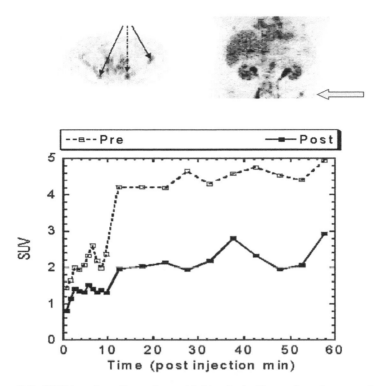

Figure 3.5 PET imaging of a patient with histologically confirmed progressive pro-state cancer that was monitored for response to high dose testosterone treatment using ^{18}F-FDHT. The top shows transaxial and coronal images of ^{18}F-FDHT uptake in three lesions prior to testosterone treatment. The bottom shows time-activity curves [activity presented as the normalized standard uptake value (SUV)] for the average of the three lesions pre- (dashed line) and posttreatment (solid line). This study demonstrates the ability to image the intracellular androgen receptor, how PET can be used to monitor therapy, and PET's ability to quantify results. Reproduced with permission from Ref. (50).

blood–brain barrier. In this regard, several [18]F- and ^{11}C-labeled ligands have been evaluated for PET imaging of the dopamine receptor (52–56). Other neu-rotransmitters that have been targeted for PET imaging include the serotonin transport system, opiate receptor, and muscarinic receptor (57–60). Most of the ligands have been radiolabeled with ^{123}I for SPECT imaging (56,61,62), however, a ^{99m}Tc-labeled agent has been successful for imaging dopamine recep-tors in the brain for the diagnosis of Parkinson's disease (63). Although a number of systems have been successfully imaged, this number is relatively small with regard to the number known to exist, and thus there are still many opportunities for the development of new imaging agents.

Some of the more widely studied tumor receptors include somatostatin receptors, vasoactive intestinal peptide (VIP) receptors, gastrin-releasing peptide (GRP) receptors, and neurotensin (NT) receptors. These are all seven-transmembrane G-protein coupled receptors that are overexpressed on a variety of tumor types and are generally rapidly internalized after binding of a peptide ligand. The peptide ligands are amenable to incorporation of a bifunctional chelating agent for radiolabeling with radiometals. Molecular imaging of somatostatin receptors [in particular somatostatin receptor subtype 2 (SSTR2)] has been the most extensively investigated group of tumor receptors. The utility of imaging somatostatin receptors with its native ligand, the 14 amino acid somatostatin peptide, is limited by the short serum half-life of this peptide. Several peptides with prolonged serum half-lives have been radiolabeled with many different radionuclides for both SPECT and PET imaging (64–77). An example of PET imaging of SSTR2-positive tumors in rats using two different somatostatin analogs is shown in Fig. 3.6. An ^{111}In-labeled somatostatin analog has been

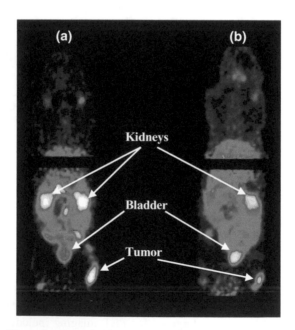

Figure 3.6 (**See color insert**) MicroPET imaging of a rat bearing a SSTR2-positive xenograft using two different ^{64}Cu-labeled somatostatin analogs. Rats were implanted with SSTR2-positive AR42J tumors in the rear flank followed by intravenous (IV) injection of the ^{64}Cu-labeled somatostatin analogs after the tumors were established. The two analogs [CB-TE2A-Y3-TATE (a) and TETA-Y3-TATE (b)] differ with regard to the chelating agent used to complex the copper. MicroPET imaging was performed 4 h after injection of the radiopharmaceuticals and shows increased tumor uptake in (a) compared with (b). This study demonstrates the ability to image SSTR2-positive tumors with PET and the effect of chelating agents on tumor uptake and distribution. This image was kindly provided by Carolyn Anderson and Jeni Sprague of Washington University in St. Louis.

approved by the FDA for SPECT imaging of neuroendocrine tumors, whereas a ^{99m}Tc-labeled analog has been approved by the FDA for SPECT imaging of non-small cell lung tumors (70,74). In addition, analogs have been radiolabeled with therapeutic radionuclides and demonstrated efficacy in somatostatin receptor positive tumors both preclinically and clinically (78–83). VIP is a 28 amino acid peptide that has been radiolabeled with ^{99m}Tc and ^{123}I for imaging colorectal cancer and cancers of the gastrointestinal tract (84,85). The 14 amino acid bombesin peptide is the amphibian homolog of the mammalian GRP and has been radiolabeled with a variety of radionuclides for both SPECT and PET imaging (86–99). A ^{99m}Tc-labeled analog has been evaluated clinically for the detection of both breast and prostate cancer (90,92,100,101). NT is a 13 amino acid peptide in which its six amino acid active fragment has been radiolabeled with ^{111}In, ^{201}Tl, and ^{99m}Tc for SPECT imaging and ^{18}F for PET imaging (102–105). These radiolabeled NT analogs have been used for the detection of pancreatic cancer (106).

Radiolabeled monoclonal antibodies, antibody fragments, and engineered antibodies have been used for imaging tumor antigens. Tumor antigens that have been targeted include prostate-specific membrane antigen (PMSA), carcinoembryonic antigen (CEA), and tumor-associated glycoprotein-72 (TAG-72). A murine monoclonal antibody that binds to an intracellular domain of PMSA and radiolabeled with ^{111}In has been approved by the FDA for the detection of prostate cancer in lymph nodes or the prostate bed (107,108). As this antibody binds to an intracellular region of PMSA, which is only accessible in cells that have a disrupted plasma membrane, monoclonal antibodies are being developed that recognize the extracellular region of PMSA (109–111). Both preclinical and clinical studies have been performed with anti-CEA antibodies, antibody fragments and engineered antibodies radiolabeled with a variety of radionuclides for both SPECT and PET imaging (112–116). It is likely that the use of engineered antibodies (diabodies and minibodies) will increase in molecular imaging studies in the future, as they can be developed against a wide array of tumor antigens and receptors and modified to optimize their pharmacokinetics for imaging purposes. An example of a ^{64}Cu-labeled anti-CEA minibody for PET imaging of CEA-positive tumors over time is shown in Fig. 3.7. The TAG-72 antigen has been the target of molecular imaging with radiolabeled antibodies in the context of both colorectal and ovarian cancer (117,118). The antibodies used in these studies have been improved over the years to increase the antibody affinity for TAG-72, reduce immunogenicity, and improve pharmacokinetics (119–122).

MDR is a major issue for cancer chemotherapy that must be overcome for the successful use of many anti-cancer agents. One member of the adenosine triphosphate (ATP)–binding cassette (ABC) superfamily of membrane transporters that has been studied extensively for molecular imaging purposes has been the 170 kDa transmembrane glycoprotein, P-glycoprotein (Pgp). Two widely studied ^{99m}Tc-labeled agents that have been used for SPECT imaging of MDR

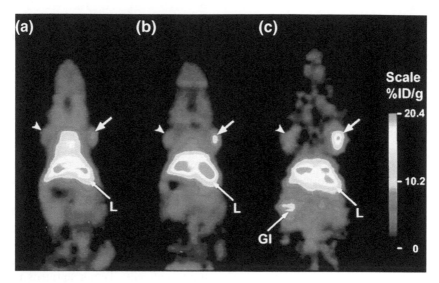

Figure 3.7 (**See color insert**) MicroPET imaging of a mouse bearing a CEA-positive xenograft using a ^{64}Cu-labeled minibody. Mice were implanted with axillary CEA-positive LS174T cells (arrow) and CEA-negative C6 cells (arrowhead). After the tumors were established, the ^{64}Cu-labeled minibody was injected intravenously (IV) and the mice were imaged 2 h (a), 6 h (b), and 24 h (c) after injection. Clear visualization of the CEA-positive tumor is observed at all time points as well as clearance through the liver (L) and the gastrointestinal (GI) tract. This study demonstrates the ability to monitor cell surface antigens over time with a radiolabeled antibody construct. It should be noted that similar studies could be performed using a gamma-emitting radionuclide and SPECT imaging. Reproduced with permission from Ref. (115).

are ^{99m}Tc-sestamibi and ^{99m}Tc-tetrofosmin (123–127). An example of imaging Pgp expression in lung cancer with ^{99m}Tc-sestamibi is shown in Fig. 3.8. Both of these agents mimic the hydrophobicity and cationic character of many chemotherapeutic agents. These agents have demonstrated clinical utility for determining MDR status in a variety of cancers and thus the ability to predict response to chemotherapy (128–131). It has also been demonstrated that ^{99m}Tc-sestamibi can be used to evaluate the effectiveness of Pgp modulators that increase the efficacy of chemotherapeutic agents (132–135). In addition to these SPECT agents, many substrates radiolabeled with PET radionuclides have been evaluated recently with some success (136–140).

C. Imaging of Exogenous Marker Genes

Reporter genes are being used to monitor the expression of genes of interest in a biological system. They are typically chimeric genes linking endogenous promoters to a gene encoding an enzyme, fluorophore, receptor, or transporter (1). Many of the conventional reporter genes utilized luciferase, β-galactosidase, alkaline phosphatase, and green fluorescent protein (141). Recently, a number

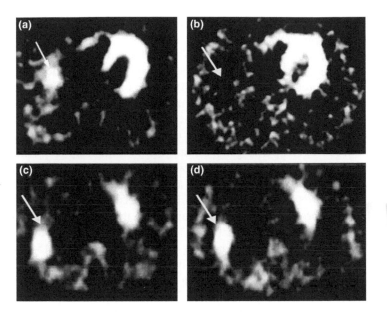

Figure 3.8 SPECT imaging of two patients with histologically confirmed lung cancer using ^{99m}Tc-sestamibi. In one patient, an early SPECT scan after ^{99m}Tc-sestamibi injection shows intense tumor uptake (a) (arrow) that is significantly decreased after a delayed scan (b). This suggests rapid washout of ^{99m}Tc-sestamibi and low expression of Pgp. In contrast, the other patient shows intense tumor uptake of ^{99m}Tc-sestamibi after an early SPECT scan (c) that does not decrease by the time of the delayed scan (d) suggesting a low level of Pgp expression. The expression levels were subsequently confirmed by immunohistochemistry on tumor biopsies. This study demonstrates the ability to image the transmembrane Pgp that has utility for predicting response to chemotherapy and efficacy of Pgp modulators. Reproduced with permission from Ref. (127).

of reporter genes have been developed that utilize PET and SPECT imaging to determine the location and magnitude of reporter gene expression. The reporter genes that will be discussed in this chapter are the herpes simplex virus-1 thymidine kinase (HSV1-TK), the sodium iodide symporter (NS), the dopamine-2 receptor (D2R), and the SSTR2. These reporter genes have been used to image gene therapy, image protein–protein interactions, monitor cell trafficking, and image transgenic mice.

Herpes Simplex Virus-1 Thymidine Kinase

The most studied nuclear imaging based reporter gene has involved the use of the HSV1-TK enzyme (or mutant versions of this enzyme) and a variety of reporter probes. In general, these probes have consisted of uracil nucleoside derivatives radiolabeled with iodine isotopes for PET and SPECT imaging or acycloguanosine derivatives radiolabeled with ^{18}F for PET imaging. These probes are transported into cells, phosphorylated by cells expressing HSV1-TK, and the phosphorylated product is trapped, leading to a signal when compared to surrounding tissue not containing HSV1-TK. This reporter has been used to image gene therapy in animal models (142), image transgenic mice (143), image protein–protein interactions (144), and monitor cell trafficking (145). Many studies involving HSV1-TK and radiolabeled probes have involved the use of cell lines stably transfected to express HSV1-TK (146–149), whereas others have used gene transfer vehicles to determine HSV1-TK expression in animal models. This reporter gene/probe system meets many of the characteristics desired for an ideal combination, however, there is a concern about the correlation between HSV1-TK expression and the accumulation of radiolabeled probes when HSV1-TK is expressed at high levels (150–152). Some studies have shown a correlation between the uptake of the acycloguanosine analogs [^{18}F]-FGCV or [^{18}F]-FHBG and HSV1-TK activity in the liver after infection of the liver with an adenovirus encoding the *HSV1-tk* gene (153,154), whereas other studies found no correlation in the liver (150). It is possible that differences in higher levels of HSV1-TK expression are not detected *in vivo* because low accumulation of the radiolabeled probes inside cells results in phosphorylation of the entire substrate. The low accumulation of the radiolabeled probes may be related to transport limitations at the cell surface that cause saturation of the signal when HSV1-TK is expressed at a high level. Zinn et al. (151) demonstrated that there was not a correlation between the tumor uptake of an iodinated uracil nucleoside derivative and the amount of adenovirus injected after intratumoral administration of an adenovirus encoding the gene for *HSV1-tk*. Richard et al. (152) has recently reported that at high viral doses, there was a poor correlation between [^{18}F]-FHBG and HSV1-TK activities in the lung after tracheal administration of an adenovirus encoding a mutant *HSV1-tk* gene. Thus, the HSV1-TK reporter has limitations for quantifying the expression level of a therapeutic gene in gene therapy protocols (see Chapter 8).

Sodium Iodide Symporter

The NIS is a transmembrane glycoprotein that is most commonly studied in the thyroid gland, where it mediates the transport of I$^-$ (155). The use of NIS as a reporter gene has been proposed after the isolation of the complementary DNA (cDNA) of rat NIS in 1996 (156). The expression of NIS in tumors after stable transfection or introduction using an adenoviral vector has been demonstrated using SPECT or PET imaging with various iodide isotopes (^{131}I$^-$, ^{123}I$^-$ for SPECT, or ^{124}I$^-$ for PET) (157–159). An example of imaging NIS expression with ^{123}I$^-$ over time in a brain tumor model is shown in Fig. 3.9. In addition, therapeutic efficacy has been demonstrated when combining NIS with the therapeutic ^{131}I$^-$ radionuclide (157,160). Another interesting aspect of NIS is that it is capable of transporting other radionuclides including ^{99m}Tc, ^{188}Re, and ^{211}At. ^{99m}Tc can be used for imaging, whereas ^{188}Re and the α-emitting ^{211}At are primarily used for

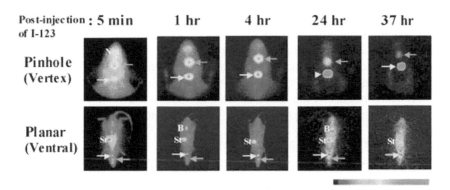

Figure 3.9 (**See color insert**) Dual headed gamma camera imaging of tumors stably transduced to express NIS using [123]I. Rats were implanted intracranially with F98 cells stably transduced to express NIS. Thirteen days later the rats were injected intravenously (IV) with ^{123}I and either whole body (planar) or cranially focused (pinhole) images were obtained at various times postinjection. The top arrow in the pinhole images (bottom arrow in the planar) indicates uptake in the NIS-expressing tumor cells and the bottom arrow in the pinhole images (top arrow in the planar) indicates thyroid uptake. Uptake and clearance was also observed in the nasal mucosa (N), stomach (St), and bladder (B). Tumor uptake is observed at 5 min postinjection and still present at 37 h. The highest tumor uptake of ^{123}I is observed at 4 h, whereas the highest thyroid uptake is observed at 24 h. These studies demonstrate that an exogenous gene (NIS) can be introduced into cells and imaged noninvasively at multiple times after administration of [123]I. Reproduced with permission from Ref. (160).

therapy (160–163). These radionuclides have an array of half-lives and energies to choose from for conducting molecular imaging or therapy studies.

Somatostatin Receptor Subtype 2

Five somatostatin receptor subtypes have been cloned (SSTR1–SSTR5), with alternate splicing of SSTR2 to yield a SSTR2A and the C-terminal truncated form, SSTR2B (164,165). The human SSTR2A (heretofore simply referred to as *hSSTR2*) has been used for imaging of gene transfer using gamma camera imaging (151,166,167). These studies used the radiolabeled somatostatin analogs, ^{111}In-DTPA-octreotide (Octreoscan), ^{99m}Tc-P829 (NeoTect) or ^{99m}Tc-P2045 to demonstrate localization in a tumor injected directly with an adenovirus (AdhSSTR2) encoding the *hsstr2* gene driven by a cytomegalovirus (CMV) promoter. It has been demonstrated that there is a strong correlation between the expression of hSSTR2 and the tumor uptake of ^{99m}Tc-P2045 after intratumoral injection of various amounts (1×10^6 plaque forming units (pfu) -3×10^8 pfu) of Ad*hsstr2* (151). While this same study showed that there was not a correlation between HSV1-TK expression and 2′-deoxy-2′-fluoro-β-D-arabinofuranosyl-5-[^{131}I]iodouracil (^{131}I-FIAU) uptake at these adenoviral doses. However, drawbacks to using hSSTR2 as a reporter of gene transfer include: (a) intracellular signaling through G proteins, (b) endogenous expression of hSSTR2 on some normal tissues and cancerous tissues, and (c) the high background radioactivity of radiolabeled somatostatin analogs due to hepatobiliary accumulation (radioiodinated analogs) and kidney accumulation (radiometal labeled analogs) (71,168,169). Therefore, modification of hSSTR2 to address these issues as well as develop novel radiopharmaceuticals that detect the modified receptor and have lower background radioactivity are necessary to optimize hSSTR2 as a reporter probe.

Dopamine-2 Receptor

As discussed earlier, the dopamine receptor is a transmembrane protein that is endogenously expressed primarily in the striatum of the brain and the pituitary gland and has been the target of PET and SPECT molecular imaging studies. The D2R has also been used as a reporter gene for imaging tumors stably expressing D2R or after gene transfer with an adenoviral vector (170). An ^{18}F-labeled spiperone derivative has been used for PET imaging of D2R expression, whereas a ^{99m}Tc-labeled ligand has been used for SPECT imaging (170,171). A plasmid consisting of both D2R and HSV1-TK with an internal ribosomal entry site has been used to transfect cells and demonstrate PET imaging of both protein products (149). Similar to SSTR2, intracellular signaling of D2R through binding of endogenous ligands may result in underlying biological problems that are not desired when utilizing this as a reporter gene. To address this issue, Liang et al. (172) used a mutant D2R that prevented ligand mediated inhibition of cyclic adenosine monophosphate, yet maintained high binding of ^{18}F-labeled spiperone.

VI. Summary

The basic principles of SPECT and PET imaging have been described to understand how these modalities can be applied for molecular imaging purposes. Each modality has strengths and weaknesses that must be considered when deciding which to use in a particular imaging study. Many of these decisions are based on the probes available for interrogating a biological target of interest. Several examples of imaging mRNA, endogenous proteins, and exogenous proteins are given for a variety of probes. It is anticipated that molecular imaging with SPECT and PET will become more widespread for the noninvasive imaging of biological processes as the technologies becomes more widely available and affordable, the number of biological hypotheses increase, and the availability of probes for testing these hypotheses increase.

Acknowledgments

I would like to thank Carolyn Anderson and Jesse Parry for their critical reading of this chapter and insightful comments. Carolyn Anderson and Jeni Sprague are thanked for providing the microPET image shown in Fig. 3.6. Finally, the Department of Radiation Oncology is thanked for financial support while writing this chapter.

References

1. Sharma V, Luker GD, Piwnica-Worms D. Molecular imaging of gene expression and protein function in vivo with PET and SPECT. J Magn Reson Imaging 2002; 16:336–351.
2. Weissleder R, Mahmood U. Molecular imaging. Radiology 2001; 219:316–333.
3. Galt JR, Faber T. Principles of single photon emission computed tomography (SPECT) imaging. In: Christian PE, Bernier D, Langan JK, eds. Nuclear Medicine and PET Technology and Techniques. 5th ed. St. Louis: Mosby, 2004:242–284.
4. Massoud TF, Gambhir SS. Molecular imaging in living subjects: seeing fundamental biological processes in a new light. Genes Dev 2003; 17:545–580.
5. Rosenthal MS, Cullom J, Hawkins W, Moore SC, Tsui BM, Yester M. Quantitative SPECT imaging: a review and recommendations by the Focus Committee of the Society of Nuclear Medicine Computer and Instrumentation Council. J Nucl Med 1995; 36:1489–1513.
6. Cullom SJ. Principles of cardiac SPECT. In: De Puey EG, Berman DS, Garcia EV, eds. Cardiac SPECT Imaging. Philadelphia: Lippincott-Raven, 1996:1–19.
7. Groch MW, Erwin WD. SPECT in the year 2000: basic principles. J Nucl Med Technol 2000; 28:233–244.
8. Schwarz SW, Anderson CJ. Radiochemistry and radiopharmacology. In: Christian PE, Bernier D, Langan JK, eds. Nuclear Medicine and PET Technology and Techniques. St. Louis: Mosby, 2004:157–183.
9. Moore ML, Murphy PH, Burdine JA. ECG-gated emission computed tomography of the cardiac blood pool. Radiology 1980; 134:233–235.
10. Christian PE. Fundamentals of molecular imaging with PET. In: Christian PE, Bernier D, Langan JK, eds. Nuclear Medicine and PET Technology and Techniques. St. Louis: Mosby, 2004:285–308.
11. Burger C, Berthold T. Physical principles and practical aspects of clinical PET imaging. In: von Schulthess GK, ed. Clinical Positron Emission Tomography. Philadelphia: Lippincott Williams and Wilkins, 2001:9–24.
12. Zanzonico P. Positron emission tomography: a review of basic principles, scanner design, and performance, and current systems. Semin Nucl Med 2004; 34:87–111.
13. Budinger T. Single photon emission computed tomography. In: Sandler M, ed. Diagnostic Nuclear Medicine. Baltimore: Williams and Wilkins, 1996:121–138.
14. Hom RK, Katzenellenbogen JA. Technetium-99m-labeled receptor-specific small-molecule radiopharmaceuticals: recent developments and encouraging results. Nucl Med Biol 1997; 24:485–498.
15. Lewis MR, Jia F. Antisense imaging: and miles to go before we sleep? J Cell Biochem 2003; 90:464–472.
16. Gambhir SS, Barrio JR, Herschman HR, Phelps ME. Imaging gene expression: principles and assays. J Nucl Cardiol 1999; 6:219–233.

17.   Miller PS. Development of antisense and antigene oligonucleotide analogs. In: Cohn WE, Moldave K, eds. Nucleic Acid Research and Molecular Biology. Vol. 52. San Diego: Academic Press, 1996:261–291.

18.   Tavitian B, Terrazzino S, Kuhnast B, Marzabal S, Stettler O, Dolle F, Deverre JR, Jobert A, Hinnen F, Bendriem B, Crouzel C, Di Giamberardino L. *In vivo* imaging of oligonucleotides with positron emission tomography. Nat Med 1998; 4:467–471.

19.   Lewis MR, Jia F, Gallazzi F, Wang Y, Zhang J, Shenoy N, Lever SZ, Hannink M. Radiometal-labeled peptide-PNA conjugates for targeting bcl-2 expression: preparation, characterization, and *in vitro* mRNA binding. Bioconjug Chem 2002; 13:1176–1180.

20.   Liu CB, Liu GZ, Liu N, Zhang YM, He J, Rusckowski M, Hnatowich DJ. Radiolabeling morpholinos with ^{90}Y, ^{111}In, ^{188}Re and ^{99m}Tc. Nucl Med Biol 2003; 30:207–214.

21.   Derossi D, Calvet S, Trembleau A, Brunissen A, Chassaing G, Prochiantz A. Cell internalization of the third helix of the Antennapedia homeodomain is receptor-independent. J Biol Chem 1996; 271:18188–18193.

22.   Frankel AD, Pabo CO. Cellular uptake of the tat protein from human immunodeficiency virus. Cell 1988; 55:1189–1193.

23.   Fawell S, Seery J, Daikh Y, Moore C, Chen LL, Pepinsky B, Barsoum J. Tat-mediated delivery of heterologous proteins into cells. Proc Natl Acad Sci USA 1994; 91:664–668.

24.   Mier W, Eritja R, Mohammed A, Haberkorn U, Eisenhut M. Preparation and evaluation of tumor-targeting peptide-oligonucleotide conjugates. Bioconjug Chem 2000; 11:855–860.

25.   Rao PS, Tian X, Qin W, Aruva MR, Sauter ER, Thakur ML, Wickstrom E. ^{99m}Tc-peptide-peptide nucleic acid probes for imaging oncogene mRNAs in tumours. Nucl Med Commun 2003; 24:857–863.

26.   Dewanjee MK, Ghafouripour AK, Kapadvanjwala M, Dewanjee S, Serafini AN, Lopez DM, Sfakianakis GN. Noninvasive imaging of c-myc oncogene messenger RNA with indium-111-antisense probes in a mammary tumor-bearing mouse model. J Nucl Med 1994; 35:1054–1063.

27.   Sato N, Kobayashi H, Saga T, Nakamoto Y, Ishimori T, Togashi K, Fujibayashi Y, Konishi J, Brechbiel MW. Tumor targeting and imaging of intraperitoneal tumors by use of antisense oligo-DNA complexed with dendrimers and/or avidin in mice. Clin Cancer Res 2001; 7:3606–3612.

28.   Tian X, Aruva MR, Rao PS, Qin W, Read P, Sauter ER, Thakur ML, Wickstrom E. Imaging oncogene expression. Ann NY Acad Sci 2003; 1002:165–188.

29.   Larson SM, Grunbaum Z, Rasey JS. Positron imaging feasibility studies: selective tumor concentration of ^{3}H-thymidine, ^{3}H-uridine, and ^{14}C-2-deoxyglucose. Radiology 1980; 134:771–773.

30.   Wahl RL, Hutchins GD, Buchsbaum DJ, Liebert M, Grossman HB, Fisher S. ^{18}F-2-deoxy-2-fluoro-D-glucose uptake into human tumor xenografts: feasibility studies for cancer imaging with positron-emission tomography. Cancer 1991; 67:1544–1550.

31.   Wahl RL, Zasadny K, Helvie M, Hutchins GD, Weber B, Cody R. Metabolic monitoring of breast cancer chemohormonotherapy using positron emission tomography: initial evaluation. J Clin Oncol 1993; 11:2101–2111.

32. Hoekstra CJ, Paglianiti I, Hoekstra OS, Smit EF, Postmus PE, Teule GJ, Lammertsma AA. Monitoring response to therapy in cancer using [^{18}F]-2-fluoro-2-deoxy-D-glucose and positron emission tomography: an overview of different analytical methods. Eur J Nucl Med 2000; 27:731–743.

33. Yang DJ, Kim CG, Schechter NR, Azhdarinia A, Yu DF, Oh CS, Bryant JL, Won JJ, Kim EE, Podoloff DA. Imaging with ^{99m}Tc ECDG targeted at the multi-functional glucose transport system: feasibility study with rodents. Radiology 2003; 226:465–473.

34. Wintersberger E, Rotheneder H, Grabner M, Beck G, Seiser C. Regulation of thymidine kinase during growth, cell cycle and differentiation. Adv Enzyme Regul 1992; 32:241–254.

35. Hannigan BM, Barnett YA, Armstrong DB, McKelvey-Martin VJ, McKenna PG. Thymidine kinases: the enzymes and their clinical usefulness. Cancer Biother 1993; 8:189–197.

36. Hengstschlager M, Knofler M, Mullner EW, Ogris E, Wintersberger E, Wawra E. Different regulation of thymidine kinase during the cell cycle of normal versus DNA tumor virus-transformed cells. J Biol Chem 1994; 269:13836–13842.

37. Rasey JS, Grierson JR, Wiens LW, Kolb PD, Schwartz JL. Validation of FLT uptake as a measure of thymidine kinase-1 activity in A549 carcinoma cells. J Nucl Med 2002; 43:1210–1217.

38. Shields AF, Grierson JR, Dohmen BM, Machulla HJ, Stayanoff JC, Lawhorn-Crews JM, Obradovich JE, Muzik O, Mangner TJ. Imaging proliferation *in vivo* with [F-18]FLT and positron emission tomography. Nat Med 1998; 4:1334–1336.

39. Buck AK, Schirrmeister H, Hetzel M, Von Der Heide M, Halter G, Glatting G, Mattfeldt T, Liewald F, Reske SN, Neumaier B. 3-Deoxy-3-[^{18}F]fluorothymidine-positron emission tomography for noninvasive assessment of proliferation in pulmonary nodules. Cancer Res 2002; 62:3331–3334.

40. Schwartz JL, Tamura Y, Jordan R, Grierson JR, Krohn KA. Effect of p53 activation on cell growth, thymidine kinase-1 activity, and 3′-deoxy-3′fluorothymidine uptake. Nucl Med Biol 2004; 31:419–423.

41. Mankoff DA, Dehdashti F, Shields AF. Characterizing tumors using metabolic imaging: PET imaging of cellular proliferation and steroid receptors. Neoplasia 2000; 2:71–88.

42. Collier TL, Lecomte R, McCarthy TJ, Meikle S, Ruth TJ, Scopinaro F, Signore A, VanBrocklin H, van De Wiele C, Waterhouse RN. Assessment of cancer-associated biomarkers by positron emission tomography: advances and challenges. Dis Markers 2002; 18:211–247.

43. Kiesewetter DO, Kilbourn MR, Landvatter SW, Heiman DF, Katzenellenbogen JA, Welch MJ. Preparation of four fluorine-18-labeled estrogens and their selective uptakes in target tissues of immature rats. J Nucl Med 1984; 25:1212–1221.

44. Mintun MA, Welch MJ, Siegel BA, Mathias CJ, Brodack JW, McGuire AH, Katzenellenbogen JA. Breast cancer: PET imaging of estrogen receptors. Radiology 1988; 169:45–48.

45. McGuire AH, Dehdashti F, Siegel BA, Lyss AP, Brodack JW, Mathias CJ, Mintun MA, Katzenellenbogen JA, Welch MJ. Positron tomographic assessment of 16 alpha-[^{18}F] fluoro-17 beta-estradiol uptake in metastatic breast carcinoma. J Nucl Med 1991; 32:1526–1531.

46. Dehdashti F, Flanagan FL, Mortimer JE, Katzenellenbogen JA, Welch MJ, Siegel BA. Positron emission tomographic assessment of "metabolic flare" to predict response of metastatic breast cancer to antiestrogen therapy. Eur J Nucl Med 1999; 26:51–56.

47. Mortimer JE, Dehdashti F, Siegel BA, Trinkaus K, Katzenellenbogen JA, Welch MJ. Metabolic flare: indicator of hormone responsiveness in advanced breast cancer. J Clin Oncol 2001; 19:2797–2803.

48. Bonasera TA, O'Neil JP, Xu M, Dobkin JA, Cutler PD, Lich LL, Choe YS, Katzenellenbogen JA, Welch MJ. Preclinical evaluation of fluorine-18-labeled androgen receptor ligands in baboons. J Nucl Med 1996; 37:1009–1015.

49. Garg PK, Labaree DC, Hoyte RM, Hochberg RB. [7alpha-18F]fluoro-17alpha-methyl-5alpha-dihydrotestosterone: a ligand for androgen receptor-mediated imaging of prostate cancer. Nucl Med Biol 2001; 28:85–90.

50. Larson SM, Morris M, Gunther I, Beattie B, Humm JL, Akhurst TA, Finn RD, Erdi Y, Pentlow K, Dyke J, Squire O, Bornmann W, McCarthy T, Welch M, Scher H. Tumor localization of 16beta-^{18}F-fluoro-5alpha-dihydrotestosterone versus ^{18}F-FDG in patients with progressive, metastatic prostate cancer. J Nucl Med 2004; 45:366–373.

51. Grasby PM. Imaging the neurochemical brain in health and disease. Clin Med 2002; 2:67–73.

52. Wagner HNJ, Burns HD, Dannals RF, Wong DF, Langstrom B, Duelfer T, Frost JJ, Ravert HT, Links JM, Rosenbloom SB, Lukas SE, Kramer AV, Kuhar MJ. Imaging dopamine receptors in the human brain by positron tomography. Science 1983; 221:1264–1266.

53. Zanzonico PB, Bigler RE, Schmall B. Neuroleptic binding sites: specific labeling in mice with ^{18}F]haloperidol, a potential tracer for positron emission tomography. J Nucl Med 1983; 24:408–416.

54. Halldin C, Farde L, Barnett A, Sedvall G. Synthesis of carbon-11 labelled SCH 39166, a new selective dopamine D-1 receptor ligand, and preliminary PET investigations. Int J Rad Appl Instrum A 1991; 42:451–455.

55. Cumming P, Gjedde A. Compartmental analysis of dopa decarboxylation in living brain from dynamic positron emission tomograms. Synapse 1998; 29:37–61.

56. Lucignani G, Frost HH. Neurochemical imaging with emission tomography: clinical applications. In: Schiepers C, ed. Diagnostic Nuclear Medicine. Berlin: Springer-Verlag, 2000:7–35.

57. Blin J, Pappata S, Kiyosawa M, Crouzel C, Baron JC. [18]F]setoperone: a new high-affinity ligand for positron emission tomography study of the serotonin-2 receptors in baboon brain *in vivo*. Eur J Pharmacol 1988; 147:73–82.

58. Frost JJ, Mayberg HS, Sadzot B, Dannals RF, Lever JR, Ravert HT, Wilson AA, Wagner HNJ, Links JM. Comparison of ^{11}C]diprenorphine and ^{11}C]carfentanil binding to opiate receptors in humans by positron emission tomography. J Cereb Blood Flow Metab 1990; 10:484–492.

59. Mulholland GK, Kilbourn MR, Sherman P, Carey JE, Frey KA, Koeppe RA, Kuhl DE. Synthesis, *in vivo* biodistribution and dosimetry of ^{11}C]*N*-methylpiperidyl benzilate (^{11}C]NMPB), a muscarinic acetylcholine receptor antagonist. Nucl Med Biol 1995; 22:13–17.

60. Madar I, Lever JR, Kinter CM, Scheffel U, Ravert HT, Musachio JL, Mathews WB, Dannals RF, Frost JJ. Imaging of delta opioid receptors in human brain by *N*1'-(^{11}C]methyl)naltrindole and PET. Synapse 1996; 24:19–28.

61. Eckelman WC, Reba RC, Rzeszotarski WJ, Gibson RE, Hill T, Holman BL, Budinger T, Conklin JJ, Eng R, Grissom MP. External imaging of cerebral muscarinic acetylcholine receptors. Science 1984; 223:291–293.

62. Newberg AB, Plossl K, Mozley PD, Stubbs JB, Wintering N, Udeshi M, Alavi A, Kauppinen T, Kung HF. Biodistribution and imaging with ^{123}I-ADAM: a serotonin transporter imaging agent. J Nucl Med 2004; 45:834–841.

63. Kung HF, Kung MP, Choi SR. Radiopharmaceuticals for single-photon emission computed tomography brain imaging. Semin Nucl Med 2003; 33:2–13.

64. Li WP, Lewis JS, Kim J, Bugaj JE, Johnson MA, Erion JL, Anderson CJ. DOTA-D-Tyr[1]-octreotate: a somatostatin analogue for labeling with metal and halogen radionuclides for cancer imaging and therapy. Bioconjug Chem 2002; 13:721–728.

65. Lubberink M, Tolmachev V, Widstrom C, Bruskin A, Lundqvist H, Westlin JE. [110m]In-DTPA-D-Phe1-octreotide for imaging of neuroendocrine tumors with PET. J Nucl Med 2002; 43:1391–1397.

66. Kowalski J, Henze M, Schuhmacher J, Macke HR, Hofmann M, Haberkorn U. Evaluation of positron emission tomography imaging using [^{68}Ga]-DOTA-D Phe[1]-Tyr[3]-octreotide in comparison to [^{111}In]-DTPAOC SPECT. First results in patients with neuroendocrine tumors. Mol Imaging Biol 2003; 5:42–48.

67. Jamar F, Barone R, Mathieu I, Walrand S, Labar D, Carlier P, de Camps J, Schran H, Chen T, Smith MC, Bouterfa H, Valkema R, Krenning EP, Kvols LK, Pauwels S. [86]Y-DOTA[0])-D-Phe[1]-Tyr[3]-octreotide (SMT487)—a phase 1 clinical study: pharmacokinetics, biodistribution and renal protective effect of different regimens of amino acid co-infusion. Eur J Nucl Med Mol Imaging 2003; 30:510–518.

68. Wester HJ, Schottelius M, Scheidhauer K, Meisetschlager G, Herz M, Rau FC, Reubi JC, Schwaiger M. PET imaging of somatostatin receptors: design, synthesis and preclinical evaluation of a novel ^{18}F-labelled, carbohydrated analogue of octreotide. Eur J Nucl Med Mol Imaging 2003; 30:117–122.

69. Uger O, Kothari PJ, Finn RD, Zanzonico P, Ruan S, Guenther I, Maecke HR, Larson SM. Ga-66 labeled somatostatin analogue DOTA-DPhe[1]-Tyr[3]-octreotide as a potential agent for positron emission tomography imaging and receptor mediated internal radiotherapy of somatostatin receptor positive tumors. Nucl Med Biol 2002; 29:147–157.

70. Bakker WH, Albert R, Bruns C, Breeman WAP, Hofland LJ, Marbach P, Pless J, Pralet D, Stolz B, Koper JW, Lamberts SWJ, Visser TJ, Krenning EP. [^{111}In-DTPA-D-Phe[1]]-octreotide, a potential radiopharmaceutical for imaging of somatostatin receptor-positive tumors: synthesis, radiolabeling and *in vitro* validation. Life Sci 1991; 49:1583–1591.

71. Krenning EP, Bakker WH, Kooij PPM, Breeman WAP, Oei HY, de Jong M, Reubi JC, Visser TJ, Bruns C, Kwekkeboom DJ, Reijs AEM, van Hagen PM, Koper JW, Lamberts SWJ. Somatostatin receptor scintigraphy with indium-111-DTPA-D-Phe-1-octreotide in man: metabolism, dosimetry and comparison with iodine-123-Tyr-3-octreotide. J Nucl Med 1992; 33:652–658.

72. Krenning EP, Kwekkeboom DJ, Bakker WH, Breeman WAP, Kooij PPM, Oei HY, van Hagen M, Postema PTE, de Jong M, Reubi JC, Visser TJ, Reijs AEM, Hofland LJ, Koper JW, Lamberts SWJ. Somatostatin receptor scintigraphy with [^{111}In-DTPA-D-Phe[1]]- and [^{123}I-Tyr[3]]-octreotide: the Rotterdam experience with more than 1000 patients. Eur J Nucl Med 1993; 20:716–731.

73. Pearson DA, Lister-James J, McBride WJ, Wilson DM, Martel LJ, Civitello ER, Taylor JE, Moyer BR, Dean RT. Somatostatin receptor-binding peptides labeled with technetium-99m: chemistry and initial biological studies. J Med Chem 1996; 39:1361–1371.

74. Vallabhajosula S, Moyer BR, Lister-James J, McBride BJ, Lipszyc H, Lee H, Bastidas D, Dean RT. Preclinical evaluation of technetium-99m-labeled somatostatin receptor-binding peptides. J Nucl Med 1996; 37:1016–1022.

75. Decristoforo C, Melendez-Alafort L, Sosabowski JK, Mather SJ. ^{99m}Tc-HYNIC-[Tyr^3]-octreotide for imaging somatostatin-receptor-positive tumors: preclinical evaluation and comparison with ^{111}In-octreotide. J Nucl Med 2000; 41:1114–1119.

76. Bangard M, Behe M, Guhlke S, Otte R, Bender H, Maecke HR, Biersack HJ. Detection of somatostatin receptor-positive tumours using the new ^{99m}Tc-tricine-HYNIC-D-Phe^1-Tyr^3-octreotide: first results in patients and comparison with ^{111}In-DTPA-D-Phe^1-octreotide. Eur J Nucl Med 2000; 27:628–637.

77. Maina T, Nock B, Nikolopoulou A, Sotiriou P, Loudos G, Maintas D, Cordopatis P, Chiotellis E. [^{99m}Tc]Demotate, a new ^{99m}Tc-based [Tyr^3]octreotate analogue for the detection of somatostatin receptor-positive tumours: synthesis and preclinical results. Eur J Nucl Med Mol Imaging 2002; 29:742–753.

78. Paganelli G, Zoboli S, Cremonesi M, Bodei L, Ferrari M, Grana C, Bartolomei M, Orsi F, De Cicco C, Macke HR, Chinol M, de Braud F. Receptor-mediated radiotherapy with ^{90}Y-DOTA-D-Phe^1-Tyr^3-octreotide. Eur J Nucl Med 2001; 28:426–434.

79. Kwekkeboom DJ, Bakker WH, Kam BL, Teunissen JJM, Kooij PPM, Herder WW, Feelders RA, Eijck CHJ, Jong M, Srinivasan A, Erion JL, Krenning EP. Treatment of patients with gastro-entero-pancreatic (GEP) tumours with the novel radio-labelled somatostatin analogue [^{177}Lu-DOTA^0,Tyr^3]octreotate. Eur J Nucl Med Mol Imaging 2003; 30:417–422.

80. Buscombe JR, Caplin ME, Hilson AJW. Long-term efficacy of high-activity ^{111}In-pentetreotide therapy in patients with disseminated neuroendocrine tumors. J Nucl Med 2003; 44:1–6.

81. Anderson CJ, Jones LA, Bass LA, Sherman ELC, McCarthy DW, Cutler PD, Lanahan MV, Cristel ME, Lewis JS, Schwarz SW. Radiotherapy, toxicity and dosimetry of copper-64-TETA-octreotide in tumor-bearing rats. J Nucl Med 1998; 39:1944–1951.

82. Anderson CJ, Dehdashti F, Cutler PD, Schwarz SW, Laforest R, Bass LA, Lewis JS, McCarthy DW. ^{64}Cu-TETA-octreotide as PET imaging agent for patients with neuroendocrine tumors. J Nucl Med 2001; 42:213–221.

83. Stolz B, Weckbecker G, Smith-Jones PM, Albert R, Raulf F, Bruns C. The somatostatin receptor-targeted radiotherapeutic [^{90}Y-DOTA-DPhe^1, Tyr^3]octreotide (^{90}Y-SMT 487) eradicates experimental rat pancreatic CA 20948 tumours. Eur J Nucl Med 1998; 25:668–674.

84. Virgolini I, Raderer M, Kurtaran A, Angelberger P, Yang Q, Radosavljevic M, Leimer M, Kaserer K, Li SR, Kornek G, Hubsch P, Niederle B, Pidlich J, Scheithauer W, Valent P. ^{123}I-vasoactive intestinal peptide (VIP) receptor scanning: update of imaging results in patients with adenocarcinomas and endocrine tumors of the gastrointestinal tract. Nucl Med Biol 1996; 23:685–692.

85. Rao PS, Thakur ML, Pallela V, Patti R, Reddy K, Li H, Sharma S, Pham HL, Diggles L, Minami C, Marcus CS. ^{99m}Tc labeled VIP analog: evaluation for imaging colorectal cancer. Nucl Med Biol 2001; 28:445–450.

86. Baidoo KE, Lin KS, Zhan Y, Finley P, Scheffel U, Wagner HN Jr. Design, synthesis, and initial evaluation of high-affinity technetium bombesin analogues. Bioconjug Chem 1998; 9:218–225.
87. Karra S, Schibli R, Gali H, Katti K, Hoffman T, Higginbotham C, Sieckman G, Volkert W. 99mTc-labeling and *in vivo* studies of a bombesin analogue with a novel water-soluble dithiadiphosphine-based bifunctional chelating agent. Bioconjug Chem 1999; 10:254–260.
88. Breeman WAP, Hofland LJ, de Jong M, Bernard BF, Srinivasan A, Kwekkeboom DJ, Visser TJ, Krenning EP. Evaluation of radiolabeled bombesin analogues for receptor-targeted scintigraphy and radiotherapy. Int J Cancer 1999; 81:658–665.
89. Breeman WAP, de Jong M, Bernard BF, Kwekkeboom DJ, Srinivasan A, van der Pluijm ME, Hofland LJ, Visser TJ, Krenning EP. Pre-clinical evaluation of [^{111}In-DTPA-Pro^1, Tyr^4]bombesin, a new radioligand for bombesin-receptor scintigraphy. Int J Cancer 1999; 83:657–663.
90. Van de Wiele C, Dumont F, Broecke RV, Oosterlinck W, Cocquyt V, Serreyn R, Peers S, Thornback J, Slegers G, Dierckx RA. Technetium-99m RP527, a GRP analogue for visualization of GRP receptor-expressing malignancies: a feasibility study. Eur J Nucl Med 2000; 27:1694–1699.
91. Van de Wiele C, Dumont F, Van Belle S, Slegers G, Peers SH, Dierckx RA. Is there a role for agonist gastrin-releasing peptide receptor radioligands in tumour imaging? Nucl Med Commun 2001; 22:5–15.
92. Van de Wiele C, Dumont F, Dierckx RA, Peers SH, Thornback JR, Slegers G, Thierens H. Biodistribution and dosimetry of ^{99m}Tc-RP527, a gastrin-releasing peptide (GRP) agonist for the visualization of GRP receptor-expressing malignancies. J Nucl Med 2002; 42:1722–1727.
93. La Bella R, Garcia-Garayoa E, Langer M, Blauenstein P, Beck-Sickinger AG, Schubiger PA. *In vitro* and *in vivo* evaluation of a ^{99m}Tc(I)-labeled bombesin analogue for imaging of gastrin releasing peptide receptor-positive tumors. Nucl Med Biol 2002; 29:553–560.
94. La Bella R, Garcia-Garayoa E, Bahler M, Blauenstein P, Schibli R, Conrath P, Tourwe D, Schubiger PAA. ^{99m}Tc-postlabeled high affinity bombesin analogue as a potential tumor imaging agent. Bioconjug Chem 2002; 13:599–604.
95. Rogers BE, Bigott HM, McCarthy DW, Della Manna D, Kim J, Sharp TL, Welch MJ. MicroPET imaging of a gastrin-releasing peptide receptor-positive tumor in a mouse model of human prostate cancer using a ^{64}Cu-labeled bombesin analog. Bioconjug Chem 2003; 14:756–763.
96. Hoffman TJ, Gali H, Smith CJ, Sieckman GL, Hayes DL, Owen NK, Volkert WA. Novel series of ^{111}In-labeled bombesin analogs as potential radiopharmaceuticals for specific targeting of gastrin-releasing peptide receptors expressed on human prostate cancer cells. J Nucl Med 2003; 44:823–831.
97. Smith CJ, Gali H, Sieckman GL, Higginbotham C, Volkert WA, Hoffman TJ. Radiochemical investigations of ^{99m}Tc-N$_3$S-X-BBN[7–14]NH$_2$: an *in vitro/in vivo* structure–activity relationship study where $X = 0$-, 3-, 5-, 8-, and 11-carbon tethering moieties. Bioconjug Chem 2003; 14:93–102.
98. Smith CJ, Volkert WA, Hoffman TJ. Gastrin releasing peptide (GRP) receptor targeted radiopharmaceuticals: a concise update. Nucl Med Biol 2003; 30:861–868.
99. Smith CJ, Sieckman GL, Owen NK, Hayes DL, Mazuru DG, Kannan R, Volkert WA, Hoffman TJ. Radiochemical investigations of gastrin-releasing

peptide receptor-specific [$^{(99m)}$Tc(X)(CO)$_3$-Dpr-Ser-Ser-Ser-Gln-Trp-Ala-Val-Gly-His-Leu-Met-(NH2)] in PC-3, tumor-bearing, rodent models: syntheses, radiolabeling, and *in vitro/in vivo* studies where Dpr = 2,3-diaminopropionic acid and X = H$_2$O or P(CH$_2$OH)$_3$. Cancer Res 2003; 63:4082–4088.

100. Scopinaro F, De Vincentis G, Varvarigou AD, Laurenti C, Iori F, Remediani S, Chiarini S, Stella S. ^{99m}Tc-bombesin detects prostate cancer and invasion of pelvic lymph nodes. Eur J Nucl Med Mol Imaging 2003; 30:1378–1382.

101. De Vincentis G, Remediani S, Varvarigou AD, Di Santo G, Iori F, Laurenti C, Scopinaro F. Role of 99mTc-bombesin scan in diagnosis and staging of prostate cancer. Cancer Biother Radiopharm 2004; 19:81–84.

102. Chavatte K, Mertens J, Van Den Winkel P. Method for effective ^{201}Tl(III) labelling of diethylenetriamine pentaacetic acid (DTPA)-functionalized peptides: radiosynthesis of ^{201}Tl(III)DTPA-neurotensin(8-13). J Labelled Cpd Radiopharm 2000; 43:1227–1234.

103. Garcia-Garayoa E, Allemann-Tannahill L, Blauenstein P, Willmann M, Carrel-Remy N, Tourwe D, Iterbeke K, Conrath P, Schubiger PA. *In vitro* and *in vivo* evaluation of new radiolabeled neurotensin(8-13) analogues with high affinity for NT1 receptors. Nucl Med Biol 2001; 28:75–84.

104. de Visser M, Janssen PJ, Srinivasan A, Reubi JC, Waser B, Erion JL, Schmidt MA, Krenning EP, de Jong M. Stabilised ^{111}In-labelled DTPA- and DOTA-conjugated neurotensin analogues for imaging and therapy of exocrine pancreatic cancer. Eur J Nucl Med Mol Imaging 2003; 30:1134–1139.

105. Bergmann R, Scheunemann M, Heichert C, Mading P, Wittrisch H, Kretzschmar M, Rodig H, Tourwe D, Iterbeke K, Chavatte K, Zips D, Reubi JC, Johannsen B. Biodistribution and catabolism of $^{(18)}$F-labeled neurotensin(8-13) analogs. Nucl Med Biol 2002; 29:61–72.

106. Buchegger F, Bonvin F, Kosinski M, Schaffland AO, Prior J, Reubi JC, Blauenstein P, Tourwe D, Garcia-Garayoa E, Bischof Delaloye A. Radiolabeled neurotensin analog, ^{99m}Tc-NT-XI, evaluated in ductal pancreatic adenocarcinoma patients. J Nucl Med 2003; 44:1649–1654.

107. Kahn D, Williams RD, Seldin DW, Libertino JA, Hirschhorn M, Dreicer R, Weiner GJ, Bushnell D, Gulfo J. Radioimmunoscintigraphy with ^{111}indium labeled CYT-356 for the detection of occult prostate cancer recurrence. J Urol 1994; 152:1490–1495.

108. Petronis JD, Regan F, Lin K. Indium-111 capromab pendetide (ProstaScint) imaging to detect recurrent and metastatic prostate cancer. Clin Nucl Med 1998; 23:672–677.

109. Liu H, Moy P, Kim S, Xia Y, Rajasekaran A, Navarro V, Knudsen B, Bander NH. Monoclonal antibodies to the extracellular domain of prostate-specific membrane antigen also react with tumor vascular endothelium. Cancer Res 1997; 57:3629–3634.

110. Holmes EH. PSMA specific antibodies and their diagnostic and therapeutic use. Expert Opin Investig Drugs 2001; 10:511–519.

111. Smith-Jones PM, Vallabhajosula S, Navarro V, Bastidas D, Goldsmith SJ, Bander NH. Radiolabeled monoclonal antibodies specific to the extracellular domain of prostate-specific membrane antigen: preclinical studies in nude mice bearing LNCaP human prostate tumor. J Nucl Med 2003; 44:610–617.

112. Erb DA, Nabi HA. Clinical and technical considerations for imaging colorectal cancers with technetium-99m-labeled antiCEA Fab' fragment. J Nucl Med Technol 2000; 28:12–18.

113. Watanabe N, Oriuchi N, Endo K, Inoue T, Kuroki M, Matsuoka Y, Tanada S, Murata H, Kim EE, Sasaki Y. CaNa2EDTA for improvement of radioimmunodetection and radioimmunotherapy with ^{111}In and ^{90}Y-DTPA-anti-CEA MAbs in nude mice bearing human colorectal cancer. J Nucl Med 2000; 41:337–344.

114. Willkomm P, Bender H, Bangard M, Decker P, Grunwald F, Biersack HJ. FDG PET and immunoscintigraphy with ^{99m}Tc-labeled antibody fragments for detection of the recurrence of colorectal carcinoma. J Nucl Med 2000; 41:1657–1663.

115. Wu AM, Yazaki PJ, Tsai S, Nguyen K, Anderson AL, McCarthy DW, Welch MJ, Shively JE, Williams LE, Raubitschek AA, Wong JYC, Toyokuni T, Phelps ME, Gambhir SS. High-resolution microPET imaging of carcinoembryonic antigen-positive xenografts by using a copper-64-labeled engineered antibody fragment. Proc Natl Acad Sci USA 2000; 97:8495–8500.

116. Sundaresan G, Yazaki PJ, Shively JE, Finn RD, Larson SM, Raubitschek AA, Williams LE, Chatziioannou AF, Gambhir SS, Wu AM. [124]I-labeled engineered anti-CEA minibodies and diabodies allow high-contrast, antigen-specific small-animal PET imaging of xenografts in athymic mice. J Nucl Med 2003; 44:1962–1969.

117. Raderer M, Becherer A, Kurtaran A, Angelberger P, Li S, Leimer M, Weinlaender G, Kornek G, Kletter K, Scheithauer W, Virgolini I. Comparison of iodine-123-vasoactive intestinal peptide receptor scintigraphy and indium-111-CYT-103 immunoscintigraphy. J Nucl Med 1996; 37:1480–1487.

118. Pinkas L, Robins PD, Forstrom LA, Mahoney DW, Mullan BP. Clinical experience with radiolabelled monoclonal antibodies in the detection of colorectal and ovarian carcinoma recurrence and review of the literature. Nucl Med Commun 1999; 20:689–696.

119. Meredith RF, Partridge EE, Alvarez RD, Khazaeli MB, Plott G, Russell CD, Wheeler RH, Liu T, Grizzle WE, Schlom J, LoBuglio AF. Intraperitoneal radioimmunotherapy of ovarian cancer with lutetium-177-CC49. J Nucl Med 1996; 37:1491–1496.

120. Tempero M, Leichner P, Baranowska-Kortylewicz J, Harrison K, Augustine S, Schlom J, Anderson J, Wisecarver J, Colcher D. High-dose therapy with [90]yttrium-labeled monoclonal antibody CC49: a phase I trial. Clin Cancer Res 2000; 6:3095–3102.

121. Kashmiri SVS, Shu L, Padlan EA, Milenic DE, Schlom J, Horan Hand P. Generation, characterization, and *in vivo* studies of humanized anticarcinoma antibody CC49. Hybridoma 1995; 14:461–473.

122. Slavin-Chiorini DC, Kashmiri SVS, Lee HS, Milenic DE, Poole DJ, Bernon E, Schlom J, Horan Hand P. A CDR-grafted (humanized) domain-deleted antitumor antibody. Cancer Biother Radiopharm 1997; 12:305–316.

123. Piwnica-Worms D, Chiu ML, Budding M, Kronauge JF, Kramer RA, Croop JM. Functional imaging of multidrug-resistant P-glycoprotein with an organotechnetium complex. Cancer Res 1993; 53:977–984.

124. Piwnica-Worms D, Rao VV, Kronauge JF, Croop JM. Characterization of multidrug resistance P-glycoprotein transport function with an organotechnetium cation. Biochemistry 1995; 34:12210–12220.

125. Cordobes MD, Starzec A, Delmon-Moingeon L, Blanchot C, Kouyoumdjian JC, Prevost G, Caglar M, Moretti JL. Technetium-99m-sestamibi uptake by human

benign and malignant breast tumor cells: correlation with *mdr* gene expression. J Nucl Med 1996; 37:286–289.

126. Chen WS, Luker KE, Dahlheimer JL, Pica CM, Luker GD, Piwnica-Worms D. Effects of MDR1 and MDR3 P-glycoproteins, MRP1, and BCRP/MXR/ABCP on the transport of $^{(99m)}$Tc-tetrofosmin. Biochem Pharmacol 2000; 60:413–426.

127. Zhou J, Higashi K, Ueda Y, Kodama Y, Guo D, Jisaki F, Sakurai A, Takegami T, Katsuda S, Yamamoto I. Expression of multidrug resistance protein and messenger RNA correlate with $^{(99m)}$Tc-MIBI imaging in patients with lung cancer. J Nucl Med 2001; 42:1476–1483.

128. Kostakoglu L, Kiratli P, Ruacan S, Hayran M, Emri S, Ergun EL, Bekdik CF. Association of tumor washout rates and accumulation of technetium-99m-MIBI with expression of P-glycoprotein in lung cancer. J Nucl Med 1998; 39:228–234.

129. Ciarmiello A, Del Vecchio S, Silvestro P, Potena MI, Carriero MV, Thomas R, Botti G, D'Aiuto G, Salvatore M. Tumor clearance of technetium 99m-sestamibi as a predictor of response to neoadjuvant chemotherapy for locally advanced breast cancer. J Clin Oncol 1998; 16:1677–1683.

130. Fukumoto M, Yoshida D, Hayase N, Kurohara A, Akagi N, Yoshida S. Scintigraphic prediction of resistance to radiation and chemotherapy in patients with lung carcinoma: technetium 99m-tetrofosmin and thallium-201 dual single photon emission computed tomography study. Cancer 1999; 86:1470–1479.

131. Nagamachi S, Jinnouchi S, Ohnishi T, Nakahara H, Flores LN, Tamura S, Yokogami K, Kawano H, Wakisaka S. The usefulness of Tc-99m MIBI for evaluating brain tumors: comparative study with Tl-201 and relation with P-glycoprotein. Clin Nucl Med 1999; 24:765–772.

132. Gottesman MM, Fojo T, Bates SE. Multidrug resistance in cancer: role of ATP-dependent transporters. Nat Rev Cancer 2002; 2:48–58.

133. Chen CC, Meadows B, Regis J, Kalafsky G, Fojo T, Carrasquillo JA, Bates SE. Detection of *in vivo* P-glycoprotein inhibition by PSC 833 using Tc-99m sestamibi. Clin Cancer Res 1997; 3:545–552.

134. Luker GD, Fracasso PM, Dobkin J, Piwnica-Worms D. Modulation of the multidrug resistance P-glycoprotein: detection with technetium-99m-sestamibi *in vivo*. J Nucl Med 1997; 38:369–372.

135. Peck RA, Hewett J, Harding MW, Wang YM, Chaturvedi PR, Bhatnagar A, Ziessman H, Atkins F, Hawkins MJ. Phase I and pharmacokinetic study of the novel MDR1 and MRP1 inhibitor biricodar administered alone and in combination with doxorubicin. J Clin Oncol 2001; 19:3130–3141.

136. Sharma V, Beatty A, Wey SP, Dahlheimer J, Pica CM, Crankshaw CL, Bass L, Green MA, Welch MJ, Piwnica-Worms D. Novel gallium(III) complexes transported by MDR1 P-glycoprotein: potential PET imaging agents for probing P-glycoprotein-mediated transport activity *in vivo*. Chem Biol 2000; 7:335–343.

137. Hendrikse NH, de Vries EG, Eriks-Fluks L, van der Graaf WT, Hospers GA, Willemsen AT, Vaalburg W, Franssen EJ. A new *in vivo* method to study P-glycoprotein transport in tumors and the blood-brain barrier. Cancer Res 1999; 59:2411–2416.

138. Levchenko A, Mehta BM, Lee JB, Humm JL, Augensen F, Squire O, Kothari PJ, Finn RD, Leonard EF, Larson SM. Evaluation of ^{11}C-colchicine for PET imaging of multiple drug resistance. J Nucl Med 2000; 41:493–501.

139. Packard AB, Kronauge JF, Barbarics E, Kiani S, Treves ST. Synthesis and biodistribution of a lipophilic 64Cu-labeled monocationic copper(II) complex. Nucl Med Biol 2002; 29:289–294.

140. Lewis JS, Dearling JL, Sosabowski JK, Zweit J, Carnochan P, Kelland LR, Coley HM, Blower PJ. Copper *bis*(diphosphine) complexes: radiopharmaceuticals for the detection of multi-drug resistance in tumours by PET. Eur J Nucl Med 2000; 27:638–646.

141. Spergel DJ, Kruth U, Shimshek DR, Sprengel R, Seeburg PH. Using reporter genes to label selected neuronal populations in transgenic mice for gene promoter, anatomical, and physiological studies. Prog Neurobiol 2001; 63:673–686.

142. Hemminki A, Zinn KR, Liu B, Chaudhuri TR, Desmond RA, Rogers BE, Barnes MN, Alvarez RD, Curiel DT. *In vivo* molecular chemotherapy and noninvasive imaging with an infectivity-enhanced adenovirus. J Natl Cancer Inst 2002; 94:741–749.

143. Green LA, Yap CS, Nguyen K, Barrio JR, Namavari M, Satyamurthy N, Phelps ME, Sandgren EP, Herschman HR, Gambhir SS. Indirect monitoring of endogenous gene expression by positron emission tomography (PET) imaging of reporter gene expression in transgenic mice. Mol Imag Biol 2002; 4:71–81.

144. Luker GD, Sharma V, Pica CM, Dahlheimer JL, Li W, Ochesky J, Ryan CE, Piwnica-Worms H, Piwnica-Worms D. Noninvasive imaging of protein–protein interactions in living animals. Proc Natl Acad Sci USA 2002; 99:6961–6966.

145. Iyer M, Barrio JR, Namavari M, Bauer E, Satyamurthy N, Nguyen K, Toyokuni T, Phelps ME, Herschman HR, Gambhir SS. 8-[^{18}F]fluoropenciclovir: an improved reporter probe for imaging HSV1-tk reporter gene expression *in vivo* using PET. J Nucl Med 2001; 42:96–105.

146. Tjuvajev JG, Stockhammer G, Desai R, Uehara H, Watanabe K, Gansbacher B, Blasberg RG. Imaging the expression of transfected genes *in vivo*. Cancer Res 1995; 55:6126–6132.

147. Tjuvajev JG, Finn R, Watanabe K, Joshi R, Oku T, Kennedy J, Beattie B, Koutcher J, Larson S, Blasberg RG. Noninvasive imaging of herpes virus thymidine kinase gene transfer and expression: a potential method for monitoring clinical gene therapy. Cancer Res 1996; 56:4087–4095.

148. Tjuvajev JG, Avril N, Oku T, Sasajima T, Miyagawa T, Joshi R, Safer M, Beattie B, DiResta G, Daghighian F, Augensen F, Koutcher J, Zweit J, Humm J, Larson SM, Finn R, Blasberg R. Imaging herpes virus thymidine kinase gene transfer and expression by positron emission tomography. Cancer Res 1998; 58:4333–4341.

149. Yu Y, Annala AJ, Barrio JR, Toyokuni T, Satyamurthy N, Namavari M, Cherry SR, Phelps ME, Herschman HR, Gambhir SS. Quantification of target gene expression by imaging reporter gene expression in living animals. Nat Med 2000; 6:933–937.

150. Narvaiza I, Barajas M, Penuelas I, Boan JF, Marti JM, Mazzolini G, Font M, Sangro B, Gambhir SS, Barrio JR, Richter JA, Qian C, Prieto J. Sensitivity of PET imaging to detect gene expression using different doses of adenovirus vector coding for herpes simplex virus thymidine kinase (AdCMVtk). Mol Ther 2002; 5:S415.

151. Zinn KR, Chaudhuri TR, Krasnykh VN, Buchsbaum DJ, Belousova N, Grizzle WE, Curiel DT, Rogers BE. Gamma camera dual imaging with a somatostatin receptor and thymidine kinase after gene transfer with a bicistronic adenovirus in mice. Radiology 2002; 223:417–425.

152. Richard JC, Zhou Z, Ponde DE, Dence CS, Factor P, Reynolds PN, Luker GD, Sharma V, Ferkol T, Piwnica-Worms D, Schuster DP. Imaging pulmonary gene expression with positron emission tomography. Am J Respir Crit Care Med 2003; 167:1257–1263.

153. Gambhir SS, Barrio JR, Phelps ME, Iyer M, Namavari M, Satyamurthy N, Wu L, Green LA, Bauer E, MacLaren DC, Nguyen K, Berk AJ, Cherry SR, Herschman HR. Imaging adenoviral-directed reporter gene expression in living animals with positron emission tomography. Proc Natl Acad Sci USA 1999; 96:2333–2338.

154. Liang Q, Gotts J, Satyamurthy N, Barrio J, Phelps ME, Gambhir SS, Herschman H. Noninvasive, repetitive, quantitative measurement of gene expression from a bicistronic message by positron emission tomography, following gene transfer with adenovirus. Mol Ther 2002; 6:73–82.

155. Dadachova E, Carrasco N. The Na/I symporter (NIS): imaging and therapeutic applications. Semin Nucl Med 2004; 34:23–31.

156. Dai G, Levy O, Carrasco N. Cloning and characterization of the thyroid iodide transporter. Nature 1996; 379:458–460.

157. Cho JY, Shen DH, Yang W, Williams B, Buckwalter TL, La Perle KM, Hinkle G, Pozderac R, Kloos R, Nagaraja HN, Barth RF, Jhiang SM. *In vivo* imaging and radioiodine therapy following sodium iodide symporter gene transfer in animal model of intracerebral gliomas. Gene Ther 2002; 9:1139–1145.

158. Groot-Wassink T, Aboagye EO, Wang Y, Lemoine NR, Reader AJ, Vassaux G. Quantitative imaging of Na/I symporter transgene expression using positron emission tomography in the living animal. Mol Ther 2004; 9:436–442.

159. Shin JH, Chung JK, Kang JH, Lee YJ, Kim KI, Kim CW, Jeong JM, Lee DS, Lee MC. Feasibility of sodium/iodide symporter gene as a new imaging reporter gene: comparison with HSV1-tk. Eur J Nucl Med Mol Imaging 2004; 31:425–432.

160. Shen DH, Marsee DK, Schaap J, Yang W, Cho JY, Hinkle G, Nagaraja HN, Kloos RT, Barth RF, Jhiang SM. Effects of dose, intervention time, and radionuclide on sodium iodide symporter (NIS)-targeted radionuclide therapy. Gene Ther 2004; 11:161–169.

161. Barton KN, Tyson D, Stricker H, Lew YS, Heisey G, Koul S, de la Zerda A, Yin FF, Yan H, Nagaraja TN, Randall KA, Jin GK, Fenstermacher JD, Jhiang S, Ho Kim J, Freytag SO, Brown SL. GENIS: gene expression of sodium iodide symporter for noninvasive imaging of gene therapy vectors and quantification of gene expression *in vivo*. Mol Ther 2003; 8:508–518.

162. Carlin S, Akabani G, Zalutsky MR. *In vitro* cytotoxicity of [211]At-astatide and ^{131}I-iodide to glioma tumor cells expressing the sodium/iodide symporter. J Nucl Med 2003; 44:1827–1838.

163. Zuckier LS, Dohan O, Li Y, Chang CJ, Carrasco N, Dadachova E. Kinetics of perrhenate uptake and comparative biodistribution of perrhenate, pertechnetate, and iodide by NaI symporter-expressing tissues *in vivo*. J Nucl Med 2004; 45:500–507.

164. Vanetti M, Kouba M, Wang X, Vogt G, Hollt V. Cloning and expression of a novel mouse somatostatin receptor (SSTR2B). FEBS Lett 1992; 311:290–294.

165. Bell G, Reisine T. Molecular biology of somatostatin receptors. Trends Neurosci 1993; 16:34–38.

166. Rogers BE, Zinn KR, Buchsbaum DJ. Gene transfer strategies for improving radio-labeled peptide imaging and therapy. Q J Nucl Med 2000; 44:208–223.

167. Zinn KR, Buchsbaum DJ, Chaudhuri T, Mountz JM, Kirkman RL, Rogers BE. Non-invasive monitoring of gene transfer using a reporter receptor imaged with a high affinity peptide radiolabeled with ^{99m}Tc or ^{188}Re. J Nucl Med 2000; 41:887–895.

168. Bakker WH, Krenning EP, Reubi JC, Breeman WAP, Setyono-Han B, de Jong J, Kooij PPM, Bruns C, Van Hagen PM, Marbach P, Visser TJ, Pless J, Lamberts SWJ. *In vivo* application of [^{111}In-DTPA-D-Phe^{1}]-octreotide for detection of somatostatin receptor-positive tumors in rats. Life Sci 1991; 49:1593–1601.

169. Bakker WH, Krenning EP, Breeman WA, Kooij PPM, Reubi JC, Lamberts SW. *In vivo* use of a radioiodinated somatostatin analogue: dynamics, metabolism, and binding to somatostatin receptor-positive tumors in man. J Nucl Med 1991; 32:1184–1189.

170. MacLaren DC, Gambhir SS, Satyamurthy N, Barrio JR, Sharfstein S, Toyokuni T, Wu L, Berk AJ, Cherry SR, Phelps ME, Herschman HR. Repetitive, non-invasive imaging of the dopamine D_2 receptor as a reporter gene in living animals. Gene Ther 1999; 6:785–791.

171. Auricchio A, Acton PD, Hildinger M, Louboutin JP, Plossl K, O'Connor E, Kung HF, Wilson JM. *In vivo* quantitative noninvasive imaging of gene transfer by single-photon emission computerized tomography. Hum Gene Ther 2003; 10:255–261.

172. Liang Q, Satyamurthy N, Barrio JR, Toyokuni T, Phelps MP, Gambhir SS, Herschman HR. Noninvasive, quantitative imaging in living animals of a mutant dopamine D2 receptor reporter gene in which ligand binding is uncoupled from signal transduction. Gene Ther 2001; 8:1490–1498.

4

Imaging Cellular and Molecular Processes in the Lung Using Bioluminescent Reporter Genes

CHRISTOPHER H. CONTAG

Stanford University School of Medicine,
Stanford, California, USA

I. Overview

A number of imaging modalities have been recently described, which allow spatiotemporal analyses of cellular and molecular changes to be monitored in living animals. These tools have been developed to enable the investigator to follow biological changes over time and in the context of intact organ systems. One of these modalities is based on the use of light emitting enzymes that, as a class, are referred to as luciferases. The light emitted from the enzymatic reactions is referred to as bioluminescence, and *in vivo* bioluminescence imaging (BLI) is based on detecting this light externally. BLI is versatile with reported applications in the fields of oncology, infectious disease, physiology, gene expression, and therapy (1–5). Moreover, this imaging modality is readily accessible to biologists because of its relative low instrumentation costs and ease of use relative to other imaging modalities. The principles and practices of this modality and representative applications for the study of lung biology and pathogenesis are the focus of this chapter.

II. Introduction

Preclinical animal models of human biology and disease are a necessary part of drug development and biological investigation. The accepted norm for the study of these models is to use serial sacrifice of animals at predetermined time points followed by conducting labor intensive assays on cell lysates and tissue homogenates from postmortem samples. The opportunities for observations to be made in real time and to assess dynamic changes and to analyze cascading pathways are lost in these approaches. Moreover, such studies are subject to artifacts due to the inherent variability in each animal, and they have required fairly large groups of animals in order to achieve statistical significance. Animal models vary in their ability to reproduce the human response, therefore achieving reproducibility and reliability are essential for interpreting data from these models. Imaging approaches that are noninvasive and enable the temporal study of lung disease have been developed (6–8) (Chapter 7) and, more recently, methods that provide cellular and molecular information have been reported (1,3,4,9–13). Application of these imaging tools to animal models of lung disease and their continued development are essential for understanding the complexity of lung disease and for effective discovery and development of new therapies.

There has been a significant amount of work devoted to development of animal models of lung disease using conventional cellular and molecular assays as the readout. These models have provided information about mechanisms of pathogenesis in lung disease. Therefore, as imaging technologies are applied to the study of these diseases, it is necessary that the imaging protocols be superimposable on existing animal models, so as to not require significant modifications to the established models and to allow the use of existing assays for validation of the molecular imaging approaches. To gain the greatest amount of information from our animal models, we need to apply multimodality approaches to these models (Chapter 8), where each modality provides different information yielding a dynamic composite of the disease states from early in the disease course to late stage disease.

There are a number of imaging modalities that have been specifically designed to take advantage of the unique characteristics of small laboratory animals such as mice and rats. Because of the small size of these animal subjects, modalities that use radiation with limited tissue penetration fit uniquely into this category. Optical imaging technologies are based on light in the visible and near-infrared (NIR) regions of the spectrum. This light can be significantly affected by the absorbing and scattering properties of mammalian tissues (reviewed in Chapter 11). These approaches are well suited for the study of rodent models of lung disease, where the depth of tissue that the radiation is required to penetrate is minimal. Light passes through tissues in a wavelength-dependent manner, which is largely a function of hemoglobin absorption which is greater for shorter wavelengths of light (<600 nm). Red and NIR light are affected less by tissue absorbtion, and use of these wavelengths allows interrogation of biological processes that are located up to several centimeters deep within living animals (14). Molecular imaging using visible and NIR light is based on the development of chemical and biological sensors with optically detectable signatures. Macroscopic approaches for detecting these signatures externally using whole body imaging have been developed and applied to rodent models.

A unique feature of optical imaging modalities, relative to other imaging methods, is that optical detectors are generally sensitive to a wide range of energies in key regions of the spectrum. As each wavelength within this range can be used with a specific reagent, it is possible to multiplex optically based systems. Twelve color flow cytometry and multiplexed fluorescent-based cell imaging are examples of multiplexed optical assays. Unfortunately, such approaches are limited in macroscopic whole body optical imaging as the different wavelengths of light are differentially affected by mammalian tissue. Light absorption due to hemoglobin and water effectively remove the blue and infrared regions of the spectrum, respectively, resulting in a window between 600 and 1300 nm where absorption of optical signals is minimal and light scattering predominates the tissue influence on the signal. Classes of reagents that can be detected in this region of the spectrum will have utility in the development of multiplexed *in vivo* assays.

BLI is a cornerstone technology in the molecular imaging field. This method is based on the idea that biological light sources that do not require excitation sources can be built into animal models of human physiology and disease as indicator lights that externally report the inner workings of mammalian biology (4). The light sources used in this modality are luciferases from a variety of different marine and terrestrial organisms. Whole body images of laboratory rodents expressing these optical tags have been used to reveal, in non-invasive assays, the relative number of labeled cells at specific sites or relative levels of gene expression (1,3,4). The high sensitivity of detection has permitted the study of small numbers of immune cells and has enabled the detection of foci arising from single engrafting stem cells (15). As such, BLI has provided an understanding of the systemic process of hematopoiesis from the early engraftment stage to full hematopoietic reconstitution (15). Multifunctional reporter genes that encode both bioluminescent and fluorescent proteins can be used to link *in vivo* cell trafficking studies to *ex vivo* assays, thus extending the versatility of this modality (15). Imaging luciferases as reporter genes in living animals provides critical spatiotemporal information about biological changes in the context of intact biological systems.

BLI is an accessible tool for biomedical investigation and provides a rapid readout. Therefore, use of this method in studies of the lung will accelerate analyses of experimental therapeutic interventions, and provide new information about lung biology, which had not been previously available in mammalian systems. Imaging leads to this information being obtained in less time using fewer animals than more conventional molecular assays. It is anticipated that animal models will become better predictors of human biology and disease through the use of imaging tools that provide real time access to cellular and molecular changes in the proper tissue and organ context.

III. Luciferase and Related Proteins

Luciferases are a class of oxygenases that produce light using chemical substrates. In contrast to fluorescent markers that require excitation light for emission, luciferases are biochemical sources of light. Luciferases have been found in a wide range of organisms from several different genera, however, only three basic biochemistries have been characterized to date (16). Luciferases that utilize each of these different chemistries have been cloned and several enzymes are used as the basis of laboratory assays including BLI. The luciferases from firefly (Coleoptera), jellyfish and sea pansies (Cnidaria), and bacteria (*Vibrio* spp. and *Photorhabdus luminescens*) are the most well characterized and all have been used *in vivo* as reporter genes. Luciferases require some form of energy, oxygen, and a specific substrate (commonly known as luciferin) for light production, and may also require co-factors. Luciferases, as extrinsic optical contrast agents, offer tremendous signal-to-noise ratios (SNR) as mammalian tissues are not generally bioluminescent. In addition, with proper targeting, these markers can be used with good predictability and versatility with the ability to evaluate a variety of different types of biological processes.

A. Coeloptera Luciferases

The luciferase that has been most commonly used in the laboratory is that obtained from the firefly (fLuc) (17). There are several other closely related insect (Coeloptera) luciferases that have more recently become available; these are derived from the click beetle (cbLuc) (18) and railroad worm (19). All of these enzymes are monomeric enzymes related to coenzyme A ligase that use a benzo-thiazole (luciferin) along with adenosine triphosphate (ATP) and oxygen to generate light (20). For use as reporter genes, the coding sequences for the fLuc and cbLuc have been optimized for expression in mammalian cells, and the sequences for the cbLuc have been further modified by removing all potential mammalian transcription factor binding sites; these sequences are commercially available (Promega Corp., Madison, WI). In the presence of luciferin, mammalian cells expressing these enzymes emit light in the visible range with emission peaks in the blue green and red regions of the spectrum. The fLuc enzyme has a broad spectral emission pattern with a significant red component. The light emission that is >600 nm is the signal that enables detection of small numbers of cells from deep within the body. The emission peak of fLuc is at 560 nm at room temperature, but is red shifted to 612 nm when used at 37°C (Zhao and Contag, unpublished data). Measurement of light production by luciferases can be rapid and performed quantitatively such that luciferases are well suited as biochemical reporters. The luciferase enzymes appear to be nontoxic to cells and their relatively short half-lives have permitted development of dynamic assays of biological activities such as gene expression and ATP levels (21–23).

As luciferases are biological reagents, their expression and activity can be manipulated for use as indicators of specific biological events. The long history of using these enzymes as reporters in cell culture has provided a solid foundation for the more recent extension into animal models of human biology and disease. The nontoxic nature of the enzymes and the apparent lack of toxicity of the substrate, luciferin, for cells and animals have been demonstrated in a number of animal models. In addition, the biodistribution of luciferin in rodents appears to be well suited for use as an *in vivo* reporter, with the substrate reaching all tissues in the body including the central nervous system (24–26). The action of luciferases on their substrates, releases light almost continually (as long as the enzyme, substrate, and cofactors are present) such that data acquisition times can be long for the detection of very weak signals from deeper within the tissue. Although useful for making sensitive measurements, this continual signal precludes the use of time resolved methods of detection where fast migrating photons can be separated from those that are multiply scattered and thus delayed from exiting the tissue. Time resolved approaches have been used for fluorescence and scatter-based imaging as the temporal differences can be used to improve resolution, enhance signal-to-noise, and provide some three-dimensional information. Another approach for improved signal resolution in optical imaging is to synchronize the signal using ultrasound, however, the relatively weak nature of bioluminescent signals does not enable such methods, as the integration times for BLI tend to be on the order of seconds to minutes, which is too long for these methods. It is fortunate that there is essentially no autoluminescence from mammalian tissues as this results in very high SNR which is a significant contributing factor to the sensitivity of BLI.

B. Luciferases from Marine Organisms

Bioluminescence is very common in marine environments, and luciferases from two marine organisms have been cloned, characterized, and used as reporter genes. These include the enzymes from the sea pansy (*Renilla reniformis*) (27–29) and the jellyfish (*Aequorea aequorea*) (30–32). As with all characterized luciferases obtained from marine organisms, both of these enzymes use coelenterazine as the substrate. The luciferase from the hydrozoan *Aequorea* (aequorin) requires a calcium ion for light production, and this has led to its use as a calcium sensor in cells and in plants (33). For use as reporter genes in mammalian cells, a codon-optimized version of the *Renilla* enzyme (hrLuc) has been developed and is commercially available. This enzyme is routinely used as a control for gene-expression assays in cell lysates and tissue homogenates, and has more recently been used *in vivo* (30,32,34–37). The advantage of having enzymes with different spectra of light emission and different chemistries is that two or more reporters may be used in the same cell line to monitor the expression of two different genes. This is the basis of the dual-color biochemical assays for cell lysates and has been extended, in a limited way, for use in animals (30,32,34–37). As rLuc does not require cofactors provided by the host cell, this protein may have the additional utility of serving as a sensor outside of the cell if expressed as a membrane bound protein.

C. Bacterial Luciferases

Several bacterial species encode luciferases that use an entirely different biochemistry than the enzymes from eukaryotic organisms. The substrates that they use include a variety of long-chain fatty aldehydes and they produce a blue-green light with a peak of 490 nm in the presence of reduced flavin mononucleotide ($FMNH_2$), as the energy source, and oxygen (38). All bacterial luciferases characterized to date are very closely related to each other and all are heterodimeric enzymes. The two genes that encode the luciferase subunits are found on the *lux* operon along with several other genes, three of which encode the biosynthetic enzymes necessary for the production of the aldehyde substrate (decanal). These five genes are called *luxA–luxE*, with *luxA* and *B* encoding the alpha and beta subunits of the luciferase, and *luxCDE* encoding biosynthetic enzymes for aldehyde production. Cloning of the *lux* operon into nonbioluminescent bacterial species results in glowing strains that do not require exogenous addition of substrate. Despite the blue light produced by bacteria expressing this operon, labeled pathogens can be tracked *in vivo* (Fig. 4.1), and this approach was the first demonstration of BLI (39).

As the bacterial enzymes are all very similar, the features of the *lux* operon from the soil organism *P. luminescens* (plLux) can be inferred from the extensive studies of the *Lux* operon from *Vibrio* spp. The plLux enzyme is ideally suited for use in mammalian animal models as the enzyme retains significant activity

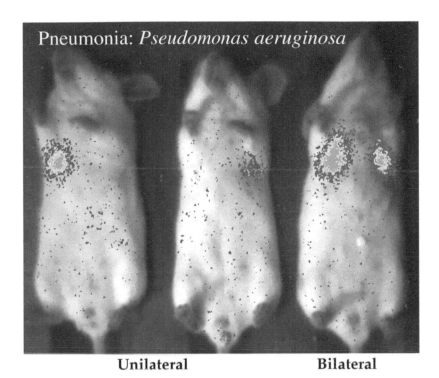

Pneumonia: *Pseudomonas aeruginosa*

Unilateral　　　　　　　**Bilateral**

Figure 4.1 (See color insert) Imaging pseudomonas infections of the lung. The bacterial *Lux* operon was integrated into the genome of *Pseudomonas*, and used to monitor lung infections following intranasal delivery. The images show evidence of unilateral and bilateral infections.

at 37°C, and has been the bacterial luciferase most commonly used in rodent models. Lux from *Vibrio* spp. has a temperature optimum which is lower than plLux. The *luxCDABE* operon from *P. luminescens* has been successfully expressed in Gram-negative bacteria (such as *Escherichia coli* and *Salmonella* spp). For expression in Gram-positive bacteria, the operon had to be redesigned (40). There are reports of further modifications to the five *lux* genes for expression in eukaryotic cells, with evidence of successful expression in the yeast *Saccharomyces cerevisiae* (41). A significant advantage of using the bacterial luciferases in mammalian cells is the ability to express the biosynthetic enzymes for substrate synthesis such that the engineered cells generate light without exogenous addition of a substrate. For this reaction, however, the enzymes must have sufficient energy in the form of $FMNH_2$, and the toxicity of the substrate has yet to be determined.

In relation to lung models of infection, it will be essential to study both the pathogen response and the host response to infection. This was demonstrated very well in a study by Sadikot et al. (42) where the p47(phox) gene product was found to regulate the NFκB response to pseudomonas infection. Here, the infection and host responses were assessed separately, using one group of animals for infection and another for host response. These studies revealed that the reduced nicotinamide adenine dinucleotide phosphate oxidase-dependent respiratory burst contributes to the defense mechanisms by modulating signaling through the NFκB pathway in pseudomonas infections. Developing the tools necessary for monitoring infection and host responses in the same animal would comprise a significant advance for these types of studies.

D. Other Luciferases

Luciferases from other marine organisms have been cloned. This includes the luciferase from the dinoflagellate *Gonyaulax*; the substrate for this reaction is a linear tetrapyrrole related to chlorophyll. The secreted luciferase of the crustacea *Vargula hilgendorfii* (vLuc), which uses an imidazopyrazine substrate similar to coelenterazine has also been cloned. The vLuc has been functionally expressed in mammalian cells and early stage embryos. As new luciferases are cloned and characterized, we may have additional tools for *in vivo* imaging; however, full characterization of these enzyme reactions and the interaction of the substrates and enzymes with mammalian cell biology is key to their successful use *in vivo*.

IV. Luciferins and Biodistribution *In Vivo*

As very few of the biosynthetic enzymes for the various substrates have been cloned and characterized, exogenous addition of these compounds is still required for their use *in vivo*. Therefore, efficient substrate delivery to the cells expressing luciferase, and knowledge of the biodistribution and clearance kinetics of these compounds are essential. The bacterial *lux* operon, obviously, has the advantage of the user being able to co-transfer the genes encoding the biosynthetic enzymes for substrate synthesis, and it is possible that this reaction can be effectively translated to mammalian cells. Even so, the effects of expressing five, or more, bacterial proteins in mammalian cells may significantly perturb the cellular physiology and present new toxicity and immunogenicity issues. Thus, even with the development of new reporter constructs, we will likely continue to use injectable luciferins for sometime. Studies of the insect luciferase substrate, luciferin, have revealed biodistribution properties and clearance kinetics that make it well suited for use in animal models. This luciferin is capable of cellular uptake through membranes (24), as well as crossing the blood–brain (43) and placental barriers (26). This compound is distributed rapidly to all organs and tissues, to the extent that this has been studied, and it appears not to have toxic effects on cells, tissues, or organs. The immunogenicity of the enzyme may be an issue but it has not been reported to date. There have been few or no reported adverse reactions to luciferin at concentrations that saturate the expressed enzyme in tissues of most rodent models.

The marine luciferases utilize coelenterazine as the chemical substrate, and the fact that there is no obvious cross-over between the two reactions these may offer the opportunity for multiplexing *in vivo* assays by using two, and perhaps more, distinct reporters (34). The *in vivo* biodistribution and kinetics of coelenterazine are not well studied, but its biodistribution is significantly different than that of luciferin (44). Coelenterazine is known to bind to serum proteins and autocatalysis of coelenterazine, due to albumin, has been documented (44). Binding of the substrate to serum proteins may prevent active substrate from reaching the luciferase expressing cells and the background noise due to catalysis of the substrate in the absence of enzyme may further reduce the sensitivity of assays based on this reaction (44). A number of coelenterazine analogs have been reported and studied, and although these compounds have different properties in both culture and *in vivo* than native coelenterazine, none of them fully overcome the limitations of this reaction *in vivo* (44).

There are many reasons, in addition to multiplexed assays, for continuing to advance the *in vivo* use of ceolenterazine-utilizing enzymes. These luciferases use energy that is present in the substrate, and the reactions do not require ATP or other sources of energy for light production (45). This means that extracellular and surface-bound luciferases could be developed for another class of *in vivo* reporters. The fact that coelenterazine is a high-energy molecule means that it is unstable, which is likely the reason that it is readily catalyzed by serum proteins. The short half-life of the substrate and its rapid clearance from the blood stream leads to very short windows of opportunity for imaging rLuc activity and it also means that the substrate is rarely in excess of the enzyme reporters. For accurate quantitation of expression levels, it is necessary that the substrate be in excess. Otherwise, there is uncertainty as to whether the signal intensity is due to substrate concentration or enzyme concentration. However, if accurate pharmacokinetic data are factored into the analyses, the substrate need not be in excess. The inability to easily use coelenterazine-utilizing enzymes in quantitative assays is a severe constraint on this reporter for *in vivo* measurements.

V. Instrumentation Used in BLI

The light emission from luciferase reactions is fairly weak and when signals originate from deep within the tissues of a rodent, the amount of light available at the surface of the animal is limited. Therefore, development of sensitive photon detectors [cooled, or intensified, charge-coupled device (CCD) cameras] (46) was necessary for advancing BLI as an imaging modality. The imaging systems consist of a dark-box imaging chamber connected to a sensitive CCD camera. There are several architectures of cameras used in low light imaging systems, and each has unique properties; the features of cooled, back-thinned CCD cameras are well suited for use in BLI (46,47). These cameras are digital and are run by a computer for both image acquisition and image analysis.

There are a large number of image analyses programs that have been used of this purpose and the key element in these programs is general user friendliness. To localize signals in the animal's body, typically two images are taken, first a grayscale reference image, then an image of the bioluminescent signal, obtained in complete darkness. The signal intensity is generally represented as a pseudocolor image and is superimposed on the reference image to facilitate localization. Depending on the camera used in the imaging system, acquisition time for the bioluminescent image is usually 1 min, but can range from several seconds to 10 min.

VI. Multifunctional Reporter Genes

Multimodality imaging by using several instruments and/or several different reporters can strengthen a study by providing both structural and multiple functional parameters. As reporter genes can be linked through genetic means, reagents can be created that are detectable by two or more modalities yielding both greater versatility than single reporters and opportunity to validate one measurement with another. The fusion of two optical reporter genes, luciferase and green fluorescent protein, was first reported in a study of gene expression in fruit flies (48). Since this report, several "flavors" of multifunctional reporters have been described. The fluorescent component of these fusions provide a link between *in vivo* measurements using luciferase and *ex vivo* assays such as flow cytometry and fluorescence microscopy (49–51). Gene fusions comprised of three reporter genes with signatures for fluorescence, bioluminescence, and nuclear imaging techniques have been reported (36,52).

There is a tremendous variety of single and multifunctional reporter genes, yet efficient transfer of these genes to key cell types in a given biological process can present a significant hurdle. Many of the studies describing these reporter genes use tumor cell lines as the target cell and evaluate these cells at subcutaneous or other superficial sites. As we move away from the artificial animal models of subcutaneous xenografts and begin to more closely model human disease by trying to study rare and difficult-to-transduce cells, we will need tools for labeling these cells. Toward this end, we have generated a transgenic donor mouse as a source of labeled cells, where multiple cell types express a dual function reporter gene (15). This animal has served as "universal donor" for studies in transplantation biology and immune cell trafficking studies. Hematopoietic stem cells from this transgenic donor have been transplanted and analyzed in recipient mice, and foci arising from single labeled hematopoietic stem cells were apparent (15). As the reporter genes are integrated into the genome of these cells, the signals are not lost over time, and as the labeled cells can be followed throughout the life of the animal, we were able to study the relative contribution of the labeled population to hematopoietic reconstitution. Transgenic animals as a source of labeled cells overcome a number of the limitations and these animals will be a useful tool for developing new therapeutic strategies and revealing the behavior of rare and difficult to transduce cells. We have begun to combine this reporter animal with knockout and transgenic animals such that we can use the transgenic reporter to study the effects of the second genetic element on cell migration and disease.

VII.   Validation of *In Vivo* Data Using *Ex Vivo* Assays

For imaging, animals are typically anesthetized (any number of anesthetics have been used) and given an intraperitoneal injection of the substrate (luciferin) at 150 mg/kg body weight. Imaging is then performed as previously described (3,49). At the end of the study, tissues can be harvested, using the images as a guide, and processed for protein or RNA extraction, or histology. Using imaging as a guide to select the ideal times and tissues for analyses can provide insight that are not available in the absence of this data. There are a number of examples where imaging has led investigators to a new tissue site or a poorly studied time point, and new information was generated (53). Luciferase activity can be determined by luminometry using conditions recommended by the vendor (Promega Corp. Madison, WI), and this serves as an excellent validation of the *in vivo* measurements. The biochemical measurements of luficerase activity in cell lysates and tissue homogenates are a simple assay that has been under-valued and under-utilized in published reports that use BLI. Relative light units per microgram of tissue protein can be recorded for each tissue sample and related to the intensity measurements made *in vivo* (26). Other assays that have been used to validate *in vivo* measurements include western blots, cytometry, and reverse transcriptase polymerase chain reaction (26). Each of these methods provides useful information that support the *in vivo* results and should be incorporated into study designs.

VIII.   Applications of BLI in the Lung

A.   Monitoring Infection of the Lung

There is a need for the development of new classes of antimicrobials, and imaging of labeled pathogens in rodents offers new opportunities for studying host–pathogen interactions. The use of engineered bioluminescent pathogens has opened the opportunity to not only localize the site of infection in an animal, but also noninvasively determine the pathogen burden without sacrificing the animal. This approach has been applied to viral, bacterial, and fungal infections (53,54), and it is important to emphasize that the models themselves are essentially unchanged as the imaging step is superimposed on the established model. Combining the standard model and imaging can provide new information, often with the use of fewer animals. Although the bacterial *lux* operon is an obvious choice of bioluminescent reporters for these pathogens, both the fLuc and the rLuc have been used to tag bacterial strains for *in vivo* bioluminescent imaging of infection. In a lung infection model, we used *Pseudomonas aerugi-nosa* labeled through the expression of the *lux* operon that had been integrated into the bacterial genome (Fig. 4.1). In this model, the bacterial load could be assessed and the disease progression monitored. This served as a foundation for a subsequent host–pathogen interaction study (42).

B. Lung Metastasis

The most common application of BLI in cancer research is the use of stably trans-fected, luciferase expressing tumor cell lines where the luciferase signal is used as a measure of tumor burden and metastasis (55). The first example of this approach used the human cervical carcinoma cell line, HeLa (56,57). HeLa cells labeled with luciferase were injected into severe combined immunodeficient mice via the tail vein, and cells were immediately apparent in the lung. This model has since been used to examine lung colonization by several tumor cell lines. These, and now many other studies, have demonstrated that luciferase expression correlates with tumor burden through the use of many *ex vivo* assays and through the use of other imaging modalities (25,56,57).

Even early studies demonstrated detection of tumor cells from internal organs, and subsequent studies have indicated that the sensitivity of BLI is as good as, or greater than, that of positron emission tomography (PET) for reporter gene detection (58). Antemortem detection of tumor cells at these deep tissue sites would previously have been detectable only by very indirect and inaccurate measurements such as weight change or development of overt signs of illness. Direct tumor examination would only have been possible following the death or sacrifice of the animal. The extraordinary sensitivity of BLI has also been demonstrated by injecting known numbers of cells, and in these studies as few as 100 cells given intraperitoneally could be visualized using a labeled prostate cancer cell line (PC3-M) (55). Studies of murine leukemia and lymphoma cell lines (A20 or BCL_1) have revealed that 1000 cells could be detected after subcu-taneous implantation, and 10,000 cells seen within the lungs following intrave-nous delivery (52). Several comparative studies have shown that BLI signals correlate well with tumor volumes as measured by magnetic resonance imaging (MRI) (25), and as that BLI detection is sensitive as PET imaging in gene transfer studies (24). The comparative ease of use and significantly lower costs of BLI, relative to these other modalities, has popularized this modality for preclinical studies. The impressive dynamic range of BLI also means that it is very unlikely that an upper limit of detection will be reached before the animal succumbs to the disease.

C. Gene Transfer to the Lung for Therapy

Rodent models are used in the development of pulmonary DNA-based therapies, however, determining the levels of gene expression in the lungs can be challenging, and real time noninvasive data are necessary for rapid development of these methods. By the way of demonstration, we used BLI to evaluate viral-mediated gene transfer to the lung (Fig. 4.2) and could use this method to repeatedly assess the levels of reporter gene expression. We used a recombinant adeno-associated viral vector, delivered into the lungs of mice, and evaluated two serotypes of AAV both containing a fusion gene encoding luciferase and yellow fluorescent protein (YFP). These viruses were introduced via tracheal intubation. After administration of luciferin, the light emitted from the luciferase reporter within animals was detected, quantified, and localized using an ultracooled CCD camera (IVIS, Xenogen Corp. Alameda, CA), at 5-day intervals over a 95-day time course. Lung tissue was collected periodically and analyzed for luciferase content and viral DNA, although confocal microscopy was performed to localize YFP within tissues. Levels of gene expression as indicated by amounts of emitted light increased from time of delivery until achieving a plateau at 15 days. BLI allowed for convenient and accurate *in vivo* assessment of the spatio-temporal pattern of gene expression in this mouse model of lung gene therapy and accelerated its optimization.

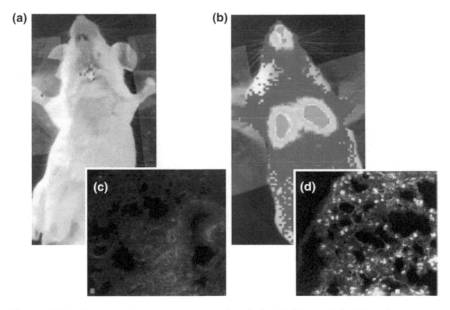

Figure 4.2   **(See color insert)** Adeno-associated viral delivery of dual function reporter gene to the lungs of Balb/c mice. Mice were treated with two different AAV vectors encoding the same dual function reporter gene comprised of Fluc and YFP (Brindle and Contag, Unpublished data). Animals were imaged for luciferase expression (a and b) and after the study fluorescence micrographs (c and d) were used to validate gene delivery to the lungs. Effective gene delivery is shown in b and d, whereas the absence of effective delivery is shown in a and b.

IX. Summary and Future Outlook

Imaging sciences and the emerging field of molecular imaging have advanced to the point where we have a variety of instruments available for imaging both structure and function in rodent models and in humans. These advances represent a convergence of cell biology, chemistry, and imaging, and the range of tools that are being developed for probing biology *in vivo* is expanding rapidly. Miniaturization of what are thought of as clinical imaging modalities, such as PET, single photon emission computed tomography (SPECT), and MRI, have enabled development of new approaches for studying animals and a new set of platforms with which we can develop the next generation of clinical imaging probes. BLI has proven to be a robust and versatile small animal imaging modality that can provide functional information about infection, gene expression, protein function, and cell migration, and as such will be a tool that is used to refine our animal models of lung development and disease. Understanding the factors that influence the generation of bioluminescent signals in animals, and those that affect the transmission of this light through mammalian tissues is essential for effective use of BLI for biological investigation.

At present, we have tools that show great promise for the detection of a wide range of functions and the availability of instruments for small animals will accelerate the development of many new tools. The great potential for advancing and refining our animal models of lung disease using *in vivo* BLI as a method of revealing biological changes has yet to be fully realized. We can study processes that were not previously accessible for investigation and begin to integrate modalities to provide more information, more rapidly than before. Full utilization of these methods to study lung biology, development, regeneration, and disease will greatly improve our ability to treat and manage lung diseases in the clinic. We will accelerate the development of new therapeutic approaches through refinement of animal models and discover the regulatory pathways that control inflammation and regeneration of lung function.

Acknowledgments

This work was supported by a grant from the NIH (R24 CA 92862) and an unrestricted gift from Philips Medical.

References

1. Doyle TC, Burns SM, Contag CH. *In vivo* bioluminescence imaging for integrated studies of infection. Cell Microbiol 2004; 6:303–317.
2. Hardy J, Edinger M, Bachmann MH, Negrin RS, Fathman CG, Contag CH. Bioluminescence imaging of lymphocyte trafficking *in vivo*. Exp Hematol 2001; 29:1353–1360.

3. Contag CH, Bachmann MH. Advances in *in vivo* bioluminescence imaging of gene expression. Annu Rev Biomed Eng 2002; 4:235–260.
4. Contag PR, Olomu IN, Stevenson DK, Contag CH. Bioluminescent indicators in living mammals. Nat Med 1998; 4:245–247.
5. Mandl S, Schimmelpfennig C, Edinger M, Negrin RS, Contag CH. Understanding immune cell trafficking patterns via *in vivo* bioluminescence imaging. J Cell Biochem Suppl 2002; 39:239–248.
6. Robinson TE, Leung AN, Northway WH, Blankenberg FG, Chan FP, Bloch DA, Holmes TH, Moss RB. Composite spirometric-computed tomography outcome measure in early cystic fibrosis lung disease. Am J Respir Crit Care Med 2003; 168:588–593.
7. Goris ML, Zhu HJ, Blankenberg F, Chan F, Robinson TE. An automated approach to quantitative air trapping measurements in mild cystic fibrosis. Chest 2003; 123:1655–1663.
8. Robinson TE, Leung AN, Moss RB, Blankenberg FG, al-Dabbagh H, Northway WH. Standardized high-resolution CT of the lung using a spirometer-triggered electron beam CT scanner. Am J Roentgenol 1999; 172:1636–1638.
9. Schuster DP, Kovacs A, Garbow J, Piwnica Worms D. Recent advances in imaging the lungs of intact small animals. Am J Respir Cell Mol Biol 2004; 30:129–138.
10. Piwnica-Worms D, Schuster DP, Garbow JR. Molecular imaging of host–pathogen interactions in intact small animals. Cell Microbiol 2004; 6:319–331.
11. Massoud TF, Gambhir SS. Molecular imaging in living subjects: seeing fundamental biological processes in a new light. Genes Dev 2003; 17:545–580.
12. Blasberg R. Imaging gene expression and endogenous molecular processes: molecular imaging. J Cereb Blood Flow Metab 2002; 22:1157–1164.
13. Blasberg R. PET imaging of gene expression. Eur J Cancer 2002; 38:2137–2146.
14. Tuchin VV. Handbook of Optical Biomedical Diagnostics. Washington: SPIE, 2002.
15. Cao YA, Wagers AJ, Beilhack A, Dusich J, Bachmann MH, Negrin RS, Weissman IL, Contag CH. Shifting foci of hematopoiesis during reconstitution from single stem cells. Proc Natl Acad Sci USA 2004; 101:221–226.
16. Hastings JW. Chemistries and colors of bioluminescent reactions: a review. Gene 1996; 173:5–11.
17. de Wet JR, Wood KV, DeLuca M, Helinski DR, Subramani S. Firefly luciferase gene: structure and expression in mammalian cells. Mol Cell Biol 1987; 7:725–737.
18. Wood KV, Lam YA, Seliger HH, McElroy WD. Complementary DNA coding click beetle luciferases can elicit bioluminescence of different colors. Science 1989; 244:700–702.
19. Viviani VR, Bechara EJ, Ohmiya Y. Cloning, sequence analysis, and expression of active *Phrixothrix* railroad-worms luciferases: relationship between bioluminescence spectra and primary structures. Biochemistry 1999; 38:8271–8279.
20. Ward WW. General aspects of bioluminescence. In: Burr JG, ed. Chemi- and Bioluminescence. New York: Marcel Dekker, 1985:321–358.
21. Rutter GA, Kennedy HJ, Wood CD, White MR, Tavare JM. Real-time imaging of gene expression in single living cells. Chem Biol 1998; 5:R285–R290.
22. Hooper CE, Ansorge RE, Rushbrooke JG. Low-light imaging technology in the life sciences. J Biolumin Chemilumin 1994; 9:113–122.
23. Hooper CE, Ansorge RE, Browne HM, Tomkins P. CCD imaging of luciferase gene expression in single mammalian cells. J Biolumin Chemilumin 1990; 5:123–130.

24. Contag CH, Spilman SD, Contag PR, Oshiro M, Eames B, Dennery P, Stevenson DK, Benaron DA. Visualizing gene expression in living mammals using a bioluminescent reporter. Photochem Photobiol 1997; 66:523–531.

25. Rehemtulla A, Stegman LD, Cardozo SJ, Gupta S, Hall DE, Contag CH, Ross BD. Rapid and quantitative assessment of cancer treatment response using *in vivo* bioluminescence imaging. Neoplasia 2000; 2:491–495.

26. Lipshutz GS, Gruber CA, Cao Y, Hardy J, Contag CH, Gaensler KM. *In utero* delivery of adeno-associated viral vectors: intraperitoneal gene transfer produces long-term expression. Mol Ther 2001; 3:284–292.

27. Karkhanis YD, Cormier MJ. Isolation and properties of *Renilla reniformis* luciferase, a low molecular weight energy conversion enzyme. Biochemistry 1971; 10:317–326.

28. Matthews JC, Hori K, Cormier MJ. Purification and properties of *Renilla reniformis* luciferase. Biochemistry 1977; 16:85–91.

29. Srikantha T, Klapach A, Lorenz WW, Tsai LK, Laughlin LA, Gorman JA, Soll DR. The sea pansy *Renilla reniformis* luciferase serves as a sensitive bioluminescent reporter for differential gene expression in *Candida albicans*. J Bacteriol 1996; 178:121–129.

30. Wang Y, Wang G, O'Kane DJ, Szalay AA. A study of protein–protein interactions in living cells using luminescence resonance energy transfer (LRET) from *Renilla* luciferase to *Aequorea* GFP. Mol Gen Genet 2001; 264:578–587.

31. Shimomura O, Johnson FH. Chemical nature of bioluminescence systems in coelenterates. Proc Natl Acad Sci USA 1975; 72:1546–1549.

32. Greer LF, Szalay AA. Imaging of light emission from the expression of luciferases in living cells and organisms: a review. Luminescence 2002; 17:43–74.

33. Plieth C. Plant calcium signaling and monitoring: pros and cons and recent experimental approaches. Protoplasma 2001; 218:1–23.

34. Bhaumik S, Gambhir SS. Optical imaging of *Renilla* luciferase reporter gene expression in living mice. Proc Natl Acad Sci USA 2002; 99:377–382.

35. Paulmurugan R, Gambhir SS. Monitoring protein–protein interactions using split synthetic renilla luciferase protein-fragment-assisted complementation. Anal Chem 2003; 75:1584–1589.

36. Ray P, De A, Min JJ, Tsien RY, Gambhir SS. Imaging tri-fusion multimodality reporter gene expression in living subjects. Cancer Res 2004; 64:1323–1330.

37. Pichler A, Prior JL, Piwnica-Worms D. Imaging reversal of multidrug resistance in living mice with bioluminescence: MDR1 P-glycoprotein transports coelenterazine. Proc Natl Acad Sci USA 2004; 101:1702–1707.

38. Frackman S, Anhalt M, Nealson KH. Cloning, organization, and expression of the bioluminescence genes of *Xenorhabdus luminescens*. J Bacteriol 1990; 172:5767–5773.

39. Contag CH, Contag PR, Mullins JI, Spilman SD, Stevenson DK, Benaron DA. Photonic detection of bacterial pathogens in living hosts. Mol Microbiol 1995; 18:593–603.

40. Francis KP, Joh D, Bellinger-Kawahara C, Hawkinson MJ, Purchio TF, Contag PR. Monitoring bioluminescent *Staphylococcus aureus* infections in living mice using a novel luxABCDE construct. Infect Immun 2000; 68:3594–3600.

41. Gupta RK, Patterson SS, Ripp S, Simpson ML, Sayler GS. Expression of the *Photorhabdus luminescens* lux genes (*luxA, B, C, D,* and E) in *Saccharomyces cerevisiae*. FEMS Yeast Res 2003; 4:305–313.

42. Sadikot RT, Zeng H, Yull FE, Li B, Cheng DS, Kernodle DS, Jansen ED, Contag CH, Segal BH, Holland SM, Blackwell TS, Christman JW. p47(phox) deficiency impairs NF-kappaB activation and host defense in *Pseudomonas pneumonia*. J Immunol 2004; 172:1801–1808.

43. Rehemtulla A, Hall DE, Stegman LD, Prasad U, Chen G, Bhojani MS, Chenevert TL, Ross BD. Molecular imaging of gene expression and efficacy following adenoviral-mediated brain tumor gene therapy. Mol Imaging 2002; 1:43–55.

44. Zhao H, Doyle TC, Wong RJ, Cao Y, Stevenson DK, Piwnica-Worms D, Contag CH. Characterization of coelenterazine analogs for measurement of *Renilla* luciferase activity in live cells and living animals. Mol Imaging 2004; 3:43–54.

45. Hori K, Anderson JM, Ward WW, Cormier MJ. *Renilla* luciferin as the substrate for calcium induced photoprotein bioluminescence. Assignment of luciferin tautomers in aequorin and mnemiopsin. Biochemistry 1975; 14:2371–2376.

46. Rice BW, Cable MD, Nelson MB. *In vivo* imaging of light-emitting probes. J Biomed Opt 2001; 6:432–440.

47. Oshiro M, Moomaw B. Cooled vs. intensified vs. electron bombardment CCD cameras—applications and relative advantages. Methods Cell Biol 2003; 72:133–156.

48. Day RN, Kawecki M, Berry D. Dual-function reporter protein for analysis of gene expression in living cells. Biotechniques 1998; 25:848–850, 852–854, 856.

49. Edinger M, Cao YA, Verneris MR, Bachmann MH, Contag CH, Negrin RS. Revealing lymphoma growth and the efficacy of immune cell therapies using *in vivo* bioluminescence imaging. Blood 2003; 101:640–648.

50. Edinger M, Hoffmann P, Contag CH, Negrin RS. Evaluation of effector cell fate and function by *in vivo* bioluminescence imaging. Methods 2003; 31:172–179.

51. Mandl S, Mari C, Edinger M et al. *In vivo* dynamics of tumor cell death: multi-modality imaging identifies key imaging times for assessing response to chemotherapy using an orthotopic mouse model of lymphoma. Mol Imaging 2004; 3:1–8.

52. Ponomarev V, Doubrovin M, Serganova I, Vider J, Shavrin A, Beresten T, Ivanova A, Ageyeva L, Tourkova V, Balatoni J, Bornmann W, Blasberg R, Gelovani Tjuvajev J. A novel triple-modality reporter gene for whole-body fluorescent, bioluminescent, and nuclear noninvasive imaging. Eur J Nucl Med Mol Imaging 2004; 31:740–751.

53. Hardy J, Francis KP, DeBoer M, Chu P, Gibbs K, Contag CH. Extracellular replication of *Listeria monocytogenes* in the murine gall bladder. Science 2004; 303:851–853.

54. Cook SH, Griffin DE. Luciferase imaging of a neurotropic viral infection in intact animals. J Virol 2003; 77:5333–5338.

55. Edinger M, Cao YA, Hornig YS, Jenkins DE, Verneris MR, Bachmann MH, Negrin RS, Contag CH. Advancing animal models of neoplasia through *in vivo* bioluminescence imaging. Eur J Cancer 2002; 38:2128–2136.

56. Edinger M, Sweeney TJ, Tucker AA, Olomu AB, Negrin RS, Contag CH. Noninvasive assessment of tumor cell proliferation in animal models. Neoplasia 1999; 1:303–310.

57. Sweeney TJ, Mailander V, Tucker AA, Olomu AB, Zhang W, Cao Y, Negrin RS, Contag CH. Visualizing the kinetics of tumor-cell clearance in living animals. Proc Natl Acad Sci USA 1999; 96:12044–12049.

58. Iyer M, Berenji M, Templeton NS, Gambhir SS. Noninvasive imaging of cationic lipid-mediated delivery of optical and PET reporter genes in living mice. Mol Ther 2002; 6:555–562.

5

Magnetic Resonance Imaging

JOEL R. GARBOW, CASSANDRA B. ORELLANA, and JEFFREY J. NEIL

Washington University,
St. Louis, Missouri, USA

I. Introduction

Magnetic resonance imaging (MRI) is a powerful and versatile imaging modality for the noninvasive, *in vivo* characterization of biological systems. The relatively low tissue density and large number of air–tissue interfaces in lung present several unique challenges to its study by magnetic resonance (MR). Nonetheless, MR techniques have been developed to provide important insights into the structure and dynamics of lungs in humans and in small-animal models of lung disease. These methods include both conventional MRI of the hydrogen atoms in water in lung tissue and imaging of air spaces using hyperpolarized helium gas. Molecular imaging can provide important insights into biological processes at the cellular or subcellular level. The linking of specific targeted molecular agents with the superb anatomical resolution provided by MRI forms a particularly powerful combination. In this chapter, we provide an overview of MR molecular imaging and MRI of lung in both humans and small animals and discuss the prospects for the development of MR-based molecular imaging techniques in lungs.

Most MRI experiments are based on the detection of MR signal from the ^{1}H atoms in water. The main reason why ^{1}H$_2$O signal is used for MRI is that the concentration of ^{1}H in water is on the order of 100 M. Although MR can be used to detect other molecules (e.g., the ^{1}H signal from lactate, the ^{31}P signal from phosphocreatine or ATP), these molecules are present in much lower—typically milli-molar—concentrations. As a result, their detection by MR requires signal averaging for long periods of time and/or evaluation of tissues at lower spatial resolution than practical for conventional imaging. Image contrast arises from differences in the properties of ^{1}H$_2$O in different tissue environments. For example, water in cerebrospinal fluid has a relatively long T_2, or transverse, relaxation time constant when compared with that of water in the adjacent white matter of brain. As a result, CSF appears brighter than white matter on T_2-weighted brain images. Conventional MRI typically exploits differences in water T_2 and T_2^* (transverse relaxation), T_1 (longitudinal relaxation), and local water concentration/^{1}H spin density and diffusion (water displacements) to obtain tissue contrast. Modifications to the MR image acquisition parameters allow development of images with different types of contrast.

The detection of water, generally present in high concentration, makes MRI different from other imaging modalities, where the actual substance to be imaged is usually an exogenous, optically active or radioactive tracer present at very low concentration. The distinction is important for the field of molecular imaging. MR does not generally directly image an exogenously administered MR-active imaging agent. Rather, MRI detects administered agents *indirectly* through their effect on the water MR signal intensity. Such MR active agents are referred to as "contrast agents" (CA) and generally must be present at $\sim$100 μM to 1 mM to be effective. This is far higher in concentration than that required for imaging optically active or radioactive tracers, ca. pico- to nano-molar. MR CAs broadly fall into two categories, those that primarily shorten the ^{1}H T_1 relaxation time constant and those that primarily shorten the T_2 or T_2^* relaxation time constants. The presence of T_1 agents causes T_1-weighted images to appear brighter, whereas the presence of T_2 and T_2^* agents causes T_2- and T_2^*-weighted images to appear darker. Under the appropriate conditions, it is possible to estimate the local CA concentration on the basis of relaxation time measurements.

As can readily be appreciated, the water content of healthy lung tissue is low relative to other tissues. Thus, the base MRI signal strength for lung parenchyma is weak. Furthermore, the large number of air–water interfaces throughout lung result in parasitic, magnetic susceptibility induced, magnetic field gradients. These lead to very short transverse (T_2) relaxation times for normal lung, further reducing the image intensity. As a consequence, MRI of normal lung tissue has not received great attention. Indeed, the MR signal intensity from normal lung tissue is so weak that it appears black with most MRI procedures. However, abnormal tissue in lung, such as tumor, edema, and inflammation, which presents greater water content and longer transverse relaxation time, can be imaged to great advantage against the black background of normal lung tissue.

II. Molecular MRI

Molecular imaging describes the visual characterization of biological processes at the cellular or subcellular level within living organisms. The development of these methods promises to provide important insights into cellular and molecular pathways and *in vivo* mechanisms of disease. A number of strategies for molecular MRI have been described recently and we begin by briefly reviewing these approaches. The reader is referred to many recent reviews of molecular imaging, and the references therein, for further discussion and detail (1–6).

A. Traditional CAs

MR CAs, built around paramagnetic centers such as gadolinium (Gd) (which shortens the T_1 relaxation time constant of water) and iron (Fe) (which primarily shortens water T_2 and T_2^* relaxation time constants), are fundamentally different than corresponding materials used in other imaging modalities. Position emission tomography (PET) tracers and optical agents can be visualized directly in corresponding imaging experiments. However, as described earlier, MR CAs act *indirectly* by affecting the relaxation properties of surrounding water molecules. These changed relaxation times, in turn, are reflected in changes in the observed intensities in MR images. Standard MR CAs, injected into the vascular system, are nonspecific and lead to changed image contrast in all tissues/organs to which they are delivered. Clinically, these CAs are used to improve the quality of anatomical images by enhancing contrast-to-noise ratio. The development of effective molecular MR methods requires the generation of specific targeted agents that recognize specific molecular and cellular processes and/or markers and then report on the physiologic status or metabolic activity of cells. One of the great strengths of MRI is its superb image resolution, and it is this image resolution that makes MR an attractive modality for the development of molecular imaging methods. At the same time, MR is a relatively insensitive method, and the successful development of MR-based molecular imaging methods requires strategies to deliver large quantities of targeted CA to the desired site in order to permit visualization of important molecular events.

B. Organ-Specific CAs

Traditional MR CAs, such as gadolinium-diethylenetriaminepenta-acetic acid (Gd-DTPA), are nonspecific molecules that are distributed widely and lead to image enhancement in many organs and tissues throughout the body. Perhaps the simplest class of specific MR agents is those that target specific organs or tissues, including blood-pool agents and those that target liver, lymph nodes, and atherosclerotic plaques. A comprehensive review of such agents has recently appeared (7).

C. Targeted CAs

A variety of targeted MR CAs have been developed for molecular imaging, including agents for imaging fibrin (8), pancreatic secretin receptors (9), and high-affinity folate receptors (10). An elegant example of the use of such targeted CAs is the imaging of angiogenesis in early stage atherosclerosis with $\alpha_v\beta_3$-integrin-targeted nanoparticles (11). Integrins, such as $\alpha_v\beta_3$, are associated with angiogenesis; atherosclerotic lesions are highly vascular compared with normal vessel tissues (12). $\alpha_v\beta_3$-targeted agents may have important clinical relevance as imaging/diagnostic agents of angiogenesis associated with the early development of atherosclerosis and may also serve as effective vehicles for drug delivery. A paramagnetic nanoparticle CA was developed that was targeted specifically to $\alpha_v\beta_3$-integrins to permit noninvasive molecular imaging of plaque-associated angiogenesis (11). The paramagnetic nanoparticles were directed to the $\alpha_v\beta_3$-integrin with a peptidomimetic vitronectin antagonist. Signal in the aortic wall of cholesterol-fed rabbits increased after the injection of this nanoparticle CA due to binding of the targeted nanoparticles to $\alpha_v\beta_3$-epitopes on the neovasculature. Further experiments established that enhancement with targeted nanoparticles greatly exceeded that of nontargeted CA. Competitive blocking of angiogenic $\alpha_v\beta_3$-integrins with targeted, nonparamagnetic nanoparticles significantly reduced the signal enhancement of $\alpha_v\beta_3$-targeted, paramagnetic nanoparticles, demonstrating the specificity of the agent.

D. Activated CAs

A second class of targetable agents can be described as activated CAs. For these agents, the physical properties of the paramagnetic complexes can be switched on or off in response to environmental changes. Examples of these include materials that are sensitive to calcium ion concentration (13,14), pH (15), and partial pressure of oxygen (pO_2) (16,17). Agents that can be activated by RF irradiation, the so-called chemical exchange saturation transfer or chemical exchange-dependent saturation transfer (CEST) agents (18–20), have also been developed. For these CAs, specificity is achieved not by a specific receptor or molecular target, but by a change in a local environmental variable.

E. Targeting Cellular Markers

The most specific and powerful molecular imaging MR CAs are those that are designed to recognize and target specific cellular markers, permitting imaging of cells that express these markers. One general strategy involves the use of specific CAs targeted to unique cell-surface molecular epitopes (specific target recognition sites), with binding provided by monoclonal antibodies (MAb) or antibody fragments. These antibodies or antibody fragments may also serve as an effective way to deliver targeted therapeutic agents. Examples of this approach include: (1) imaging of 9L glioma cells following introduction of a Gd-DTPA-labeled MAb against these glioma cells (21); (2) *in vivo* studies of human MM-138 melanoma xenografts in nude mice targeted with antimelanoma MAb (22); (3) targeting of paramagnetic, polymerized liposomes (23) or Gd-perfluorocarbon nanoparticles (24) to $\alpha_v\beta_3$-integrin receptor via biotin–avidin linkers; and (4) imaging of breast cancer cells expressing HER-2/neu receptors, imaged via a two-step labeling protocol using biotinylated Herceptin MAb and avidin-Gd-DTPA conjugates (25).

Similar approaches have been described using targeted CAs composed of superparamagnetic iron oxide (SPIO) particles conjugated with MAb or MAb fragments. Molecular imaging MR experiments have been performed to image the protein E-selectin in human endothelial cells using the $F(ab)_2$ fragment of antihuman E-selectin MAb conjugated to cross-linked iron oxide (CLIO) particles (26). Imaging of the HER-2/neu receptors on the surface of human breast cancer cells has been achieved using Herceptin MAb and SPIO complexes (27). *In vivo* imaging of inflammation sites has recently been described with human polyclonal immunoglobulin G (IgG) attached to monocrystalline iron oxide nanoparticles (MION). A concern in the development of *in vivo*-targeted nonpeptide-based imaging probes is that the large molecular size of conjugates may prevent their effective delivery to target sites.

F. Imaging Transgene Expression

Labeling of cells with SPIO particles has enabled numerous recent studies of cell migration and trafficking, including studies using T-cells (28–30), T-lymphocytes (31), and stem cells (32–34). A particularly exciting area for the development of targeted CAs is the imaging of gene expression. The goal of these experiments is to detect gene expression before phenotypic changes occur. In detecting gene expression, a common strategy is the imaging of marker genes. In this approach, a marker gene is included along with the gene of interest and the detection of its expression demonstrates expression of the gene of interest. Two different classes of marker genes can be employed in these experiments: marker genes that encode for intracellular enzymes and those that encode for cell-surface proteins and receptors. The former have the advantages of simple expression strategies and that the expression products are not recognized by the immune system. The latter have favorable reaction kinetics and are amenable to the development of synthetic receptors that can be engineered to recognize established imaging agents. The detection of imaging marker genes *in vivo* requires imaging probes with sufficient specificity for the desired target. Imaging probes developed thus far fall into two broad categories. The first are those that target a specific cell structure and are then bound to or internalized into a cell. The second are those that are processed by an enzyme, leading to either a change in the signal characteristics of the imaging probe or trapping of the probe inside the cell.

Weissleder et al. provided perhaps the first demonstration that MRI can noninvasively visualize transgene expression *in vivo* with engineered transferrin receptor (ETR), a cell-surface receptor that shuttles superparamagnetic nanoparticles into cells (35). ETR is rapidly internalized and recycled, allowing a single receptor to shuttle many nanoparticles into each cell. In culture, cells stably transfected to overexpress high levels of the receptor protein bind five times the normal levels of halotransferrin, a natural ligand of the receptor. The receptor-targeted MR CA consists of a MION to which human halotransferrin is covalently conjugated (Tf-MION). In transfected 9L glioma cells, ETR expression correlated with increases in internalized Tf-MION as measured by staining for iron levels, and expression levels of the receptor correlated with MR signal intensities in T_2-weighted images. To visualize transgene expression in a live animal, ETR^+ cells were implanted in one flank of a mouse and ETR^- cells in the other flank. The mouse was injected with a superparamagnetic Tf conjugate and imaged 24 h later. The resulting uptake of MION particles lowered the signal intensity in the ETR^+ flank relative to the ETR^- flank, a change that typically persists for 3–14 days.

High-efficiency internal labeling of cells can also be achieved by attaching a peptide bearing the HIV-Tat protein translocation sequence to dextran CLIO superparamagnetic particles (36). The uptake of peptide-bearing CLIO particles into lymphocytes is increased by greater than 100-fold relative to untagged particles (36). Similar uptake is observed into human CD34+ progenitor cells, mouse neural progenitor cells, human CD4+ lymphocytes, and mouse splenocytes. One strategy for using such labeled cells is to label them outside the animal and then inject them back into the animal. In this fashion, CLIO-Tat particles have been used for tracking *in vivo* targeting of lymphocytes to tumors, resulting from implant of 9L tumor cells, in murine brain. MRI allowed clear visualization of the CLIO-Tat labeled lymphocytes in the 9L tumor.

G. Switchable CAs

An elegant example of a switchable CA is (4,7,10-tri[acetic acid]-1-[2-β-galactopyranosylethoxy]-1,4,7,10-tetraazacyclododecane) gadolinium, the so-called EgadMe molecule, developed by Louie et al. (37). β-Galactosidase is used frequently as a marker enzyme in molecular biology and the functionality of the triggerable EgadMe molecule is based on β-galactosidase activity. EgadMe has a Gd center whose accessibility to water is blocked by a covalently attached galactopyranose molecule. Cleavage of galactopyranose by β-galactosidase activates the CA by exposing the paramagnetic center to water protons, thereby shortening the local water ^1H T_1 relaxation time constant. The feasibility of detecting EgadMe activation by β-galactosidase has been demonstrated in a *Xenopus laevis* embryo model (37).

H. Imaging Gene Products

Another strategy for detecting gene expression is to exploit the inherent imageability of gene products to enhance MR signals within cells. An example of this approach is provided by monitoring changes in MR intensities resulting from the activity of tyrosinase. Tyrosinase catalyzes the hydroxylation of tyrosine to dioxyphenyl alanine (DOPA) and the subsequent oxidation of DOPA to DOPA-quinone that eventually leads to melanin formation. Melanin itself has a high-binding capacity for metals, such as iron, which causes cells rich in melatonin to accumulate iron. The resulting enhancement of MR signals thus serves as a marker of tyrosinase activity (38). Cells transfected with a vector containing a gene for human tyrosinase yielded signal intensity eight times greater than that of control cells (39). Recently, a number of tyrosine mutants have been generated that have higher enzyme activity and lower endogenous toxicity. These mutants have been transfected successfully into a variety of different nontumorigenic human cells and tumor cells and hold great promise as potential imaging markers.

III. MRI of Lung

MRI of the lung presents a unique set of challenges. In this section, we describe the features of lung that make it a particularly difficult organ to successfully image and we summarize recent MR studies of lung in both small animals and human. These studies can be divided into two broad categories: (1) ^1H MR studies, which are focused on lung pathology, including edema, tumor, and fibrotic lesions; (2) hyperpolarized ^3He gas imaging to assess ventilation and measure diffusion in both healthy and diseased lung parenchyma. In addition, we describe oxygen-sensitive ^{3}He MRI experiments to measure alveolar oxygen partial pressure (pAO_2) and perfusion imaging measurements to evaluate pulmonary blood flow.

A. Proton Imaging

Although the opportunities for characterization are significant, lungs present unique challenges for MRI (40), requiring the development of new and innovative methods. A review of small-animal MRI of lungs has recently appeared (41). Among the complicating factors for the study of lungs by ^{1}H MR methods are (1) low tissue density and low water content within the lung severely limiting signal-to-noise; (2) variations in magnetic susceptibility associated with the many air–tissue interfaces of the alveoli and bronchioles resulting in short T_2^* and T_2 relaxation times; (3) respiratory and cardiac motions leading to significant image blurring in the absence of motion-synchronized data acquisition.

In response to these challenges, researchers generally use very fast gradient-echo imaging sequences with short echo times (TEs) (to overcome variations in magnetic susceptibility) or spin-echo sequences with respiratory synchronization (42,43). In addition, static magnetic field strength, gradient strength, and RF coil performance can all affect sensitivity and spatial resolution in MRI experiments. For small-animal imaging studies, 4.7–9.4 tesla MR scanners (^{1}H resonance frequencies of 200–400 MHz) are commonly used, compared with the 1.5–3 tesla magnetic fields (^{1}H resonance frequencies of 60–120 MHz), typical of clinical scanners. For animal work, high gradient strengths, for example, 15–100 G/cm, compared with 2–3 G/cm on most clinical human scanners, are also typical. Experiments in small animals are performed with respiratory gating (43–45) as breath holding is often not an option. Data collection varies from minutes to one or more hours per animal, depending upon the nature of the experiments being performed.

Many pulmonary studies in small animals have focused on edema (46,47) or other disease states, including lungs affected with tumors or fibrotic lesions, in which the density of tissue increases and the corresponding susceptibility broadening due to air–tissue interfaces is decreased. In general, a good correlation has been observed between MRI-determined estimates of lung water and the gold standard gravimetric method (40,48). MRI has been used to assess edema and inflammation in the lungs following allergen or endotoxin challenges (49,50), after exposure to an 85% diatomic oxygen (O_2) atmosphere, and after treatment with paraquat (43). Figure 5.1 shows respiratory-gated spin-echo ^{1}H-MR images of a healthy mouse and one whose lungs are filled with fibrotic lesions after administration of intratracheal bleomycin.

A recent study described MRI characterization of lung tumors in mice (51). Aimed at understanding the genetic modifiers of lung cancer induction and therapy, MRI was used to detect small tumors in the lungs of mice treated with the tobacco-specific carcinogen, benzo(a)pyrene. Figure 5.2 shows representative

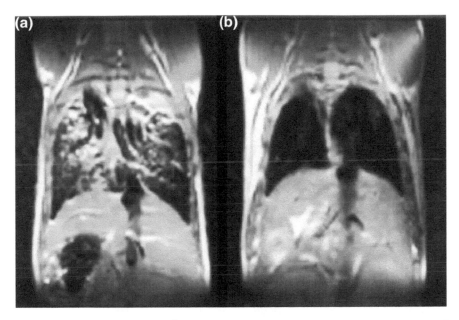

Figure 5.1 Respiratory-gated ^{1}H spin-echo images of: (a) fibrotic mouse lung and (b) healthy mouse lung. Images were collected with TR $\sim$3 s, TE $= 20$ ms, FOV $=$ 2.5 cm, slice thickness $= 1$ mm, 128 $\times$ 128 data matrix, four averages. [From Ref. (41).]

respiratory-gated, spin-echo MR images and photographs taken of the lungs after sacrifice of the same mice. The overall correspondence between the tumors seen in the photograph and those shown in the MR image is excellent.

B. Hyperpolarized Gas Imaging

MR methods can be used to image airways and create ventilation maps of the lung through the administration of an inhaled gas. MRI of normal gases suffers from very poor signal-to-noise ratios due to the extremely low density of gas. However, with hyperpolarized noble gases (52), such as ^{3}He and ^{129}Xe (53), magnetic moments can be $10^5\times$ those at thermal equilibrium. These extremely high nuclear spin polarizations more than compensate for the 10^3 lower density of the gaseous state relative to that of liquid water, yielding images that are, in many cases, of higher sensitivity than observed in ^{1}H-MR images of tissue water.

In its most straightforward application, hyperpolarized gas can be used as a gaseous inhaled contrast agent. Regions of the lung that are well ventilated appear bright in images following inhalation of hyperpolarized ^{3}He; regions of impaired ventilation appear darker (53–56). Measurement of signal intensity in a single, multislice set of rapidly collected images produces a ventilation map. T_1 relaxation of ^{3}He in lungs is due almost entirely to interaction with

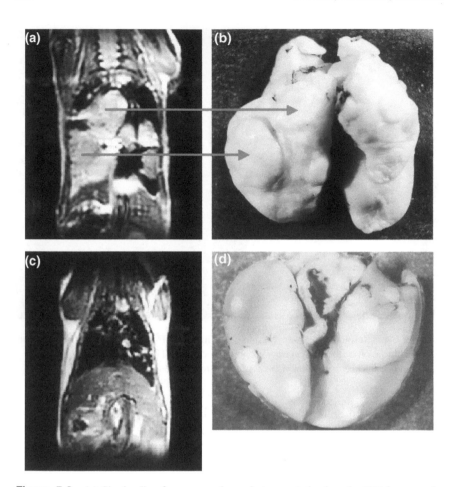

Figure 5.2 (a) Single slice from coronal, respiratory-gated spin-echo MR images of a p53$^{+/-}$Ink4a/Arf$^{+/-}$ mouse, 6 months following treatment with benzo(a)pyrene, showing a heavy tumor burden. Imaging parameters are TR ∼3 s; TE = 20 ms; FOV = 2.5 cm; slice thickness = 0.5 mm, 128 × 128 data matrix, four averages. Under these experimental conditions, the images of healthy mouse lung parenchyma are completely black and the bright spots visible in these images are due to lung tumors. (b) Photograph of the lungs from the same mouse. The red arrows highlight the correspondence between the tumors visible in the MR image and those in the photograph. (c) Single slice from coronal, respiratory-gated spin-echo MR images of a p53$^{+/+}$Ink4a/Arf$^{+/+}$ mouse, following treatment with benzo(a)pyrene, showing a lighter tumor burden. (d) Corresponding photograph of lungs from this mouse. [From Ref. (51).]

oxygen in the gas phase. However, given the relatively small variations in pO_2 in lungs (57), the effects of minor variations in T_1 on image intensity can be minimized by collecting data on a time scale that is short compared with typical ^{3}He T_1s (20 s).

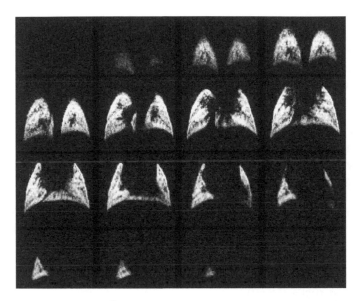

Figure 5.3 Hyperpolarized [3]He mouse-lung ventilation images collected using an asymmetric gradient echo multislice imaging sequence. 15 consecutive, 1 mm thick coronal slices are shown. Imaging parameters are FOV = 2.6 cm, resolution = 0.203 mm/pixel, ~6 ms between RF pulses, TE = 1.2 ms, number of scans = 2. Acquisition of these images, scanning one line of k-space on each slice per breath, takes ~2 min. [From Ref. (91).]

[3]He imaging of small animals requires higher spatial resolution than corresponding studies in humans, so that a single breathhold of hyperpolarized [3]He, as typically performed in clinical studies, does not yield adequate signal-to-noise ratio. Instead, small volumes of hyperpolarized gas are repetitively delivered using a ventilator, and data are collected over periods of many minutes. Figure 5.3 shows one slice from a multislice, hyperpolarized [3]He ventilation image of a mouse lung collected in our laboratory. Several recent studies have focused on generating high-resolution lung ventilation maps in small animals using hyperpolarized [3]He gas (57–60), whereas Johnson et al. (61) recently described a combined [3]He/^{1}H imaging study of rat lung.

MRI using hyperpolarized [3]He gas has been used in several studies to detect ventilation defects in humans. [3]He imaging has been compared to spirometry measurements for observing small-airway obstruction and decreased pulmonary ventilation in asthmatics before and after bronchodilator therapy, thereby providing a direct method for evaluating therapeutic response (62). In a recent study, [3]He gas imaging was compared to ventilation scintigraphy for imaging ventilation defects in smokers. The results of this study demonstrated that MRI can consistently identify known ventilatory abnormalities with better spatial resolution than scintigraphy (54). Gas imaging has been employed successfully to study cystic fibrosis patients, proving sensitive to both morphologic and ventilation abnormalities when compared with thin section CT (63). Hyperpolarized ^{3}He has also been used to identify ventilatory abnormalities in lung transplant recipients with bronchiolitis obliterans syndrome (64). ^{3}He methods can also be used to measure lung volumes, and MR-determined volumes correlate well with the results of pulmonary function tests (PFTs). In fact, MRI has a better correlation with PFTs than CT, possibly because CT identifies air-filled lung and does not provide a direct assessment of the distribution of ventilation (65). Hyperpolarized ^{3}He methods have been applied to patients with single lung transplant, emphysema, and idiopathic pulmonary fibrosis (66).

Dynamic imaging experiments using hyperpolarized gas, in which a series of time-resolved intensities are measured during the inspiration/expiration cycle, can provide information about functional lung ventilation and ventilation distribution that is absent from static imaging experiments (67). Dynamic imaging is achieved by selecting experimental conditions to observe either recently inhaled fresh gas only or all of the gas within the lung. It is also possible to obtain a simultaneous regional assessment of both lung ventilation and perfusion by monitoring ^{3}He image intensity as a function of time following an IV bolus injection of SPIO nanoparticles (68,69).

MRI with hyperpolarized ^{3}He has demonstrated the ability to identify and quantify impaired distribution of ventilation in lung transplant patients, in whom preferential distribution of the graft is observed (70). In patients with emphysema, patterns of irregular and delayed ^{3}He entry with redistribution and air trapping were observed. This abnormal movement was not noted in healthy patients (71–73).

C. Diffusion

MRI measurement of hyperpolarized gas diffusion is another important source of information about lung morphology and disease. The diffusion of gas is restricted by the microstructure of the lung—its small airways and alveolar walls—making diffusion sensitive to microstructural features on an alveolar distance scale, well below the spatial—resolution limits of conventional MRI. These properties can be quantified as a gas apparent diffusion coefficient (ADC), complementing information about the uniformity of gas transport derived from ventilation images.

In healthy lungs, gas diffusion, as measured by ADC, is homogeneous, reflecting the uniformity of tissue within the lungs. A typical ADC value in the alveolar spaces in healthy rodent lung is $0.16 \text{ cm}^2/\text{s}$, more than an order of magnitude smaller than the ADC in trachea ($2.4 \text{ cm}^2/\text{s}$), where diffusion is relatively unrestricted (43). In an elastase-induced model of emphysema in rats, Chen et al. recently demonstrated that the breakdown of elastic components leads to an overall enlargement of alveolar volume, lessening restrictions to diffusion and increasing diffusivity as measured by ADC (74).

The local cylindrical geometry of the airways not only reduces the average diffusion rate, but also produces local, orientation-dependent effects with diffusion along (parallel to) the long axis of an airway being significantly faster than diffusion across (radial or perpendicular to) the long axis. Yablonskiy et al. recently proposed a theoretical model that provides a basic explanation of ^{3}He diffusivity measurements (75). These authors showed that analysis of the non-exponential signal decay on a voxel-by-voxel basis yields separate values for ADC along and across the acinar airways, despite the fact that individual airways are too small to be resolved directly. This model links the transverse ADC and the mean airway radius, R. In healthy lungs, an anisotropy-derived estimate of the mean radius for acinar airways is in excellent agreement with results of histology on excised lungs. The results demonstrate substantial differences between healthy and emphysematous lung at the acinar level and may provide new insights into emphysema progression. These methods can now be extended to longitudinal studies characterizing changes in mean small-airway radius in animal models of lung disease.

Increased ADC values have been measured in humans with diseases that lead to alveolar tissue destruction, such as emphysema. As airspace size increases, ADC values greater than two times those found in healthy lungs are measured (56). In patients with emphysema, there is a strong correlation between ADC and FEV1 (75).

The diffusion studies described earlier involve measurement of random gas-atom displacements over times of milliseconds, so that most atoms remain in a single, small airway. Thus, these measurements reveal sizes or average diameters of the small airways. Measurements of displacements $>2-10$ s have recently been reported (76), covering distances of a few centimeters, by following the decay of tagged ("striped") longitudinal magnetization (Fig. 5.4). In this case, the connectivity of the airways is explored. To travel centimeters, gas atoms starting in one small airway (commonly an alveolar duct) must go up and back down many levels of airway branching. Navigation of this tortuous path is difficult, and the measured ADC over centimeter distances in healthy lungs is much smaller (by a factor of 10) than the ADC measured over milliseconds and ~ 0.5 mm distances.

D. Ventilation Imaging

Molecular oxygen has paramagnetic properties and can be used as a CA in ^{1}H MRI (77). For oxygen enhancement imaging, a scan is acquired with the patient breathing room air and compared to a scan with the patient breathing 100% oxygen delivered by facemask (77). Oxygen alters the MRI signal of blood and other fluids by two mechanisms. The first is a reduction in local deoxyhemoglobin concentration. Deoxyhemoglobin is paramagnetic and reduces the T_2^* relaxation time constant of local water, which is detectable via T_2^*-weighted ^{1}H imaging. The second is an increase in the amount of O_2 directly dissolved in blood water. This has the effect of shortening the local water T_1 relaxation time constant, which is detectable by T_1-weighted ^{1}H imaging (78). The increase in

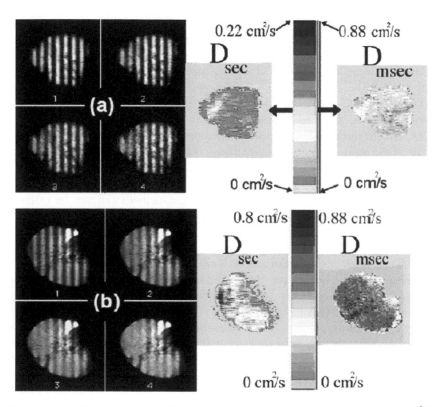

Figure 5.4 **(See color insert)** Measurement of the displacement of hyperpolarized ^{3}He gas over distances of a few centimeters achieved by following the decay of tagged ("striped") longitudinal magnetization. In (a), each grayscale image of this healthy lung advances 1.96 s (the first being immediately after initial tagging pulses). Little decay of modulation is evident, and the resultant map of D_{sec} has an average of 0.017 cm^2/s, about 12× smaller than D_{msec}. In (b), each grayscale image advances only 0.38 s; decay is apparent beginning at image no. 2. D_{sec} approaches D_0 in the apex—an increase of 50× over healthy lung. [From Ref. (76).]

blood signal intensity for patients breathing oxygen compared with breathing room air is about 15% (79). In the clinical setting, oxygen enhancement can be used to aid in diagnosis of pulmonary embolism by identifying areas of decreased signal where vessels have poor oxygen uptake. This method can also be used to evaluate regional oxygen distribution for lung diseases such as asthma or emphysema. In emphysema, affected areas have decreased oxygen enhancement due to a decrease in direct diffusion of molecular oxygen to the capillary bed (78). This oxygen-enhancement technique is much less complex and less expensive than that of hyperpolarized gas. However, unlike hyperpolarized gas, dynamic imaging of ventilation cannot be performed, nor are diffusion images available.

E. Intrapulmonary pAO_2

Oxygen-sensitive ^{3}He MRI can be used to measure alveolar pAO_2 due to the paramagnetic properties of oxygen, which allow oxygen to cause depolarization of hyperpolarized ^{3}He (80). The relationship between the pAO_2 and the loss of oxygen is linear and can be measured by calculating the T_1 relaxation time of ^{3}He (81,82). A close correlation has been observed between pAO_2 calculated via ^{3}He T_1 and measurements of end-tidal pAO_2 (83). The ^{3}He MR technique shows promise for estimating oxygen uptake by the lung and monitoring V/Q mismatch.

F. Perfusion Imaging

Pulmonary emboli can be diagnosed with MR angiography using intravenous Gd injection. Gd increases signal intensity on T_1-weighted images by reducing the T_1 relaxation time constant of blood (77). Imaging during the first pass of the CA (prior to its egress from the circulation) shows a signal defect in the area of the clot. Blood pool agents such as ultrasmall SPIO particles have also been used. As the half-life of SPIO particles in blood is longer than Gd-based CAs, their use allows a more prolonged investigation time in areas of slow or complex blood flow. Another technique for evaluating pulmonary embolism is by imaging pulmonary perfusion using arterial spin tagging. In this case, no CA is necessary. The water in pulmonary arterial water is "labeled" with an RF pulse and detected as it enters the lung. The spatial resolution and signal-to-noise ratio are lower for this technique than for methods involving administration of CA (84).

In an attempt to learn more about the pathophysiology of certain diseases, perfusion imaging with Gd has been used to evaluate pulmonary blood flow in conditions such as pneumonia and chronic obstructive pulmonary disease (COPD) (85). CAs are also being used to evaluate perfusion in lungs of patients with known ventilation defects, such as emphysema, while ventilation is measured using hyperpolarized gas and/or oxygen. This information is especially helpful for severe emphysema patients (86–89), who may require lung volume reduction surgery to improve shortness of breath and help lung function (90).

The combination of contrast blood-flow measurements and ventilation MRI has several advantages over scintigraphy. These include greater spatial resolution, incorporation of functional and anatomical information, and the ability to visualize pulmonary vasculature without ionizing radiation. However, drawbacks of using gadolinium chelates as CA include the necessity of acquiring information with the first pass of the CA and leakage of Gd into the extracellular space. These combine to cause the first-pass signal to reflect perfusion and first-pass extraction fraction. As a result, an absolute quantification of perfusion cannot be obtained (85). To date, studies on this method have included only small groups of subjects; larger studies are needed to prove efficacy.

IV. Future Prospects

In summary, the use of MR methods for molecular imaging is a relatively new and rapidly advancing area, as substantiated by the myriad strategies currently under development. These methods are just now finding their way into evaluation of lung (e.g., imaging of oxygen status via ^{3}He T_1 measurements). This delay is likely related to the technical difficulties inherent in lung MRI. With time, a variety of unique lung-specific approaches, including agents and methods that target lung tumors and fibrotic lesions, will be developed to meet these challenges.

Acknowledgment

We thank Professor Joseph J. H. Ackerman, Washington University in St. Louis, for encouragement and helpful discussions.

References

1. Allport J, Weissleder R. *In vivo* imaging of gene and cell therapies. Exp Hematol 2001; 29:1237–1246.
2. Bremer C, Weissleder R. *In vivo* imaging of gene expression. Acad Radiol 2001; 8:15–23.
3. Gillies R. *In vivo* molecular imaging. J Cell Biochem Suppl 2002; 39:231–238.
4. Artemov D. Molecular magnetic resonance imaging with targeted contrast agents. J Cell Biochem 2003; 90:518–524.
5. Blankenberg F. Molecular imaging: the latest generation of contrast agent and tissue characterization techniques. J Cell Biochem 2003; 90:443–453.
6. Piwnica-Worms D, Schuster DP, Garbow JR. Molecular imaging of host–pathogen interactions in intact small animals. Cell Microbiol 2004; 6:319–331.
7. Weinmann H-J, Ebert W, Misselwitz B, Schmitt-Willich H. Tissue-specific MR contrast agents. Eur J Radiol 2003; 46:33–44.
8. Flacke S, Fischer S, Scott M et al. Novel MRI contrast agent for molecular imaging of fibrin: implications for detecting vulnerable plaques. Circulation 2001; 104:1280–1285.
9. Konda S, Aref M, Wang S, Brechbiel M, Wiener E. Specific targeting of folate-dendrimer MRI contrast agents to the high affinity folate receptor expressed in ovarian tumor xenografts. Magma 2001; 12:104–113.
10. Shen T, Bogdanov A, Bogdanova A, Poss K, Brady T, Weissleder R. Magnetically labeled secretin retains receptor affinity to pancreas acinar cells. Bioconjugate Chem 1996; 7:311–316.
11. Winter P, Morawksi A, Caruthers S et al. Molecular imaging of angiogenesis in early-stage atherosclerosis with $\alpha_v\beta_3$-antegrin-targeted nanoparticles. Circulation 2003; 108:2270–2274.
12. Brooks P, Montgomery A, Rosenfeld M et al. Integrin $\alpha_v\beta_3$ antagomists promote tumor regression by inducing apoptosis of angiogenic blood vessels. Cell 1994; 79:1157–1164.

13. Li W-H, Fraser S, Meade T. A calcium-sensitive magnetic resonance imaging contrast agent. J Am Chem Soc 1999; 121:1413–1414.
14. Li W-H, Parigi G, Fragai M, Luchinat C, Meade T. Mechanistic studies of a calcium-dependent MRI contrast agent. Inorg Chem 2002; 41:4018–4024.
15. Aime S, Barge A, Delli Castelli D et al. Paramagnetic lanthanide(III) complexes as pH-sensitive chemical exchange saturation transfer (CEST) contrast agents for MRI applications. Magn Reson Med 2002; 47:639–648.
16. Aime S, Botta M, Gianolio E, Terreno E. A $p(O_2)$-responsive MRI contrast agent based on the redox switch of manganese(II/III)-porphyrin complexes. Angew Chem Int Ed Engl 2000; 39:747–750.
17. Zhang S, Winter P, Wu K, Sherry A. A novel europium(III)-based MRI contrast agent. J Am Chem Soc 2001; 123:1517–1518.
18. Aime S, Delli Castelli D, Fedeli F, Terreno E. A paramagnetic MRI-CEST agent responsive to lactate concentration. J Am Chem Soc 2002; 124:9364–9365.
19. Zhang S, Merritt M, Woessner DE, Lenkinski RE, Sherry AD. PARACEST agents: modulating MRI contrast via water proton exchange. Acc Chem Res 2003; 36:783–790.
20. Zhang S, Trokowski R, Sherry AD. A paramagnetic CEST agent for imaging glucose by MRI. J Am Chem Soc 2003, 125.15288–15289.
21. Matsumura A, Shibata Y, Nakagawa K, Nose T. MRI contrast enhancement by Gd-DTPA-monocolonal antibody in 9L glioma rats. Acta Neurochir Suppl 1994; 60:356–358.
22. Shahbazi-Gahrouei D, Williams M, Rizvi S, Allan B. *In vivo* studies of Gd-DTPA-monoclonal antibody and Gd-porphyrins: potential magnetic resonance imaging contrast agents for melanoma. J Magn Reson Imaging 2001; 14:169–174.
23. Sipkins D, Cheresh D, Kazemi M, Nevin L, Bednarski M, Li K. Detection of tumor angiogenesis *in vivo* by $\alpha_v\beta_3$-targeted magnetic resonance imaging. Nat Med 1998; 4:623–626.
24. Anderson S, Rader R, Westin W et al. Magnetic resonance contrast enhancement with $\alpha_v\beta_3$ targeted nanoparticles. Magn Reson Medicine 2000; 44:433–439.
25. Artemov D, Mori N, Ravi R, Bhujwalla Z. Magnetic resonance molecular imaging of the Her-2/neu receptor. Cancer Res 2003; 63:2723–2727.
26. Kang H, Josephson L, Petrovsky A, Weissleder R, Bogdanov A Jr. Magnetic resonance imaging of inducible E-selectin expression in human endothelial cell culture. Bioconjugate Chem 2002; 13:122–127.
27. Artemov D, Mori N, Okollie B, Bhujwalla Z. MR molecular imaging of the Her-2/neu receptor in breast cancer cells using targeted iron oxide nanoparticles. Magn Reson Med 2003; 49:403–408.
28. Dodd CH, Hsu HC, Chu WJ et al. Normal T-cell response and *in vivo* magnetic resonance imaging of T cells loaded with HIV transactivator-peptide-derived superparamagnetic nanoparticles. J Immunol Methods 2001; 256:89–105.
29. Sundstrom JB, Mao H, Santoianni R et al. Magnetic resonance imaging of activated proliferating rhesus macaque T cells labeled with superparamagnetic monocrystalline iron oxide nanoparticles. J Acquir Immune Defic Syndr 2004; 35:9–21.
30. Anderson SA, Shukaliak-Quandt J, Jordan EK et al. Magnetic resonance imaging of labeled T-cells in a mouse model of multiple sclerosis. Ann Neurol 2004; 55:654–659.

31. Kircher MF, Allport JR, Graves EE et al. *In vivo* high resolution three-dimensional imaging of antigen-specific cytotoxic T-lymphocyte trafficking to tumors. Cancer Res 2003; 63:6838–6846.

32. Jendelova P, Herynek V, DeCroos J et al. Imaging the fate of implanted bone marrow stromal cells labeled with superparamagnetic nanoparticles. Magn Reson Med 2003; 50:767–776.

33. Jendelova P, Herynek V, Urdzikova L et al. Magnetic resonance tracking of transplanted bone marrow and embryonic stem cells labeled by iron oxide nanoparticles in rat brain and spinal cord. J Neurosci Res 2004; 76:232–243.

34. Arbab AS, Jordan EK, Wilson LB, Yocum GT, Lewis BK, Frank JA. *In vivo* trafficking and targeted delivery of magnetically labeled stem cells. Hum Gene Ther 2004; 15:351–360.

35. Weissleder R, Moore A, Mahmood U et al. *In vivo* magnetic resonance imaging of transgene expression. Nat Biotechnol 2000; 6:351–354.

36. Lewin M, Carlesso N, Tung C et al. Tat peptide-derivatized magnetic nanoparticles allow *in vivo* tracking and recovery of progenitor cells. Nat Biotechnol 2000; 18:410.

37. Louie A, Huver M, Ahrens E et al. *In vivo* visualization of gene expression using magnetic resonance imaging. Nat Biotechnol 2000; 18:321–325.

38. Enochs W, Petherick P, Bogdanova A, Mohr U, Weissleder R. Paramagnetic metal scavenging by melanin: MR imaging. Radiology 1997; 204:417.

39. Weissleder R, Simonova M, Bogdanova A, Bredow S, Enochs W, Bogdanov A Jr. MR imaging and scintigraphy of gene expression through melanin induction. Radiology 1997; 204:425–429.

40. Hedlund L, Dewalt S, Cofer G, Johnson G. MR microscopy of the lung. In: Cutillo A, ed. Application of Magnetic Resonance to the Study of the Lung. Futura Press, 1996; 401–415.

41. Schuster D, Kovacs A, Garbow JR, Piwnica-Worms D. Recent advances in imaging the lungs of intact small animals. Am J Respir Cell Molecular Biol 2004; 30:129–138.

42. Beckman N, Tigani B, Mazzoni L, Fozard J. MRI of lung parenchyma in rats and mice using a gradient-echo sequence. NMR Biomed 2001; 14:297–306.

43. Hedlund L, Johnson G. Mechanical ventilation for imaging the small animal lung. ILAR 2002; 43:159–174.

44. Garbow JR, Dugas J, Conradi M. Respiratory gating for MRI and MRS in rodents. IEEE Symp Bioinformatic Bioeng 2003; 3:126–129.

45. Garbow JR, Dugas J, Song S-K, Conradi M. A Simple, Robust hardware device for passive or active respiratory gating in MRI and MRS experiments. Concepts Magn Reson, Part B: Magn Reson Eng 2004; 21B:40–48.

46. Caruthers S, Paschal C, Pou N, Harris T. Relative quantification of pulmonary edema with non-contrast enhanced MRI. J Magn Reson Imaging 1997; 7:544–550.

47. Caruthers S, Paschal C, Pou N, Roselli J, Harris T. Regional measurements of pulmonary edema by using magnetic resonance imaging. J Appl Physiol 1998; 84:2143–2153.

48. Cutillo A, Goodrich K, Krishnamurthy G et al. Lung water measurement by nuclear magnetic resonance: correlation with morphometry. J Appl Physiol 1995; 79:2163–2168.

49. Beckmann N, Tigani B, Ekatodramis D, Borer R, Mazzoni L, Fozard J. Pulmonary edema induced by allergen challenge in the rat: noninvasive assessment by magnetic resonance imaging. Magn Reson Med 2001; 45:88–95.

50. Tigani B, Schaeublin E, Sugar R, Jackson A, Rozard J, Beckmann N. Pulmonary inflammation monitored noninvasively by MRI in freely breathing rats. Biochem Biophys Res Commun 2002; 292:216–221.

51. Garbow JR, Zhang Z, You M. Detection of primary lung tumors in rodents by magnetic resonance imaging. Cancer Res 2004; 64:2740–2742.

52. Moller H, Chen X, Saam B et al. MRI of the lungs using hyperpolarized noble gases. Magn Reson Med 2002; 47:1029–1051.

53. Leawoods JC, Yablonskiy DA, Saam B, Gierada DS, Conradi MS. Hyperpolarized ^{3}He gas production and MR imaging of the lung. Concepts Magn Reson 2001; 13:277–293.

54. de Lange E, Mugler J III, Brookeman J et al. Lung air spaced: MR imaging evaluation with hyperpolarized ^{3}He Gas. Radiology 1999; 210:851–857.

55. Salerno M, Altes T, Brookeman J, de Lange E, Mugler J III. Dynamic spiral MRI of pulmonary gas flow using hyperpolarized ^{3}He: preliminary studies in healthy and diseased lungs. Magn Reson Med 2001; 46:667–677.

56. Salerno M, de Lange E, Altes T, Truwit J, Brookeman J, Mugler J III. Emphysema: hyperpolarized helium 3 diffusion MR imaging of the lungs compared with spirometric indexes-initial experience. Radiology 2002; 222:252–260.

57. Deninger A, Mansson S, Petersson J et al. Quantitative measurement of regional lung ventilation using ^{3}He MRI. Magn Reson Med 2002; 48:223–232.

58. Chen X, Chawla M, Hedlund L, Moller H, MacFall J, Johnson G. MR microscopy of lung airways with hyperpolarized ^{3}He. Magn Reson Med 1998; 39:79–84.

59. Moller H, Chen X, Chawla M et al. Sensitivity and resolution in 3D NMR microscopy of the lung with hyperpolarized noble gases. Magn Reson Med 1999; 41:800–808.

60. Viallon M, Cofer G, Suddarth S et al. Functional MR microcopy of the lung using hyperpolarized ^{3}He. Magn Reson Med 1999; 41:787–792.

61. Johnson G, Cofer G, Hedlund L, Maronpot R, Suddarth S. Registered ^{1}H and ^{3}He magnetic resonance microscopy of the lung. Magn Reson Med 2001; 45:365–370.

62. Altes T, Powers P, Knight-Scott J et al. Hyperpolarized ^{3}He MR lung ventilation imaging in asthmatics: preliminary findings. J Magn Reson Imaging 2001; 13:378–384.

63. Donnelly L, MacFall J, McAdams H et al. Cystic fibrosis: combined hyperpolarized ^{3}He-enhanced and conventional proton MR imaging in the lung—preliminary observations. Radiology 1999; 212:885–889.

64. McAdams HP, Palmer SM, Donnelly LF, Charles HC, Tapson VF, MacFall JR. Hyperpolarized ^{3}He-enhanced MR imaging of lung transplant recipients: preliminary results. AJR Am J Roentgenol 1999; 173:955–959.

65. Kauczor HU, Markstaller K, Puderbach M et al. Volumetry of ventilated airspaces by 3He MRI: preliminary results. Invest Radiol 2001; 36:110–114.

66. Zaporozhan J, Ley S, Gast KK et al. Functional analysis in single-lung transplant recipients: a comparative study of high-resolution CT, ^{3}He-MRI, and pulmonary function tests. Chest 2004; 125:173–181.

67. Chen B, Brau A, Johnson G. Measurement of regional lung function in rats using hyperpolarized ^{3}He dynamic MRI. Magn Reson Med 2003; 49:78–88.

68. Cremillieux Y, Berthezene Y, Humblot H et al. A combined ^{1}H perfusion/^{3}He ventilation NMR study in rat lungs. Magn Reson Med 1999; 41:645–648.

69. Viallon M, Berthezene Y, Decorps M et al. Laser-polarized ^{3}He as a probe for dynamic regional measurements of lung perfusion and ventilation using magnetic resonance imaging. Magn Reson Med 2000; 44:1–4.

70. Gast KK, Puderbach MU, Rodriguez I et al. Distribution of ventilation in lung transplant recipients: evaluation by dynamic ^{3}He-MRI with lung motion correction. Invest Radiol 2003; 38:341–348.

71. Iwasawa T, Yoshiike Y, Saito K, Kagei S, Gotoh T, Matsubara S. Paradoxical motion of the hemidiaphragm in patients with emphysema. J Thorac Imaging 2000; 15:191–195.

72. Iwasawa T, Kagei S, Gotoh T et al. Magnetic resonance analysis of abnormal diaphragmatic motion in patients with emphysema. Eur Respir J 2002; 19:225–231.

73. Suga K, Tsukuda T, Awaya H et al. Impaired respiratory mechanics in pulmonary emphysema: evaluation with dynamic breathing MRI. J Magn Reson Imaging 1999; 10:510–520.

74. Chen X, Hedlund L, Moller H, Chawla M, Maronpot R, Johnson G. Detection of emphysema in rat lungs by using magnetic resonance measurements of ^{3}He diffusion. PNAS 2000; 97:11478–11481.

75. Yablonskiy D, Sukstanskii A, Leawoods J et al. Quantitative *in vivo* assessment of lung microstructure at the alveolar level with hyperpolarized ^{3}He diffusion MRI. PNAS 2002; 99:3111–3116.

76. Leawoods J, Yablonskiy D, Choong C et al. Short- and long-range diffusivities of ^{3}He in healthy and emphysematous, excised human lungs. Proceedings of the 12th International Society for Magnetic Resonance in Medicine, 2004; 12:1683.

77. Kauczor HU, Chen XJ, van Beek EJ, Schreiber WG. Pulmonary ventilation imaged by magnetic resonance: at the doorstep of clinical application. Eur Respir J 2001; 17:1008–1023.

78. Ohno Y, Hatabu H, Takenaka D, Van Cauteren M, Fujii M, Sugimura K. Dynamic oxygen-enhanced MRI reflects diffusing capacity of the lung. Magn Reson Med 2002; 47:1139–1144.

79. Loffler R, Muller CJ, Peller M et al. Optimization and evaluation of the signal intensity change in multisection oxygen-enhanced MR lung imaging. Magn Reson Med 2000; 43:860–866.

80. Eberle B, Weiler N, Markstaller K et al. Analysis of intrapulmonary O_2 concentration by MR imaging of inhaled hyperpolarized helium-3. J Appl Physiol 1999; 87:2043–2052.

81. Deninger AJ, Eberle B, Ebert M et al. Quantification of regional intrapulmonary oxygen partial pressure evolution during apnea by ^{3}He MRI. J Magn Reson 1999; 141:207–216.

82. Deninger AJ, Eberle B, Bermuth J et al. Assessment of a single-acquisition imaging sequence for oxygen-sensitive ^{3}He-MRI. Magn Reson Med 2002; 47:105–114.

83. Durand E, Guillot G, Darrasse L et al. CPMG measurements and ultrafast imaging in human lungs with hyperpolarized helium-3 at low field (0.1 T). Magn Reson Med 2002; 47:75–81.

84. Wielopolski P, Oudkerk M, van Ooijen P. Magnetic resonance imaging and angiography of the pulmonary vascular system. In: Oudkerk M, van Beek E, ten Cate I, eds. Pulmonary Embolism. Berlin: Blackwell Science, 1999:250–329.

85. Amundsen T, Torheim G, Waage A, Bjermer L, Steen PA, Haraldseth O. Perfusion magnetic resonance imaging of the lung: characterization of pneumonia and chronic obstructive pulmonary disease. A feasibility study. J Magn Reson Imaging 2000; 12:224–231.

86. Sergiacomi G, Sodani G, Fabiano S et al. MRI lung perfusion 2D dynamic breath-hold technique in patients with severe emphysema. In Vivo 2003; 17:319–324.

87. Haraldseth O, Amundsen T, Rinck PA. Contrast-enhanced pulmonary MR imaging. Magma 1999; 8:146–153.

88. Hatabu H, Chen Q, Levin DL, Tadamura E, Edelman RR. Ventilation-perfusion MR imaging of the lung. Magn Reson Imaging Clin N Am 1999; 7:379–392.

89. Johkoh T, Muller NL, Kavanagh PV et al. Scintigraphic and MR perfusion imaging in preoperative evaluation for lung volume reduction surgery: pilot study results. Radiat Med 2000; 18:277–281.

90. Gierada DS, Hakimian S, Slone RM, Yusen RD. MR analysis of lung volume and thoracic dimensions in patients with emphysema before and after lung volume reduction surgery. AJR Am J Roentgenol 1998; 170:707–714.

91. Dugas J, Garbow JR, Kobayashi D, Conradi M. Hyperpolarized ^{3}He MRI of mouse lung. Magn Reson Med 2004; 52:1310–1317.

6

Imaging the Mouse Lung with Micro-CT

**WOLFGANG RECHEIS, GEOFFREY McLENNAN,
ALAN F. ROSS, and ERIC A. HOFFMAN**

University of Iowa,
Iowa City, Iowa, USA

ANN V. Clough

Marquette University,
Milwaukee, Wisconsin, USA

STEVEN T. HAWORTH

Medical College of Wisconsin,
Milwaukee, Wisconsin, USA

I. Introduction

Computed tomography (CT) of the lung has made major advances in hardware and software over the last decade. The human lung can now be imaged rapidly and volumetrically, with digital information easily transported, stored, reviewed, and then both subjectively and objectively analyzed (1,2). Figure 6.1 depicts examples that span anatomic segmentation (3–8), automatic labeling (9), image based lung modeling (10,11), ventilation (12,13) and perfusion imaging (14,15), a morphometric correlation to *in vivo* imaging (16), and a large animal model of evolving lung inflammation. In large animal models, functional imaging demonstrates early changes in pathology (17). Our methods demonstrate that measures of both structure and function provide early signs of pathologic processes (2). Still, there remains a need to correlate pathologic phenotypes with genotypes and to phenotype diversity at the alveolar/bronchiolar and arteriolar levels *in vivo* and *in situ*.

It is our view that micro-CT will have a profound influence on the documentation of anatomical and physiological phenotypic changes in many genetic mouse models. The mapping of the human genome, together with that of other animals and plants, is providing an enormous amount of new information, the full extent of which will still emerge over the next several decades. The mouse has become the prototypic animal model for the study of genetic based diseases. Frequently, however, abnormalities are noted within the animals, beyond the specifically induced biological defect or outside the targeted organ. Thus, the full phenotype of these animals may include a variety of unexpected anatomical and physiological abnormalities, in addition to biochemical and genetic changes. Describing these abnormalities fully is critical to understanding the complex interaction of different genetic influences. Although individual animals are relatively inexpensive, the cost of developing a model can be very significant. This expense is amplified when animals must be sacrificed and studied at multiple time points during growth or during the development of a disease. Determining such time points is somewhat arbitrary, and important information may not be recorded if complete observations are not made. Micro-CT scanning will allow numerous experiments in mouse models to be planned with greater precision. The cost of exploring the complex phenotypic expression of genetic changes will be reduced, and longitudinal studies will be greatly facilitated by allowing a more complete and accurate description of events. As shown in Fig. 6.2, mouse imaging using conventional CT scanners lacks the spatial resolution needed. To maximize the potential of micro-CT to quantitatively evaluate the mouse lung, imaging protocols, reconstruction algorithms, and image analysis methods all must be established and specifically tailored to *in vivo*, *in situ*, and *ex vivo* imaging of lung tissue.

The normal mouse lung differs from the human lung in overall size, alveolar size, lung segmentation into different lobes, and respiratory rate (18). Thus, understanding phenotypic lung expression may be facilitated by the development of a CT derived structural lung atlas of the normal adult mouse, such a reference image library for the mouse lung currently does not exist. Of great importance to micro-imaging, however, is the fact that alveolar size does not scale with the rest of the animal, and thus it is possible to image alveolar level structure with a resolution in reach of current micro-CT scanners.

In addition to the normal lung, mouse models of human disease create the opportunity to evaluate structural and functional characteristics that cannot easily be assessed in the human. For example, reasonable mouse models of pulmonary emphysema exist that develop from either smoking or various induced genetic abnormalities. Many mouse models, however, do not faithfully replicate human pathophysiology. For example, the mouse model of cystic fibrosis does not develop the same type of lung disease as the human counterpart (19). Therefore, a full characterization of these models will require the development of specific mouse ventilators and pulmonary function testing equipment (18), the development of micro-CT scanners built specifically for mouse studies, and the development of 3D microscopy/pathology techniques. These three complementary techniques will then allow information-rich cross-sectional and longitudinal studies in the normal animal as well as relevant environmentally induced and genetic lung disease models.

We are establishing methods which will allow imaging of the respiratory system of a mouse (*in vivo*, *in situ*, and *ex vivo*) by micro-CT with repeatable accuracy. The acquired spatial and density information will establish a normative atlas against which early pathologic processes can be detected and followed. The information provided subsequently is a summary of that process in relation to methods of X-ray imaging in general and micro-CT specifically. The use of micro-CT, however, is not limited only to small rodent imaging. There is also increasing interest in studying structures from biopsy probes of humans and large animals, and these same methods will be appropriate for these applications as well.

II. Technical Principals and Overview of Micro-CT

The basic principles of micro-CT or cone-beam CT have been described by a number of papers. The topics range from mathematical theories on cone-beam reconstruction, or detector and X-ray source design, to practical applications. Jorgensen et al. (20), Ritman (21,22), and Rüegsegger et al. (23) give a good overview of the technical basis for micro-CT, and micro-CT continues to advance with improving hardware and software.

A. Micro-CT Introduction

Micro-CT scanners have inherent system limitations in their signal-to-noise ratio (SNR) performance due to their small voxel size and relatively low X-ray exposure level, but they can be used effectively to scan the bony structures of a small animal (24–26). *In vivo* soft tissue imaging is still a challenge, however, because long exposure times cause motion artifacts, which limit

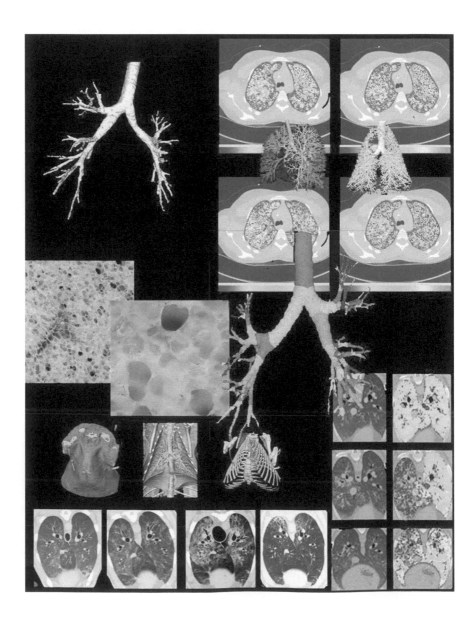

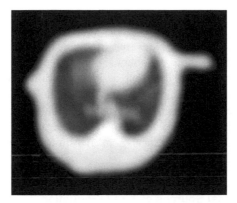

Figure 6.2 A conventional medical CT scanner provides a spatial resolution at best of roughly 100 μm × 100 μm × 750 μm voxels. In this example, a mouse lung was scanned with a state-of-the-art Siemens system. In contrast to micro-CT, the scanning time is much faster the whole data volume was acquired in ~2 s. It is obvious that these methods cannot be used to study small structures in the lung down to alveolar level.

spatial resolution and the SNR. The first commercially available micro-CT devices came to market only a few years ago (27). The invention and introduction of high-resolution CCD detectors (up to 4k by 4k matrix and more) together with X-ray sources having small and variable focal spots, combined with relatively

---

Figure 6.1 **(See color insert)** Shown is a composite representing several methods for quantifying the lung, including airway segmentation (upper left), airway segment labeling (center), and color coding of blood flow parameters (upper and lower right) from a time series analysis of the passage of a bolus of iodinated contrast agent. Super-imposed on the upper right blood flow images, we display a mathematical model of the airway tree for both humans (left) and sheep (right). This model actually extends out to the terminal bronchi and is generated from a starting segmentation of the lungs and airway tree using CT scanning, providing a subject specific, complete airway tree model (work in collaboration with Merryn Tawhai and Peter Hunter, Auckland, New Zealand). In the lower portion of the image, we demonstrate a sheep model of lung inflammation leading to emphysema. Cross-sectional images with and without superposition of blood flow are shown in the lower right. Color coded images of perfusion at day 16 (lower row of this grouping) demonstrate the emergence of flow pattern abnormalities in the left lung which match the blood flow patterns in the treated right lung. Matching gray scale images showed no signs of pathology either visually or through a quantitative evaluation of the lung density histogram. The volumetric images one row from the bottom demonstrate that we are able to image the sheep (and humans) volumetrically in great detail. In the middle left, we depict our ability to harvest lungs to establish pathologic correlates with the CT images. Micro-CT, as discussed in this chapter, provides the link between these large animal and human imaging studies to the micro-CT evaluation of the mouse lung at the very interface of gas exchange (see text for references to works represented by this composite image).

high power, have made *in vivo* lung scanning of small animals possible. Table 6.1 gives an overview of some commercially available micro-CT systems that are designed for *in vivo* studies. Note that this table is not complete and only a few parameters of the various scanners are presented.

Figure 6.3 shows two different design possibilities of micro-CT. In the upper panel (developed at Marquette University), the system rotates the animal or specimen. In the lower panel, the system rotates the X-ray tube and detector around the animal. An important trade-off is the cumulative dose exposure during the scan when long-term survival *in vivo* studies are considered (discussed subsequently) (28).

B. Micro-Focal Sources of X-ray Production

In general, micro-CT scanners use micro-focal X-ray sources, except in very special cases where other X-ray sources are applied, such as synchrotron radiation, laser-induced X-ray production, or conventional X-ray tubes (29,30).

The focal spot is the region of an X-ray tube anode from which X-rays emanate as a result of electron impact. The size of the focal spot is a critical parameter in many X-ray imaging systems, including projection radiography and computed tomography, and certainly in micro-CT. Newer generations of X-ray tubes for cone-beam micro-CT have a focal spot size of <1 μm. A smaller focal spot size generally allows better resolution. This effect, sometimes called geometric unsharpness, depends on the location of the object in the source-to-detector direction. The impact of the focal spot on resolution increases with geometric magnification, that is, increasing distance between the object and the detector for a fixed source-to-detector distance. Thus, a small focal spot is desired to optimize spatial resolution.

The power of micro-focal X-ray tubes ranges between 4 and 100 W. X-ray tubes $>10-20$ W need to have a variable focal spot to prevent the (tungsten) anode from melting or evaporating, because the electron impact for X-ray production is focused on a small area. Therefore, if an X-ray tube is operating at its power limit, decreasing the size of the focal spot will require a decrease in the tube current. There is, therefore, a trade-off between increased spatial resolution due to the smaller size of the focal spot and increased image noise in a fixed exposure time due to the necessary decrease in X-ray intensity.

C. Filters

Commercially available micro-CT systems utilize X-ray sources with tungsten as the anode material, which has a characteristic X-ray emission spectrum. This spectrum has a significant peak at $\sim$60 kV and a second peak at 67 kV at a typical maximum kinetic energy of the electrons of 100 kV (Fig. 6.4). Tissue absorbs X-rays better with lower energy photons (about energy^3 dependence in regions <25 kV) (31).

Table 6.1 Some Performance Characteristics of Commercially Available Micro-CT Scanners

	Scanco	Skyscan	Imtek	EVS/GE	Stratec	BIR
Scanner product	VivaCT 40	Skyscan 1076	MicroCAT 2	Explore RS	XCT Research M	Actis Volume CT
X-ray source	Focal spot: 5–7 μm, 30–70 kV, 160 μA	Focal spot: 5 μm, 20–100 kV, 40–200 μA	Focal spot: 9 μm, 20–130 kV, 400 μA	Focal spot: 2–90 kV, 180 μA	Focal spot: 50 μm, 45–60 kV, 0.2–500 μA	Focal spot: 3 μm, 10–225 kV, 0.01–300 μA
Detector size	2048 × 255	4000 × 2300	4096 × 4096	2048 × 2048	12 detectors	1408 × 1888
Field of view (mm)	20–40	35 or 38	35–110	40	50	300
Spatial resolution (μm)	10	9–35	15	27–90	70–500	12.5
Scan speed	360 s	5 fps	5 fps	180–900 s	80 s	1–30 fps

(a)

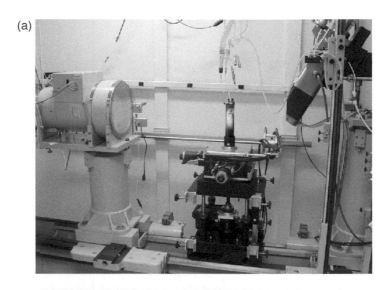

(b)

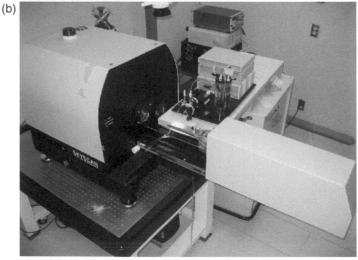

Figure 6.3 There are two basic methods for constructing a micro-CT either the X-ray source–detector system remains fixed and the object rotates (a) or the source–detector system rotates around the fixed object (b). Method (b) is normally used for *in vivo* scanners. Figure (a) represents the X-ray imaging system with the detector (left), source (right), and stage (center) supporting a mouse or rat. This technique is suitable for very high spatial resolutions down to 1 μm. In special cases (described in the text), CT imaging is performed by rotating the specimen within the beam using a typical total scan time of ∼2 min. Dynamic angiographic projection imaging can be performed at 60 frames/s during the passage of a bolus of X-ray contrast medium. Figure (a) shows a commercially available *in vivo* scanning system with physiologic monitoring and gating possibilities (Skyscan 1076).

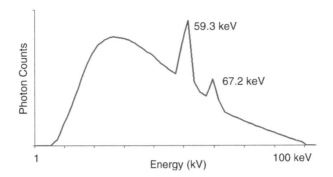

Figure 6.4 X-ray emission spectrum of tungsten at a maximum electron energy of 100 kV with its characteristic peaks at 59.3 kV and 67.2 kV.

There are attempts to create more mono-energetic X-rays by using the characteristic $K\alpha$ emission radiation of certain anode metals like copper, silver, or molybdenum. Generally, however, tungsten is used most commonly, especially for *in vivo* scanning which demands shorter acquisition and higher X-ray energies, especially for the measurement of bony structures.

These factors have a significant influence on imaging soft tissues. Profiles of tissues with rather similar attenuations cannot be resolved effectively, resulting in similar gray values after image reconstruction. One way to optimize these profiles, and to improve the image resolution of tissues with similar gray scales, is to use metal filters to block specific ranges of the X-ray spectrum. The filter quality is dependent on the material used and on its thickness. For example, 0.5 mm aluminum significantly filters the emission spectrum from <10 kV to ~25 kV. In contrast, titanium (25 µm thickness) shows a significant peak at 7 kV (Fig. 6.5). Other materials used are copper, tin, and other metals in various thicknesses depending on the energy to be eliminated. For any soft tissue imaging, including the lung, the right choice of filter and of scanning parameters (kilovolt and microampere) must be determined empirically.

D. Some Detector Characteristics

The physical parameters of the detectors/cameras are also of critical importance. These determine the resolution of the scanner. The field of view (FOV) that can be covered, namely the x–y field of view and the z-axis coverage, is also determined by the detectors. Modern high resolution CCD cameras are composed of an element size of a few micrometers. The CCD matrix ranges up to 4k × 4k in the newest generation of commercially available micro-CT scanners. A typical system comprises a 10 megapixel CCD camera (4000 × 2300 effective pixels), with a 12 bit dynamic output and a 6.7 µm pixel size at the CCD surface. The CCD is coated with a thin layer of a material that is capable of converting X-ray photons into visible light. In many cases, gadolinium oxide is used, this

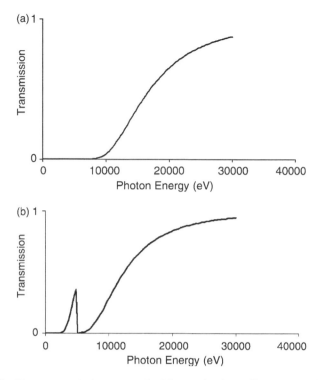

Figure 6.5 X-ray transmission curve of a 0.5 mm aluminum filter (a) at the lower end of the energy spectrum, transmission decreases, and then gets X-ray transparent >30 kV. The lower image shows the different transmission capabilities of a 25 μm titanium filter with a significant peak at 7 kV (data from: http://www.cxro.lbl.gov/).

has a very specific sensitivity curve (Fig. 6.6). Another material used for X-ray to light conversion is cesium iodine.

Yet another critical parameter is the read-out time of the signals. The shorter the read-out time, the better the temporal resolution between single exposures. A typical CCD system has a minimum read-out time of 100–200 ms. The read-out time is of importance for *in vivo* scanning of moving targets such as the lung. A mouse breathes with a rate up to 180 times/min. Even with sedation, the respiratory rate is ~60 times/min. Even if a detector with a very fast read-out time is available (in the range of milliseconds), a significant number of photons is required to create reasonable images, thus dictating a minimum aperture time for a single exposure. Therefore, this situation presents another significant trade-off: to improve image quality for a given single exposure the X-ray dose has to be increased. In many cases, the X-ray tube is not capable of delivering the necessary amount of photons or the applied dose will have a significant impact on the animal's health when long term repeated *in vivo* scanning is needed (Section E). One way of scanning the breathing

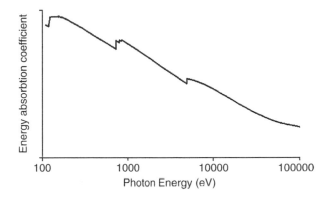

Figure 6.6 X-ray energy absorption curve of gadolinium oxide which converts X-ray photons into visible light. CCD cameras or other light sensitive devices measure emitted photons. Note there is a significant impact on detector sensitivity as a function of photon energy (data from http://physics.nist.gov/PhysRefData/XrayMassCoef/ElemTab).

lung is to gate the micro-CT scanner to the respiratory cycle whereby each angle of view is acquired at a fixed portion of the respiratory cycle. Of course, a respiratory gated scan can take significantly longer than a nongated scan since time is spent for each gate signal. This time extension may be minimized in the case of a mechanically ventilated animal where the respirator and the scanner can be optimally synchronized.

One generation of *in vivo* scanners now commercially available is capable of a read-out time of 20 ms but with a correspondingly limited spatial resolution (≥ 100 μm). These scanners are typically used in combination with functional imaging methods, like micro-PET and other nuclear imaging methods, or to make dynamic measurements.

On the basis of the physical principles just discussed, we may conclude that the total X-ray sensitivity of a micro-CT system is a function of electron energy (X-ray production), filtering (to enhance or delete certain X-ray spectra), and finally the X-ray absorption sensitivity of the X-ray converter at the CCD detector.

E. Comments on Dose Exposure

As described in a paper on quality limits of micro-CT (32), the linear attenuation coefficient is proportional to $(\text{dose})^{-1/2}$ and to the (isotropic voxel size)$^{-2}$ in the reconstructed volume. Therefore an improvement in precision can only be achieved by increasing the isotropic voxel size (thereby decreasing the resolution of the image) or by increasing the X-ray dose. A lower spectral energy will provide a higher contrast image with a micro-CT system, but there will be fewer photons reaching the detector to form the image.

This dose is ~1% of LD50/30 for a mouse (9 Gy). The LD50/30 is a measure of lethal dose to 50% of the population after 30 days. The influence of dose exposure in an experimental situation is not well explored, and there are questions regarding the possible changes that X-ray exposure could have on long term *in vivo* studies. Certainly, however, the frequency and duration of micro-CT studies have the potential to have a significant influence on mouse biology in the living animal.

F. Resolution of the Systems

In medical computed tomography, as well as with micro-CT, we distinguish between spatial and contrast resolution (i.e., the ability to distinguish between different densities). Spatial resolution is generally quantified in terms of smallest separation at which two points can be distinguished as separate entities. The limiting value of the resolution is determined by the design and construction of the system and by the amount of data and sampling method. There are methods available to measure the spatial resolution directly, and indirect methods to calculate the resolution of a system. The indirect methods are somewhat more objective compared with the direct ones.

The geometrical resolution can be represented by the modulation transfer function (MTF). Basically, the MTF is the ratio between the true dimension of the object and the resolution of the images acquired. It is usually calculated from the measurements of a thin wire phantom which provides the point spread function of the system. A given point spread function is used to calculate the MTF. The MTF curves describe the ratio of the contrast in the CT or micro-CT image to the contrast in the object with respect to the spatial frequency. The MTF demonstrates the frequency components of a structure in line pairs per millimeter (lp/mm). Normally, the MTF, and therefore the resolution of a CT system, is evaluated at 10% contrast difference (Fig. 6.7).

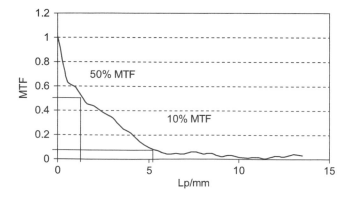

Figure 6.7 MTF of a typical micro-CT system: note the 10% threshold, that is, the frequency at which the contrast has dropped to 10% of the maximum value obtained by 0 lp/mm. This system would be capable of resolving 5 lp/mm.

G. Tomographic Reconstruction

Micro-CT typically utilizes cone-beam geometry and is thus true "volume CT". The term "volume CT" or "volumetric CT" has been used in association with the Mayo Clinic effort to build the dynamic spatial reconstructor (DSR) (33). The recent development of multislice row (MDCT) scanners represents a significant movement toward the use of true cone-beam geometry. Micro-CT offers a unique opportunity to test the mathematics and image processing needs of clinical scanners.

Early spiral-CT scanners (34) provided stacks of cross-sectional CT sections. However, the slices were separated in time. The DSR acquired all the slices simultaneously but cone-beam reconstructions required a prohibitive amount of computation time. Tomography slices in medical CT have, until recently, been generated from one-dimensional projections via fan-beam methods.

A "true" volume scanner uses two-dimensional radiographic projections that are collected via CCD cameras or other high-resolution detector arrays. The projection images are collected from different angles of view to generate the necessary volume dataset for the subsequent slice reconstruction. There are two different methods to do this: either the object rotates and the x-ray source and the detectors remain fixed or the X-ray detector unit rotates and the scanned object remains fixed. Thus, in micro-CT, the fan-beam geometry is opened to a "pyramid like" or cone-beam geometry (Fig. 6.8). This new geometry needs a much more elaborate reconstruction algorithm to calculate slices from the shadow image volume data set: the so-called cone-beam algorithm [Feldkamp algorithm, (35)]. As the volume data set is acquired via two-dimensional projections, a much higher resolution (Fig. 6.9) can be achieved when compared with fan-beam geometry. Basically, the reconstructed slices are all of the same resolution in all three spatial dimensions. This serves to accommodate oblique reconstructions and other approaches to volumetric exploration of the data.

Even today, image reconstruction remains a problem in micro-CT scanning as it is very computationally expensive. On a conventional PC (3 GHz processor, 1 Gb RAM), a reconstruction of a $1000 \times 1000 \times 1000$ cube can take several hours. Various companies are now providing workstation clusters with highly effective programs and algorithms to reconstruct high-resolution volumes in a reasonable time, thus reducing the reconstruction time to a few minutes for a $1000 \times 1000 \times 1000$ cube. To maximize the utility of micro-CT to evaluate animals over time, under multiple physiologic conditions and to explore many animals in a short period of time, it is critical that reconstruction times be, at worst, on the order of hours not days. There must also be the facility to reconstruct image data at low resolution in near real time if one is to be able to adjust experimental protocols based on the observations made at the time of the study.

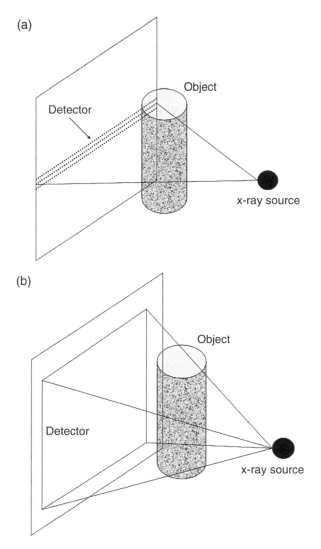

Figure 6.8 (a) The principle geometry of a "fan-beam" system: only one slice is acquired at a time. This acquisition technique is used in clinical CT scanners. In modern multi-detector CT scanners a modified fan-beam algorithm is used. (b) Principle geometry of a "cone-beam" system: this method uses full 2D X-ray profiles (shadow images) to generate a volume data set, a method typical for micro-CT.

H. Ring Artifact Reduction

Ring artifacts in the images can appear because of defective detectors or nonlinearities of the detector system. Another reason can be drift of the detector sensitivity between white field calibrations and small misalignments in the

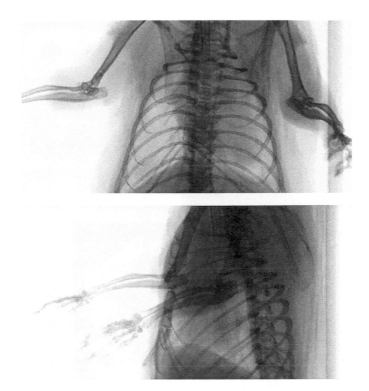

Figure 6.9 Radiographic projections or shadow images of a mouse acquired with a cone-beam micro-CT at two different angles.

scanner's center of rotation. These artifacts are undesirable because they may interfere with the qualitative and quantitative analysis of images.

Additional processing of the shadow images before the tomographic image reconstruction process can help to reduce ring artifacts (36). Examples of such artifacts are shown in Fig. 6.10.

I. Beam Hardening

As a consequence of the polychromatic X-ray source used in micro-CT and in medical CT, attenuation of X-rays is not a linear function of absorber thickness. If this nonlinear beam hardening effect is not compensated for, the reconstructed images will be corrupted by cupping artifacts. The effect causes different gray-scale value attenuation on normally homogeneous objects (such as phantoms) or the wrong determination of gray-scale values (Fig. 6.11). Especially in lung imaging, the exact determination of gray values is of critical interest as it is the only method to gain access to structural changes caused by diseases when structure *per se* is not visible. In the case of *in vivo* scanning, because of scan

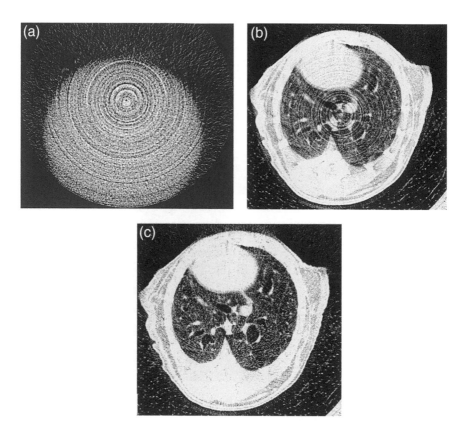

Figure 6.10   Example of ring artifacts in an image of a water phantom (a). During the reconstruction process, most of these artifacts can be reduced. (b) Mouse lung scan reconstructed without ring artifact reduction. (c) Mouse lung scan reconstructed with ring artifact reduction which results in significant improvement in image quality.

time and physiologic motion, it is not likely that one will see alveolar level structures (discussed subsequently). Reconstruction algorithms can compensate for or limit the beam hardening effect. This turns out to be a crucial step: a too low or too high chosen parameter can lead to misleading gray value distribution that can lead to a wrong quantification of tissue types.

It is essential to compensate for the beam hardening effect when analyzing gray values quantitatively because beam hardening will influence the gray value calibration significantly. Medical CT scanners offer sophisticated methods for automated Hounsfield Unit [(HU) X-ray attenuation estimates] calibration depending on the imaging protocols used. A current project in our lab deals with automation of HU calibration for micro-CT scanners, taking into account various scan protocols and the related necessary beam hardening corrections.

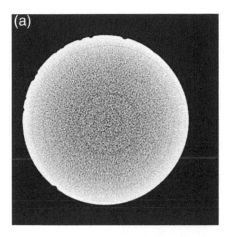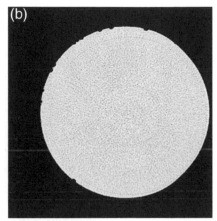

Figure 6.11 Beam hardening correction: a plastic syringe filled with water was scanned with a conventional micro-CT protocol used in *in vivo* studies. The image in (a) was calculated without beam hardening correction. Note that gray values vary from light near the surface of the syringe to darker in the middle. This effect is not caused by varying attenuation factors of the phantom itself but by the beam hardening effect. It is possible to correct this artifact during the reconstruction process (b). In this case, the gray values distribute more evenly across the reconstructed image.

J. Hounsfield Unit Calibration

Although a micro-CT is capable of having a resolution of a few micrometers or less, this may not be sufficient to image the structures of interest. For instance, in Fig. 6.12, we demonstrate the effect of imaging with a voxel size of 35, 18, and 9 μm. Furthermore, with *in vivo* scanning, both image acquisition time and spatial resolution are critical. Under these circumstances, the images may not be highly detailed, but can still provide an average gray value that is representative of the underlying structure. These data may still be very informative with regards to the presence or absence of disease. Thus, HU calibration is an important prerequisite for meaningful data analysis. Even so, the noise inherent in any one system makes HU calibration a great challenge. Typical gray value distributions are in the range of ± 50 HU or worse depending on the system and protocol used. Currently, HU calibration is a time-consuming project that cannot be performed automatically by several commercial manufacturers of micro-CT scanners. This lack of attention to HU calibration is in part historic. Micro-CT scanners were initially built for the micro-chip industry and for orthopaedic research where detection of high contrast structures, and not accurate density measurements, was the primary goal.

K. Commercially Available Systems

Currently, there are six major manufactures of micro-CT scanners including Bio-Imaging Research (http://www.bio-imaging.com), Enhanced Vision Systems

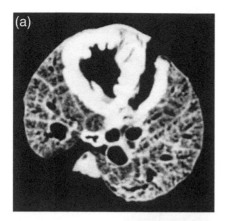
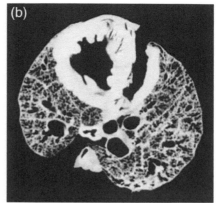

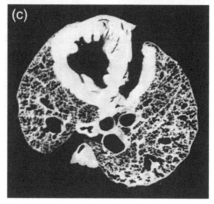

Figure 6.12 A fixed mouse lung was scanned with different scan protocols and reconstructions were calculated at the same position. Different scan resolutions, related reconstruction times, and the required memory per slice (for half field of view reconstruction) are shown: (a) 35 μm/voxel, 500 × 500 × 16 bit matrix, 0.5 MB/slice, 30 min volume acquisition time, 1 min back projection time per slice. (b) 18 μm/voxel, 1000 × 1000 × 16 bit matrix, 2 MB/slice, 90 min volume acquisition time, 2 min back projection time/slice. (c) 9 μm/voxel, 2000 × 2000 × 16 bit matrix, 8 MB/slice, 270 min volume acquisition time, 7 min back projection time/slice.

(http://www.gemedical.com/Preclinical_Imaging) recently acquired by GE Medical Systems, ImTek (http://www.imtekinc.com) recently aligned with Philips Medical, ScancoMedical (http://www.scanco.ch/), SkyScan (http://www.skyscan.be), and Stratec (http://www.stratec-med.com/) (see Table 6.1). Numerous investigators have also built their own custom designed systems.

III. Small Animal Lung Imaging

Micro-CT is becoming a very important tool for small animal imaging including imaging of mice. Different techniques have been proposed to image small anatomic structures using micro-CT and synchrotron X-ray CT. Synchrotron radiation X-ray sources offer high photon intensity, good collimation, and a broad continuous energy range from which any desired spectral region can be selected. A scanner based on a synchrotron source, which provides monochromatic and parallel X-ray beams, gives performance close to the theoretical limits, thereby opening new directions for medical imaging. With the use of mono-energetic X-rays at high doses, this method is capable of spatial resolution which is superior to conventional micro-CT. However, at present, there are only a few studies in which synchrotron-CT has been used for analysis of lung structures (37–40).

Likewise, only a few papers have dealt specifically with micro-CT imaging of the lung. Areas of interest include the evaluation of chemically fixed lungs, such as sheep or pig lungs, to analyze the 3D morphology of alveolar structures (41). Another group has developed a special lung airway contrasting method in excised rat lungs (42,43). Three-dimensional reconstructions showed branching and merging bronchi ranging from 500 to 150 μm (8–16 airway generations). The morphometry of the small airways (diameter, length, branching angle, and gravity angle between the gravity direction and the airway vector) was analyzed using a three-dimensional thinning algorithm. The diameter and length exponentially decreased with airway generation. These results are comparable to those found by our own group. Another research group has focused on micro-CT analyses of lung nodules, in particular micro-architectural features which may distinguish benign from malignant nodules (44). As preliminary results, they have shown a correlation between light microscopy and micro-CT images, suggesting potential as a clinical examination tool. Another study has examined pulmonary arterial distensibility in excised rat lungs imaged with micro-CT (45,46). The researchers used perfluorooctyl bromide to enhance X-ray absorbance. The vessel diameters were obtained by fitting a functional form to the image of the vessel circular cross-section. The diameter measurements obtained over a range of vascular pressures were used to characterize the distensibility of the rat pulmonary arteries.

A different and new challenge is soft tissue imaging, especially *in vivo* lung imaging with micro-CT (47). If motion artifact reduction technologies can be incorporated to solve problems caused by the long scan times required for *in vivo* micro-CT, soft tissue imaging of the lung and microvessels may be possible. Indeed, our goal is to establish micro-CT, its image reconstruction, protocol optimization, and image analysis and post-processing as a validated tool in small animal lung imaging. A major interest of our group is imaging the small airways using *in vivo* scanning techniques as well as evaluating changes in chronic asthma and in various emphysema mouse models. We expect to develop a mouse lung atlas to compliment our growing human lung atlas based on micro-CT imaging data. As shown in Figs. 6.13 and 6.14, it is possible to create impressive volumetric images of the lung with volume visualization techniques. It is important that these techniques are quantitatively accurate and that methods be developed that can make use of such quantitative accuracy.

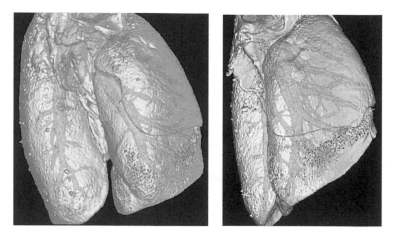

Figure 6.13 Volume rendering of a fixed mouse lung including the segmented bronchial tree in different angles of view. The airways were segmented using in-house developed software (5) (35 μm pixel resolution scan, Skyscan 1076 scanner, AnalyzeAVW software for visualization).

A.   Optimized *In Situ* and *In Vivo* Mouse Lung Protocol

In Situ Scanning Protocols

We have developed methodology for scanning the murine lung *in situ* and *in vivo*, including optimizing micro-CT acquisition and reconstruction parameters, using

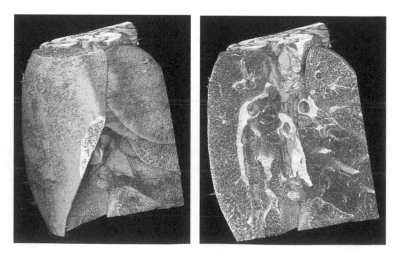

Figure 6.14   Volume rendering of fixed mouse lungs (25 μm effective resolution scan, Imtek micro-CT). The renderings were generated with the Amira software package.

in situ scans on recently sacrificed mice. Scanning has been performed using the Skyscan 1076 *in vivo* micro-CT scanner. Mice, following sacrifice, were intubated tracheally and the lungs inflated with a positive airway pressure of 20 cm H_2O. For scanning, each mouse was placed in a customized bed constructed of expanded polystyrene foam of medium density (Styrotech, Wolverhampton, UK) so as to minimize extraneous and asymmetric X-ray absorption and beam hardening associated with the sample holder.

One objective of scanning the lungs of mice is the assessment of emphysema on the basis of measured HU density within specified volumes of the lung. Protocols for scanning and reconstruction have been developed for accurate measurement of HU density regardless of location inside or outside the mouse thorax, unbiased by beam hardening artifacts. The procedure has been validated by checking for equal HU measurements of air in tracheal cavities and outside the thorax, on the reconstructed cross-section images.

Beam hardening has been minimized by several means. An X-ray voltage of 50 kV and filtration by 0.5 mm aluminum, in combination with the X-ray absorption efficiency profile of the gadolinium oxide scintillator at energies <50 kV (exponential-like increase with decreasing energy), combine to produce an effective energy spectrum (as measured by the camera) which is reasonably thin and approximately normal. Software correction of beam hardening (the application of a power-law density response curve) in the reconstruction process has been calibrated by scanning a tube of water approximating the width of the mouse thorax (2 cm). Employing these scanning and reconstruction parameters, two protocols have been established, one at 35 μm and other at 18 μm nominal resolution (pixel size), with acquisition times of 20 and 40 min, respectively. The scanning acquisition is >360°, and the rotation steps for the 35 μm pixel and 18 μm pixel scans are 0.45° and 0.6°, respectively. Recall that contrast resolution of low density structures is enhanced by using the lower kilovolt range.

More work is still necessary to identify optimal trade-offs between improved image quality and scanning times. Furthermore, an iterative approach to scan protocol development will have to take into consideration methods which can accommodate image reconstruction noise and increased or decreased spatial resolution.

Micro-CT appears a useful tool for scanning *ex vivo*, fixed mouse lungs with sufficient spatial resolution and tolerable levels of noise because there are no temporal constraints on image acquisition. There are no motion artifacts or fluid shifts which can occur with *in situ* lung scans. Thus, for instance, it is possible to use the 9 μm pixel resolution protocol of the Skyscan 1076 scanner. Optimized protocols for fixed mouse lung with different spatial resolutions are also being developed. The basic characteristics of the 9 μm protocol are: scanning time ~120 min, no filter, 50 kV and 200 μA.

Scan protocols are also under development to follow *in vivo* changes in the mouse lung over time. Varying degrees of spatial and density resolution are utilized, depending on the course of disease progression, and these are guided by pulmonary function measures obtained through technology such as the Scireq ventilator/pulmonary function system. Of particular note, *in situ* lungs of freshly sacrificed mice do not remain stationary when one is working on the micron scale. Tissues continue to relax and decay and fluid volumes continuously shift. To minimize this problem, the lung is maintained in the inflated state with continuous positive pressure at the trachea during scanning. Images of lungs in frozen mice have been unsatisfactory to date. We suspect that this is due to crystallization of water in the alveoli.

In Vivo Scanning Protocols

In vivo scanning is much more complicated and involved than *ex vivo* or *in situ* scanning. The necessary setup includes full anesthesia, physiologic monitoring, and the capacity for respiratory gating of the scanner. The physiologic monitoring and control system may consist of some or all of the following components:

1. Camera for real-time visualization of the animal during scanning.
2. Real-time local body movement detection to ensure noncontact synchronization of scanning with breathing.
3. Air/gas flow sensor for synchronization of scanning with breathing.
4. Sensor for animal temperature measurement.
5. Animal heating by airflow on the object bed.
6. ECG-amplifier.
7. Signals derived from a mechanical ventilator.

In vivo lung scanning requires the shortest possible scan times to avoid motion artifacts. There are also minimal requirements for the radiation dose needed to minimize image noise if gray-scale values are to be estimated. Currently available micro-CT systems require significant trade-offs in these matters. For instance, the dose exposure may significantly affect the animal's health during long term *in vivo* studies with repeated imaging sessions.

Micro-CT protocols need to be optimized in terms of scan time, SNR, and spatial resolution. Many parameters have to be taken into account to obtain "best possible" images. Figure 6.15 shows an 18 μm and a 35 μm *in vivo* respiratory gated scan. When one is able to identify a signal sufficiently representative of the respiratory cycle (such as chest wall motion detected from a video camera or gas flow through an endotracheal tube), it is possible to gate the scanner to spontaneous breathing (Figs. 6.16 and 6.17). Careful HU calibration and estimates of partial volume averaging artifacts are required if the purpose of the study is to determine and quantify parenchymal changes by estimating densities within image voxels.

B. Examination of Lung Tissue Samples from Larger Animals

Micro-CT can also be used to examine lung tissue samples obtained from larger animals or humans. Structure and gray-scale derived texture can be assessed. For example, emphysema was induced with papain instillation into sheep lung.

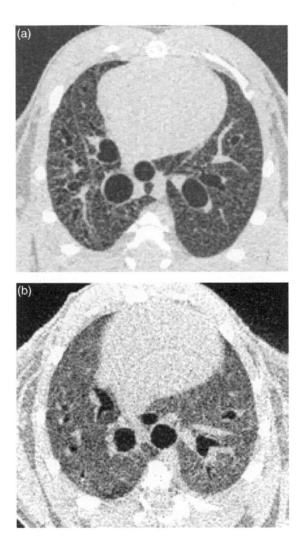

Figure 6.15 Comparison of resolution achieved (a) *in situ* (dead mouse with lung inflated at constant PEEP level) vs. an *in vivo* [gated to end expiration (b)] scan. Isotropic reconstructed voxel size was 18 µm. The worse SNR in the *in vivo* scan is mostly the result of reduced exposure time, that is, 1770 ms for the *in situ* scan and 295 ms for the *in vivo* scan. The reduced exposure time was necessary to minimize motion artifacts.

In a medical MDCT scanner, histogram methods were used to evaluate emphysematous regions. After lung fixation, samples of various regions of the lung suspected of being either emphysematous or normal were taken and then scanned via micro-CT. The resultant micro-CT data are shown in Fig. 6.17.

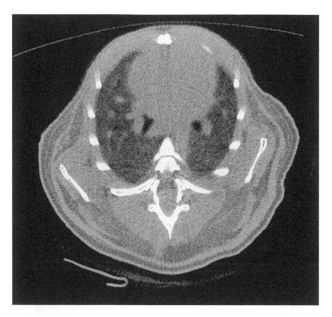

Figure 6.16   A 35 μm *in vivo* scan is shown, gated to spontaneous breathing of the mouse. Here the exposure time per single frame was 158 ms.

C.   Dynamic Imaging: Microfluoroscopy Coupled to Micro-CT

Because of the long scanning time needed to image the lungs by micro-CT, it is not possible to image dynamic processes such as blood flow or ventilation, in contrast to current MDCT scanners whose rotation times are on the order of 0.33 s for a full 360° rotation. An alternative approach is to simply utilize a single view from the micro X-ray imaging system to study physiological processes and then to relate these processes to 3D anatomy by imaging the many angles of view needed for CT reconstruction at the completion of the single view study.

This strategy has been used by members of the Keck Imaging Laboratory at Marquette University to study structural and functional consequences related to hypoxic pulmonary vasoconstriction. For example, the group has examined how the geometric and mechanical properties of the pulmonary vasculature respond to both acute hypoxia and chronic exposure to hypoxia resulting in vascular remodeling (48–50). Of particular interest is how the changes in these properties affect the longitudinal and parallel distributions of stresses and strains on and within vessel walls (46,50,51). The overall strategy has been to combine dynamic planar angiographic imaging at several resolutions with high-resolution micro-CT imaging of vascular structure.

The scanning instrumentation is illustrated in the upper panel of Fig. 6.3. The spatial capabilities are illustrated in Fig. 6.18, showing projection images

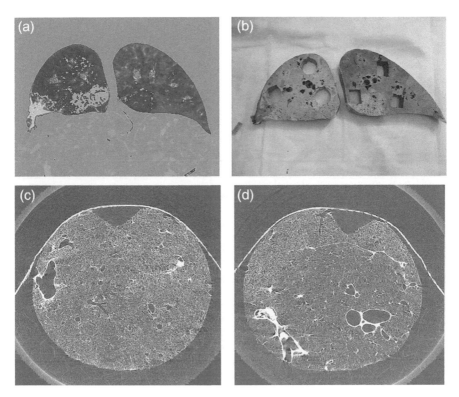

Figure 6.17 **(See color insert)** A sheep was scanned in a conventional CT scanner in order to measure regional blood flow with a dynamic CT protocol. (a) CT of a sheep lung with subsequent histogram analysis: the lung area marked in green was suspected of being emphysemateous as its overall density was slightly lower than the rest of the lung. (b) After lung fixation, samples were taken at the same level as the CT slices. (c) Micro-CT of a nonemphysemateous region, 25 μm pixel resolution, 40 min scan, 45 kV, 400 μA: the lung tissue structure is relatively homogeneous. (d) Micro-CT of the emphysemateous region, 25 μm pixel resolution, 40 min scan, 45 kV, 400 μA: the sample shows a lower density. A subsequent histological examination corroborated that the regions of lower density in the micro-CT images were emphysemateous.

of an isolated rat lung with the arterial tree filled with perfluorooctyl bromide (providing X-ray contrast) at three magnification levels. The ability to image and quantify vascular structure of the entire lung as well as particular regions at very high resolution is shown. Although this approach is extremely useful for examining vessels as small as 20 μm in the periphery of the lung, the overlap of vessels in the projection images renders this approach problematic for reliably measuring all visible vessels. However, rotation of the specimen within the beam enables acquisition of projection images that are used for 3D

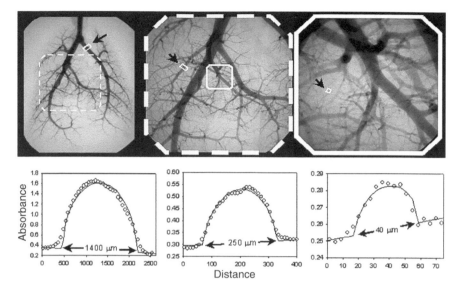

Figure 6.18   Projection images of a rat lung at three magnification levels. The white dashed box on the left image encloses the middle image and the solid white box on the middle image encloses the right image. The small white rectangles designated by the arrows are the boxes across which the line scans were taken for vessel diameter estimation in the respective lower panels. The solid lines in the lower panels indicate a model fit to the line scan data obtained from the vessel cross section.

volumetric CT reconstruction as shown in Fig. 6.19. These images have then been used to characterize the morphometric structure of vessel trees by measuring vessel lengths, branching angles, and diameters. In addition, limited functional information is also obtainable. For example, modulating the vascular and airway pressures can characterize distensibility via pressure–diameter relationships (45,50). Examination of the response of different segments of the vasculature to various pulmonary vasodilators or vasoconstrictors (52,53) is also possible.

Overall and regional pulmonary vascular function has been assessed using dynamic projection angiography (54). Fig. 6.20 illustrates three time frames extracted from a sequence of images of a region of dog lung obtained during passage of a bolus of X-ray contrast medium. Regions-of-interest positioned over artery and vein pairs as well as the surrounding microvasculature, yield time–absorbance curves that were used to determine the effects of alveolar hypoxia on pulmonary microvascular volume (49). Absorbance data during both normoxic (alveolar gas 15% O_2) and hypoxic (5% O_2) conditions were collected and analyzed to obtain arterial inlet and venous outlet time–absorbance curves from which total pulmonary vascular volume was calculated. Microvascular regions (vessels smaller than ~40 μm) were measured from high

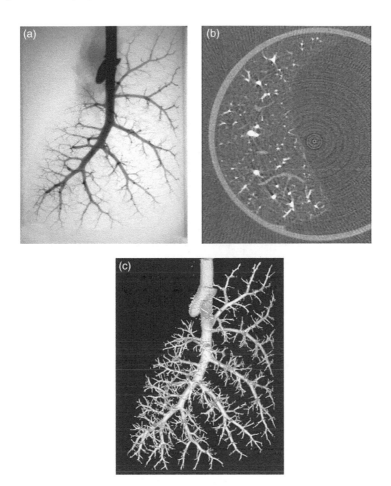

Figure 6.19 (a) A projection image of a rat lung with arteries enhanced by filling with perfluorooctyl bromide. (b) A transaxial slice through the reconstructed 3D volume. (c) A surface shaded rendering of the three-dimensional volume of the same rat left lung at about the same viewing angle and with the threshold set to eliminate the smallest vessels so the basic tree structure can be seen.

magnification image sequences and the fractional change in microvascular volume from normoxia to hypoxia was determined from the area under the microvascular absorbance curves. Hypoxia decreased total lobar volume by $\sim 13\%$ and microvascular volume by $\sim 26\%$. Given the morphometry of the lung vasculature, this suggests that capillary volume was substantially decreased by hypoxia. The physical explanation for this change is not apparent, but as flow was held constant, simple narrowing of arteries would not be expected to decrease capillary pressure, although an active change in capillary dimensions may be possible.

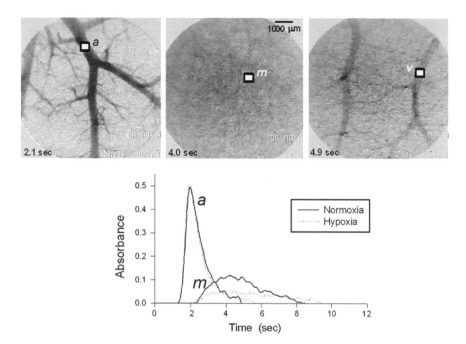

Figure 6.20 (Top) Angiographic images acquired during the passage of a bolus of contrast medium through a field of view through a dog lung perfused at constant flow. The indicated times are when the change in opacification was maximum in the regions indicated by the artery, a, vein, v, and microvascular, m, boxes. On the left the bolus fills the arteries but has barely begun to reach the capillaries. The background in the middle panel is dark because the bolus has virtually left the arteries and is spread throughout the capillary bed. By 4.9 s, the bolus has reached the veins, but it has not yet completely left the capillaries. (Bottom) Absorbance curves a and v represent the concentration of contrast material passing through the respective detection sites during normoxic ($PO_2 = 116$ Torr) conditions whereas m represents the residue curve obtained from the indicated microvascular region during normoxia and hypoxia ($PO_2 = 39$ Torr). Thus m represents the amount of contrast material residing in the microvessels at a given time so that the area under m is proportional to the microvascular volume, which is substantially decreased by hypoxia.

Angiographic studies were also used to address the question of how the complex routes blood can take through the lungs actually produce the overall pulmonary vascular transport function (distribution of transit times), which is important for studies of organ function. A common visualization of transit time dispersion in conducting trees has been based on the assumption that flow through of any connecting segment is proportional to the number of terminals subtended by that segment, and that the transit time through each segment is its volume divided by its flow. One consequence of these assumptions is that short pathways would have short transit times and long pathways would have long transit times, so that the transit time distribution would be close to a scaled distribution of path lengths. The contribution of the pulmonary arterial and venous trees to the whole lung transport function was examined by measuring time–absorbance curves from selected pulmonary arteries and veins; these studies revealed that path length contributed remarkably little to the dispersion of lung transit times (55). This result appears to indicate that the bolus arrives at arteries of a given diameter at about the same time regardless of the wide range in distances it had to travel to reach each vessel of that diameter. This observation can be explained by assuming that despite the apparent complexity of the arterial branching pattern, at each asymmetric bifurcation, the faster streamlines tend to pass through the larger diameter daughter branch, whereas the smaller daughter receives the slower streamlines. In other words, the streamlines with low velocity at the inlet, which are also closest to the vessel wall, pass into small branches serving short pathways, whereas the higher midstream velocity streamlines continue on through the larger branches to long pathways. Thus, the arterial transit time distribution is not a reflection of the path length distribution, but instead the path length distribution and branching pattern are matched to the vessel velocity profiles so that near uniformity in arterial transit times is achieved.

Progress is being made toward combining static micro-CT data, which provide vessel structure and distensibility, with dynamic projection angiography at high resolution for measuring the contribution of vessel tone, regardless of the interaction of tone and vascular remodeling on hemodynamic function. Future enhancements of micro-CT scanners are moving in the direction of improved spatial resolution but also perhaps more importantly towards increased temporal resolution for improved functional applications.

A tour-de-force example of dynamic micro X-ray-based imaging is demonstrated in Fig. 6.21. Here a ground beetle was scanned via a synchrotron X-ray source and the projection data allowed researchers to follow the dynamic properties of the tubular respiratory apparatus. (56)

D. Conclusions

Imaging the *in situ* mouse lung is a feasible task although specific scanning parameters have to be taken into account. Significant compromises between spatial resolution and scan time are currently required. We discuss methods of achieving optimal images over a reasonable scan time, that is, within the time before the lung undergoes postmortem destruction. Quantification issues are still being resolved. *In vivo* scanning is also more challenging procedure which includes anesthesia to be maintained throughout the scan, triggering of the CT, physiologic monitoring, and so on. We present recent results in our laboratory indicating

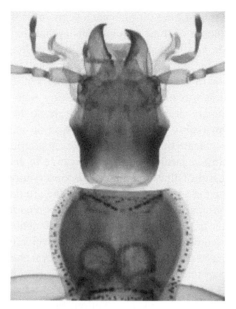

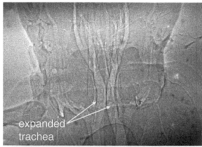

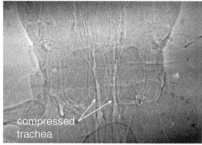

Figure 6.21 (a) Ground beetle, *Platynus decentis*, family Carabidae. X-ray images from the beamline at the Advanced Photon Source, Argonne National Laboratory. Beetle specimen scanned at four points during tracheal compression (two times ~0.5 s apart). These images demonstrate that beetles rapidly compress and expand the tracheal system in a manner superficially similar to the inflation of lungs. (b) Upper right: beetle tracheal tubes fully expanded. (c) Lower right: beetle tracheal tubes fully compressed. Beetles and other insects can inhale and exhale 1/2 the volume of the large trachea, similar to the volume of human lungs during mild exercise. [Reproduced by kind permission of Westneat et al. (56).]

that meaningful *in vivo* imaging is feasible, allowing for longitudinal studies in the same mouse. These recommendations are summarized subsequently in relation to our current experience with a Skyscan 1076 system.

1.   Imaging with 35 and 18 μm voxel spatial resolution *in vivo* is possible in an anesthetized mouse, with recovery.
2.   If HUs are well calibrated, 35 μm scans *in vivo* will be useful to estimate underlying structural changes using density and texture information, despite inherent physiologic motion artifacts.
3.   *In situ* (postmortem) imaging with 18 μm scan provides anatomic detail suitable for airway wall measurements.
4.   *Ex vivo* imaging with 9 μm scan provides anatomic detail suitable for alveolar level visualization.
5.   *In vivo* imaging can provide detail suitable for lung volume measurements and may provide detail suitable for lung density measurements.

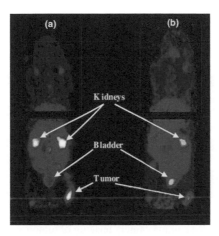

Figure 3.6 MicroPET imaging of a rat bearing a SSTR2-positive xenograft using two different ^{64}Cu-labeled somatostatin analogs. Rats were implanted with SSTR2-positive AR42J tumors in the rear flank followed by intravenous (IV) injection of the ^{64}Cu-labeled somatostatin analogs after the tumors were established. The two analogs [CB-TE2A-Y3-TATE (a) and TETA-Y3-TATE (b)] differ with regard to the chelating agent used to complex the copper. MicroPET imaging was performed 4 h after injection of the radiopharmaceuticals and shows increased tumor uptake in (a) compared with (b). This study demonstrates the ability to image SSTR2-positive tumors with PET and the effect of chelating agents on tumor uptake and distribution. This image was kindly provided by Carolyn Anderson and Jeni Sprague of Washington University in St. Louis.

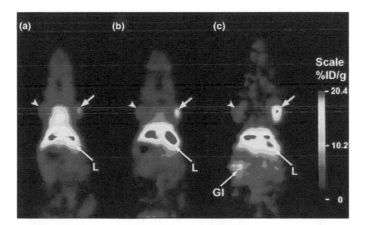

Figure 3.7 MicroPET imaging of a mouse bearing a CEA-positive xenograft using a ^{64}Cu-labeled minibody. Mice were implanted with axillary CEA-positive LS174T cells (arrow) and CEA-negative C6 cells (arrowhead). After the tumors were established, the ^{64}Cu-labeled minibody was injected intravenously (IV) and the mice were imaged 2 h (a), 6 h (b), and 24 h (c) after injection. Clear visualization of the CEA-positive tumor is observed at all time points as well as clearance through the liver (L) and the gastrointestinal (GI) tract. This study demonstrates the ability to monitor cell surface antigens over time with a radiolabeled antibody construct. It should be noted that similar studies could be performed using a gamma-emitting radionuclide and SPECT imaging. Reproduced with permission from Ref. (115).

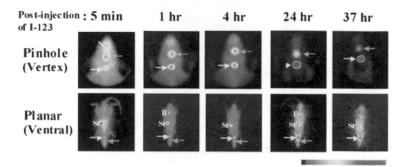

Post-injection : **5 min**   **1 hr**   **4 hr**   **24 hr**   **37 hr**
of I-123

**Pinhole
(Vertex)**

**Planar
(Ventral)**

Figure 3.9 Dual headed gamma camera imaging of tumors stably transduced to express NIS using [123]I. Rats were implanted intracranially with F98 cells stably transduced to express NIS. Thirteen days later the rats were injected intravenously (IV) with ^{123}I and either whole body (planar) or cranially focused (pinhole) images were obtained at various times postinjection. The top arrow in the pinhole images (bottom arrow in the planar) indicates uptake in the NIS-expressing tumor cells and the bottom arrow in the pinhole images (top arrow in the planar) indicates thyroid uptake. Uptake and clearance was also observed in the nasal mucosa (N), stomach (St), and bladder (B). Tumor uptake is observed at 5 min postinjection and still present at 37 h. The highest tumor uptake of ^{123}I is observed at 4 h, whereas the highest thyroid uptake is observed at 24 h. These studies demonstrate that an exogenous gene (NIS) can be introduced into cells and imaged noninvasively at multiple times after administration of [123]I. Reproduced with permission from Ref. (160).

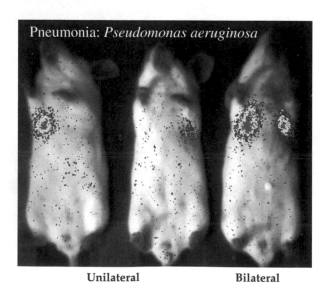

Unilateral   **Bilateral**

Figure 4.1 Imaging pseudomonas infections of the lung. The bacterial *Lux* operon was integrated into the genome of *Pseudomonas*, and used to monitor lung infections following intranasal delivery. The images show evidence of unilateral and bilateral infections.

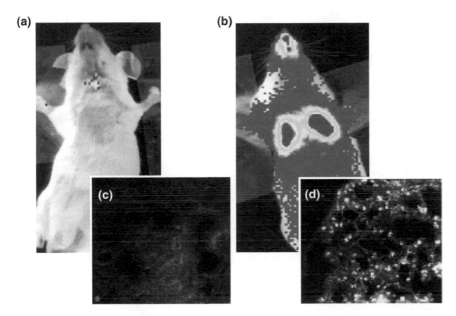

Figure 4.2 Adeno-associated viral delivery of dual function reporter gene to the lungs of Balb/c mice. Mice were treated with two different AAV vectors encoding the same dual function reporter gene comprised of Fluc and YFP (Brindle and Contag, Unpublished data). Animals were imaged for luciferase expression (a and b) and after the study fluorescence micrographs (c and d) were used to validate gene delivery to the lungs. Effective gene delivery is shown in b and d, whereas the absence of effective delivery is shown in a and b.

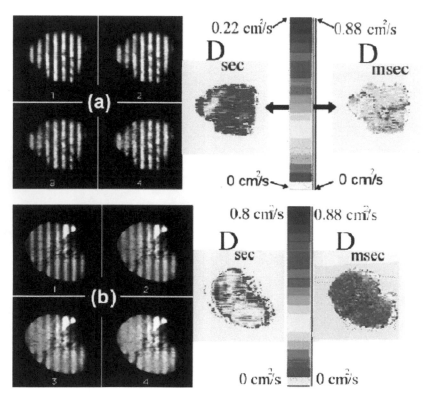

Figure 5.4 Measurement of the displacement of hyperpolarized ^{3}He gas over distances of a few centimeters achieved by following the decay of tagged ("striped") longitudinal magnetization. In (a), each grayscale image of this healthy lung advances 1.96 s (the first being immediately after initial tagging pulses). Little decay of modulation is evident, and the resultant map of D_{sec} has an average of 0.017 cm^2/s, about 12× smaller than D_{msec}. In (b), each grayscale image advances only 0.38 s; decay is apparent beginning at image no. 2. D_{sec} approaches D_0 in the apex—an increase of 50× over healthy lung. [From Ref. (76).]

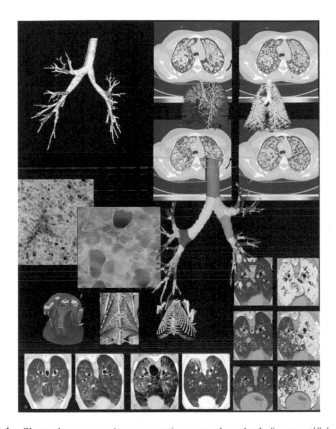

Figure 6.1 Shown is a composite representing several methods for quantifying the lung, including airway segmentation (upper left), airway segment labeling (center), and color coding of blood flow parameters (upper and lower right) from a time series analysis of the passage of a bolus of iodinated contrast agent. Super-imposed on the upper right blood flow images, we display a mathematical model of the airway tree for both humans (left) and sheep (right). This model actually extends out to the terminal bronchi and is generated from a starting segmentation of the lungs and airway tree using CT scanning, providing a subject specific, complete airway tree model (work in collaboration with Merryn Tawhai and Peter Hunter, Auckland, New Zealand). In the lower portion of the image, we demonstrate a sheep model of lung inflammation leading to emphysema. Cross-sectional images with and without superposition of blood flow are shown in the lower right. Color coded images of perfusion at day 16 (lower row of this grouping) demonstrate the emergence of flow pattern abnormalities in the left lung which match the blood flow patterns in the treated right lung. Matching gray scale images showed no signs of pathology either visually or through a quantitative evaluation of the lung density histogram. The volumetric images one row from the bottom demonstrate that we are able to image the sheep (and humans) volumetrically in great detail. In the middle left, we depict our ability to harvest lungs to establish pathologic correlates with the CT images. Micro-CT, as discussed in this chapter, provides the link between these large animal and human imaging studies to the micro-CT evaluation of the mouse lung at the very interface of gas exchange (see text for references to works represented by this composite image).

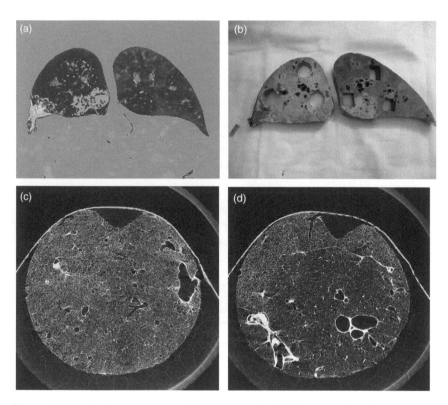

Figure 6.17 A sheep was scanned in a conventional CT scanner in order to measure regional blood flow with a dynamic CT protocol. (a) CT of a sheep lung with subsequent histogram analysis: the lung area marked in green was suspected of being emphysemateous as its overall density was slightly lower than the rest of the lung. (b) After lung fixation, samples were taken at the same level as the CT slices. (c) Micro-CT of a nonemphysemateous region, 25 μm pixel resolution, 40 min scan, 45 kV, 400 μA: the lung tissue structure is relatively homogeneous. (d) Micro-CT of the emphysemateous region, 25 μm pixel resolution, 40 min scan, 45 kV, 400 μA: the sample shows a lower density. A subsequent histological examination corroborated that the regions of lower density in the micro-CT images were emphysemateous.

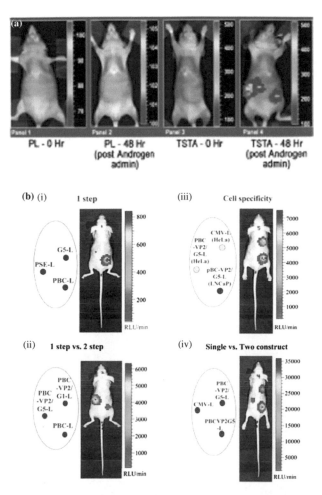

Figure 7.3 (a) *In vivo* optical imaging of mice carrying LNCaP cells transiently transfected with vectors representing the TSTA system. (Panel 1) LNCaP cells were transiently transfected with the vector, PSE-*fl* (PL) wherein an enhanced prostate-specific antigen promoter (PSE) directly drives *fl* expression and the cells were implanted intraperitoneally. The mouse was imaged using D-luciferin (substrate for *fl*, 150 mg/kg). (Panel 2) The same mouse in Panel 1 was reimaged 48 h following implantation of an androgen pellet. (Panel 3) LNCaP cells transiently transfected with the TSTA vectors (PSE-GAL4VP16 and G5-E4T-*fl*) were implanted in a nude mouse. The mouse was imaged using D-Luciferin. (Panel 4) The same mouse in Panel 3 was reimaged 48 h after implantation of an androgen pellet. Pictures shown in the figure represent bioluminescent images superimposed on gray-scale photographs. Reporter gene expression is detected in the cells representing the TSTA system, whereas *fl* expression using the one-step vector is at basal levels. [Reproduced with permission from Iyer et al. (42)]. (b) Optical imaging of one-step and TSTA system in living athymic nude mice. (i–iv) Pictures shown in the figure represent bioluminescent images superimposed on gray-scale photographs with a scale in relative light units (RLU) per minute. A map representing the dorsal surface of the mice is on the left; the circles denote the relative position of the three injection sites, with the transfected vectors labeled over each circle. The representative groups are indicated on the top of each panel. [Reproduced with permission from Zhang et al. (43)].

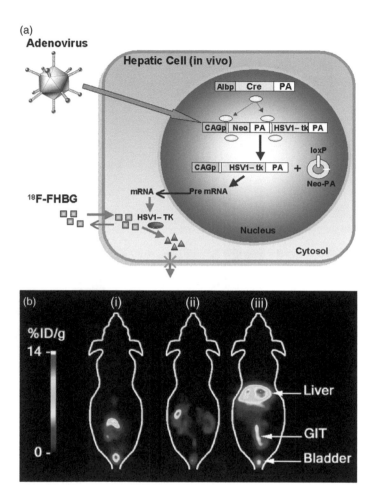

Figure 7.4 Imaging Cre–loxP activation. (a) Schematic of the Cre–loxP system. An adenovirus carrying the silent PET reporter gene delivers its genetic information (CAGp-loxP-Neo-PA-loxP-*HSV1-tk*-PA) into the hepatic cells. In the livers of transgenic mice, the albumin promoter drives the Cre recombinase expression. The Cre recombinase acts upon the adenoviral DNA causing excision of the Neo-PA cassette and recombination at the loxP sites leading to the *HSV1-tk* mRNA formation. The expressed *HSV1-TK* protein acts on the reporter probe ([^{18}F-FHBG]) and consequently its metabolite is trapped within the hepatic cells leading to a detectable PET signal. [Reproduced with permission from Sundaresan et al. (52)]. (b) MicroPET imaging shows *HSV1-tk* expression in the liver as seen by accumulation of the tracer [^{18}F-FHBG] in the hepatic region: (i) Cre– animal 48 h after virus injection; (ii) Cre+ animal before virus injection; and (iii) Cre+ animal 48 h after virus injection. The color scale (%ID/g) indicates the percentage of injected dose that accumulates per gram of liver. In the images shown, the maximum accumulation of [^{18}F-FHBG] was 14% ID/g in the liver of transgenic mice (c) infected with the adenovirus. [Reproduced with permission from Sundaresan et al. (52).]

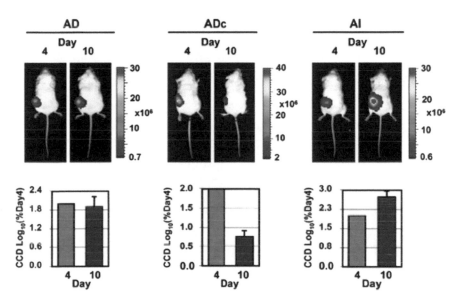

Figure 7.5 Imaging AR signaling in LAPC-9 tumors. SCID mice implanted with LAPC-9 prostate tumor xenografts (androgen dependent, AD and androgen independent, AI groups) were injected with 10^7 plaque forming units (pfu) of an adenovirus carrying the TSTA system (Ad-TSTA) and the mice were imaged every 3–4 days over a 14-day period. Representative mice at day 4 and day 10 after virus injection from the AD group, the castrated AD group (Adc), and the stable AI group. The bar graph summarizes a cohort of three or more animals and summarizes the log of the percentage change in signal from day 4 to day 10. Color images of visible light are superimposed on photographic images of mice with a scale in photons per second per square centimeter per steradian (sr). [Reproduced with permission from Zhang et al. (95).]

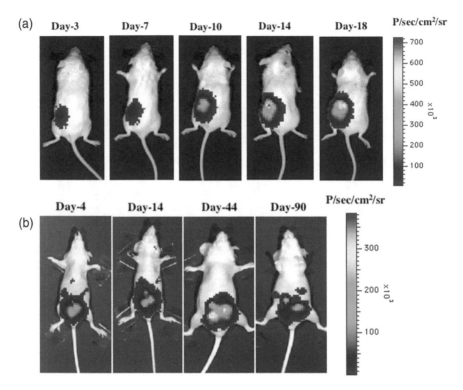

Figure 7.6 Tumor-specific expression of *fl* reporter gene in male, SCID mice following intratumoral injection of a lentivirus carrying the TSTA system. (a) Six-week-old male, SCID mice were implanted with prostate tumor LAPC-9 xenografts in the left, bottom flank. When the tumor size reached 0.5–0.6 cm in diameter, lentivirus carrying the TSTA system (LV-TSTA) was injected directly into the tumor. The mice were imaged using a charge coupled device (CCD) camera on days 3, 7, 10, 14 and 18 using D-Luciferin as the substrate (150 mg/kg, i.p.). Color images of visible light are superimposed on photographic images of mice with a scale in photons per second per square centimeter per steradian (sr). A significantly high level of *fl* gene expression is observed in the tumor, which continues to persist to day 18. (b) *In vivo* optical imaging of mice following direct intraprostatic delivery of LV-TSTA. [Reproduced with permission from Iyer et al. (124).] (b) Six-week-old male, nude mice were injected with the lentivirus in the dorsal lobe of the prostate. The mice were imaged using the CCD camera 2–4 days after virus injection. Subsequent imaging was performed every 3–4 days till day 21, then once a week until day 90. By day 4, a high level of bioluminescence signal is observed in the prostate (2.2×10^5 photons/s per cm^2 per sr). The *fl* expression shows strong persistence with time. [Reproduced with permission from Iyer et al. (124).]

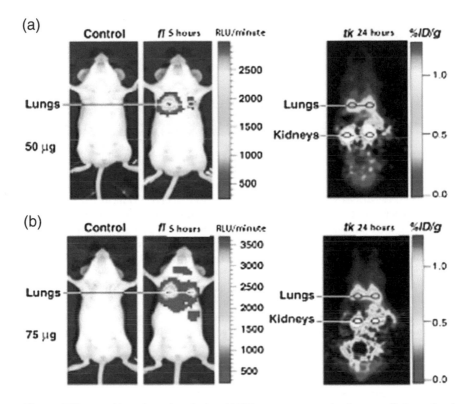

Figure 7.7 Dual imaging of optical and PET reporter genes in the same living animal using cationic liposomes. CD-1 mice were first imaged 5 h after injection using the CCD camera in the absence of D-Luciferin (control) and then imaged again following injection of D-Luciferin. The same mice were imaged 24 h later with [^{18}F]-FHBG using microPET. (a) A CD-1 mouse injected with 50 µg each of *fl* and *HSV1-sr39tk* DNA–DOTAP–cholesterol complex via tail-vein. Pictures shown in the figure represent bioluminescent images superimposed on gray-scale photographs with a scale in relative light units per minute (RLU/min). The control image shows background levels of *fl* expression in the lungs (<50 RLU/min). At 5 h, the *fl* gene expression is significantly greater than that of the control (2958 RLU/min). The same mouse imaged at 24 h shows low levels of *HSV1-sr39tk* gene expression in the lung (percent injected dose per gram, 0.46%ID/g). [Reproduced with permission from Iyer et al. (133).] (b) A CD-1 mouse was injected with 75 µg each of *fl* and *HSV1-sr39tk* DNA–DOTAP–cholesterol complex via tail-vein. The control image shows background levels of *fl* expression (<50 RLU/min). In contrast, the image acquired after injection of D-luciferin shows a high level of *fl* expression in the lungs (3668 RLU/min). MicroPET imaging using [^{18}F]-FHBG shows increased levels of *HSV1-sr39tk* gene expression in the lungs at 24 h (1.0%ID/g). [Reproduced with permission from Iyer et al. (133).]

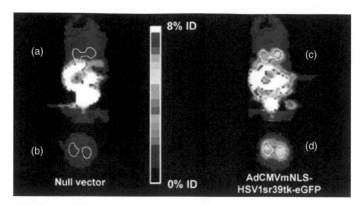

Figure 7.8 Reporter gene expression with PET in a control mouse infected with a null vector (left) and a mouse expressing mutant *HSV1-sr39tk* gene (right). Ad-CMVmNLS-*HSV1-sr39tk-eGFP*, adenovirus-cytomegalovirus promoter-, mutated nuclear localization signal – *HSV1-sr39tk-eGFP* vector. Three days after adenovirus-mediated intratracheal gene transfer, 10 μCi/g of body weight of [^{18}F]-FHBG was intravenously injected into both mice. PET imaging was performed after 1 h over 15-min acquisition time. (a, c) Coronal views of mice. (b, d) Corresponding transverse slices obtained at midlung level. In both mice, regions of interest are drawn to indicate lung boundaries (white lines), and tracer uptake was expressed as percentage of injected dose (ID/g). Although there was significant pulmonary uptake of tracer in mice expressing viral thymidine kinase, pulmonary activity was not different from background in control mice. High levels of activity in abdomen are due to a combination of urinary excretion and biliary excretion into the gastrointestinal tract. [Reproduced with permission from Richard et al. (146).]

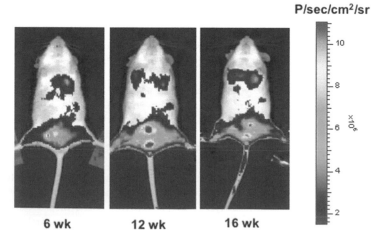

Figure 7.9 Repetitive optical imaging of TSTA-*fl* transgenic mice. A transgenic male mouse was imaged in the CCD camera at 8 weeks of age, then subsequently reimaged at 12 and 16 weeks. Color images of visible light are superimposed on photographic images of mice with a scale in photons per second per square centimeter per steradian (sr). Gene expression is primarily observed in the prostate tissue and shows persistence with time ($2–3 \times 10^6$ p/s per cm^2 per sr). [Reproduced with permission from Iyer M and Gambhir SS (Transgenic Research, 2005, in press).]

6. Efforts must be made to provide accurate HU calibration for *in vivo* study to be of maximum utility.
7. In Table 6.2, we provide our method for lung fixation for postmortem/*ex vivo* imaging of the lung such that the lung maintains its *in vivo* geometric structural characteristics. This fixation method has been developed through an iterative process, comparing *in vivo* and *ex vivo*/postfixation images of the same lungs.

Note: all values above represent isotropic voxel dimensions.

Micro-CT imaging not only allows study of lung anatomy down to the alveolar level, but also it provides a testing ground for improved cone-beam algorithms which can then be translated up to future clinical scanners. Micro-CT imaging has seen a rapid transition from one-of-a-kind laboratory instruments to commercially developed systems which have moved from use in the study of high contrast static structures (such as postmortem specimens of bone) towards

Table 6.2 Protocol for Lung Fixation

I. *Mouse preparation*	**III. *Tracheal dissection***
(a) Inject mouse with ~0.4 cc anesthetic (ketamine/xylazine mixture with 17.5 mg/cc ketamine and 2.5 mg/cc xylazine) and test reflexes on pain	(a) Dissect tissue with curved hemostats. After dissection of tissue surrounding trachea, a loose knot must be in position to secure placement of 20/22 gage angiocath
(b) Inject barbituate (pentobarbital) to euthanize ~0.15 cc and pin mouse limbs back to begin dissection	(b) Cut knick into trachea superior to 2.0 silk string, insert angiocath, and tighten knot
II. *Accessing internal organs*	**IV. *Lung removal***
(a) Snip skin inferior to xyphoid process (thoracic cavity) and cut in strait line to lateral sides	Pull tightly and gently on both strings and cut connective tissue surrounding lungs
(b) Pull liver downward with small forceps and cut vessels and connective tissue, locate diaphragm and make small puncture on each side	**V. *Lung fixation***
	(a) Use modified Heitzman's solution: 25% polyethylene glycol (PEG), 10% ethanol (95%), 10% formaldehyde (37%), and 55% distilled water.
(c) Cut diaphragm along ribcage	(b) Inject trachea with 1 cc modified Heitzman's solution. Then, immerse lungs in modified Heitzman's solution with a 20 cm above ground tracheal drip for 24 h.
(i) Start at puncture mark and cut towards sternum on both sides	
(ii) Do not complete cut-leave tissue posterior to sternum	
(d) Cut sternum and pin back ribs to expose lungs and heart	(c) Air dry with 20 cm H_2O continuous airway pressure for 24 h.
(e) Administer right ventricular injection to perfuse the tissue with 20 cc phosphate buffered saline	(d) After lungs are fixed and dried, place them in sealed container at room temperature.

more recent interest in imaging structural changes over time *in vivo*. A small but growing number of applications have now sought to study soft tissue structures and a number of manufacturers have begun to market what they call *in vivo* scanners. It has become clear that much work is necessary to develop the scanners and the image handling to accommodate the special needs of soft tissue imaging and particularly soft tissue imaging *in vivo*. If we are to rely on imaged gray scale and gray scale texture to assess changes in the lung periphery *in vivo* as a marker of microstructural changes over time (with eventual postmortem imaging to verify microstructural changes), we must be able to rely on the accuracy of the soft tissue attenuation coefficients and the scanner's gray scale sensitivity.

The combination of micro X-ray fluoroscopy and micro-CT, offers the potential for new insights into structure–function relationships in the lung. This will be further enhanced with the introduction of multi-modality protocols utilizing various combinations of technology, as outlined in other chapters of this book.

Data management and image processing of micro-CT images remain challenging: one volumetric image of the mouse lung in 9 μm pixel resolution can be as large as 30 GB. The visualization and meaningful analysis of data would be facilitated by a move to PC-based software development on a 64 bit processor platform with maximized RAM. New strategies in image processing and analysis will have to be defined by close collaboration with investigators in computer science and biology. Imaging on a regular basis with subsequent analysis and storage will require the addition of large disc farms. Nevertheless, with anticipated progress in hardware and software technology, mouse micro-CT imaging will become a common reality.

References

1. Hoffman EA, McLennan G. Assessment of pulmonary structure–function relationships and clinical outcomes measures: quantitative volumetric CT of the lung. Acad Radiol 1997; 4(11):758–776.
2. Hoffman EA, Reinhardt JM, Sonka M, Simon BA, Guo J, Saba O, Chon D, Samrah S, Shikata H, Tschirren J, Palagyi K, Beck KC, McLennan G. Characterization of the interstitial lung diseases via density-based and texture-based analysis of computed tomography images of lung structure and function. Acad Radiol 2003; 10(10):1104–1118.
3. Hoffman EA, Sinak LJ, Robb RA, Ritman EL. Noninvasive quantitative imaging of shape and volume of lungs. J Appl Physiol 1983; 54(5):1414–1421.
4. Shikata H, Hoffman EA, Sonka M. Automated segmentation of pulmonary vascular tree from 3D CT images. Prog Biomed Optics Imaging 2004; 5(23):107–116.
5. Tschirren J, Hoffman E, McLennan G, Sonka M. Airway tree segmentation using adaptive regions of interest. Prog Biomed Optics Imaging 2004; 5(23):117–124.
6. Bilgen D, Hoffman EA, Reinhardt JM. Segmentation and analysis of human airway tree from 3D X-ray CT images. IEEE Trans Med Imaging. In press.

7. Hu S, Hoffman EA, Reinhardt JM. Automatic lung segmentation for accurate quantitation of volumetric X-ray CT images. IEEE Trans Med Imaging 2001; 20(6):490–498.

8. Wood S, Hoford J, Zerhouni E, Hoffman E, Mitzner W. Quantitative 3-D reconstruction of airway and pulmonary vascular trees using HRCT. Biomed Image Process Biomed Visual 1993; 1905:316–323.

9. Tschirren J, Palágyi K, Hoffman EA, Sonka M. Segmentation, skeletonization, and branchpoint matching—a fully automated quantitative evaluation of human intrathoracic airway trees. In: Dohi T, Kikinis R, eds. Proceedings of Fifth International Conference on Medical Image Computing and Computer Assisted Intervention; 2002; Tokyo, Japan: Springer-Verlag Berlin Heidelberg, 2002: 12–19.

10. Hoffman EA, Acharya RS, Wollins JA. Computer-aided analysis of regional lung air content using three-dimensional computed tomographic images and multinomial models. Int J Mathem Model 1986; 7:1099–1116.

11. Tawhai MH, Hunter P, Tschirren J, Reinhardt J, McLennan G, Hoffman EA. CT-based geometry analysis and finite element models of the human and ovine bronchial tree. J Appl Physiol 2004; 97(6):2310–2321.

12. Hoffman EA, Ritman EL. Effect of body orientation on regional lung expansion in dog and sloth. J Appl Physiol 1985; 59(2):481–491.

13. Tajik JK, Chon D, Won C, Tran BQ, Hoffman EA. Subsecond multisection CT of regional pulmonary ventilation. Acad Radiol 2002; 9(2):130–146.

14. Chon D, Beck K, Shikata H, Larsen R, Hoffman EA. Regional pulmonary blood flow by dynamic multi-slice X-ray CT. J Appl Physiol. In press.

15. Chulho W, Chon D, Tajik J, Tran B, Robinswood G, Beck K, Hoffman EA. CT-based assessment of regional pulmonary microvascular blood flow parameters. J Appl Physiol 2003; 94:2483–2493.

16. Tomimitsu S, Samrah S, Hoffman E, Beck K, McLennan G. Lung preparation technique for computed tomography-pathologic correlation. Am J Resp Crit Care Med 2003; 167(7):A875.

17. Samrah S, McLennan G, Chon D, Beck KC, Ross A, Hoffman EA. Multi-row detector CT-based measures of microvascular mean transit times and parenchymal texture as an early marker of inflammatory processes leading to emphysema. Am J Respir Crit Care Med 2003; 167(7):A874.

18. Irvin CG, Bates JH. Measuring the lung function in the mouse: the challenge of size. Respir Res 2003; 4(1):4.

19. Shapiro SD. Animal models for chronic obstructive pulmonary disease: age of klotho and marlboro mice. Am J Respir Cell Mol Biol 2000; 22(1):4–7.

20. Jorgensen S, Demirkaya O, Ritman EL. Three-dimensional imaging of vasculature and parenchyma in intact rodent organs with X-ray micro-CT. Am J Physiol 1998; 275(3, Pt 2):H1103–H1114.

21. Ritman EL. Molecular imaging in small animals—roles for micro-CT. J Cell Biochem Suppl 2002; 39:116–124.

22. Ritman E. Micro-computed tomography-current status and developments. Ann Rev Biomed Eng 2004; 6:185–208.

23. Rüegsegger P. Imaging of Bone Structure. 2nd ed. Boca Raton: CRC Press, 2001:1–24.

24. Paulus M, Gleason S, Kennel S, Hunsicker P, Johnson D. High resolution X-ray computed tomography an emerging tool for small animal cancer research. Neoplasia 2000; 2(1–2):62–70.

25. Paulus M, Sari-Sarraf H, Gleason S, Bobrek M, Hicks J, Johnson D, Behel J, Thompson L, Allen W. A new X-ray computed tomography system for laboratory mouse imaging. IEEE Trans Nucl Sci 1999; 46(3):558–564.

26. Durand EP, Rüegsegger P. High contrast resolution of computed tomography images for bone structure analysis. Med Phys 1992; 19:569–573.

27. Sasov A, Van Dyck D. Desktop X-ray microscopy and microtomography. J Microsc 1998; 191(2):151–158.

28. Marxen M, Thornton M, Chiarot C, Klement G, Koprivnikar J, Sled J, Henkelman R. Micro CT scanner performance and considerations for vascular specimen imaging. Med Phys 2004; 31(2):305–313.

29. Chen LM, Forget P, Toth R, Kieffer JC, Krol A et al. Laser-based intense hard X-ray source for mammography. Proc SPIE 2003; 5030:923–928.

30. Bonse U, Busch F. X-ray computed microtomography (microCT) using synchrotron radiation (SR). Prog Biophys Mol Biol 1996; 65(1–2):133–169.

31. Grodzins L. Optimum energies for x-ray transmission tomography of small samples: applications of synchrotron radiation to computerized tomography I. Nucl Instrum Methods Phys Res, 1983; 206(3): 541–545.

32. Ford N, Thornton M, Holdsworth D. Fundamental image quality limits for micro-computed tomography in small animals. Med Phys 2003; 30(11):2869–2877.

33. Robb RA, Hoffman EA, Sinak LJ, Harris LD, Ritman EL. High-speed three-dimensional X-ray computed tomography: the dynamic spatial reconstructor. Proc IEEE 1983; 71:308–319.

34. Kalender W, Seissler W, Klotz E, Vock P. Spiral volumetric CT with single-breath-hold technique, continuous transport, and continuous scanner rotation. Radiology 1990; 176(1):181–183.

35. Feldkamp LA, Davis LC, Kress JW. Practical cone-beam algorithm. J Opt Soc Am 1984; 1(A):612–619.

36. Tang X, Ning R, Yu R, Conover D. Cone beam volume CT image artifacts caused by defective cells in X-ray flat panel imagers and the artifact removal using a wavelet-analysis-based algorithm. Med Phys 2001; 28(5):812–825.

37. Fujimoto S, Johkoh T, Koyama M, Ueguchi O, Honda H, Nakamura H. Analysis of three-dimensional microanatomy of the human lung tissue specimens using ultra high-resolution CT with a monochromatic synchrotron radiation system. In: RSNA. Supplement to Radiology 226. 2003: A259.

38. Bayat S, Le Duc G, Porra L, Berruyer G, Nemoz C, Monfraix S, Fiedler S, Thomlinson W, Suortti P, Standertskjold-Nordenstam CG, Sovijarvi AR. Quantitative functional lung imaging with synchrotron radiation using inhaled xenon as contrast agent. Phys Med Biol 2001; 46(12):3287–3299.

39. Porra L, Monfraix S, Berruyer G, Le Duc G, Nemoz C, Thomlinson W, Suortti P, Sovijarvi AR, Bayat S. Effect of tidal volume on distribution of ventilation assessed by synchrotron radiation CT in rabbit. J Appl Physiol 2004; 96(5):1899–1908.

40. Ikura H, Shimizu K, Ikezoe J, Nagareda T, Yagi N. *In vitro* evaluation of normal and abnormal lungs with ultra-high-resolution CT. J Thorac Imaging 2004; 19(1):8–15.

41. Litzlbauer H, Moell C, Neuhauser C, Nachtmann S, Greschus W. Three-dimensional assessment of alveolar tissue by micro-computed tomography. In: RSNA. Supplement to Radiology 226. 2003: A259.

42. Sera T, Fujioka H, Yokota H, Makinouchi A, Himeno R, Schroter R, Tanishita K. Three-dimensional visualization and morphometry of small airways from microfocal X-ray computed tomography. J Biomech 2003; 36(11):1587–1594.

43. Sera T, Fujioka H, Yokota H, Makinouchi A, Himeno R, Schroter R, Tanishita K. Localized compliance of small airways in excised rat lungs using microfocal X-ray computed tomography. J Appl Physiol 2004; 96(5):1665–1673.

44. Niki N, Kawata Y. Image analysis of pulmonary nodules using micro-CT. Proc SPIE; 2001; 718–725.

45. Karau KL, Johnson RH, Molthen RC, Dhyani AH, Haworth ST, Hanger CC, Roerig DL, Dawson CA. Microfocal X-ray CT imaging and pulmonary arterial distensibility in excised rat lungs. Am J Physiol Heart Circ Physiol 2001; 281(3):H1447–H1457.

46. Karau KL, Molthen RC, Dhyani A, Haworth ST, Hanger CC, Roerig DL, Johnson RH, Dawson CA. Pulmonary arterial morphometry from microfocal X-ray computed tomography. Am J Physiol Heart Circ Physiol 2001; 281(6):H2747–H2756.

47. Cavanaugh D, Johnson E, Price R, Kurie J, Travis E, Cody D. *In vivo* respiratory-gated micro-CT imaging in small-animal oncology models. Mol Imaging 2004; 3(1):55–62.

48. Dawson CA, Krenz GS, Karau KL, Hanger ST, Hanger C, Linehan JH. Structure–function relationships in the pulmonary arterial tree. J Appl Physiol 1998; 86:569–583.

49. Clough AV, Haworth ST, Ma W, Dawson CA. Effects of hypoxia on pulmonary microvascular volume. Am J Physiol Heart Circ Physiol 2000; 279(3):H1274–H1282.

50. Molthen RC, Wietholt C, Haworth ST, Dawson CA. Estimation of pulmonary arterial volume changes in the normal and hypertensive fawn-hooded rat from 3D micro-CT data. In: Chen C-T, Clough A, eds. Physiology and Function from Multidimensional Images. Proc SPIE, 4683. 2002:266–275.

51. Johnson RH. Analysis of 3D pulmonary microangiograms. In: Doi K, MacMahon H, Giger M, Hoffman K, eds. Computer-aided Diagnosis in Medical Imaging. Amsterdam: Elsevier, 1999:369–376.

52. Guarin M, Dawson CA, Nelin LD. The arterial site of action of nitric oxide in the neonatal pig lung determined by microfocal angiography. Lung 2001; 179(1):43–55.

53. Bentley J, Rickaby D, Haworth ST, Hanger CC, Dawson CA. Pulmonary arterial dilation by inhaled NO: arterial diameter, NO concentration relationship. J Appl Physiol 2001; 91(5):1948–1954.

54. Clough AV, Linehan JH, Dawson C. Regional perfusion parameters from pulmonary microfocal angiograms. Am J Physiol 1997; 272(3 Pt 2):H1537–H1548.

55. Clough AV, Haworth ST, Hanger CC, Wang J, Roerig DL, Linehan JH, Dawson CA. Transit time dispersion in the pulmonary arterial tree. J Appl Physiol 1998; 85(2):565–574.

56. Westneat MW, Betz O, Blob RW, Fezzaa K, Cooper WJ, Lee WK. Tracheal respiration in insects visualized with synchrotron X-ray imaging. Science 2003; 299(5606):558–560.

7

Noninvasive Imaging Strategies to Visualize Tissue-Specific Gene Expression Using Transcriptional Amplification Approaches

MEERA IYER

David Geffen School of Medicine at UCLA, Los Angeles, California, USA

SANJIV S. GAMBHIR

Stanford University School of Medicine, Stanford, California, USA

I. Introduction

Selective expression of therapeutic genes in tissues of interest is an essential requirement in gene therapy applications. This is due to the adverse effects of therapeutic genes on normal cells during therapy. Selective targeting of cells in patients will lead to increased treatment efficacy and safety. There are several ways to achieve targeted expression of transgenes in cells. For instance, one approach involves transcriptional targeting with tissue-specific regulatory elements and enhancers. These regulatory elements may be induced to restrict gene expression specifically to the tissue of interest.

Transcriptional activation is a key phenomenon during DNA transcription to messenger RNA and subsequent translation to a protein. Transcription is regulated through interaction between the promoter in the DNA and several transcription factors. For gene therapy applications, it is essential for the activity of a promoter to be upregulated in the target tissue. In this context, strength and tissue specificity of a promoter are important considerations. Virus-based promoters exhibit strong activity but have limited use because of a possible silencing of gene expression *in vivo* and lack of specificity. Therefore, recent interest has been focused on using promoters that carry regulatory elements that are either tissue-specific or inducible (1). However, many of the known tissue-specific promoters are poor activators of transcription. Hence, it has become evident that such promoters would find better utility if the issue of their weak transcriptional activity could be overcome. This has been made possible by linking such promoters to transactivating elements. One of the most extensively used and studied transactivator is the GAL4–VP16 fusion protein. The GAL4–VP16 transactivator has the ability to augment transgene expression from a weak promoter several hundred-fold, while maintaining tissue specificity.

In the recent past, noninvasive molecular imaging has emerged as a powerful tool to monitor cellular and molecular events *in vivo*. Rapid advances in small animal imaging instrumentation combined with the development of new imaging reporter probes have contributed to an exponential spurt of *in vivo* imaging assays. Thus, it is now possible to noninvasively monitor biologic processes such as cell trafficking, gene expression, inflammation, apoptosis, and signal transduction pathways (2). Furthermore, noninvasive imaging with vectors carrying tissue-specific gene expression systems holds significant promise and will lead to a better understanding of the efficacy and safety of selective tumor-targeting approaches.

II. GAL4 Transactivating System

Transcriptional activation is one of the fundamental means of regulating gene expression in eukaryotes and is governed by an ensemble of multi subunit transcription factor complexes. These multicomponent complexes that assemble on the promoters of genes include DNA-binding proteins, transcriptional activators, coactivators, adaptors, and other accessory proteins (3–6). Formation of a preinitiation complex at the right time and at the right promoter is a prerequisite for mRNA synthesis.

Clinical gene therapy research is faced with the key question of how to regulate the expression of therapeutic genes in a patient. The expression of many eukaryotic genes is directed by responses to environmental, hormonal, or metabolic stimuli. Studies in animal models using constitutive promoters to drive gene expression find limited use because of the continuous expression of the transferred genes. Gene expression in a constitutive manner eventually leads to downregulation of gene expression and toxicity. The solution to this problem lies in using regulatory elements in the promoter that can be activated only upon introducing an exogenous chemical or ligand. At the same time, the regulatory elements should not activate other endogenous genes. Inducible gene expression systems have been demonstrated to be extremely useful to elucidate the biological functions of genes in bacteria, yeast, and *Drosophila* species. Regulated gene expression in mammalian cells is highly desirable and bears special significance when the gene product is likely to be cytotoxic. For mammalian cells, the commonly used induction systems comprise promoters that are controlled by endogenous transcription factors by way of response to heat shock (7), heavy metal (8), or glucocorticoid hormone (9). The use of such promoters has been limited because of their high basal activity and the endogenous gene expression that is elicited by the inducing agents, which affect the expression of cellular genes along with the gene being studied.

Transcriptional regulation of gene expression has also been accomplished by using transactivators carrying DNA-binding and activation domains from bacteria, yeast, and mammalian proteins. Activating regions of different transcriptional activators are grouped on the basis of their amino acid compositions. Activating regions that are rich in acidic residues include GAL4, GCN4, and VP16. GAL4 mediates transcription in yeast, plant, insect, and mammalian cells. GAL4 is a universal activator; when introduced into any of a wide array of eukaryotic cells, it activates transcription of a gene bearing Gal4-binding sites nearby. The key to the universal action of GAL4 is that it bears two functions on a single peptide: a DNA-binding surface and an acidic activating region that interacts with a target protein. Because the mammalian cells lack Gal4-like activity and the yeast GAL4 protein recognizes a complex palindromic sequence of 17 base pairs, which is unlikely to occur by chance in mammalian cells, the GAL4 transactivator selectively mediates induction of gene expression in mammalian cells. Figure 7.1 illustrates the different functional domains of GAL4. Note that GAL4 refers to the transactivator and Gal4 denotes the binding sites positioned upstream of the reporter gene.

The role of the GAL4 transactivator was first discovered in yeast in the late 1970s. When yeast (*Saccharomyces cerevisiae*) were grown on a medium

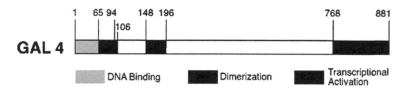

Figure 7.1 Functional domains of GAL4 containing several separable functional regions, including a DNA-binding domain (1–65), a dimerization domain (65–94), and three activating regions (94–106, 148–196, and 768–881).

containing galactose, transcription of the galactose metabolic genes, GAL1 and GAL10, was induced several thousand-fold (10–12). Induction of these divergently transcribed genes requires a short DNA sequence located between them, the GAL4 upstream-activating sequence (UAS$_G$), as well as the specific activator protein, GAL4. GAL4 is a yeast regulatory protein that binds to four sites in the UAS to activate transcription of the adjacent GAL1 and GAL10 genes (13–15). The four related 17-base pair dyad symmetrical sequences within the UAS$_G$ are responsible for GAL4-specific binding and transcriptional activation. The DNA-binding and transcriptional activation functions of GAL4 are separable. In the presence of galactose, GAL4 is freed from GAL80, an inhibitor that covers GAL4's activating region (16). This results in a significant increase in transcriptional activation. Giniger and Ptashne (10) have shown that binding of GAL4 protein to the UAS sites is cooperative *in vivo*. They found that binding sites that have a low affinity for GAL4 protein *in vitro* have little UAS activity when present as single sites but combine their activities synergistically when the two are cloned adjacent to each other. In parallel research, a synthetic GAL4-responsive promoter containing Gal4-binding sites and a TATA box with minimal transcriptional activity in mammalian cells was found to be efficiently transactivated in the presence of a GAL4 transactivator. In early experiments with yeast, it was not apparent whether GAL4 bound DNA at all. *In vivo* footprinting by Ptashne and colleagues (17) with wild-type and mutant GAL4 yeast indicated that GAL4 was responsible for generating a DMS footprint over the four DNA sites of the UAS$_G$. This prompted an analysis of various deletions of GAL4 synthesized in *Escherichia coli* as fusions to β-gal. It was found that fragments bearing the amino terminal 74 or 147 amino acids of GAL4 bound the UAS *in vitro* by footprinting analysis. Derivatives containing the amino terminus but lacking the carboxy terminus failed to activate *in vivo*. The hypothesis was that these derivatives were bound *in vivo* but lacked the activation domain. To prove this hypothesis, a wide range of heterologous activation domains, including VP16, were fused to the DNA-binding domain and were found to restore the ability of the DNA-binding region to activate transcription (18).

In other experiments with *Drosophila* species, Fischer et al. (19) have shown that GAL4, when expressed in particular tissues of *Drosophila* larvae, stimulates tissue-specific transcription of a *Drosophila* promoter linked to

Gal4-binding sites. The effector construct used in the study contained a *Drosophila* Adh promoter driving transcription of the yeast GAL4 coding sequence. The reporter construct consisted of a TATA box of *Drosophila* heat shock protein (HSP) 70 gene with four Gal4 17-mers placed upstream, driving transcription of the *E. coli* gene encoding β-galactosidase (β-gal). To facilitate binding *in vivo*, the minimal DNA-binding domain of GAL4 was fused to a heterologous activation domain such as VP16. The three components of VP16 activator complex on herpes simplex virus (HSV) early genes include Oct-1, the host cell factor (HCF), and the HSV–VP16 protein, which contains the activation domain. VP16 is a transactivator that activates the immediate early (IE) genes of HSV-1. Fusing the DNA-binding fragment of GAL4 to a highly acidic portion of the HSV–VP16 leads to significantly more activation than with GAL4 itself (20). The hybrid protein activates transcription in a highly efficient manner when bound close to, or at large distances from the gene. The VP16 domain encodes one of the most potent acidic activating functions known and works in species from yeast to man. VP16 is a 65 kd polypeptide that mediates its action through cis-regulatory elements located in regions adjacent to each IE gene (21). The protein is a structural component of the viral capsid, and its action does not require viral protein synthesis during initial infection. After infection and viral uncoating, VP16 binds to early viral promoters in a complex with cellular proteins. The original assumption was that the VP16 transactivation domain was localized to the carboxy-terminal 78 amino acids of the 490-amino-acid protein. Subsequent fusion of the carboxy-terminal region to the GAL4 DNA-binding domain gave rise to a chimera, GAL4–VP16, which was found to activate transcription from a Gal4 site-responsive reporter template (22).

There are different schools of thought as to why GAL4–VP16 is a potent activator. Some investigators believe that GAL4 forms stable dimers that efficiently fill the GAL4 DNA-binding sites *in vivo* (10). Others suggest that the acidic region of VP16 interacts with unusual avidity with certain components of the transcriptional apparatus, such as the TATA-binding factor TFIID (22). Gill and Ptashne (23) have demonstrated that GAL4 derivatives, when expressed in high levels in yeast, inhibit transcription of certain genes lacking Gal4-binding sites and derivatives bearing stronger activating regions inhibited even more efficiently. They also found that simultaneous expression of the negative regulator GAL80 at high levels relieves the inhibitory effect. This inhibition, called *squelching*, has been attributed to the interaction between an activating region and a transcription factor and can also occur freely in solution. At high activator concentrations, this reaction would sequester the transcription factor and inhibit transcription. The inhibitory effect was initially observed in genes lacking the DNA-binding domain, but at high activator concentrations, genes that carried DNA-binding domains were also inhibited (23).

In parallel work, Triezenberg and colleagues (22) found that VP16 inhibits transcription of genes lacking appropriate binding sites. This inhibitory effect is the unavoidable outcome of expression of a strong activating region. Continuous expression at high levels of this activator can be detrimental to cells. Yueh et al. (24) have shown that expression of the HSV protein VP16 is toxic to preimplantation mouse embryo but is better tolerated at later developmental stages. They observed the lethal effect to be exerted during transition from the two-cell to the four-cell stage, thereby reducing survival to the blastocyst stage. The authors speculate that the observed toxicity may occur through binding of VP16 to cellular proteins, leading to reduced availability of these proteins for essential cellular processes. Inducible gene expression systems are valuable tools for elucidating the biologic function of a wide variety of genes in bacteria, yeast, and *Drosophila* species, but one must exert a certain degree of caution to sustain the balance between optimal activation and minimal toxicity.

III. Tissue-Specific Promoters

Interaction between enhancer and promoter elements embedded within the DNA and protein transcription factors results in regulation of transcription. Promoters can be constitutive (e.g., cytomegalovirus or CMV), which are active in a wide range of cell types or tissue-specific. Important measures for promoter selection include size, strength, and tissue specificity. Constitutive promoters find limited use in targeted gene transduction because of their broad range of expression and the frequency of being silenced *in vivo*. Therefore, the use of tissue-specific promoters to achieve transduction in the desired cell/tissue is of considerable interest.

Several tissue-specific promoters have been well characterized and used in clinical gene therapy applications. Their utility has been limited because of their natural activity in normal tissues. Therefore, they are mainly used in tissues that are dispensable such as breast, prostate, melanocytes, and endocrine tissues. A 209-base pair segment of the human tyrosinase promoter linked to two enhancer elements was shown to drive high-level, melanoma-specific expression of a reporter gene in transient transfection assays (25). An adenoviral vector carrying the murine tyrosinase promoter-enhancer expression cassette was demonstrated to maintain transcriptional specificity for pigment cell lineages. In hepatocarcinomas, *in vitro* transcriptional targeting was achieved with α-fetoprotein (AFP) and carcinoembryonic antigen (CEA) promoters (26,27). AFP is specifically expressed in hepatocellular carcinomas. The AFP promoter was inserted into a retroviral vector to infect and kill hepatoma cells in a selective manner (26). CEA is a common tumor marker and is expressed in colon, hepatic, lung, and pancreatic cancers. Targeted expression and tumor regression were demonstrated in CEA-positive tumor bearing mice using adenoviral vectors carrying a therapeutic gene driven by CEA promoter (1,28,29).

Tissue-specific expression in the lung was demonstrated using the human surfactant SP-B promoter (30). This promoter was shown to be active in the adult type II alveolar epithelial cells and bronchial epithelial cells, thereby rendering it suitable for lung cancer targeting. Osteocalcin (OC) is a noncollagenous bone matrix protein and is highly expressed in osteoblasts. The OC promoter was shown to drive osteoblast-specific expression of the herpes simplex virus type I thymidine kinase gene (*HSV1-tk*) and resulted in the suppression of murine osteosarcoma *in vivo* after ganciclovir administration (31). The vector carrying the OC promoter was also studied in a model of osteosarcoma lung metastases (32). Gene therapy approaches to treat breast and prostate cancer assume significant importance because of their long-lasting nature and metastatic potential. Adenoviral vectors containing either the β-gal or *HSV1-tk* genes driven by breast tissue-specific promoters carrying regulatory sequences from the human α-lactalbumin (*hALA*) gene or the ovine β-lactoglobulin (*oBLG*) gene, were used to target expression to breast cancer cells *in vitro* and *in vivo* (33).

From the preceding discussion, it is clear that tissue-specific promoters play a key role in restricting gene expression to cancer cells. Although many of these promoters are able to maintain high levels of expression in target cells and are cell-type-specific, others suffer from weak transcriptional activity. The prostate-specific antigen (*PSA*) gene is expressed in the epithelial cells of normal and cancerous prostate. PSA is a known tumor marker and is used in the diagnosis of prostate cancer. Because of its highly tissue-specific nature, the PSA promoter has been extensively used in developing new approaches to prostate cancer gene therapy (34,35). But, the native PSA promoter, while being highly tissue-specific, demonstrates weak transcriptional activity. Therefore, for use in the development of highly efficient gene delivery vectors for prostate cancer, it is essential to amplify levels of the PSA promoter-driven gene expression. There are several strategies for increasing the transcriptional activating ability of weak promoters for gene therapy and molecular imaging applications. These are discussed in the following section.

IV. Strategies to Enhance Transcriptional Activation of Weak, Tissue-Specific Promoters

There are several strategies to augment the transcriptional activity of weak promoters. The first of these entails the use of short-length promoters that are devoid of regions not contributing to the transcriptional potency and multimerization of positive regulatory or enhancer sequences. This approach was demonstrated by using the CEA, PSA, and tyrosinase promoters (25,26,35). The limitation with this approach is that it is not a generalizable strategy because each promoter has to be optimized for maximal expression. Another approach makes use of promoters that contain activating point mutations, such as the AFP (36) and the multidrug resistance 1 (MDR1) promoters (37).

Ishikawa et al. (36) used a retroviral vector in which the variant type of the 0.3 kb human AFP promoter carried a G-to-A substitution at nucleotide − 119, a point mutation relevant to human AFP promoter regulated *HSV1-tk* gene expression. This strategy was adopted from an earlier study that showed only a G-to-A substitution at nucleotide − 119 in the human AFP promoter was responsible for the hereditary persistence of human AFP (38). In another study, chloramphenicol acetyltransferase (CAT) reporter gene expression was used to determine the MDR1 promoter efficiency and drug inducibility (37). MDR drug sensitive cell lines were transfected with constructs in which the reporter gene expression was driven by wild-type and point-mutated MDR1 promoter regions. In both cell types, the point-mutated promoter regions significantly enhanced basal and drug-induced CAT expression.

A third strategy involves randomly combing multiple tissue-specific elements, and then subsequently identifying the optimal construct. The value of this strategy was demonstrated in a muscle-specific promoter in which 5–20 DNA elements were assembled in random order (39). These cassettes were then linked to a minimal chicken α-actin promoter. One of these constructs was shown to be more potent in differentiating muscle cells than the CMV IE promoter. Yet another approach involves the use of recombinant transcriptional activators (RTAs). The structure of RTAs is based on bringing together DNA-binding domains and transactivating areas resulting from different proteins. Nettelbeck et al. (40) have used the von Willebrand factor (vWF) promoter, an endothelial cell-type-specific promoter, to drive the expression of the desired effector/reporter gene and a strong artificial transcriptional activator. The transcriptional activator consists of a DNA-binding domain of LexA and the HSV–VP16 transactivator. The transactivator fuels transcription through LexA-binding sites placed on the promoter. Using this strategy, Nettelbeck et al. showed that the transcriptional activity of the vWF promoter can be enhanced 14- to 100-fold while maintaining cell-type specificity.

A related approach makes use of a tissue-specific promoter driving the expression of a GAL4–VP16 fusion protein. This chimeric transcription factor then activates the gene of interest through Gal4-binding sites positioned upstream of a TATA region from the minimal adenovirus E1b promoter. This strategy is commonly referred to as the two-step transcriptional amplification (TSTA) system and falls under the category of two-tiered approaches for transcriptional activation (Fig. 7.2). A potent transcriptional activator, which is driven by a tissue-specific promoter, acts on a second expression plasmid, encoding the reporter/therapeutic gene. This two-step approach results in tissue-specific amplification of gene expression. Gene activation by GAL4 requires a Gal4-binding site (UAS_G) in front of the gene, whereas activation by the LexA fusion protein requires a suitably positioned LexA operator.

Between the GAL4–VP16 and LexA–VP16 fusion proteins, the Gal4–VP16 transactivator is the more commonly used system to achieve signal amplification from weak, tissue-specific promoters. Easy availability and

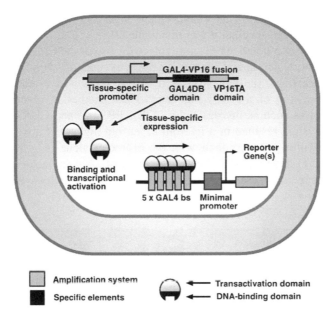

Figure 7.2 Schematic diagram of the TSTA system. The first step consists of activation of the GAL4–VP16 transactivator by a tissue-specific promoter. This is followed by binding of the transactivator complex to five Gal4-binding sites placed upstream of the target gene and a minimal promoter. Transcription of the reporter gene leads to reporter protein, which in turn leads to a detectable signal in the presence of a reporter probe.

manipulation of GAL4–VP16 vectors have contributed to its wide use. Segawa et al. (41) initially demonstrated prostate-specific amplification by utilizing the TSTA system. They used the TSTA system to drive an expanded polyglutamine to induce apoptosis selectively in PSA-positive cancer cells. In our laboratory, we have demonstrated the use of the TSTA system to enhance the transcriptional activity of the prostate-specific promoter in cell culture and in living mice [Fig. 7.3(a)] (42). In our initial studies, the effector template consisted of a GAL4 DNA-binding domain fused to a single VP16 activation domain, the reporter component comprised the TATA region from the adenovirus E1b promoter fused to the *fl* gene, bearing five 17-base pair Gal4-binding sites upstream from the TATA box. In our attempts to further augment the transcriptional activity of the PSA promoter, we demonstrated that the increase in activity could be titrated over an 800-fold range (43). This ability to achieve the desired level of gene expression by modifying the number of activation domains and the number of Gal4-binding sites illustrates the enormous potential of the TSTA system. The effector and reporter components of the TSTA system were further cloned into a single vector, resulting in levels of *fl* gene expression that were two- to threefold higher than those driven by the CMV promoter

[Fig. 7.3(b)]. This significant enhancement in reporter gene expression was attained while tissue specificity was maintained.

A second two-tiered approach involves the use of the Cre–loxP system to facilitate temporal and spatial control of gene activation (44–46). In suicide gene therapy applications, the Cre–loxP system has been used to enhance tissue-specific expression of the *HSV1-tk* gene. These studies involved the use of weak promoters such as thyroglobulin (47), AFP (48), and CEA (49,50). The use of this system resulted in a fivefold to tenfold higher cytotoxic effect with the thyroglobulin promoter than with the promoter alone (47). Kaczmarczyk and Green (51) have reported the development of a single vector containing a modified Cre recombinase and loxP sites (51). Using a prostate-specific probasin

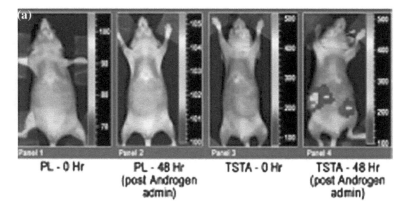

PL - 0 Hr   PL - 48 Hr   TSTA - 0 Hr   TSTA - 48 Hr
                   (post Androgen   (post Androgen
                   admin)   admin)

Figure 7.3   (**See color insert**) (a) *In vivo* optical imaging of mice carrying LNCaP cells transiently transfected with vectors representing the TSTA system. (Panel 1) LNCaP cells were transiently transfected with the vector, PSE-*fl* (PL) wherein an enhanced prostate-specific antigen promoter (PSE) directly drives *fl* expression and the cells were implanted intraperitoneally. The mouse was imaged using D-luciferin (substrate for *fl*, 150 mg/kg). (Panel 2) The same mouse in Panel 1 was reimaged 48 h following implantation of an androgen pellet. (Panel 3) LNCaP cells transiently transfected with the TSTA vectors (PSEGAL4VP16 and G5-E4T-*fl*) were implanted in a nude mouse. The mouse was imaged using D-Luciferin (Panel 4) The same mouse in Panel 3 was reimaged 48 h after implantation of an androgen pellet. Pictures shown in the figure represent bioluminescent images superimposed on gray-scale photographs. Reporter gene expression is detected in the cells representing the TSTA system, whereas *fl* expression using the one-step vector is at basal levels. [Reproduced with permission from Iyer et al. (42)]. (b) Optical imaging of one-step and TSTA system in living athymic nude mice. (i–iv) Pictures shown in the figure represent bioluminescent images superimposed on gray-scale photographs with a scale in relative light units (RLU) per minute. A map representing the dorsal surface of the mice is on the left; the circles denote the relative position of the three injection sites, with the transfected vectors labeled over each circle. The representative groups are indicated on the top of each panel. [Reproduced with permission from Zhang et al. (43)].

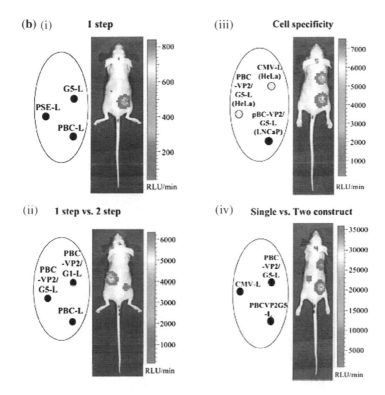

Figure 7.3 *Continued.*

promoter, they demonstrated a 300-fold increase in promoter activity. In our laboratories, we have demonstrated that the conditional activation of a PET reporter gene, *HSV1-tk*, by the Cre–loxP system can be repetitively imaged in living mice (52). An adenovirus carrying a silent *HSV1-tk* was injected intravenously into transgenic mice that express Cre recombinase in their liver (Cre+) and in control mice (Cre−) (Fig. 7.4A). Liver-specific *HSV1-tk* expression was detected in a micro positron emission tomography (PET) scanner after injection of the reporter probe, 9-[4-fluoro-3-(hydroxymethyl) butyl] guanine ([^{18}F]-FHBG [Fig. 7.4(b)]. However, a major drawback of the Cre–loxP system is that once the Cre recombinase cuts specific sites, this process cannot be reversed, thereby making it difficult to modulate the levels of gene expression.

V. Role of Molecular Imaging in the Noninvasive Monitoring of Gene Expression *In Vivo*

One of the main challenges facing the clinical gene therapy community is in the design and development of highly efficient gene delivery vectors. In light of

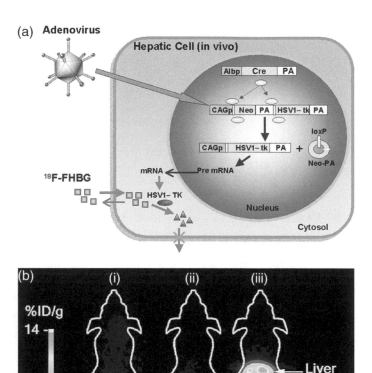

Figure 7.4 (See color insert) Imaging Cre–loxP activation. (a) Schematic of the Cre–loxP system. An adenovirus carrying the silent PET reporter gene delivers its genetic information (CAGp-loxP-Neo-PA-loxP-*HSV1-tk*-PA) into the hepatic cells. In the livers of transgenic mice, the albumin promoter drives the Cre recombinase expression. The Cre recombinase acts upon the adenoviral DNA causing excision of the Neo-PA cassette and recombination at the loxP sites leading to the *HSV1-tk* mRNA formation. The expressed *HSV1-TK* protein acts on the reporter probe ([^{18}F-FHBG]) and consequently its metabolite is trapped within the hepatic cells leading to a detectable PET signal. [Reproduced with permission from Sundaresan et al. (52)]. (b) MicroPET imaging shows *HSV1-tk* expression in the liver as seen by accumulation of the tracer [^{18}F-FHBG] in the hepatic region: (i) Cre– animal 48 h after virus injection; (ii) Cre+ animal before virus injection; and (iii) Cre+ animal 48 h after virus injection. The color scale (%ID/g) indicates the percentage of injected dose that accumulates per gram of liver. In the images shown, the maximum accumulation of [^{18}F-FHBG] was 14% ID/g in the liver of transgenic mice (c) infected with the adenovirus. [Reproduced with permission from Sundaresan et al. (52).]

the recent failure of clinical trials using viral vectors, risk assessment becomes all the more significant when dealing with viral vectors. This is where *in vivo* molecular imaging will play a key role in gene therapy research. The goals in gene therapy are to replace a damaged gene with a functional gene, introduce a gene whose product will cause the death of an unwanted tumor population, or introduce a new function into a target cell population. Before one can achieve these objectives, several questions come to mind. How does one follow the path the gene takes after delivery *in vivo*? Does the gene reach its target? Is the gene product of interest being expressed at the target? How much of it is expressed at the target site? How long does the expression persist? Can the magnitude of gene expression be regulated? The answers to all these questions lie in our ability to perform *in vivo* imaging studies. Researchers use small animal models to answer many of these questions. Mice are preferred because of their short breeding time and well-characterized genetics. They have been used to study routes of administration, dose and time effects, and alterations in vector design.

Conventional methods to monitor reporter gene expression include tissue biopsy, followed by immunohistochemistry and *in situ* hybridization with probes targeted for reporter gene mRNA. These methods are limited by their lack of ability to determine the location and magnitude of therapeutic gene expression in a noninvasive manner. In this context, the use of a reporter gene coupled to a therapeutic gene allows for *indirect* monitoring of therapeutic gene expression. The beauty of noninvasive molecular imaging lies in the ability to repetitively and quantitatively assess gene expression levels in living subjects. Repetitive imaging allows the same animal to be followed for extended periods, thereby improving the quality of the data set and reducing the number of animals required for each study. An overview of molecular imaging and its applications is provided in a recent review (2). Successful visualization of exogenous gene expression at the protein level requires marker or reporter genes that encode either cell-surface receptors or intracellular enzymes. These approaches are described in detail in an earlier publication (53). Radionuclide imaging techniques can be used to monitor the location, magnitude, and persistence of reporter gene expression in animals and humans (54). Several molecular imaging methods that are in use include single-photon emission computed tomography (SPECT) (55), PET (56), magnetic resonance imaging (MRI) (57), optical imaging (58,59), and computed tomography (CT) (60).

PET technology allows measurement of the temporal and spatial biodistribution of a molecular probe in the same animal. Another advantage is the availability of a direct link between the animal model and human studies (61). The recent development of small-animal PET cameras (microPET) has fueled the growth of molecular imaging assays. These approaches permit rapid testing of human cell targets implanted in mice and optimization of the imaging signal. Early generation microPET scanners had a spatial resolution of 2 mm^3 (62), but newer models claim to be even better with a resolution of 1 mm^3 (63).

We have reported the noninvasive monitoring of *HSV1-tk* reporter gene expression with carbon 14–labeled ganciclovir (64). In our efforts to improve the sensitivity of the PET imaging assay, we validated other reporter probes and mutant reporter genes *in vivo* (65–68). The combination of the mutant *HSV1-sr39tk* reporter gene and [^{18}F]-FHBG reporter probe offered the highest sensitivity in PET imaging assays. Furthermore, we also evaluated the dosimetry and pharmacokinetics of [^{18}F]-FHBG in healthy human volunteers (69). We found that [^{18}F]-FHBG has the desirable *in vivo* characteristics of stability, rapid blood clearance, biosafety, and acceptable radiation dosimetry in humans.

In vivo bioluminescence imaging involves the emission of visible photons at certain wavelengths based on energy-dependent reactions catalyzed by luciferases. The emitted photons are measured by using highly sensitive charge couple device (CCD) cameras. The use of the firefly luciferase (*fl*) reporter gene for monitoring gene expression has been widely reported (59,70–72). Early studies have shown the number of transfected cells that can be detected using the CCD cameras was found to be as low as 100 cells in the peritoneal cavity and 1000 cells in a subcutaneous location (73). This technique was also used to monitor the growth and regression of human cervical carcinoma cells engrafted into immunodeficient mice (74). In our laboratories, bioluminescence imaging was first used to demonstrate *fl* reporter gene expression in the skeletal muscles of living mice (75). Since then, we have come to rely heavily on this technique for the noninvasive monitoring of reporter gene expression in living animals. Using the TSTA system, we demonstrated significant augmentation in the activity of the prostate-specific promoter (42,43). Noninvasive imaging of protein–protein interactions was demonstrated in living mice by using transiently transfected cells and bioluminescence imaging with the yeast two-hybrid system (76). Recently, split reporter technology has also been used to image protein–protein interactions in living mice (77). We have also demonstrated the utility of multimodality imaging using both bioluminescence and microPET imaging to monitor cardiac-specific reporter gene expression (78).

The bioluminescence imaging technique is easy to perform, costs less than other imaging modalities, requires short acquisition times, and can be used to image several mice at a given time. Moreover, it does not require radiolabeled probes and has a high signal-to-background ratio. All these features make it a very attractive and powerful tool for *in vivo* imaging applications. However, because there is no suitable clinical equivalent of the CCD camera, bioluminescence imaging, for now, is limited to small-animal imaging research.

Indirect imaging of therapeutic gene expression based on the expression of a reporter gene can be accomplished in several ways (79). These include the use of vectors wherein the imaging and the therapeutic gene are linked by an internal ribosomal entry site (IRES) (80) or bidirectional promoter elements that drive the expression of two separate genes (81). The ability to noninvasively monitor gene expression *in vivo* will greatly aid in the development of therapeutic strategies.

Molecular imaging will have far-reaching implications in cancer gene therapy by facilitating the early detection of tumors, monitoring the effects of pharmacologic intervention in disease states, and visualizing long-term transgene expression in preclinical and clinical models.

VI. Gene Therapy Vectors

The goal in gene therapy is to develop efficient, nontoxic gene delivery vehicles that can deliver exogenous genetic material into specific cells or tissues. If successful, it will offer a powerful means to provide highly selective therapy for a wide range of diseases without having to worry about toxicity issues. For the past several years, the field of cancer gene therapy has been under active research (82,83). The gene therapy community is mainly divided into two groups: those who believe that viral vectors are the ideal vehicles for gene delivery *in vivo* and those who believe that nonviral vectors will become the mainstay in gene therapy applications. The design of vectors is also dependent on the type of gene therapy being studied. There is no universally applicable ideal vector available today. In certain applications, gene transfer to a large population of cancer cells may be required, whereas in others, regulated expression of the transferred gene may be needed. Currently, there are several clinical trials using viral vectors (84–86). In this section, we briefly discuss the different types of viral and nonviral vectors, their advantages and limitations.

A. Adenoviruses

Adenoviruses are popular as gene therapy vectors because of their high-transfection efficiencies and their ability to generate high-titer viral stocks. They represent double-stranded DNA viruses that have the ability to infect both dividing and nondividing cells (87). Recombinant adenoviruses were initially used as gene transfer vehicles in clinical trials for cystic fibrosis (88). Subsequently, adenoviruses were used to achieve gene transfer into a variety of cell types cancer therapy applications (89–92).

Wu et al. (93) have demonstrated the use of an adenoviral vector carrying a modified PSA promoter for selective expression in prostate tumors. To demonstrate the potential of the TSTA system in a gene therapy paradigm, we incorporated the system into a replication-deficient adenovirus (Ad-TSTA) (94). We found that Ad-TSTA-mediated *fl* gene expression was greater than that of the CMV promoter. The Ad-TSTA system was also used to study androgen receptor (AR) dynamics in prostate cancer progression in living mice (Fig. 7.5) (95). Noninvasive imaging with Ad-TSTA in live mice was used to monitor the AR function during tumor progression from an androgen-dependent (AD) to an androgen-independent (AI) state. The loss and recovery of AR activity during tumor growth was also visualized *in vivo* (95). The results were suggestive of AR's fully functional role in recurrent cancer.

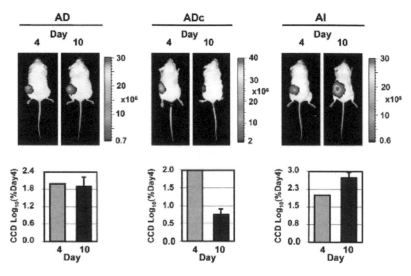

Figure 7.5 (**See color insert**) Imaging AR signaling in LAPC-9 tumors. SCID mice implanted with LAPC-9 prostate tumor xenografts (androgen dependent, AD and androgen independent, AI groups) were injected with 10^7 plaque forming units (pfu) of an adenovirus carrying the TSTA system (Ad-TSTA) and the mice were imaged every 3–4 days over a 14-day period. Representative mice at day 4 and day 10 after virus injection from the AD group, the castrated AD group (Adc), and the stable AI group. The bar graph summarizes a cohort of three or more animals and summarizes the log of the percentage change in signal from day 4 to day 10. Color images of visible light are superimposed on photographic images of mice with a scale in photons per second per square centimeter per steradian (sr). [Reproduced with permission from Zhang et al. (95).]

In adenovirus-mediated transfection, gene expression is transient because the viral DNA does not integrate permanently into the host cell genome. Therefore, in applications in which a high level of persistent expression is warranted, repeated administration of the adenovirus becomes essential. This constitutes one of the several drawbacks of using adenoviral vectors for gene therapy. A second limitation is the cellular and humoral immune response to these viruses (96,97). Adenoviral vectors are being looked at more closely now than ever before following the first reported death in clinical trials in which these vectors were used (98). Efforts to find ways to make these viruses safer and less toxic have led to the development of second- and third-generation vectors with many of the viral genes deleted (99). An adenoviral vector expressing β-gal from the strong major IE murine cytomegalovirus (MIEmCMV) promoter was used to achieve 100% gene transfer efficiency and expression in the adult rat brain (100,101). When low doses of the vector were used, transgene expression was observed in relatively large areas of the brain at high levels with complete absence of any cellular inflammation or cytotoxicity. Further improvements in coming years are likely to make these viruses even safer to use.

B. Adeno-Associated Virus

Adeno-associated viruses (AAV) are single-stranded DNA viruses that can infect both dividing and nondividing cells (102,103). Transfection with these viruses results in DNA incorporation into the host cell genome. These viruses have several advantages as gene-delivery vectors. The parental virus does not cause disease; they can transduce both dividing and nondividing cells and persist for the lifetime of the cell (104), nor do they induce inflammatory responses. The main limitations of AAV vectors include a limited payload capacity (4.5 kb) and need for helper viruses for their production. The latter requirement often results in contamination of the AAVs during production. Efforts to overcome this limitation include induction of viral replication through genotoxic stimuli such as heat shock, chemicals, or irradiation (105). These viruses have been used to attain long-term gene expression *in vivo*. AAV vectors have been shown to be capable of expressing the human cystic fibrosis transmembrane conductance regulator (CFTR) cDNA in the airway epithelium of rabbits (106). Prolonged expression of reporter genes for up to 18 months has been achieved in immunocompetent mice by direct intramuscular injection of AAV vectors (107). Therapeutic levels of expression of the human erythropoietin have been attained by intramuscular injection of an AAV vector (108). With improvements in AAV vectors, it is plausible that these vectors will find increasing use in therapeutic applications.

C. Retroviruses

Retroviruses are lipid-enveloped particles containing a homodimer of linear, single-stranded RNA genomes of 7–11 kb. After transfection, the RNA genome is retro-transcribed into linear double-stranded DNA and integrated into the cell chromatin (109). The ability of retroviruses to integrate into the host genome significantly increases their utility for *in vivo* study of gene expression for extended periods. The family of retroviruses includes the mammalian and avian C-type retroviruses, lentiviruses, and spumaviruses. Retroviruses can be used to insert up to 8 kb of foreign DNA. The first use of retroviruses to deliver exogenous DNA was reported in 1981 (110,111). Retroviral vectors carrying multiple genes (human interleukin-2 and *HSV1-tk*) were used to demonstrate regression in tumor size in gene therapy of thyroid cancer (112). Insertion of multiple genes in a retrovirus is difficult to achieve because of the size limitation of DNA insertion. Also, most retroviruses only infect actively dividing cells during mitosis (113,114). This poses a serious drawback because tumors contain cells that are in the resting phase, which can escape therapy. In this regard, lentiviruses specifically hold an edge over the retroviruses by virtue of their ability to infect nondividing cells.

D. Lentiviruses

Lentiviruses are promising vectors for gene delivery *in vivo* with many in preclinical development for gene therapy (115). The mechanism of nuclear targeting (by transport of the preinitiation complex through the nucleophore) confers the ability to infect nondividing cells. Replication-defective vectors were originally derived from human immunodeficiency virus 1 (HIV-1) to transduce lymphocytes, but it was the development of a vesicular stomatitis virus glycoprotein (VSV-G) pseudotyped lentiviral vector with broad tropism that drove their use in gene therapy (116). Over the years, lentiviruses have undergone several modifications aimed at increasing their biosafety. Vigna and Naldini (115) found that the genetic information required to package a functional lentiviral core in the vector comprises only a fraction of the parental genome. New generations of lentiviruses are made up of minimal packaging constructs; these are the self-inactivating (SIN) lentiviral vectors. They contain a deletion in the 3′ long terminal repeat (LTR) that results in transcriptional inactivation of the LTR. This feature considerably reduces the risk of vector recombination (117).

Further improvements in transduction efficiency and transgene expression have been achieved by incorporating a central polypurine tract (cPPT) and a post-transcriptional regulatory element (PRE) into the lentivirus vectors (118). From our laboratories, we have recently reported the noninvasive imaging of lentivirus-mediated reporter gene expression in living mice (119). We demonstrated the use of both bioluminescence and microPET imaging to monitor the expression of *fl* and *HSV1-sr39tk* reporter genes, respectively. The expression of the reporter genes was driven by a constitutive CMV promoter. The utility of constitutive promoters for long-term monitoring of gene expression is limited because of the inability to control gene expression and potential toxicity. In this context, transcriptional targeting using lentivirus vectors carrying tissue-specific promoters is an attractive approach to visualize expression of transgenes in specific cells or tissues (120–123).

We have recently demonstrated the noninvasive imaging of the TSTA system-based prostate-specific expression of *fl* reporter gene in living mice using bioluminescence imaging [Fig. 7.6(a)] (124). We observed that *fl* gene expression could be monitored longitudinally after injection of the lentivirus into the prostate [Fig. 7.6(b)]. We also demonstrated cell-type specificity *in vivo* using an AD prostate tumor model. The combined use of a SIN lentivirus vector and the TSTA amplification strategy makes this approach very attractive for use with other weak, tissue-specific promoters. In addition, the reporter gene cassette can also be modified to include multiple reporter genes or a reporter gene and a therapeutic gene leading to multimodality imaging approaches for long-term, tissue-specific, noninvasive monitoring of gene expression.

E. Nonviral Vectors

Because of the immunogenicity and biosafety issues associated with viral vectors, a significant number of researchers in the gene therapy community believe that nonviral gene delivery vehicles will be the vectors of choice in clinical gene therapy applications. Nonviral vectors are less immunogenic, can be

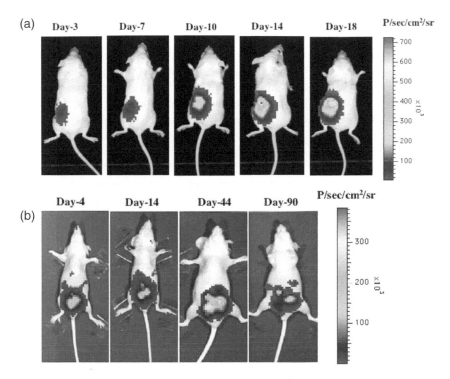

Figure 7.6 (**See color insert**) Tumor-specific expression of *fl* reporter gene in male, SCID mice following intratumoral injection of a lentivirus carrying the TSTA system. (a) Six-week-old male, SCID mice were implanted with prostate tumor LAPC-9 xenografts in the left, bottom flank. When the tumor size reached 0.5–0.6 cm in diameter, lentivirus carrying the TSTA system (LV-TSTA) was injected directly into the tumor. The mice were imaged using a charge coupled device (CCD) camera on days 3, 7, 10, 14 and 18 using D-Luciferin as the substrate (150 mg/kg, i.p.). Color images of visible light are super-imposed on photographic images of mice with a scale in photons per second per square centimeter per steradian (sr). A significantly high level of *fl* gene expression is observed in the tumor, which continues to persist to day 18. (b) *In vivo* optical imaging of mice following direct intraprostatic delivery of LV-TSTA. [Reproduced with permission from Iyer et al. (124).] (b) Six-week-old male, nude mice were injected with the lentivirus in the dorsal lobe of the prostate. The mice were imaged using the CCD camera 2–4 days after virus injection. Subsequent imaging was performed every 3–4 days till day 21, then once a week until day 90. By day 4, a high level of bioluminescence signal is observed in the prostate (2.2×10^5 photons/s per cm^2 per sr). The *fl* expression shows strong persistence with time. [Reproduced with permission from Iyer et al. (124).]

produced in large quantities, and can be targeted effectively to organs (125). However, a major limitation of nonviral vectors is the low efficiency of gene transfer *in vivo*. The last several years have seen tremendous improvements in the formulation and design of these vectors, leading to significant improvements in transfection efficiency. Nonviral vectors, like liposomes and polymers, are usually cationic in nature and interact with the negatively charged DNA through electrostatic interactions. The net positive charge on the complex enables interaction with the cell membrane, followed by internalization by endocytosis (126). Several factors influence the stability and efficiency of liposome–DNA complexes such as particle size, zeta potential, and the ratio of DNA and liposome used (127). With continued improvements in the design of such vectors, one can hope to be able to increase their usage in clinical gene therapy applications.

Felgner et al. (128) first introduced liposomes as vehicles for gene transfer in 1987. They used the cationic lipid, *N*-[1-(2,3-dioleyloxy) propyl]-*N,N,N*-trimethylammonium chloride (DOTMA) to form complexes with DNA, thereby facilitating fusion of the complex with the plasma membrane of cells resulting in uptake and expression. Since then, different formulations of cationic lipids have been evaluated for their gene transfer ability *in vivo* (129–131). The most notable of these is 1,2-dioleoyl-3-trimethylammonium-propane (DOTAP). DOTAP consists of two unsaturated diacyl side chains, an ester linker, and a propyl ammonium group (132). DOTAP was used along with cholesterol as the helper lipid to achieve CAT gene delivery in mice (131). DOTAP–cholesterol formulations were found to be the most efficient, producing high levels of gene expression, predominantly in the lung. In our laboratories, we used DOTAP–cholesterol to demonstrate noninvasive imaging of *fl* DNA using both bioluminescence and microPET imaging (Fig. 7.7) (133). Reporter gene expression (*fl* and *HSV1-sr39tk*) was observed primarily in the lungs after systemic administration of the plasmid DNA–liposome complex.

The second class of nonviral vectors are synthetic cationic polymers which, when combined with DNA, form a polyplex. Their synthetic origin makes it convenient to modify their structure and molecular weight. The most popular and extensively studied cationic polymer is polyethylenimine (PEI). PEI displays efficient transfection characteristics because of its ability to protonate, bind, protect, and deliver DNA *in vivo* (134). PEI has also been conjugated with antibodies, vitamins, and receptor ligands for tumor targeting. Pegylated PEI polyplexes have conjugated with transferrin, to achieve tumor-specific expression with highly stable polyplexes (134). We have used bioluminescence imaging to demonstrate noninvasive imaging of transferrin targeted PEI/*fl* DNA complexes in living mice (135). Like cationic liposomes, the overall efficiency of PEI polyplexes depends on several factors (molecular weight, zeta potential, particle size).

VII. Imaging Pulmonary Gene Expression *In Vivo*

Recent advances in vector development and promoter enhancement have extended the potential of gene therapy from hereditary to acute diseases (136).

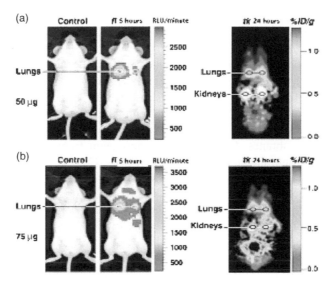

Figure 7.7 **(See color insert)** Dual imaging of optical and PET reporter genes in the same living animal using cationic liposomes. CD-1 mice were first imaged 5 h after injection using the CCD camera in the absence of D-Luciferin (control) and then imaged again following injection of D-Luciferin. The same mice were imaged 24 h later with [^{18}F]-FHBG using microPET. (a) A CD-1 mouse injected with 50 μg each of *fl* and *HSV1-sr39tk* DNA–DOTAP–cholesterol complex via tail-vein. Pictures shown in the figure represent bioluminescent images superimposed on gray-scale photographs with a scale in relative light units per minute (RLU/min). The control image shows background levels of *fl* expression in the lungs (<50 RLU/min). At 5 h, the *fl* gene expression is significantly greater than that of the control (2958 RLU/min). The same mouse imaged at 24 h shows low levels of *HSV1-sr39tk* gene expression in the lung (percent injected dose per gram, 0.46%ID/g). [Reproduced with permission from Iyer et al. (133).] (b) A CD-1 mouse was injected with 75 μg each of *fl* and *HSV1-sr39tk* DNA–DOTAP–cholesterol complex via tail-vein. The control image shows background levels of *fl* expression (<50 RLU/min). In contrast, the image acquired after injection of D-luciferin shows a high level of *fl* expression in the lungs (3668 RLU/min). MicroPET imaging using [^{18}F]-FHBG shows increased levels of *HSV1-sr39tk* gene expression in the lungs at 24 h (1.0%ID/g). [Reproduced with permission from Iyer et al. (133).]

The field of gene therapy for acute diseases encompasses maladies such as asthma, cardiogenic and noncardiogenic pulmonary edema, and acute myocardial infarction. It is now possible to visualize the use of gene therapy for the treatment of lung disorders that include pulmonary hypertension and acute respiratory distress syndrome. For example, Weiss et al. (137) have demonstrated the successful transfer of HSP-70 gene to rat lungs after experimental lung injury. This led to a significant decrease in lung interstitial and alveolar edema and mortality. Although the previous study did not use imaging, noninvasive imaging of pulmonary gene transfer in preclinical models will be a valuable tool to evaluate the success of therapeutic gene transfer to the lung in gene therapy applications. Gene transfer to the lung allows for specific targeting of gene expression to lung airway and alveolar epithelium but has been hampered by physical and immunologic barriers (138,139). Physical barriers to pulmonary gene transfer include mucins and surfactants lining the airways and alveolar spaces and glycocalyceal proteins on the apical surface of airway epithelial cells. The tight junctions between the epithelial cells limit access of vectors to receptors on basolateral cell surface membranes. Immunologic barriers stem from the innate immune response to the introduction of exogenous vectors. Current work in the area of pulmonary gene therapy is focused on overcoming these barriers and includes removal of the transmembrane mucin glycoprotein by treatment with neuraminidase (140). In a related study using sheep trachea in organ culture, removal of mucin resulted in a 25-fold increase in cationic liposome-mediated gene transfer (141).

Current methods to deliver genes to the airway and alveolar epithelium include nasal deposition, direct instillation into the trachea with a catheter or bronchoscope, and inhalation of vectors (142–144). The use of nasal deposition of vector in humans has been limited to the nasal epithelia (142). Direct vector instillation often leads to heterogeneous delivery in limited areas of the lung, thereby necessitating the need for multiple instillations. The inhalation approach leads to gene transfer in all areas of the lung but requires large amounts of the vector. Additionally, the aerosolization process has been shown to disrupt cationic liposomes (145).

To assess the efficiency of cationic liposome-mediated gene transfer *in vivo*, we used DOTAP–cholesterol complexed with plasmid DNA (*fl* and *HSV1-sr39tk*) in a mouse model. After systemic delivery of the DNA–liposome complex in CD-1 mice, bioluminescent and PET imaging were performed using D-Luciferin and [^{18}F]-FHBG, respectively (133). Gene expression was observed predominantly in the lungs because the pulmonary vasculature is the first capillary bed encountered by the lipid complexes after systemic administration (Fig. 7.7). Gene expression in the lungs was detected as early as 5 h and persisted until 24 h. Gene expression was found to be higher in the right lung across several mice. *Ex vivo* analysis of the lung tissue confirmed this differential gene expression. The observed asymmetry in the lung signal may be related to physiologic events within the animal, such as blood flow. Gene delivery to the lung has also been demonstrated in a rat model using a replication-incompetent adenovirus carrying a fusion gene of the mutant *HSV1-sr39tk* and green fluorescent protein (*GFP*) (146). After intratracheal administration of the virus, *HSV1-sr39tk* gene expression was detected in the lungs using [^{18}F]-FHBG as the reporter substrate (Fig. 7.8). Among the different techniques used to increase gene expression in the lungs, cationic lipid-based gene delivery leads to expression in the pulmonary endothelial cells. Intratracheal administration of adenoviral vectors yields transgene expression in the alveolar epithelial cells.

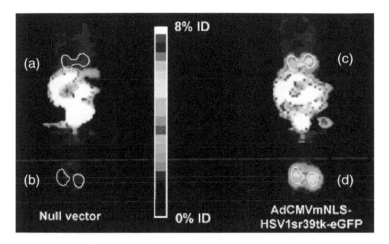

Figure 7.8 **(See color insert)** Reporter gene expression with PET in a control mouse infected with a null vector (left) and a mouse expressing mutant *HSV1-sr39tk* gene (right). Ad-CMVmNLS-*HSV1-sr39tk*-e*GFP*, adenovirus-cytomegalovirus promoter-, mutated nuclear localization signal – *HSV1-sr39tk*-e*GFP* vector. Three days after adeno-virus-mediated intratracheal gene transfer, 10 μCi/g of body weight of [^{18}F]-FHBG was intravenously injected into both mice. PET imaging was performed after 1 h over 15-min acquisition time. (a, c) Coronal views of mice. (b, d) Corresponding transverse slices obtained at midlung level. In both mice, regions of interest are drawn to indicate lung boundaries (white lines), and tracer uptake was expressed as percentage of injected dose (ID/g). Although there was significant pulmonary uptake of tracer in mice expressing viral thymidine kinase, pulmonary activity was not different from background in control mice. High levels of activity in abdomen are due to a combination of urinary excretion and biliary excretion into the gastrointestinal tract. [Reproduced with permission from Richard et al. (146).]

A comparative study using surfactant vs. saline solution to improve adenovirus-based reporter gene transfer to rat lungs showed that an increase in gene transfer efficiency was achieved with surfactant (147).

    With continued improvement in the design of vectors, it should now be possible to achieve high levels of transgene expression in the lungs and to monitor gene expression over an extended period. The reporter gene expression observed in the studies described earlier was driven by a constitutive CMV promoter. As major limitations of using constitutive promoters include the inability to modulate the levels of gene expression, potential silencing effects, and toxicity, the use of lung-specific promoters will allow targeted expression specifically to the lung tissue. Further, the use of lung-specific promoters in a TSTA system will significantly enhance the transcriptional activities of such promoters, leading to a highly amplified signal in the lung. With increased use of gene therapy approaches to treat lung disorders, the TSTA system carrying lung-specific promoters will be a powerful tool for *in vivo* monitoring of pulmonary gene expression.

VIII. Transgenic Mouse Models

Transgenic mouse models constitute an important platform to study gene function, regulation, and the evaluation of transgene expression during growth and development. Transgenic mouse models allow visualization of gene expression patterns in a longitudinal manner. Several groups have used transgenic models to monitor gene expression, developmental regulation, and response to therapy. For instance, Green et al. (148) demonstrated repetitive imaging of the endogenous albumin gene in transgenic mice using microPET. The expression of the reporter gene, *HSV1-tk*, was driven by an albumin promoter. Bioluminescence imaging has been used extensively to monitor gene expression in transgenic mouse models. Lee et al. (149) used bioluminescence imaging to demonstrate intestine-specific expression of the lactase gene. The goal in this study was to identify regions of the lactase gene involved in the spatiotemporal expression in the intestine of developing transgenic mice. A transgenic mouse model has been used to study factors controlling bone morphogenetic protein 4 (Bmp 4) expression during primordial and mature tissue development (150). The activity of nuclear factor κB (NF-κB) promoter has been imaged in transgenic mice using a bioluminescent reporter (*fl*) (151). Voojs et al. (152) have studied retinoblastoma suppressor gene-dependent pituitary cancer development with coexpression of the *fl* gene. Using bioluminescence imaging, they demonstrated both long-term monitoring of gene expression and the ability to assess therapeutic response.

The hormonal and tissue-specific regulation of the PSA promoter has made it an attractive model for the study of gene function. With the significant levels of amplification attained by using the prostate-specific TSTA system, the development of transgenic mouse models carrying prostate-specific promoters should facilitate the study of tissue specificity and developmental regulation of gene expression. Tissue-specific transgenic mouse models carrying the TSTA system can be single- or two-tiered. The single-tiered system incorporates a single vector carrying the effector and reporter cassettes, whereas in the two-tiered approach, the effector and reporter cassettes are placed in two different vectors, which are then used to generate two different lines of transgenic mice. The gene of interest is activated in the offspring by crossing the effector and reporter mice. Because of concerns regarding the potential deleterious effects of the transactivators in a single-tiered system, several investigators have resorted to using the two-tiered approach to generate and study transgenic mouse models (153,154).

The two-tiered system circumvents the problem of excessive expression and toxicity caused by the transactivators and the expressed transgenes. Ornitz et al. (154) have reported the development of a two-tiered transgenic system that activated an otherwise silent transgene in the progeny arising from genetic crossing. The transactivator strain carried a *GAL4* gene driven by a mouse mammary tumor virus (MMTV) LTR. The target gene studied was int-2 cDNA inserted between the UAS/elastase promoter and the *hGH* gene. Similarly, Byrne and Ruddle (153) have demonstrated the use of a transactivator strain carrying the HSV1–VP16 transactivator and an effector strain carrying a CAT reporter gene regulated by the HSV1-1E promoter element. One advantage of using the two-tiered system is the ability to combine different promoter and transgene pairs by simple mating.

In continuation with our work on the prostate-specific TSTA system, we have recently developed a transgenic mouse model carrying the *fl* reporter gene (155). The *fl* gene expression is rendered prostate-specific through the use of a prostate-specific promoter-driven TSTA system (Fig. 7.9). Our previous studies revealed that the use of a single vector carrying the two transcriptional units leads to a significant enhancement in *fl* bioluminescence signal *in vivo* (43). In this study, we also demonstrated the highly titratable nature of the TSTA system, leading to an ~800-fold increase in reporter gene expression. This work led to the development of the TSTA transgenic mouse model to monitor amplified prostate-specific gene expression using bioluminescence imaging and to explore the deleterious effects, if any, from the potent transactivator. No deleterious effects were observed in the transgenic offspring. The founder animals and their progeny were healthy, bred well, and demonstrated no signs of spontaneous tumor development. In an earlier report, a single expression

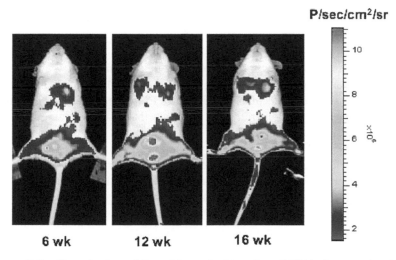

Figure 7.9 (**See color insert**) Repetitive optical imaging of TSTA-*fl* transgenic mice. A transgenic male mouse was imaged in the CCD camera at 8 weeks of age, then subsequently reimaged at 12 and 16 weeks. Color images of visible light are superimposed on photographic images of mice with a scale in photons per second per square centimeter per steradian (sr). Gene expression is primarily observed in the prostate tissue and shows persistence with time ($2-3 \times 10^6$ p/s per cm^2 per sr). [Reproduced with permission from Iyer M and Gambhir SS (Transgenic Research, 2005, in press).]

vector carrying the two transcriptional cassettes was used to demonstrate tissue-specific gene expression in muscle, notochordal, and neuronal tissues (156). The authors found that the high frequency of GAL4–VP16-amplified transgene expression was maintained in the single vector and low to moderate levels of the vector were well tolerated. However, some toxicity was observed at high concentrations of the vector resulting in malformed embryos. Further to the TSTA transgenic mouse model, we have recently demonstrated amplification of *fl* gene expression from the vascular endothelial growth factor (VEGF) promoter in a transgenic model (157,158).

The development of a prostate-specific transgenic mouse model provides a platform for developing other transgenic mouse models using relatively weak tissue-specific promoters. These models should have significant applications in prostate cancer gene therapy by marrying them with other models that possess the ability to develop spontaneous malignancies. The use of spontaneous tumor models will enable the study of key targets during disease progression and better characterization of early events. Transgenic mouse models of lung cancer using lung-specific promoters will allow the regulation of gene expression in the lung and the development of diagnostic and therapeutic approaches for the treatment of lung cancer. Such models, combined with sensitive imaging modalities, will play a vital role in accelerating the development of more effective therapies.

IX. Conclusion

The use of tissue-specific amplification strategies will likely play a key role in gene therapy and in molecular imaging. With signal amplification being a critical parameter in *in vivo* molecular imaging, the TSTA strategy described in this chapter is a useful and generalizable approach that will allow the use of any weak, tissue-specific promoter to be used in targeted gene therapy imaging. This strategy should continue to find applications for highly amplified gene expression in many areas, including pulmonary gene therapy. With further refinements in vector development and molecular imaging techniques, many models are likely to benefit from this strategy.

References

1. Nettelbeck DM, Jerome V, Muller R. Gene therapy: designer promoters for tumour targeting. Trends Genet 2000; 16:174–181.
2. Massoud TF, Gambhir SS. Molecular imaging in living subjects: seeing fundamental biological processes in a new light. Genes Dev 2003; 17:545–580.
3. Martin KJ. The interactions of transcription factors and their adaptors, coactivators and accessory proteins. Bioessays 1991; 13:499–503.

4. Ptashne M, Gann A. Transcriptional activation by recruitment. Nature 1997; 386:569–577.
5. Gaudreau L, Adam MA, Ptashne M. Activation of transcription *in vitro* by recruitment of the yeast RNA polymerase II holoenzyme. Mol Cell 1998; 1:913–916.
6. Keaveney M, Struhl K. Activator-mediated recruitment of the RNA polymerase II machinery is the predominant mechanism for transcriptional activation in yeast. Mol Cell 1998; 1:917–924.
7. Wurm FM, Gwinn KA, Kingston RE. Inducible overproduction of the mouse c-myc protein in mammalian cells. Proc Natl Acad Sci USA 1986; 83:5414–5418.
8. Mayo KE, Warren RS, Palmiter RD. The mouse metallothionein-I gene is transcriptionally regulated by cadmium following transfection into human or mouse cells. Cell 1982; 29:99–108.
9. Hynes NE, Kennedy N, Rahmsdorf U, Groner B. Hormone-responsive expression of an endogenous proviral gene of mouse mammary tumor virus after molecular cloning and gene transfer into cultured cells. Proc Natl Acad Sci USA 1981; 78:2038–2042.
10. Giniger E, Ptashne M. Cooperative DNA binding of the yeast transcriptional activator GAL4. Proc Natl Acad Sci USA 1988; 85:382–386.
11. Hopper JE, Broach JR, Rowe LB. Regulation of the galactose pathway in *Saccharomyces cerevisiae*: induction of uridyl transferase mRNA and dependency on GAL4 gene function. Proc Natl Acad Sci USA 1978; 75:2878–2882.
12. St John TP, Davis RW. The organization and transcription of the galactose gene cluster of *Saccharomyces*. J Mol Biol 1981; 152:285–315.
13. Bram R, Kornberg R. Specific protein binding to far upstream activating sequences in polymerase II promoters. Proc Natl Acad Sci USA 1985; 82:43–47.
14. Keegan L, Gill G, Ptashne M. Separation of DNA binding from the transcription-activating function of a eukaryotic regulatory protein. Science 1986; 231:699–704.
15. Selleck SB, Majors JE. *In vivo* DNA-binding properties of a yeast transcription activator protein. Mol Cell Biol 1987; 7:3260–3267.
16. Zenke FT, Engles R, Vollenbroich V, Meyer J, Hollenberg CP, Breunig KD. Activation of gal4p by galactose-dependent interaction of galactokinase and gal80pinteraction of galactokinase and Gal80p. Science 1996; 272:1662–1665.
17. Giniger E, Varnum SM, Ptashne M. Specific DNA binding of GAL4, a positive regulatory protein of yeast. Cell 1985; 40:767–774.
18. Ma J, Ptashne M. Deletion analysis of GAL4 defines two transcriptional activating segments. Cell 1987; 48:847–853.
19. Fischer JA, Giniger E, Maniatis T, Ptashne M. GAL4 activates transcription in *Drosophila*. Nature 1988; 332:853–856.
20. Triezenberg SJ, LaMarco KL, McKnight SL. Evidence of DNA:protein interactions that mediate HSV-1 immediate early gene activation by VP16. Genes Dev 1988; 2:730–742.
21. Carey M, Smale ST. Transcriptional Regulation in Eukaryotes. New York: Cold Spring Harbor Laboratory Press, 2000:640.
22. Sadowski I, Ma J, Triezenberg S, Ptashne M. GAL4-VP16 is an unusually potent transcriptional activator. Nature 1988; 335:563–564.

23. Gill G, Ptashne M. Negative effect of the transcriptional activator GAL4. Nature 1988; 334:721–724.

24. Yueh YG, Yaworsky PJ, Kappen C. Herpes simplex virus transcriptional activator VP16 is detrimental to preimplantation development in mice. Mol Reprod Dev 2000; 55:37–46.

25. Siders WM, Halloran PJ, Fenton RG. Transcriptional targeting of recombinant adenoviruses to human and murine melanoma cells. Cancer Res 1996; 56:5638–5646.

26. Richards CA, Austin EA, Huber BE. Transcriptional regulatory sequences of carcinoembryonic antigen: identification and use with cytosine deaminase for tumor-specific gene therapy. Hum Gen Ther 1995; 6:881–893.

27. Kanai F, Lan KH, Shiratori Y, Tanaka T, Ohashi M, Okudaira T, Yoshida Y, Wakimoto H, Hamada H, Nakabayashi H, Tamaoki T, Omata M. *In vivo* gene therapy for alpha-fetoprotein-producing hepatocellular carcinoma by adenovirus-mediated transfer of cytosine deaminase gene. Cancer Res 1997; 57:461–465.

28. Lan KH, Kanai F, Shiratori Y, Ohashi M, Tanaka T, Okudaira T, Yoshida Y, Hamada H, Omata M. *In vivo* selective gene expression and therapy mediated by adenoviral vectors for human carcinoembryonic antigen-producing gastric carcinoma. Cancer Res 1997; 57:4279–4284.

29. Haviv YS, Curiel DT. Conditional gene targeting for cancer gene therapy. Adv Drug Deliv Rev 2001; 53:135–154.

30. Bohinski RJ, Huffman JA, Whitsett JA, Lattier DL. cis-Active elements controlling lung cell-specific expression of human pulmonary surfactant protein B gene. J. Biol Chem 1993; 268:11160–11166.

31. Ko SC, Cheon J, Kao C, Gotoh A, Shirakawa T, Sikes RA, Karsenty G, Chung LW. Osteocalcin-promoter based toxic gene therapy for the treatment of osteosarcoma in experimental models. Cancer Res 1996; 56:4614–4619.

32. Shirakawa T, Ko SC, Gardner TA, Cheon J, Miyamoto T, Gotoh A, Chung LW, Kao C. *In vivo* suppression of osteosarcoma pulmonary metastasis with intravenous osteocalcin promoter-based toxic gene therapy. Cancer Gene Ther 1998; 5:274–280.

33. Anderson LM, Swaminathan S, Zackon I, Tajuddin AK, Thimmapaya B, Weitzman SA. Adenovirus-mediated tissue-targeted expression of the HSV-tk gene for the treatment of breast cancer. Gene Ther 1999; 6:854–864.

34. Rodriguez R, Schuur ER, Lim HY, Henderson GA, Simons JW, Henderson DR. Prostate attenuated replication competent adenovirus (ARCA) CN706: a selective cytotoxic for prostate-specific antigen-positive prostate cancer cells. Cancer Res 1997; 57:2559–2563.

35. Pang S, Dannull J, Kaboo R, Xie Y, Tso CI, Michel K, deKernion JB, Belldegrun A, Wu L. Identification of a positive regulatory element responsible for tissue-specific expression of prostate-specific antigen. Cancer Res 1997; 57:495–499.

36. Ishikawa H, Nakata K, Mawatari F, Ueki T, Tsuruta S, Ido A, Nakao K, Kato Y, Ishii N, Eguchi K. Utilization of variant-type of human alpha-fetoprotein promoter in gene therapy targeting for hepatocellular carcinoma. Gene Ther 1999; 6:465–470.

37. Stein U, Walther W, Shoemaker RH. Vincristine induction of mutant and wild-type human multidrug-resistance promoters is cell-type-specific and dose-dependent. J Cancer Res Clin Oncol 1996; 122:275–282.

38. McVey JH, Michaelides K, Hansen LP, Ferguson-Smith M, Tilghman S, Krumlauf R, Tuddenham EG. A G → A substitution in an HNF I binding site in the human alpha-fetoprotein gene is associated with hereditary persistence of alpha-fetoprotein (HPAFP). Hum Mol Genet 1993; 2:379–384.

39. Li X, Eastman EM, Schwartz RJ, Draghia-Akli R. Synthetic muscle promoters: activities exceeding naturally occurring regulatory sequences. Nat Biotechnol 1999; 17:241–245.

40. Nettelbeck DM, Jerome V, Muller R. A strategy for enhancing the transcriptional activity of weak cell type-specific promoters. Gene Ther 1998; 5:1656–1664.

41. Segawa T, Takebayashi H, Kakehi Y, Yoshida O, Narumiya S, Kakizuka A. Prostate-specific amplification of expanded polyglutamine expression: a novel approach for cancer gene therapy. Cancer Res 1998; 58:2282–2287.

42. Iyer M, Wu L, Carey M, Wang Y, Smallwood A, Gambhir SS. Two-step transcriptional amplification as a method for imaging reporter gene expression using weak promoters. Proc Natl Acad Sci USA 2001; 98:14595–14600.

43. Zhang L, Adams JY, Billick E, Ilagan R, Iyer M, Le K, Smallwood A, Gambhir SS, Carey M, Wu L. Molecular engineering of a two-step transcription amplification (TSTA) system for transgene delivery in prostate cancer. Mol Ther 2002; 5:223–232.

44. Lakso M, Sauer B, Mosinger B, Lee EJ, Manning RW, Yu SH, Mulder KL, Westphal H. Targeted oncogene activation by site-specific recombination in transgenic mice. Proc Natl Acad Sci USA 1992; 89:6232–6236.

45. Sauer B. Manipulation of transgenes by site-specific recombination in transgenic mice. Methods Enzymol 1993; 225:890–900.

46. Voziyanov I, Pathania S, Jayaram M. A general model for site-specific recombination by the integrase family recombinases. Nucleic Acid Res 1999; 27:930–941.

47. Nagayama Y, Nishihara E, Iitaka M, Namba H, Yamashits S, Niwa M. Enhanced efficacy of transcriptionally targeted suicide gene/prodrug therapy for thyroid carcinoma with the Cre–loxP system. Cancer Res 1999; 59:3049–3052.

48. Sakai Y, Kaneko S, Sato Y, Kanegae Y, Tamaoki T, Saito I, Kobayashi K. Gene therapy for hepatocellular carcinoma using two recombinant adenovirus vectors with alpha-fetoprotein and cre–loxP system. J Virol Methods 2001; 92:5–17.

49. Kijima T, Osaki T, Nishino K, Kumagai T, Funakoshi T, Goto H, Tachibana I, Tanio Y, Kishimoto T. Application of the Cre recombinase/loxP system further enhances antitumor effects in cell type-specific gene therapy against antigen-producing cancer. Cancer Res 1999; 59:4906–4911.

50. Goto H, Osaki T, Kijima T, Nishino K, Kumagai T, Funakoshi T, Kimura M, Takeda Y, Yoneda T, Tachibana I, Hayashi S. Gene therapy utilizing the Cre/loxP system selectively suppresses tumor growth of disseminated carcinoembryonic antigen-producing cancer cells. Int J Cancer 2001; 94:414–419.

51. Kaczmarczyk SJ, Green JE. A single vector containing modified cre recombinase and LOX recombination sequences for inducible tissue-specific amplification of gene expression. Nucleic Acids Res 2001; 29:E56–6.

52. Sundaresan G, Paulmurugan R, Berger F, Stiles B, Nagayama Y, Wu H, Gambhir SS. MicroPET imaging of Cre–loxP-mediated conditional activation of a herpes simplex virus type I thymidine kinase reporter gene. Gene Ther 2004; 11:609–618.

53. Gambhir SS, Barrio JR, Herschman HR, Phelps ME. Assays for noninvasive imaging of reporter gene expression. Nucl Med Biol 1999; 26:481–490.

54. Gambhir SS, Barrio JR, Herschman HR, Phelps ME. Imaging gene expression: principles and assays. J Nucl Cardiol 1999; 6:219–233.

55. Budinger TF. Critical review of PET, SPECT and neuroreceptor studies in schizophrenia. J Neural Transm 1992; 36:3–12.

56. Phelps ME. PET: the merging of biology and imaging into molecular imaging. J Nucl Med 2000; 41:661–681.

57. Jackson EF, Ginsberg LE, Schomer DF, Leeds NE. A review of MRI pulse sequences and techniques in neuroimaging. Surg Neurol 1997; 47:185–199.

58. Yang M, Baranov E, Moossa AR, Penman S, Hoffman RM. Visualizing gene expression by whole-body fluorescence imaging. Proc Natl Acad Sci USA 2000; 97:12278–12282.

59. Contag PR, Olomu IN, Stevenson DK, Contag CH. Bioluminescent indicators in living mammals. Nat Med 1998; 4:245–247.

60. Hopper KD, Singapuri K, Finkel A. Body CT and oncologic imaging. Radiology 2000; 215:27–40.

61. Chatziioannou A. Molecular imaging of small animals with dedicated PET tomographs. Eur J Nucl Med 2002; 29:98–114.

62. Cherry SR, Gambhir SS. Use of positron emission tomography in animal research. Ilar J 2001; 42:219–232.

63. Chatziioannou A, Tai YC, Doshi N, Cherry SR. Detector development for micro-PET II: a 1 micron resolution PET scanner for small animal imaging. Phys Med Biol 2001; 46:2899–2910.

64. Gambhir SS, Barrio JR, Wu L, Iyer M, Namavari M, Satyamurthy N, Bauer E, Parrish C, MacLaren DC, Borghei AR, Green LA, Sharfstein S, Berk AJ, Cherry SR, Phelps ME, Herschman HR. Imaging of adenoviral-directed herpes simplex virus type 1 thymidine kinase reporter gene expression in mice with radio-labeled ganciclovir. J Nucl Med 1998; 39:2003–2011.

65. Gambhir SS, Bauer E, Black ME, Liang Q, Kokoris MS, Barrio JR, Iyer M, Namavari M, Phelps ME, Herschman HR. A mutant herpes simplex virus type 1 thymidine kinase reporter gene shows improved sensitivity for imaging reporter gene expression with positron emission tomography. Proc Natl Acad Sci USA 2000; 97:2785–2790.

66. MacLaren DC, Gambhir SS, Satyamurthy N, Barrio JR, Sharfstein S, Toyokuni T, Wu L, Berk AJ, Cherry SR, Phelps ME, Herschman HR. Repetitive, non-invasive imaging of the dopamine D2 receptor as a reporter gene in living animals. Gene Ther 1999; 6:785–791.

67. Iyer M, Barrio JR, Namavari M, Bauer E, Satyamurthy N, Nguyen K, Toyokuni T, Phelps ME, Herschman HR, Gambhir SS. 8-[18F]Fluoropenciclovir: an improved reporter probe for imaging HSV1-tk reporter gene expression *in vivo* using PET. J Nucl Med 2001; 42:96–105.

68. Min JJ, Iyer M, Gambhir SS. Comparison of [18F]FHBG and [14C]FIAU for imaging of HSV1-tk reporter gene expression: adenoviral infection vs stable transfection. Eur J Nucl Med 2003; 30:1547–1560.

69. Yaghoubi S, Barrio JR, Dahlbom M, Iyer M, Namavari M, Goldman R, Herschman HR, Phelps ME, Gambhir SS. Human pharmacokinetic and dosimetry

studies of [F-18]FHBG: a reporter probe for imaging herpes simplex virus type-1 thymidine kinase reporter gene expression. J Nucl Med 2001; 42:1225–1234.

70. Thompson EM, Adenot P, Tsuji FI, Renard JP. Real time imaging of transcriptional activity in live mouse preimplantation embryos using a secreted luciferase. Proc Natl Acad Sci USA 1995; 92:1317–1321.

71. Contag CH, Jenkins D, Contag PR, Negrin RS. Use of reporter genes for optical measurements of neoplastic disease *in vivo*. Neoplasia 2000; 2:41–52.

72. Contag CH, Bachmann MH. Advances in *in vivo* bioluminescence imaging of gene expression. Annu Rev Biomed Eng 2002; 4:235–260.

73. Edinger M, Sweeney TJ, Tucker AA, Olomu AB, Negrin RS, Contag CH. Noninvasive assessment of tumor cell proliferation in animal models. Neoplasia 1999; 1:303–310.

74. Sweeney TJ, Mailander V, Tucker AA, Olomu AB, Zhang W, Cao Y, Negrin RS, Contag CH. Visualizing the kinetics of tumor-cell clearance in living animals. Proc Natl Acad Sci USA 1999; 96:12044–12049.

75. Wu JC, Sundaresan G, Iyer M, Gambhir SS. Noninvasive optical imaging of firefly luciferase reporter gene expression in skeletal muscles of living mice. Mol Ther 2001; 4:297–306.

76. Ray P, Pimenta H, Paulmurugan R, Berger F, Phelps ME, Iyer M, Gambhir SS. Noninvasive quantitative imaging of protein–protein interactions in living subjects. Proc Natl Acad Sci USA 2002; 99:3105–3110.

77. Paulmurugan R, Umezawa Y, Gambhir SS. Noninvasive imaging of protein–protein interactions in living subjects by using reporter protein complementation and reconstitution strategies. Proc Natl Acad Sci USA 2002; 99:15608–15613.

78. Wu JC, Chen IY, Sundaresan G, Min JJ, De A, Qiao JH, Fishbein MC, Gambhir SS. Molecular imaging of cardiac cell transplantation in living animals using optical bioluminescence and positron emission tomography. Circulation 2003; 108:1302–1305.

79. Ray P, Bauer E, Iyer M, Barrio JR, Satyamurthy N, Phelps ME, Herschman H, Gambhir SS. Monitoring gene therapy with reporter gene imaging. Semin Nucl Med 2001; 31:312–320.

80. Yu Y, Annala AJ, Barrio JR, Toyokuni T, Satyamurthy N, Namavari M, Cherry SR, Phelps ME, Herschman HR, Gambhir SS. Quantification of target gene expression by imaging reporter gene expression in living animals. Nat Med 2000; 6:933–937.

81. Sun X, Annala AJ, Yaghoubi SS, Barrio JR, Nguyen KN, Toyokuni T, Satyamurthy N, Namavari M, Phelps ME, Herschman HR, Gambhir SS. Quantitative imaging of gene induction in living animals. Gene Ther 2001; 8:1572–1579.

82. Marshall E. Gene therapy on trial. Science 2000; 288:951–957.

83. McCormick F. Cancer gene therapy: fringe or cutting edge. Nat Rev Cancer 2001; 1:130–141.

84. Schuler M, Herrmann R, De Greve JL, Stewart AK, Gatzemeier U, Stewart DJ, Laufman L, Gralla R, Kuball J, Buhl R, Heussel CP, Kommoss F, Perruchoud AP, Shepherd FA, Fritz MA, Horowitz JA, Huber C, Rochlitz C. Adenovirus-mediated wild-type p53 gene transfer in patients receiving chemotherapy for advanced non-small-cell lung cancer: results of a multicenter phase II study. J Clin Oncol 2001; 19:1750–1758.

85. Reid T, Galanis E, Abbruzzese J, Sze D, Andrews J, Romel L, Hatfield M, Rubin J, Kim D. Intra-arterial administration of a replication-selective adenovirus (dl1520) in patients with colorectal carcinoma metastatic to the liver: a phase I trial. Gene Ther 2001; 8:1618–1626.

86. Kuball J, Wen SF, Leissner J, Atkins D, Meinhardt P, Qiuijano E, Engler H, Hutchins B, Maneval DC, Grace MJ, Fritz MA, Storkel S, Thuroff JW, Huber C, Schuler M. Successful adenovirus-mediated wild-type p53 gene transfer in patients with bladder cancer by intravesical vector instillation. J Clin Oncol 2002; 20:957–965.

87. Li Q, Kay MA, Finegold M, Stratford-Perricaudet LD, Woo SL. Assessment of recombinant adenoviral vectors for hepatic gene therapy. Hum Gen Ther 1993; 4:403–409.

88. Brody SL, Crystal RG. Adenovirus-mediated *in vivo* gene transfer. Ann NY Acad Sci 1994; 716:90–101.

89. Kovesdi I, Brough DE, Bruder JT, Wickham TJ. Adenoviral vectors for gene transfer. Curr Opin Biotechnol 1997; 8:583–589.

90. Benihoud K, Yeh P, Perricaudet M. Adenovirus vectors for gene delivery. Curr Opin Biotechnol 1999; 10:440–447.

91. Anderson SC, Johnson DE, Engler H, Hancock W, Huang W, Wills KN, Gregory RJ, Sutjipto S, Wen SF, Lofgren S, Shepard HM, Maneval DC. p53 Gene therapy in a rat model of hepatocellular carcinoma: intra-arterial delivery of recombinant adenovirus. Clin Cancer Res 1998; 4:1649–1659.

92. Roy I, Holle L, Song W, Holle E, Wagner T, Yu X. Efficient translocation and apoptosis induction by adenovirus encoded VP22-p53 fusion protein in human tumor cells *in vitro*. Anticancer Res 2002; 22:3185–3189.

93. Wu L, Matherly J, Smallwood A, Belldegrun AS, Carey M. Chimeric PSA enhancers exhibit augmented activity in prostate cancer gene therapy vector. Gene Ther 2001; 8:1416–1426.

94. Sato M, Johnson M, Zhang L, Zhang B, Le KH, Gambhir SS, Carey M, Wu L. Optimization of adenoviral vectors to direct highly amplified prostate-specific gene expression for imaging and gene therapy. Mol Ther 2003; 8:726–737.

95. Zhang J, Johnson M, Le KH, Sato M, Ilagan R, Iyer M, Gambhir SS, Wu L, Carey M. Interrogating androgen receptor function in recurrent prostate cancer. Cancer Res 2003; 63:4552–4560.

96. Yang Y, Nunes F, Berencsi K, Furth E, Gönczöl E, Wilson J. Cellular immunity to viral antigens limits E1-deleted adenoviruses for gene therapy. Proc Natl Acad Sci USA 1994; 91:4407–4411.

97. Mack C, Song WR, Carpenter H, Wickham TJ, Kovesdi I, Harvey BG, Magovern CJ, Isom OW, Rosengart T, Falck-Pedersen E, Hackett NR, Crystal RG, Mastrangeli A. Circumvention of anti-adenovirus neutralizing immunity by administration of an adenoviral vector of an alternate serotype. Hum Gen Ther 1997; 8:99–109.

98. Raper SE, Yudkoff M, Chirmule N, Gao GP, Nunes FA, Haskal ZJ, Furth EE, Propert KJ, Robinson MB, Magosin S, Simoes L, Speicher J, Hughes J, Tazelaar J, Wivel NA, Wilson JM, Batshaw ML. A pilot study of *in vivo* liver-directed gene transfer with an adenoviral vector in partial ornithine transcarbamylase deficiency. Hum Gen Ther 2002; 13:163–175.

99. Schiedner G, Morral N, Parks RJ, Wu Y, Koopmans SC, Langston C, Graham FL, Beaudet AL, Kochanek S. Genomic DNA transfer with a high-capacity adenovirus vector results in improved *in vivo* gene expression and decreased toxicity. Nat Genet 1998; 18:180–183.

100. Gerdes CA, Castro MG, Lowenstein PR. Strong promoters are the key to highly efficient, noninflammatory and noncytotoxic adenoviral-mediated transgene delivery into the brain *in vivo*. Mol Ther 2000; 2:330–338.

101. Thomas CE, Schiedner G, Kochanek S, Castro MG, Lowenstein PR. Preexisting antiadenoviral immunity is not a barrier to efficient and stable transduction of the brain, mediated by novel high-capacity adenovirus vectors. Hum Gen Ther 2001; 12:839–846.

102. Kotin RM. Prospects for the use of adeno-associated virus as a vector for human gene therapy. Hum Gen Ther 1994; 5:793–801.

103. Flotte TR, Carter BJ. Adeno-associated virus vectors for gene therapy. Gene Ther 1995; 2:357–362.

104. Templeton NS, Lasic DD. Gene Therapy, Therapeutic Mechanisms and Strategies. New York: Marcel Dekker, 2000:584.

105. Yakinoglu AO, Heilbronn R, Burkle A, Schlehofer JR, zur Hausen H. DNA amplification of adeno-associated virus as a response to cellular genotoxic stress. Cancer Res 1988; 48:3123–3129.

106. Flotte IR, Afione SA, Solow R, McGrath SA, Conrad C, Zeitlin PL, Guggino WB, Carter BJ. *In vivo* delivery of adeno-associated vectors expressing the cystic fibrosis transmembrane conductance regulator to the airway epithelium. Proc Natl Acad Sci USA 1993; 93:10163.

107. Xiao X, Li J, Samulski RJ. Efficient long-term gene transfer into muscle tissue of immunocompetent mice by adeno-associated virus vector. J Virol 1996; 70:8098–8108.

108. Kessler PD, Podsakoff GM, Chen X, McQuiston SA, Colosi PC, Matelis LA, Kurtzman GJ, Byrne B. Gene delivery to skeletal muscle results in sustained expression and systemic delivery of a therapeutic protein. Proc Natl Acad Sci USA 1996; 93:14082–14087.

109. Miller AD. Development and applications of retroviral vectors. In: Coffin JM, Hughes SH, Varmus HE, eds. Retroviruses. New York: CSHL Press, 1997.

110. Shimotohno K, Temim HM. Formation of infectious progeny virus after insertion of herpes simplex thymidine kinase gene into DNA of an avian retrovirus. Cell 1981; 26:67–77.

111. Wei CM, Gibson M, Spear PG, Scolnick EM. Construction and isolation of a transmissible retrovirus containing the *src* gene of Harvey murine sarcoma virus and the thymidine kinase gene of herpes simplex virus type I. J Virol 1981; 39:935–944.

112. Barzon L, Bonaguro R, Castagliuolo I, Chilosi M, Franchin E, Del Vicchio C, Giaretta I, Boscaro M, Palu G. Gene therapy of thyroid cancer via retrovirally-driven combined expression of human interleukin-2 and herpes simplex virus thymidine kinase. Eur J Endocrinol 2003; 148:73–80.

113. Miller DG, Adam MA, Miller AD. Gene transfer by retrovirus vectors occurs only in cells that are actively replicating at the time of infection. Mol Cell Biol 1990; 10:4239–4242.

114. Lewis PF, Emerman M. Passage through mitosis is required for oncoretroviruses but not for the human immunodeficiency virus. J Virol 1994; 68:510–516.
115. Vigna E, Naldini L. Excellent tools for experimental gene transfer and promising candidates for gene therapy. J Gene Med 2000; 5:308–316.
116. Naldini L, Blomer U, Gallay P, Ory D, Mulligan R, Gage RH, Verma IM, Trono D. *In vivo* gene delivery and stable transduction of nondividing cells by a lentiviral vector. Science 1996; 272:263–267.
117. Bukovsky AA, Song JP, Naldini L. Interaction of human immunodeficiency virus-derived vectors with wild-type virus in transduced cells. J Virol 1999; 73:7087–7092.
118. Barry SC, Harder B, Brzezinski M, Flint LY, Seppen J, Osborne WR. Lentivirus vectors encoding both central polypurine tract and posttranscriptional regulatory element provide enhanced transduction and transgene expression. Hum Gen Ther 2001; 12:1103–1108.
119. De A, Lewis XZ, Gambhir SS. Noninvasive imaging of lentiviral mediated reporter gene expression in living mice. Mol Ther 2003; 7:681–691.
120. Naldini L, Blomer U, Gage FH, Trono D, Verma IM. Efficient transfer, integration, and sustained long-term expression of the transgene in adult rat brains injected with a lentiviral vector. Proc Natl Acad Sci USA 1996; 93:11382–11388.
121. Blomer U, Naldini L, Kafri T, Trono D, Verma IM. Highly efficient and sustained gene transfer in adult neurons with a lentivirus vector. J Virol 1997; 71:6641–6649.
122. Kafri T, Blomer U, Peterson DA, Gage FH, Verma IM. Sustained expression of genes delivered directly into liver and muscle by lentiviral vectors. Nat Genet 1997; 17:314–317.
123. Park PK, Ohashi K, Chui W, Naldini L, Kay MA. Efficient lentiviral transduction of liver requires cell cycling *in vivo*. Nat Genet 2000; 24:49–52.
124. Iyer M, Salazar FB, Lewis X, Zhang L, Carey M, Wu L, Gambhir SS. Non-invasive imaging of enhanced prostate-specific gene expression using a two-step transcriptional amplification-based lentivirus vector. Mol Ther 2004; 10:545–552.
125. Huang L, Viroonchaatapan E. Introduction. In: Huang L, Hung M-C, Wagner E, eds. Nonviral Vectors for Gene Therapy, Chapter 1. London: Academic Press, 1999:4–22.
126. Behr JP. Gene transfer with synthetic cationic amphiphiles: prospects for gene therapy. Bioconjug Chem 1994; 5:382–389.
127. Pedroso de Lima MC, Simoes S, Pires P, Faneca H, Duzgunes N. Cationic lipid–DNA complexes in gene delivery: from biophysics to biological applications. Adv Drug Deliv Rev 2001; 47:277–294.
128. Felgner PL, Gadek TR, Holm M, Roman R, Chan HW, Wenz M, Northrop JP, Ringold GM, Danielsen M. Lipofection: a highly efficient, lipid-mediated DNA-transfection procedure. Proc Natl Acad Sci USA 1987; 84:7413–7417.
129. Felgner JH, Kumar R, Sridhar CN, Wheler CJ, Tsai YJ, Border R, Ramsey P, Martin M, Felgner PL. Enhanced gene delivery and mechanism studies with a novel series of cationic lipid formulations. J Biol Chem 1994; 269:2550–2561.
130. Li S, Huang L. *In vivo* gene transfer via intravenous administration of cationic lipid–protamine–DNA (LPD) complexes. Gene Ther 1997; 4:891–900.

131. Templeton NS, Lasic DD, Frederik PM, Strey HH, Roberts DD, Pavlakis GN. Improved DNA : liposome complexes for increased systemic delivery and gene expression. Nat Biotechnol 1997; 15:647–652.

132. Lasic DD. Liposomes in Gene Delivery. Boca Raton, FL: CRC Press, 1997.

133. Iyer M, Berenji M, Templeton NS, Gambhir SS. Noninvasive imaging of cationic lipid-mediated delivery of optical and PET reporter genes in living mice. Mol Ther 2002; 6:555–562.

134. Boussif O, Lezoualc'h F, Zanta MA, Mergny MD, Scherman D, Demeneix BA, Behr JP. A versatile vector for gene and oligonucleotide transfer into cells in culture and *in vivo*: polyethylenimine. Proc Natl Acad Sci USA 1995; 92:7297–7301.

135. Hildebrandt IJ, Iyer M, Wagner E, Gambhir SS. Optical imaging of transferrin targeted PEI'DNA complexes in living subjects. Gene Ther 2003; 10:758–764.

136. Factor P. Gene therapy for acute diseases. Mol Ther 2001; 4:515–524.

137. Weiss YG, Maloyan A, Tazelaar J, Raj N, Deutschman CS. Adenoviral transfer of HSP-70 into pulmonary epithelium ameliorates experimental acute respiratory distress syndrome. J Clin Invest 2002; 110:801–806.

138. Bromberg JS, Debruyne LA, Qin L. Interactions between the immune system and gene therapy vectors: bidirectional regulation of response and expression. Adv Immunol 1998; 69:353–409.

139. Look DC, Brody SL. Engineering viral vectors to subvert the airway defense response. Am J Respir Cell Mol Biol 1999; 20:1103–1106.

140. Arcasoy SM, Latoche J, Gondor M, Watkins SC, Henderson RA, Hughey R, Finn OJ, Pilewski JM. MUC1 and other sialoglycoconjugates inhibit adenovirus-mediated gene transfer to epithelial cells. Am J Respir Cell Mol Biol 1997; 17:422–435.

141. Kitson C, Angel B, Judd D, Rothery S, Severs NJ, Dewar A, Huang L, Wadsworth SC, Cheng SH, Geddes DM, Alton EW. The extra- and intracellular barriers to lipid and adenovirus-mediated pulmonary gene transfer in native sheep airway epithelium. Gene Ther 1999; 6:534–546.

142. Zabner J, Ramsey BW, Meeker DP, Aitken ML, Balfour RP, Gibson RL, Launspach J, Moscicki RA, Richards SM, Standaert TA, Williams-Warren J, Wadsworth SC, Smith AE, Welsh MJ. Repeat administration of an adenovirus vector encoding cystic fibrosis transmembrane conductance regulator to the nasal epithelium of patients with cystic fibrosis. J Clin Invest 1996; 97:1504–1511.

143. Harvey BG, Leopold PL, Hackett NR, Grasso TM, Williams PM, Tucker AL, Kaner RJ, Ferris B, Gonda I, Sweeney TD, Ramalingam R, Kovesdi I, Shak S, Crystal RG. Airway epithelial CFTR mRNA expression in cystic fibrosis patients after repetitive administration of a recombinant adenovirus. J Clin Invest 1999; 194:1245–1255.

144. Katkin JP, Gilbert BE, Langston C, French K, Beaudet AL. Aerosol delivery of a beta-galactosidase adenoviral vector to the lungs of rodents. Hum Gen Ther 1995; 6:985–995.

145. Brown AR, Chowdhury SI. Propellant-driven aerosols of DNA plasmids for gene expression. J Aerosol Med 1997; 10:129–146.

146. Richard J-C, Chen DL, Ferkol T, Schuster DP. Molecular imaging of pediatric lung diseases. Pediatr Pulmonol 2004; 37:286–296.

147. Richard J-C, Factor P, Welch LC, Schuster DP. Imaging the spatial distribution of transgene expression in the lungs with positron emission tomography. Gene Ther 2003; 10:2074–2080.

148. Green LA, Yap CS, Nguyen K, Barrio JR, Namavari M, Satyamurthy N, Phelps ME, Sandgren EP, Herschman HR, Gambhir SS. Indirect monitoring of endogenous gene expression by positron emission tomography (PET) imaging of reporter gene expression in transgenic mice. Mol Imaging Biol 2002; 4:71–81.

149. Lee SY, Wang Z, Lin CK, Contag CH, Olds LC, Cooper AD, Sibley E. Regulation of intestine-specific spatiotemporal expression by the rat lactase promoter. J Biol Chem 2002; 277:13099–13105.

150. Zhang J, Tan X, Contag CH, Lu Y, Guo D, Harris SE, Feng JQ. Dissection of promoter control modules that direct Bmp4 expression in the epithelium-derived components of hair follicles. Biochem Biophys Res Commun 2002; 293:1412–1419.

151. Carlsen H, Moskaug JO, Fromm SH, Blomhoff R. *In vivo* imaging of NF-kappa B activity. J Immunol 2002; 168:1441–1446.

152. Vooijs M, Jonkers J, Lyons S, Berns A. Noninvasive imaging of spontaneous retinoblastoma pathway-dependent tumors in mice. Cancer Res 2002; 62: 1862–1867.

153. Byrne GW, Ruddle FH. Multiplex gene regulation: a two-tiered approach to transgene regulation in transgenic mice. Proc Natl Acad Sci USA 1989; 86:5473–5477.

154. Ornitz DM, Randall WM, Leder P. Binary system for regulating transgene expression in mice: targeting int-2 gene expression with yeast GAL4/UAS control elements. Proc Nat Acad Sci USA 1991; 88:698–702.

155. Iyer M, Salazar F, Lewis X, Zhang L, Wu L, Carey M, Gambhir SS. Noninvasive imaging of a transgenic mouse model using a prostate-specific two-step transcriptional amplification strategy. 2005; In press.

156. Fraser SE, Koster RW. Tracing transgene expression in living zebrafish embryos. Dev Biol 2001; 233:329–346.

157. Wang Y, Iyer M, Wu L, Carey M, Gambhir SS. A two-step transcriptional approach for imaging vascular endothelial growth factor (VEGF) gene expression using a bioluminescent reporter gene. Mol Imaging Biol 2002; 4:S42.

158. Wang Y, Iyer M, Wu L, Carey M, Gambhir SS. A transgenic mouse model incorporating a two-step transcriptional approach for imaging of vascular endothelial growth factor (VEGF) gene expression, Second Annual Meeting of the Society for Molecular Imaging, San Fransisco, CA, 2003.

Section 2: Application to the Lungs

8

Pulmonary Transgene Expression Imaging

DANIEL P. SCHUSTER

Washington University School of Medicine,
St. Louis, Missouri, USA

I. Introduction

The possibility and promise of being able to follow the expression of biology modifying genes noninvasively in whole animals, including humans, is one of the most exciting aspects of the developing revolution in "molecular imaging." So far, most studies of "gene expression imaging" follow the expression of target genes via visualization of *in vivo* gene "reporters" (1–4). Already these techniques have begun to impact the fields of cancer research and gene therapeutics (1,5–8). A relatively small number of studies also show how these imaging methods can be used to study the expression of genes within the lungs.

II. Platforms for Gene Expression Imaging

Radionuclide-based methods, optical techniques, and magnetic resonance imaging (MRI) have each been used as platforms for gene expression imaging. Thus far, studies in the lungs have almost exclusively been limited to radionuclide-based methods.

A. Radionuclide-Based Methods

These platforms include planar gamma scintigraphy, single-photon emission computed tomography (SPECT), and positron emission tomography (PET). They differ in their availability, cost, need for specialized infrastructure and technical expertise, and ability to accurately quantify tissue radioactivity noninvasively (9).

PET

Most gene expression imaging studies have employed PET, arguably the most sensitive (level of detection approaches 10^{-11} M of tracer) and accurate (can accurately quantify tissue radioactivity regardless of tissue depth) radionuclide-based method (10,11). Another advantage is that PET uses isotopes, which are often very short-lived (half-lives from minutes to hours). Of special importance, human dosimetry data are already available for one radiopharmaceutical used in transgene expression imaging with PET (12), and a recent case report demonstrates the feasibility of using PET to monitor gene transfer in humans (13). Reviews of the instrumentation and physics underlying PET imaging technology can be found elsewhere (14).

Until recently, limitations in spatial resolution made PET studies in small animals impossible. For instance, most PET scanners in clinical use have an image spatial resolution of 10–15 mm (although more recent instruments can achieve resolution approaching 1–2 mm); the mouse lung, in contrast, is ~10 mm wide. Other issues such as scanner sensitivity (i.e., the fraction of radioactive events actually detected by the device) and the amount of radioactivity that can be injected without causing physiologic disturbances (a function of tracer-specific activity) also have limited PET applications to small animals. Recent improvements in radiation detector technology and electronics, however, now make it possible to perform PET imaging studies even in mice (9,15), as will be discussed subsequently.

Non-PET

Less complex and more widely available systems include planar gamma scintigraphy and SPECT imaging (16,17). Disadvantages include a loss of sensitivity (tomographic displays require collimation, which reduces radioactivity counts available for quantitation); accuracy (it is difficult or impossible to correct radioactivity measurements for the attenuation of emitted radiation by tissue); and, in the case of planar gamma scintigraphy, a loss of spatial information (these images emphasize events near the body surface and are not tomographic "slices" of tissue within the organ).

Overall, the fairest assessment of both PET and non-PET systems is that their use to monitor gene expression in living animals is still new and incompletely developed. Therefore, the advantages of one over another are still theoretical and systematic studies are needed to determine each method's relative benefits and drawbacks.

B. Optical Imaging

Bioluminescence is the principal form of optical imaging that has been used for gene expression imaging studies, including studies of various genetic regulatory elements in transgenic mice (18), and in studies of *in vivo* gene transfer (19–21). As mammalian tissues do not emit significant levels of intrinsic light, bioluminescence can be used to generate images with virtually no background noise.

Optical imaging offers several key benefits over PET. PET radiopharmaceuticals generally need to be made on-site and require appropriate radiation safety precautions. In contrast, bioluminescence studies are simpler to conduct because the substrates are commercially available and readily prepared. Furthermore, multiple animals can be studied at the same time, and they can be studied quickly because image acquisition times are typically short. The interval between studies that involve repetitive imaging is also short, unlike radionuclide-based methods, which require time for radioactive decay. Finally, both the reporter gene products and substrates used in bioluminescence studies (e.g., luciferases and D-luciferin) appear to be nontoxic to mammalian cells. This is a theoretical advantage over radionuclide-based methods, which depend on the use of ionizing radiation (22).

The sensitivity of detecting light emitted from within an organism depends on many factors including the level of reporter gene expression used to generate the bioluminescence signal; the distance light must travel through tissue from source to detector; and the sensitivity of the detection system. As a general rule, photon intensity at the detectors falls ~10-fold for each centimeter of tissue depth (23). Not only does this mean that quantitative accuracy may be compromised, but also that the images are surface-weighted so that light sources closer to the surface of the animal appear brighter compared to deeper sources (24). A related problem is that the images are planar instead of the tomographic or three-dimensional images produced by techniques like PET. Thus, at present, bioluminescent images lack depth information. Finally, highly vascular organs such as the lungs suffer a further reduction in signal because of light absorption by hemoglobin.

C. Magnetic Resonance Imaging

Although the exquisite anatomic detail afforded by MRI is well documented, novel approaches using MRI for gene expression imaging have also been developed in recent years (5,25).

MR images can be generated when nuclides (e.g., ^{1}H and ^{3}He) in an individual lying within a magnetic field are subjected to a radio-frequency (rf) pulse applied at a "resonant" frequency. These nuclides absorb energy, generating a detectable signal. The signal strength depends upon the nuclide concentration; its frequency depends on the nuclide's identity and the strength of the local magnetic field. By applying magnetic field gradients in well-defined directions, the frequency of the proton signal is made dependent upon spatial position. Altering the sequence of rf pulses, and then collecting and processing the signal data produces a map of MR signal intensity vs. position (i.e., an image). Tissue contrast is provided by weighting the signal, according to the time required for the MR-active nuclides to return to equilibrium ("relaxation"), or by administering contrast agents that alter MR signal intensity, such as chelated gadolinium or superparamagnetic nanoparticles.

Although MRI can achieve images with a spatial resolution on the order of 10–50 mm (as opposed to PET images with a spatial resolution of 1–2 mm at best), it is also several orders of magnitude less sensitive than either radionuclide- or optical-based techniques. Therefore, various amplification strategies must be employed to enhance signal generation for the purposes of gene expression imaging (6). These amplification strategies may require that mass amounts of imaging probe be administered, with potentially harmful intrinsic pharmacologic effects.

MRI studies of the lungs can be especially challenging (26). The lungs' relatively low tissue density (reducing the concentration of MR-active nuclides) and its magnetic field inhomogeneities (a result of the air–tissue interfaces within the lungs) are obstacles not encountered in MRI studies of other organ systems. Thus far, these problems have precluded the use of MRI as a method for gene expression imaging of the lungs.

III. Strategies for Gene Expression Imaging

Technically, imaging can be used to monitor both endogenous genes and the transfer of exogenous genes ("transgenes"). The latter, however, has received considerably more attention. In both cases, "direct" as well as "indirect" imaging strategies can be used to detect gene expression.

Direct approaches depend on probes of various types that either accumulate in tissues by binding directly to the DNA, to the RNA message, to the gene product itself (e.g., when that product is a receptor), or are trapped intracellularly as they are modified by the gene product (e.g., when that product is an enzyme).

With indirect approaches, similar strategies are employed to visualize the expression of a suitable reporter gene that is simultaneously linked to the target gene of interest by a common promoter. The principal advantage of this strategy is that a new specific probe does not have to be synthesized and evaluated for each new gene of interest. On the other hand, care must be taken to ensure that expression of the reporter gene correlates strongly with expression of the target gene.

A. Endogenous Gene Expression

Endogenous gene expression can be evaluated at both the transcriptional (messenger RNA) and translational (protein) level. The most direct strategy for monitoring mRNA levels with imaging is to synthesize a radiolabeled antisense oligodeoxynucleotide (RASON) that is directed against a specific (usually 10–15 base pair) sequence within the mRNA (27,28). This strategy of "*in vivo* hybridization" is analogous to the commonly employed microscopic method of "*in situ* hybridization." Given current techniques, the chemical synthesis per se of such radiolabeled probes is straightforward, but production of sufficient quantities for whole animal imaging is still a significant challenge.

There are at least two other major limitations with the RASON approach (27). For one, RASON penetration across cell membranes into the appropriate target cell is often quite limited. Even more problematic is that the concentration of mRNA copies within a given cell may be quite low (sometimes a few hundred to a few hundred thousand copies). Thus, the imaging signal from RASON binding to target mRNA would usually be expected to be weak. To actually employ imaging to detect specific RASON binding, the oligodeoxynucleotide would have to be synthesized and radiolabeled at a very high specific activity. In addition, clearance from blood would have to be rapid, and nonspecific binding to nontarget tissues or other intracellular components would have to be minimal to ensure a high target-to-background signal. Altogether, these restrictions have made it difficult to pursue the RASON approach for gene expression imaging so far.

Endogenous gene expression can also be monitored using radiolabeled probes that bind directly to the gene product. This strategy has the advantage of amplifying the imaging signal compared to the RASON approach (many protein molecules can be produced from each mRNA). However, as previously noted, the principle disadvantage is that a new specific probe would have to be synthesized and evaluated for each new target gene. An alternative indirect approach to monitoring endogenous gene expression would require the development of genetically modified animals ("transgenics") to visualize the expression of a suitable reporter transgene that has been introduced into the cell and linked to the target gene by a common promoter.

B. Exogenous Gene Expression

In contrast to monitoring endogenous gene expression, imaging can also be used to monitor therapeutic or biology-modifying transgenes that are introduced into tissues via a variety of vector technologies, including viruses, liposome-encapsulated DNA, or naked DNA. To visualize the delivery of these transgenes, the vector itself or the viral capsid can be labeled, for instance, with a radioactive tag (25,29,30). However, this approach requires radiolabeling of the vector genome or viral protein and may not correlate with transgene function. Nevertheless, a recent study using gamma scintigraphy and a technetium-99m labeled adenovector carrying the human cystic fibrosis transmembrane regulator (*CFTR*) gene delivered to the lungs of baboons via aerosolization demonstrates that this approach is feasible (30,31).

Instead of attempting to visualize the accumulation of vector itself in a given tissue, other direct approaches can be used to visualize the expression of exogenously delivered transgenes using probes specific to the gene or gene product. However, as previously noted, a different suitable ligand or substrate is then required for each new gene of interest.

"Reporter gene" strategies have been pursued to overcome this (32). One needs to only develop assays to measure the expression of a few reporters that can then be linked using standard molecular biology methods to any number of different target genes. The reporter gene strategy can be used to evaluate gene expression in whole animals as well as in *in vitro* systems, but traditional methods of assaying reporter gene expression (enzymatic, immunohistochemical, or *in situ* hybridization) all require tissue retrieval via biopsy or after sacrificing the animal. Classic examples of reporter genes include β-galactosidase, alkaline phosphatase, or luciferase. Thus, to evaluate the location, magnitude, and/or timing of gene expression with these methods, one must perform assays on multiple individual animals at each time-point in each tissue of interest. Obviously, this requirement makes the evaluation of transgene expression in humans difficult and sometimes impossible.

C. PET Imaging for Reporter Gene Expression

The use of imaging to monitor reporter gene expression can theoretically overcome the disadvantages associated with tissue-based techniques. The concepts underlying the use of PET imaging to monitor a reporter transgene are illustrated in Fig. 8.1. The reporter transgene ("PET reporter gene, PRG"), capable of trapping or binding a suitable positron-emitting radionuclide-labeled tracer ("PET reporter probe, PRP"), must be introduced into a target tissue, for instance via a viral vector. A PET imaging signal is generated as the PRP accumulates over time in tissues expressing the PRG.

Tjuvajev et al. (33) were the first to show that PET imaging could be used to monitor tissue transgene expression in this way. Since then, a number of different PRG–PRP reporter systems have been described (4,34–36), including exogenous enzymes (37,38), membrane-bound receptors (39), or cell-membrane transporters (40). Of these, enzyme-based strategies have the theoretical advantage of additional signal amplification because each reporter protein can metabolize and trap many molecules of radioactive probe. In contrast, receptor-based systems, while providing no additional signal amplification, do have the advantage of not requiring possibly rate-limiting intracellular transport of

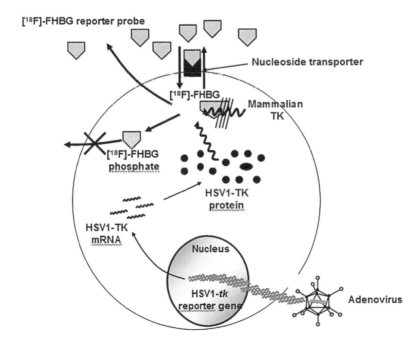

Figure 8.1 Schematic illustrating principles underlying reporter transgene expression imaging with PET. An adenoviral vector is used to introduce a PET reporter gene [e.g., HSV1-*thymidine kinase (tk)*] into a target cell, such as the lung airway epithelium. The gene is transcribed and translated into the thymidine kinase (TK) protein. The viral TK enzyme has a relaxed substrate specificity compared to mammalian TK, allowing it to phosphorylate (and trap) the radiolabeled reporter probe [^{18}F]-FHBG. [Reproduced with permission from Richard et al. (85).]

the radioactive probe into the cell interior in order to be trapped as a result of reporter enzyme metabolism.

To date, the optimal PRG–PRP system is still a matter of debate, and may differ depending on the tissue or process under study. Even so, the use of PET imaging to monitor exogenous gene transfer in pulmonary tissue by measuring the expression of a suitable enzyme is already proving to be a fruitful experimental strategy (41–43).

So far, mutant variants of the *Herpes simplex* virus type 1-*tk* (mHSV1-*tk*) have been the only reporter genes successfully detected in the lungs with PET imaging (43,44), using 9-(4-[^{18}F]-fluoro-3-hydroxymethylbutyl)guanine ([^{18}F]-FHBG), an imaging substrate for the mutant *tk* (45,46) as the PET reporter probe. Examples of images obtained in a rat and a mouse infected after intratracheal administration with adenovector carrying the mHSV1-*tk* gene are shown in Fig. 8.2. Using this PRG–PRP combination, very low levels of viral TK expression have been detected, even below the sensitivity of detection by fluorescence imaging of green fluorescent protein (GFP) expression (Fig. 8.3) (47). In comparison to *in vitro* techniques, PET imaging's apparent higher sensitivity is plausible given its exquisite sensitivity (48,49).

Alternative combinations of imaging reporter genes and/or reporter probes may be useful, especially given recent concerns about quantitation of the imaging signal with TK as a reporter gene (discussed subsequently). The human somatostatin type 2 receptor gene (*hSSTr2*) may be one such alternative PRG (50). Figure 8.4 shows an image from the lungs of a rat infected with an adenovector carrying the *hSSTr2* gene. [^{64}Cu]-1,4,8,11-tetraazacyclotetradecacne-*N,N',N'',N'''*-tetraacetic acid octreotide (TETA-OC) was used as the PET tracer ligand for this receptor (51,52).

High levels of gene expression in the lungs have been achieved in these studies by administering the adenoviral vectors intratracheally. This method of gene delivery targets the pulmonary epithelium, which may not always be optimal for diseases involving the pulmonary vasculature. Unfortunately, the intravenous administration of viral vectors does not produce high levels of transgene expression in the lungs because the liver, with its high concentration of the coxsackie-adenovirus receptor (CAR, which is required for adenoviral entry into cells), limits adenovector delivery to the lungs.

Several alternative strategies have recently been explored to circumvent this problem. In one, so-called "transductional" retargeting is used to redirect adenovirus toward the lungs, for example, by using bi-specific antibodies capable of binding both to the adenovirus itself and to molecules such as angiotensin converting enzyme, which are expressed at high concentrations in pulmonary endothelium. Reynolds et al. (16) used this approach to detect increased lung expression (via gamma scintigraphic imaging of the accumulation of a technetium 99m-labeled peptide ligand for the receptor) of the *hSSTr2* after intravenous adenovector administration in rats. Further enhancements may be possible via "transcriptional" targeting involving the use of cell-specific promoters (53).

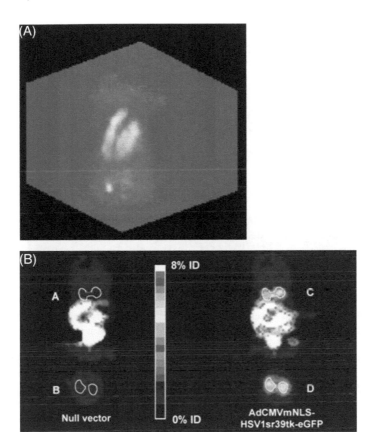

Figure 8.2 **(See color insert)** (A) Three-dimensional views of the lungs in a rat infected with 1×10^{11} viral particles (VP) of AdCMV-mNLS-HSV1sr39*tk-egfp*. A movie version of this figure is available at: http://ccs.wustl.edu/schuster_avifile/avi.htm. Reproduced with permission from Ref. (43). (B) Reporter gene expression imaging with PET in a control mouse infected with a null vector (A and B) and a mouse expressing the mutant HSV1-*tk* gene (C and D). Panels A and C are coronal views of the mice, whereas B and D are corresponding transverse slices obtained at the mid-lung level. In both mice, regions-of-interest (ROIs) are drawn to indicate lung boundaries (white lines) and tracer uptake was expressed as a percentage of injected dose (ID). There was significant pulmonary uptake of the tracer in the mouse expressing the viral TK when compared with the control mouse. High levels of activity in the abdomen are due to a combination of urinary excretion and of biliary excretion into the gastrointestinal tract.

However, this particular strategy has not yet been evaluated with imaging methods (16,53).

In contrast to viral vectors, encapsulating naked DNA in cationic lipids is another strategy for increasing the relative expression of intravenously

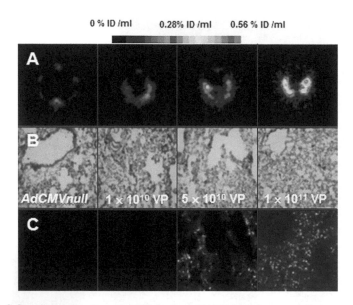

Figure 8.3 (**See color insert**) PET images (A), light microscopic micrographs (B), and corresponding fluorescence micrographs (C) obtained in one rat infected with AdCMVnull (left panel) and three rats, respectively, infected with 1×10^{10}, 5×10^{10}, and 1×10^{11} viral particles (VP) of AdCMV-mNLS-sr39*tk-egfp* (panel 2, 3, and 4 from left to right). The PET images are transverse slices obtained at the mid-chest level. Light and fluorescent micrographs ($10\times$ magnification) represent identical lung areas in the left lung from adjacent sections. Exposure time for each fluorescent micrograph was the same (960 ms). Fluorescence was mainly seen in distal parenchymal (alveolar) cells rather than in airway epithelium or microvessel endothelium. [Reproduced with permission from Richard et al. (43).]

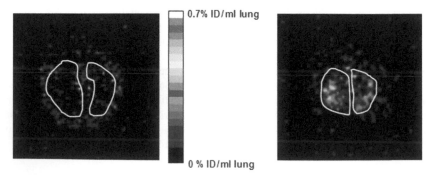

Figure 8.4 (**See color insert**) (Left) Transverse image taken 1 h after IV administration of [^{64}Cu]-TETA-OC from a rat after null vector administration. (Right) Three days after intratracheal administration of adenovectors containing *hSSTr2*. The image is at the mid-thoracic level. The white lines on each figure depict lung ROIs. The color bar shows units of percentage of injected dose (ID) per gram.

administered transgenes to the lungs instead of other organs like the liver. Recently, several groups have shown that this strategy can be employed effectively with optical imaging (Fig. 8.5), PET, and gamma scintigraphy (29,30,44).

IV. Gene Expression Studies of the Lungs with PET

A. PET Imaging to Detect the Time-Course of Transgene Expression in the Lungs

The possibility of using noninvasive imaging to study the onset and duration of transgene expression is obviously an attractive one, both for gene therapeutics and for studies that seek to determine relationships between the effectiveness of gene transfer and the biological effects of the gene product. In a recent study (42), we found that significant levels of the transgene could be detected in the lungs as early as 4–6 h after gene transfer (Fig. 8.6). The imaging results were validated with two *in vitro* assays of transgene expression. Dumasius et al. (54) have also reported physiologically significant levels of human β_2-adrenergic receptor in the lungs within hours after adenovirus-mediated gene transfer. Together, these results confirm the high efficiency of adenoviral vectors, and suggest that they may be particularly appropriate for therapeutic gene transfer during acute diseases such as acute lung injury and acute respiratory distress syndrome (ARDS). They also demonstrate the usefulness of this imaging strategy to determine the onset of transgene expression.

In this same study (42), peak levels of gene expression were obtained 4 days after infection with the adenovector and increased by a factor of 2–3 over baseline measurements (Fig. 8.6). In contrast, *in vitro* assays of gene

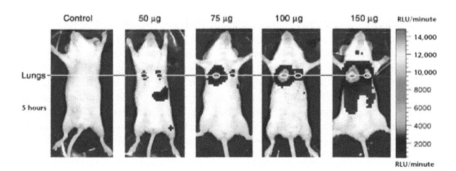

Figure 8.5 Optical imaging of mice following injection of the firefly luciferase gene *fl* conjugated to DOTAP: cholesterol liposomal complexes. All images shown consist of a visible light image superimposed on an image of the mouse with a scale in relative light units (RLU)/min. Each animal received an injection of D-luciferin 10 min before imaging. Images were obtained 5 h after injection of the complexes. Mice injected with increasing amounts of DNA show increasing levels of *fl* gene expression in the lungs. [Reproduced with permission from Iyer et al. (44).]

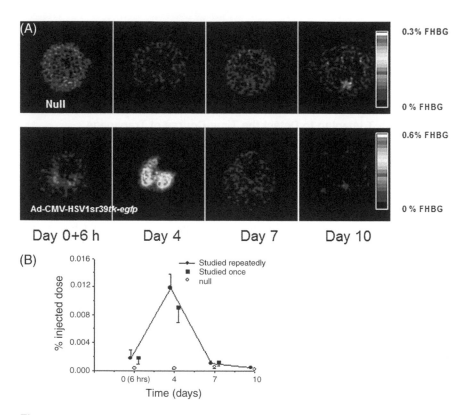

Figure 8.6 (A) Transverse PET images obtained at the mid-chest level in two rats studied serially. (A, top row) Rat administered null vector;. (A, bottom row) rat administered the adenovectors AdCMV-mNLS-HSV1*sr39tk-egfp*, a fusion gene of a mHSV1-*tk* (the mutation was to a nuclear localization sequence, NLS) and the enhanced green fluorescent protein gene (*egfp*), driven by the cytomegalovirus promoter (CMV). Note the different scales. Also note tracer uptake is detected within 6 h of vector administration, intensifies significantly by day 4, is barely detectable by day 7, and is negligible by day 10. (B) Summary data from 16 rats, including those studied serially ($n = 4$), studied once at the same time-points (then sacrificed for lung TK activity analyses) ($n = 4$ at each time-point), or studied at same time-points after null vector administration ($n = 4$). Temporally, the measurements of percentage of ID of [^{18}F]-FHBG closely followed the measurements of lung tissue TK activity. [Reproduced with permission from Richard et al. (42).]

expression increased 50–150-fold. This observation suggests that PET imaging of this particular PRG–PRP may not fully track the magnitude of gene expression, especially in tissues with high levels of expression.

In any given study, the duration of transgene expression will be a function of several factors, including the species used, tissue transduced, and the extent to which an inflammatory response is invoked by the adenovector. For instance, relatively transient transgene expression after adenovirus-mediated gene transfer has been linked to a cytotoxic T cell response to major histocompatibility complex 1 (MHC-1) adenoviral antigens, which leads to rapid clearance of trans-duced cells. A more prolonged expression of virally delivered transgenes is pos-sible in immune-deficient mice (55–57) or in immune-competent animals after infection with newer generation adenovectors that are deleted of all adenoviral genes ("gutless," or helper dependant) (58–60). Imaging provides a convenient way to follow the duration of gene expression with these newer vector technol-ogies. As an example, in the study discussed earlier, transgene expression was no longer detectable, by imaging or by *in vitro* assays, 10 days after infection with the adenovector. Inubushi et al. (61) made a similar observation when they used an analogous imaging strategy to follow myocardial reporter gene expression in rats.

To some extent, of course, the apparent duration of transgene expression will be determined by the sensitivity of the biological method used to quantify it. Low-sensitivity methods will underestimate the apparent duration of reporter gene expression whereas high-sensitivity methods may detect physiologically insignificant levels of the transgene. As already noted, the PET PRG–PRP repor-ter system used in our studies is at least as sensitive as *in vitro* assessments of TK enzymatic activity or GFP quantitation by ELISA (43). However, the biological significance of the different detection thresholds of these three techniques is unknown. One advantage of the imaging strategy employed in our studies, however, is that they will only detect functional reporter proteins, whereas other methods (e.g., northern-blots, western-blots, ELISA) may detect nonfunc-tional copies of transcript or proteins. Thus, a variety of factors, both technical and biological, can affect the evaluation of transgene expression kinetics.

B. PET Imaging to Evaluate Methods of Vector Delivery to the Lungs

Optimal vector delivery is a critical issue in developing gene therapy protocols for lung diseases in humans. To deliver transgenes to the airways or to alveolar epithelial cells, vectors are usually administered intratracheally. Surfactant has been proposed as one means of improving adenovector delivery, based on its bio-physical properties, which should result in a more rapid distal dispersion of vector than with saline. Furthermore, surfactant re-uptake by alveolar type 2 epithelial cells as part of normal surfactant metabolism might result in the co-transport of both surfactant and the adenovector into these cells, providing another possible mechanism to improve gene transfer efficiency to lung tissue (62).

Although surfactant-based vehicles have been reported to allow more effi-cient adenovirus-mediated gene transfer and to facilitate vector dispersion in the lungs (62–65), the experimental evidence supporting this perception has not been especially strong. For instance, an increase in gene transfer efficiency may be obtained with surfactant-based vehicles when a low volume of delivery medium is used (65), whereas a superiority of surfactant over saline-based vehicles was not found at higher delivery volumes (4 mL/kg) (65). In addition, numerous other factors may interfere with the efficiency of vehicle delivery (e.g., lung instillation technique, surfactant concentration in the vehicle, etc.).

To determine whether PET imaging could be used to evaluate different methods of vector delivery, we studied rats administered an adenovector carrying the same mutant HSV1-*tk* gene as used in previously described studies (41). We found that the surfactant vehicle improved transfection efficiency of the mutant *tk* gene into the lungs of rats with normal lungs by at least 40%, providing evidence that PET imaging could be used as a new tool to evaluate methods of vector delivery to the lungs noninvasively—a method that could eventually be applied to humans.

C. PET Imaging to Evaluate the Intrapulmonary Distribution of Transgene Expression

Many lung diseases such as pulmonary edema are regionally heterogeneous. Therefore, the effectiveness of gene transfer as a means of studying lung biology may depend in part on whether transgenes can be delivered to the most severely affected parts of the lungs. PET imaging is ideal for displays of intra-organ regional data.

Several techniques have been proposed to increase transgene expression following direct airway instillation of vectors (e.g., exogenous surfactant, perfluorochemical liquids), but their impact on vector spatial distribution has been unclear (62). Although the direct instillation of vector results in a heterogeneous deposition within limited portions of the lungs (62), inhalation of aerosolized vector solutions can result in more diffuse transgene distribution throughout the lungs. However, aerosolization is relatively inefficient, as only 10–30% of aerosolized particles reach the lower airways. As the surface active properties of surfactant should lead to rapid dispersion and deposition of vector into the alveolar spaces, administration of viral vectors in a surfactant vehicle could be another means of enhancing gene delivery to the alveolar epithelium (65).

In our study, comparing surfactant and saline vehicles for airway delivery of adenovector (41), a slightly increased tracer concentration in the peripheral regions of the lungs in the surfactant group was consistently observed when compared with tracer concentration in similar regions of the lungs of rats in a saline group. Although the magnitude of this redistribution is low and its biological signification may not be great, it demonstrates that biologically significant differences in future studies should be easily detected by PET imaging.

A frequency distribution of gene expression (expressed as percentage of ID of radiotracer uptake in each picture element) showed that the increased uptake of vector using surfactant as a vehicle could be explained by the 24% of lung volume elements that showed uptake of 0.3%/mL of lung or higher (top half of all values) after vector delivery with surfactant as the vehicle vs. only 4%

of the lung after vector delivery with a saline vehicle. Furthermore, the location of the picture elements with high levels of expression (>0.3%ID/mL) in the surfactant group were evenly distributed throughout the lung (i.e., there was no ventral–dorsal or rostral–caudal gradients). (Fig. 8.7).

Several technical issues should be mentioned when considering the results for such studies. For instance, lung boundaries are not easily detected on PET images without an attenuation scan (allowing the chest wall to be defined by creating a regional map of tissue density). Unfortunately, attenuation images of sufficient quality are not yet readily available with the current generation of microPET devices (a problem not present in clinical PET studies). Therefore, ROIs have been identified in these studies by drawing them on tomographic chest slices where radioactivity is greater than background. The result is that low-activity pixels at the periphery of the lung may be excluded from the analysis. This problem should be reduced as multimodal imaging with combinations of PET and X-ray computed tomography (CT) become more readily available (Chapter 7).

A related problem can result from the influence of so-called partial-volume averaging on estimates of lung radioactivity with PET. Given the relatively limited spatial resolution of PET, the activity measurements in picture elements representing regions within the lungs can be influenced by nearby low-activity regions (e.g., outside the thorax). The result will be an underestimation of signal intensity/distribution. Even so, for whole lung ROIs, image-derived radioactivity measurements obtained after the accumulation of a PRP in the presence of a viral PRG such as TK have been strongly and linearly correlated to direct

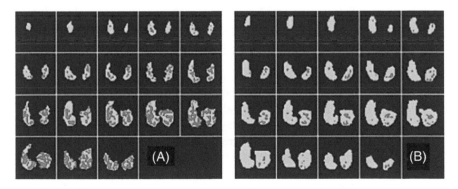

Figure 8.7 **(See color insert)** Parametric images of lung [^{18}F]-FHBG distribution in a rat administered adenovectors in a surfactant vehicle (A) or a saline vehicle (B). The pixels within each ROI drawn on each slice were colored in pale blue. Pixels with radioactivity values greater than 0.3% of [^{18}F]-FHBG ID/mL were colored in red. [^{18}F]-FHBG = 9-(4-[^{18}F]-fluoro-3-hydroxymethylbutyl)guanine. Note that higher levels of expression with the surfactant vehicle are apparent, without any specific spatial dependence. [Reproduced with permission from Richard et al. (41).]

measurements of tissue radioactivity obtained with a gamma counter, even in small animals (43). A major reason for this strong correlation is that as the viral vector is administered intratracheally, the lung is the only organ to express TK, and therefore, the only tissue to retain high levels of the PRP. For smaller ROIs (e.g., at the periphery of the lung), some partial-volume averaging effect must be present. In addition, respiratory variation due to tidal breathing will produce a similar effect.

D. Quantitation of Reporter Gene Expression in the Lungs with PET Imaging

A key premise underlying the use of imaging to monitor and quantify transgene expression is that, over a relevant physiologic range, the level of reporter-gene expression is directly related to the imaging signal, which in turn depends on the tissue accumulation of the reporter probe (1,4). However, although the sensitivity of imaging to detect reporter gene expression has been confirmed in several studies (43,66), the strength of the correlation between tissue-tracer uptake and tissue-based assays of *tk* as the reporter gene has been variable (43,61). For instance, several studies suggest that the imaging signal may plateau as high levels of HSV1-*tk* are achieved in target tissue (43,61), whereas others report highly linear correlations between *in vitro* assays of gene expression and the tissue accumulation of both pyrimidine [such as 2′-fluoro-2′-deoxy-1-β-D-arabinofuranosyl-5-iodouracil (FIAU)] and acycloguanosine derivatives (such as the [^{18}F]-FHBG) (55,67). Studies by Zinn et al. (17,50,68) suggest that the correlation of imaging signal with *in vitro* assays of gene expression may be more reliable when hSSTr2 is used as the reporter gene. (In this case, however, there is concern that radioligand binding to this mammalian receptor may trigger unwanted physiologic effects.)

The issue of how best to quantify gene expression via imaging has received relatively little attention. The most common approach is to simply express the accumulation of tracer in organs such as the lungs (i.e., tissue radioactivity) as a percentage of the dose of injected radioactivity (%ID). Although straightforward, this approach has the disadvantage of being influenced by factors such as the time-point at which it is measured, body mass, and the fraction of total tissue radioactivity which is resident in the blood rather than in cells specifically expressing the reporter protein. This latter factor may be especially important in lung studies as 50% of the normal lung parenchymal tissue density is due to blood.

The accuracy of tissue radioactivity measurements with PET, however, makes it possible to use potentially more robust methods of quantitation. For instance, a commonly used method of quantifying tracers that are irreversibly trapped within tissues (at least during the scan) is to calculate a so-called "net influx rate constant," K_i. An example of a reporter protein that functions this way would be TK, which via phosphorylation traps radioactive substrates such as $[^{18}F]$-FHBG (Fig. 8.1) (1).

More generally, compartmental modeling of tracer kinetics can be used to analyze the time-activity data in both tissue and blood perfusing the organ-of-interest during the scan period. For a standard three-compartment model in which tracer is irreversibly trapped in tissue (Fig. 8.8), a set of rate constants describing the movement of tracer between blood and tissue can be obtained by fitting the experimental data points obtained from imaging (Fig. 8.9) to the following equation:

$$C_T(t) = \frac{K_1}{\alpha_2 - \alpha_1} \times [(k_3 + k_4 - \alpha_1)e^{-\alpha_1 t} + (\alpha_2 - k_3 - k_4)e^{-\alpha_2 t}]$$

$$\otimes C_A(t) + BV C_A(t)$$

where $\alpha_{2,1} = (1/2)(k_2 + k_3 + k_4 \pm \sqrt{(k_2 + k_3 + k_4)^2 - 4k_2 k_4})$, $\otimes$ is the convolution operator, BV is the blood volume component, and K_1, k_2, k_3, and k_4 represent the individual rate constants.

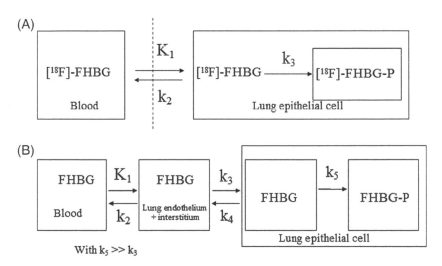

Figure 8.8 (A) Diagram of a three compartment model representing $[^{18}F]$-FHBG kinetics within the lungs. In this model, K_1 and k_2 are rate constants representing transport of $[^{18}F]$-FHBG into and out of cells, and k_3 represents the rate of phosphorylation of $[^{18}F]$-FHBG in cells expressing the viral TK (Fig. 8.1). Since $[^{18}F]$-FHBG-P is assumed to be trapped intracellularly, k_4 (a rate constant representing $[^{18}F]$-FHBG dephosphorylation) was not included in the model. $[^{18}F]$-FHBG = 9-(4-$[^{18}F]$-fluoro-3-hydroxymethylbutyl)-guanine. (B) Revised (four compartment) model of $[^{18}F]$-FHBG kinetics within the lungs. [Reproduced with permission from Richard et al. (71).]

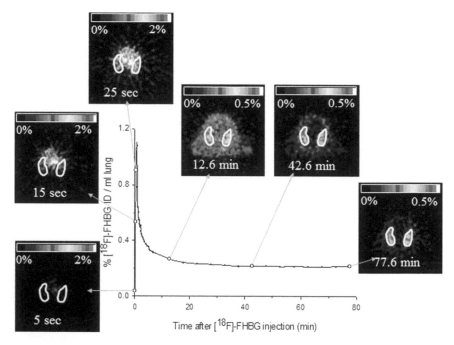

Figure 8.9 Example of how a pulmonary time-activity curve is generated from a multiple-image dataset. Pulmonary ROIs are drawn on multiple transverse slices of a PET image, and subsequently merged to obtain a measurement of pulmonary radioactivity originating from the whole lung volume at the time of PET image data acquisition. These ROIs are then superimposed on images obtained at each of the sampling times with PET, to generate the lung time-activity curve. For clarity, only one of the multiple transverse thoracic slices is displayed at six of 37 time-points. Color scale is shown on top of each PET image, and expressed as a percentage of [^{18}F]-FHBG ID. [^{18}F]-FHBG = 9-(4-[^{18}F]-fluoro-3-hydroxymethylbutyl)guanine; ID = indected dose. [Reproduced with permission from Richard et al. (71).]

As [^{18}F]-FHBG is assumed to be trapped in cells after phosphorylation by TK, k_4 is set to zero and dropped from the equation. K_1, k_2, k_3, and BV are then estimated by nonlinear regression.

The influx constant K_i is then calculated as:

$$K_i \, (\text{mL blood/mL lung/min}) = K_1 \frac{k_3}{(k_2 + k_3)}$$

A simple graphical method of calculating K_i was introduced by Patlak (69,70), in which the experimental data points obtained after tracer equilibration are fit to the following linear equation:

$$\frac{C_T(t)}{C_A(t)} = K_i \times \frac{\int_0^t C_A(\tau)\, d\tau}{C_A(t)} + B$$

where $C_T(t)$ and $C_A(t)$ are tissue and blood radioactivity, respectively, at each sample time-point (t), τ is the integration variable, K_i, the influx constant, and B, the parameter representing the initial volume of distribution of the tracer (the intercept when plotted graphically).

Recently, we undertook a comprehensive evaluation of these various forms of image quantitation in gene expression imaging studies of the lungs and compared the results with *in vitro* assays of the expression of TK enzyme activity (71). In this analysis, we found that the pulmonary uptake of [^{18}F]-FHBG increased as TK enzyme activity increased only at low levels of HSV1-*tk* expression and then plateaued as TK activity continued to increase [Fig. 8.10(A)]. Compartmental modeling failed to improve the correlation with *in vitro* assays of transgene expression.

Several factors might account for this apparent plateau effect. Competition for phosphorylation between [^{18}F]-FHBG and cellular thymidine is one possibility, as recently noted by Min et al. (66). Another possible cause is that tracer availability to the viral transgene was restricted in some way. For instance, [^{18}F]-FHBG was recently shown to accumulate much more slowly in mammalian cells expressing the wild type HSV1-*tk in vitro* than other radiolabeled pyrimidine nucleoside derivatives (13), and it was hypothesized that [^{18}F]-FHBG uptake might be limited by cell membrane transport (13).

A related possibility is that transport into target cells per se might not be rate-limiting, whereas transport into the immediate extracellular environment of these tissues might be. As the viral vector was administered intratracheally in our studies, infection and gene transfer occurred primarily in alveolar epithelial cells. However, the PET reporter probe is administered intravenously. It must therefore cross pulmonary vascular endothelial and interstitial compartments before it can gain access to alveolar epithelial cells. Trapping of tracer that makes it to this point might indeed be a function of transgene expression, but overall uptake might be limited by the barrier posed by the endothelium/interstitium. Indeed, we found that a linear relationship could be obtained when the pulmonary uptake of [^{18}F]-FHBG and *in vitro* assays of TK activity were correlated in rats after treatment with the thiourea ANTU, an agent known to increase pulmonary vascular permeability [Fig. 8.10(B)].

These results suggest that the pulmonary endothelium can act as a critical barrier, limiting access of reporter probe to target cells expressing the viral reporter transgene *tk*. Accordingly, in normal rat lungs, uptake of the reporter probe [^{18}F]-FHBG appears to be a function of both transport into tissues expressing the transgene and the level of transgene expression itself.

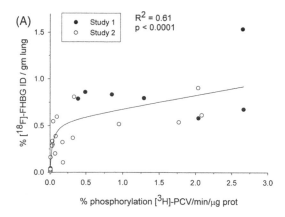

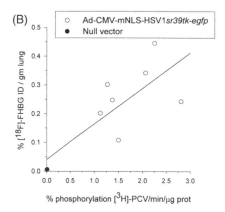

Figure 8.10 (A) Relationship between the lung uptake of [^{18}F]-FHBG and *in vitro* enzyme activity of a mutant HSV1-TK. Data are were combined from two studies and were fitted to a hyperbolic equation and corresponding regression curve and R^2 are displayed. (B) Relationship between the lung uptake of [^{18}F]-FHBG and mutant HSV1-TK enzyme activity in rats with ANTU-induced increases in pulmonary vascular permeability. [^{18}F]-FHBG = 9-(4-[^{18}F]-fluoro-3-hydroxymethylbutyl)guanine, ID = injected dose, mHSV1-TK = mutant *Herpes simplex* virus-1 thymidine kinase, PCV = penciclovir. [Reproduced with permission from Richard et al. (71).]

As the pulmonary endothelium/interstitium appears to pose a barrier for intravenously administered [^{18}F]-FHBG uptake by pulmonary epithelial cells expressing a reporter imaging transgene, it is possible that inhalational delivery of the radiotracer might improve the correlation between imaging signal and *in vitro* assays of reporter transgene expression. However, although this strategy might work well in normal lungs, it would be difficult to ensure that all portions of the lungs were equally exposed to radiotracer (a necessary condition if quantitation is to be meaningful) during disease states where regional ventilation would be expected to vary considerably. Of course, the kinetics of [^{18}F]-FHBG uptake or other reporter probes by the lungs after intravenous administration of the radiotracer might be quite different if endothelial cells rather than epithelial cells were transduced by the gene vector.

These studies indicate that the interpretation of the imaging signal in terms of transgene expression will require careful evaluation, involving factors such as species used, the target organ, and the disease state. The results do not mean that the concept of using imaging to monitor the expression of reporter transgenes is invalid. For instance, as has been described, these strategies can clearly be used to determine the onset and duration of gene expression, as well as to study the intrapulmonary distribution of vector delivery, and to compare different vector vehicles (41,43,47). Furthermore, alternative combinations of imaging reporter genes and/or reporter probes, possibly applied in different tissues or different species, could well yield different results with respect to *in vitro* assays of gene expression. The field is still nascent and much is yet to be learned about how best to optimize the promise of noninvasive gene expression imaging.

V. Applications

There are potentially multiple applications of reporter gene imaging in the lungs. For instance, the evaluation of pulmonary transcriptional expression of an endogenous gene in transgenic animals is now achievable by using the corresponding promoter/enhancer of the endogenous gene to drive expression of the reporter gene (72,73). Alternatively, by linking a "therapeutic" or "biology-modifying" gene with an imaging reporter gene, one should be able to infer the level of expression of the therapeutic gene from the expression level of the reporter. The potential for this strategy to monitor pulmonary gene therapy *in vivo* is obvious, but the relationship between the imaging signal and the physiologic effect of any "therapeutic" gene is yet to be demonstrated.

Several approaches are available for linking the expression of the reporter gene to the target/therapeutic gene, and a limited number of studies demonstrate feasibility by various imaging methods: creating a fusion of target and reporter genes, positioning each gene independently on a single vector (both downstream of an identical promoter), co-administration of identical vectors with one carrying the target gene while the other carries the reporter, use of a bicistronic vector containing an internal ribosomal entry site, or a bidirectional promoter system to inducibly coexpress a target gene and a reporter gene under the control of an exogenously administered drug such as tetracycline (12,74–76). To be useful, any one of these strategies must yield a reliable direct relationship between the expression of the reporter and the target gene over a physiologically relevant range of expression levels. Each approach has its own set of potential advantages and disadvantages; it is still too early to tell which approach is preferable under the greatest number of circumstances appropriate for both experimental and clinical studies.

The evaluation of gene therapeutics will probably be one of the first clinical applications for gene expression imaging. Several approaches have been developed for therapeutic gene transfer, including a variety of recombinant viruses (adenovirus and adeno-associated virus) (77–79), liposomes (80), and molecular conjugates (81), each of which has its own advantages and disadvantages (82–84). However, a significant limitation to evaluating gene therapeutics in patients with lung disease is a lack of clinical endpoints. Obtaining portions of the lungs that have been targeted for genetic correction (e.g., the distal airways in patients with cystic fibrosis) has been difficult, making it virtually impossible, for instance, to directly detect effective transfer and expression of the *CFTR* gene at those sites. Surrogate markers, like inflammatory indices and bacterial clearance from the lung, have been proposed, but are nonspecific and may be epiphenomena related more to the vector than the gene payload. Imaging provides a very promising alternative surrogate marker for effective gene transfer.

Another critical factor in determining the effectiveness of gene therapy is the duration of transgene expression. Many of the vectors currently applied introduce foreign genes as episomes, resulting in transient expression of the transgene. Some viral vectors will insert the foreign gene into the host cell's genome, but the duration of transgene expression depends on the survival of the type of cell transfected. Consequently, gene transfer in such cases would need to be repeated. Once again, imaging provides a noninvasive strategy to address this issue.

Thus, noninvasive, molecular imaging of reporter gene expression, delivered concurrently with *CFTR* or other therapeutic genes, could provide information regarding the onset and duration of transgene expression, of gene delivery systems, and of vector dose–response relationships (85). Clearly, gene expression imaging holds considerable promise as a method for monitoring the effectiveness of gene therapy protocols.

References

1. Massoud T, Gambhir S. Molecular imaging in living subjects: seeing fundamental biological processes in a new light. Genes Dev 2003; 17:545–580.
2. Blasberg R. Imaging gene expression and endogenous molecular processes: molecular imaging. J Cereb Blood Flow Metab 2002; 22(10):1157–1164.
3. Blasberg RG, Gelovani-Tjuvajev J. *In vivo* molecular-genetic imaging. J Cell Biochem Suppl 2002; 39:172–183.
4. Blasberg RG, Tjuvajev JG. Molecular-genetic imaging: current and future perspectives. J Clin Invest 2003; 111(11):1620–1629.
5. Weissleder R. Scaling down imaging: molecular mapping of cancer in mice. Nat Rev Cancer 2002; 2:11–18.
6. Weissleder R, Mahmood U. Molecular imaging. Radiology 2001; 219(2):316–333.
7. Sharma V, Luker GD, Piwnica-Worms D. Molecular imaging of gene expression and protein function *in vivo* with PET and SPECT. J Magn Reson Imaging 2002; 16:336–351.

8. Piwnica-Worms D. Perspectives in imaging: present and future prospects of clinical molecular imaging. In: Kufe D, Pollock RE, Weichselbaum RR, Bast RC, Gansler TS, Holland JF, Frei E, eds. Cancer Medicine. Hamilton, Ontario: BC Decker, Inc., 2003:2764–2769.

9. Schuster DP, Kovacs A, Garbow J, Piwnica-Worms D. Recent advances in imaging the lungs of intact small animals. Am J Respir Cell Mol Biol 2004; 30:129–138.

10. Schuster DP. Positron emission tomography: theory and its application to the study of lung disease. Am Rev Respir Dis 1989; 139(3):818–840.

11. Schuster DP. The evaluation of lung function with PET. Semin Nucl Med 1998; 28(4):341–351.

12. Yaghoubi S, Barrio JR, Dahlbom M, Iyer M, Namavari M, Satyamurthy N, Goldman R, Herschman HR, Phelps ME, Gambhir SS et al. Human pharmacokinetic and dosimetry studies of [(18)F]FHBG: a reporter probe for imaging herpes simplex virus type-1 thymidine kinase reporter gene expression. J Nucl Med 2001; 42(8):1225–1234.

13. Jacobs A, Voges J, Reszka R, Lercher M, Gossmann A, Kracht L, Kaestle C, Wagner R, Wienhard K, Heiss WD et al. Positron-emission tomography of vector-mediated gene expression in gene therapy for gliomas. Lancet 2001; 358:727–729.

14. Bailey D, Karp J, Surti S. Physics and instrumentation in PET. In: Bailey D, Townsend DV, Valk P, Maisey M, eds. Positron Emission Tomography: Principles and Practice. London: Springer-Verlag, 2003:41–68.

15. Chatziioannou A. Molecular imaging of small animals with dedicated PET tomographs. Eur J Nucl Med 2002; 29:98–114.

16. Reynolds PN, Zinn KR, Gavrilyuk VD, Balyasnikova IV, Rogers BE, Buchsbaum DJ, Wang MH, Miletich DJ, Grizzle WE, Douglas JT, Danilov SM, Curiel DT et al. A targetable, injectable adenoviral vector for selective gene delivery to pulmonary endothelium in vivo. Mol Ther 2000; 2(6):562–578.

17. Zinn K, Chaudhuri T. The type 2 human somatostatin receptor as a platform for reporter gene imaging. Eur J Nucl Med 2002; 29:388–399.

18. Ciana P, Raviscioni M, Mussi P. In vivo imaging of transcriptionally active estrogen receptors. Nat Med 2003; 9:82–86.

19. Contag C, Ross B. In vivo bioluminescence imaging as an eyepiece into biology. J Mag Reson Imaging 2002; 16:378–387.

20. Lipshutz G, Gruber C, Cao Y, Hardy J, Contag C, Gaensler K. In utero delivery of adeno-associated viral vectors: intraperitoneal gene transfer produced long-term expression. Mol Ther 2001; 3:284–292.

21. Wu JC, Sundaresan G, Iyer M, Gambhir SS. Noninvasive optical imaging of firefly luciferase reporter gene expression in skeletal muscles of living mice. Mol Ther 2001; 4(4):297–306.

22. Sweeney T, Mailander V, Tucker A. Visualizing the kinetics of tumor-cell clearance in living animals. Proc Natl Acad Sci USA 1999; 96:12044–12049.

23. Contag C, Contag P, Mullins J, Spilman S, Stevenson D, Benaron D. Photonic detection of bacterial pathogens in living hosts. Mol Microbiol 1995; 18:593–603.

24. Weissleder R. A clearer vision for in vivo imaging. Nat Biotechnol 2001; 19(4):316–317.

25. Bogdanov A, Weissleder R. In vivo imaging of gene delivery and expression. Trends Biotechnol 2002; 20(8):S11–S18.

26. Hedlund L, Dewalt S, Cofer G, Johnson G. Application of magnetic resonance to the study of the lung. In: Cutillo A, ed. Application of Magnetic Resonance to the Study of the Lung. Futura Press, 1996:401–415.

27. Piwnica-Worms D. Making sense out of anti-sense: challenges of imaging gene translation with radiolabeled oligonucleotides. J Nucl Med 1994; 35:1064–1065.

28. Gambhir SS, Barrio J, Herschman H, Phelps M. Imaging gene expression: principles and assays. J Nucl Cardiol 1999; 6:219–233.

29. Delepine P, Montier T, Guillaume C, Vaysse L, Le Pape A, Ferec C. Visualization of the transgene distribution according to the administration route allows prediction of the transfection efficacy and validation of the results obtained. Gene Ther 2002; 9(11):736–739.

30. Lerondel S, Le Pape A, Sene C, Faure L, Bernard S, Diot P, Nicolis E, Mehtali M, Lusky M, Cabrini G, Pavirani A et al. Radioisotopic imaging allows optimization of adenovirus lung deposition for cystic fibrosis gene therapy. Hum Gene Ther 2001; 12(1):1–11.

31. Lerondel S, Vecellio None L, Faure L, Sizaret PY, Sene C, Pavirani A, Diot P, Le Pape A et al. Gene therapy for cystic fibrosis with aerosolized adenovirus-CFTR: characterization of the aerosol and scintigraphic determination of lung deposition in baboons. J Aerosol Med 2001; 14(1):95–105.

32. Naylor L. Reporter gene technology: the future looks bright. Biochem Pharmacol 1999; 58:749–757.

33. Tjuvajev JG, Stockhammer G, Desai R, Uehara H, Watanabe K, Gansbacher B, Blasberg RG et al. Imaging the expression of transfected genes *in vivo*. Cancer Res 1995; 55(24):6126–6132.

34. MacLaren DC, Toyokuni T, Cherry SR, Barrio JR, Phelps ME, Herschman HR, Gambhir SS et al. PET imaging of transgene expression. Biol Psychiat 2000; 48(5):337–348.

35. Gambhir SS, Bauer E, Black ME, Liang Q, Kokoris MS, Barrio JR, Iyer M, Namavari M, Phelps ME, Herschman HR et al. A mutant herpes simplex virus type 1 thymidine kinase reporter gene shows improved sensitivity for imaging reporter gene expression with positron emission tomography. Proc Natl Acad Sci USA 2000; 97(6):2785–2790.

36. Massoud TF, Gambhir SS. Molecular imaging in living subjects: seeing fundamental biological processes in a new light. Genes Dev 2003; 17(5):545–580.

37. Haberkorn U, Oberdorfer F, Gebert J, Morr I, Haack K, Weber K, Lindauer M, van Kaick G, Schackert HK et al. Monitoring gene therapy with cytosine deaminase: *in vitro* studies using tritiated-5-fluorocytosine. J Nucl Med 1996; 37(1):87–94.

38. Gambhir SS, Barrio JR, Wu L, Iyer M, Namavari M, Satyamurthy N, Bauer E, Parrish C, MacLaren DC, Borghei AR, Green LA, Sharfstein S, Berk AJ, Cherry SR, Phelps ME, Herschman HR et al. Imaging of adenoviral-directed herpes simplex virus type 1 thymidine kinase reporter gene expression in mice with radiolabeled ganciclovir. J Nucl Med 1998; 39(11):2003–2011.

39. MacLaren DC, Gambhir SS, Satyamurthy N, Barrio JR, Sharfstein S, Toyokuni T, Wu L, Berk AJ, Cherry SR, Phelps ME, Herschman HR et al. Repetitive, non-invasive imaging of the dopamine D2 receptor as a reporter gene in living animals. Gene Ther 1999; 6(5):785–791.

40. Groot-Wassink T, Aboagye EO, Glaser M, Lemoine NR, Vassaux G. Adenovirus biodistribution and noninvasive imaging of gene expression *in vivo* by positron emission tomography using human sodium/iodide symporter as reporter gene. Hum Gene Ther 2002; 13:1723–1735.
41. Richard JC, Factor P, Welch LC, Schuster DP. Imaging the spatial distribution of transgene expression in the lungs with positron emission tomography. Gene Ther 2003; 10(25):2074–2080.
42. Richard J, Factor P, Ferkol T, Ponde D, Zhou Z, Schuster D. Repetitive imaging of reporter gene expression in the lungs. Mol Imaging 2003; 2:1–8.
43. Richard JC, Zhou Z, Ponde DE, Dence CS, Factor P, Reynolds PN, Luker GD, Sharma V, Ferkol T, Piwnica-Worms D, Schuster DP et al. Imaging pulmonary gene expression with positron emission tomography. Am J Respir Crit Care Med 2003; 167:1257–1263.
44. Iyer M, Berenji M, Templeton NS, Gambhir SS. Noninvasive imaging of cationic lipid-mediated delivery of optical and PET reporter genes in living mice. Mol Ther 2002; 6(4):555–562.
45. Alauddin MM, Conti PS. Synthesis and preliminary evaluation of 9-(4-[18F]-fluoro-3-hydroxymethylbutyl)guanine ([18F]FHBG): a new potential imaging agent for viral infection and gene therapy using PET. Nucl Med Biol 1998; 25(3):175–180.
46. Ponde DE, Dence CS, Schuster DP, Welch MJ. Microwave mediated rapid and reproducible radiosynthesis of [18F]FHBG. Nucl Med Biol 31:133 138.
47. Richard JC, Factor P, Welch LC, Schuster DP. Imaging the spatial distribution of transgene expression in the lungs with positron emission tomography. Gene Ther 2003; 10:2074–2080.
48. Herschman HR, MacLaren DC, Iyer M, Namavari M, Bobinski K, Green LA, Wu L, Berk AJ, Toyokuni T, Barrio JR, Cherry SR, Phelps ME, Sandgren EP, Gambhir SS et al. Seeing is believing: non-invasive, quantitative and repetitive imaging of reporter gene expression in living animals, using positron emission tomography. J Neurosci Res 2000; 59(6):699–705.
49. Phelps ME. PET: a biological imaging technique. Neurochem Res 1991; 16(9):929–940.
50. Zinn KR, Chaudhuri TR, Krasnykh VN, Buchsbaum DJ, Belousova N, Grizzle WE, Curiel DT, Rogers BE et al. Gamma camera dual imaging with a somatostatin receptor and thymidine kinase after gene transfer with a bicistronic adenovirus in mice. Radiology 2002; 223(2):417–425.
51. Anderson C, Pajeau T, Edwards W, Hserman E, Rogers B, Welch M. *In vitro* and *in vivo* evaluation of copper-64-labeled octreotide conjugates. J Nucl Med 1995; 36:2315–2325.
52. Anderson CJ, Dehdashti F, Cutler PD, Schwarz SW, Laforest R, Bass LA, Lewis JS, McCarthy DW, Anderson C, Dehdashti F, Cutler P et al. 64Cu-TETA-octreotide as a PET imaging agent for patients with neuroendocrine tumors. J Nucl Med 2001; 42:213–221.
53. Reynolds PN, Nicklin SA, Kaliberova L, Boatman BG, Grizzle WE, Balyasnikova IV, Baker AH, Danilov SM, Curiel DT et al. Combined transductional and transcriptional targeting improves the specificity of transgene expression *in vivo*. Nat Biotechnol 2001; 19(9):838–842.

54. Dumasius V, Jameel M, Burhop J, Meng FJ, Welch LC, Mutlu G GM, Factor P et al. *In vivo* timing of onset of transgene expression following adenoviral-mediated gene transfer. Virology 2003; 308(2):243–249.

55. Liang Q, Gotts J, Satyamurthy N, Barrio J, Phelps ME, Gambhir SS, Herschman HR et al. Noninvasive, repetitive, quantitative measurement of gene expression from a bicistronic message by positron emission tomography, following gene transfer with adenovirus. Mol Ther 2002; 6(1):73–82.

56. Zsengeller ZK, Wert SE, Hull WM, Hu X, Yei S, Trapnell BC, Whitsett JA et al. Persistence of replication-deficient adenovirus-mediated gene transfer in lungs of immune-deficient (nu/nu) mice. Hum Gene Ther 1995; 6(4):457–467.

57. Yang Y, Nunes FA, Berencsi K, Gonczol E, Engelhardt JF, Wilson JM. Inactivation of E2a in recombinant adenoviruses improves the prospect for gene therapy in cystic fibrosis. Nat Genet 1994; 7(3):362–369.

58. Schiedner G, Morral N, Parks RJ, Wu Y, Koopmans SC, Langston C, Graham FL, Beaudet AL, Kochanek S et al. Genomic DNA transfer with a high-capacity adeno-virus vector results in improved *in vivo* gene expression and decreased toxicity. Nat Genet 1998; 18(2):180–183.

59. Morsy M, Gu M, Motzel S, Zhao J, Lin J, Su Q, Allen H, Franlin L, Parks RJ, Graham FL, Kochanek S, Bett AJ, Caskey CT et al. An adenoviral vector deleted for all viral coding sequences results in enhanced safety and extended expression of a leptin transgene. Proc Natl Acad Sci USA 1998; 95:7866–7871.

60. Andrews JL, Kadan MJ, Gorziglia MI, Kaleko M, Connelly S. Generation and characterization of E1/E2a/E3/E4-deficient adenoviral vectors encoding human factor VIII. Mol Ther 2001; 3(3):329–336.

61. Inubushi M, Wu JC, Gambhir SS, Sundaresan G, Satyamurthy N, Namavari M, Yee S, Barrio JR, Stout D, Chatziioannou AF, Wu L, Schelbert HR et al. Posi-tron-emission tomography reporter gene expression imaging in rat myocardium. Circulation 2003; 107(2):326–332.

62. Weiss D. Delivery of gene transfer vectors to lung: obstacles and the role of adjunct techniques for airway administration. Mol Ther 2002; 6(2):148–152.

63. Jobe AH, Ikegami M, Yei S, Whitsett JA, Trapnell B. Surfactant effects on aeroso-lized and instilled adenoviral-mediated gene transfer. Hum Gene Ther 1996; 7(6):697–704.

64. Jobe AH, Ueda T, Whitsett JA, Trapnell BC, Ikegami M. Surfactant enhances adenovirus-mediated gene expression in rabbit lungs. Gene Ther 1996; 3(9):775–779.

65. Katkin JP, Husser RC, Langston C, Welty SE. Exogenous surfactant enhances the delivery of recombinant adenoviral vectors to the lung. Hum Gene Ther 1997; 8(2):171–176.

66. Min JJ, Iyer M, Gambhir SS. Comparison of [(18)F]FHBG and [(14)C]FIAU for imaging of HSV1-tk reporter gene expression: adenoviral infection vs stable trans-fection. Eur J Nucl Med Mol Imaging 2003; 30(11):1547–1560.

67. Tjuvajev JG, Avril N, Oku T, Sasajima T, Miyagawa T, Joshi R, Safer M, Beattie B, DiResta G, Daghighian F, Augensen F, Koutcher J, Zweit J, Humm J, Larson SM, Finn R, Blasberg R et al. Imaging herpes virus thymidine kinase gene transfer and expression by positron emission tomography. Cancer Res 1998; 58(19):4333–4341.

68. Zinn KR, Buchsbaum DJ, Chaudhuri TR, Mountz JM, Grizzle WE, Rogers BE. Noninvasive monitoring of gene transfer using a reporter receptor imaged with a high-affinity peptide radiolabeled with 99mTc or 188Re. J Nucl Med 2000; 41(5):887–895.

69. Patlak C, Blasberg R, Fenstermacher J. Graphical evaluation of blood-to-brain transfer constants from multiple-time uptake data. J Cereb Blood Flow Metab 1983; 3(1):1–7.

70. Patlak C, Blasberg R. Graphical evaluation of blood-to-brain transfer constants from multiple-time uptake data. J Cereb Blood Flow Metab 1985; 5(4):584–590.

71. Richard J-C, Zhou Z, Chen DL, Mintun MA, Piwnica-Worms D, Factor P, Ponde DE, and Schuster DP. Quantitation of pulmonary transgene expression with PET imaging. J Nucl Med 2004; 45:644–654.

72. Doubrovin M, Ponomarev V, Beresten T, Balatoni J, Bornmann W, Finn R, Humm J, Larson S, Sadelain M, Blasberg R, Gelovani Tjuvajev J et al. Imaging transcriptional regulation of p53-dependent genes with positron emission tomography *in vivo*. Proc Natl Acad Sci USA 2001; 98(16):9300–9305.

73. Green LA, Yap CS, Nguyen K, Barrio JR, Namavari M, Satyamurthy N, Phelps ME, Sandgren EP, Herschman HR, Gambhir SS et al. Indirect monitoring of endogenous gene expression by positron emission tomography (PET) imaging of reporter gene expression in transgenic mice. Mol Imag Biol 2002; 4(1):71–81.

74. Yu Y, Annala AJ, Barrio JR, Toyokuni T, Satyamurthy N, Namavari M, Cherry SR, Phelps ME, Herschman HR, Gambhir SS et al. Quantification of target gene expression by imaging reporter gene expression in living animals. Nat Med 2000; 6(8):933–937.

75. Tjuvajev JG, Chen SH, Joshi A, Joshi R, Guo ZS, Balatoni J, Ballon D, Koutcher J, Finn R, Woo SL, Blasberg RG et al. Imaging adenoviral-mediated herpes virus thymidine kinase gene transfer and expression *in vivo*. Cancer Res 1999; 59(20):5186–5193.

76. Sun X, Annala AJ, Yaghoubi S, Barrio JR, Nguyen KN, Toyokuni T, Satyamurthy N, Namavari M, Phelps ME, Herschman HR, Gambhir SS et al. Quantitative imaging of gene induction in living animals. Gene Ther 2001; 8(20):1572–1579.

77. Wagner J, Moran M, Messner A, Daifuku R, Conrad CK, Reynolds T, Guggino WB, Moss RB, Carter BJ, Wine JJ, Flotte TR, Gardner P et al. A phase I/II study of tgAAV-CF for the treatment of chronic sinusitis in patients with cystic fibrosis. Hum Gene Ther 1998; 9(6):889–909.

78. Flotte T, Virella-Lowell I, Chesnut K. Adeno-associated viral vectors for CF gene therapy methods. Methods Mol Med 2002; 70:599–608,

79. Crystal RG, McElvaney NG, Rosenfeld MA, Chu CS, Mastrangeli A, Hay JG, Brody SL, Jaffe HA, Eissa NT, Danel C et al. Administration of an adenovirus containing the human CFTR cDNA to the respiratory tract of individuals with cystic fibrosis. Nat Genet 1994; 8(1):42–51.

80. Noone P, Hohneker K, Zhou Z, Johnson LG, Foy C, Gipson C, Jones K, Noah TL, Leigh MW, Schwartzbach C, Efthimiou J, Pearlman R, Boucher RC, Knowles MR et al. Safety and biological efficacy of a lipid-CFTR complex for gene transfer in the nasal epithelium of adult patients with cystic fibrosis. Mol Ther 2000; 1:105–114.

81. Ziady A, Kelley T, Milliken E, Ferkol T, Davis P. Partial correction of the nasal chloride transport defect in CF mice after apical application of serpin enzyme complex receptor targeted DNA complexes. Mol Ther 2002; 5:413–419.
82. Griesenbach U, Ferrari S, Geddes D, Alton E. Gene therapy progress and prospects: cystic fibrosis. Gene Ther 2002; 9:1344–1350.
83. Ferrari S, Moro E, Pettenazzo A, Behr JP, Zacchello F, Scarpa M. ExGen 500 is an efficient vector for gene delivery to lung epithelial cells *in vitro* and *in vivo*. Gene Ther 1997; 4(10):1100–1106.
84. Flotte T, Ferkol T. Genetic Therapy: past present and future. Pediatr Clin N Am 1997; 44:153–178.
85. Richard JC, Chen DL, Ferkol T, Schuster DP. Molecular imaging for pediatric lung diseases. Ped Pulmonol 2004; 37:286–296.

9

Inflammation Imaging in the Lungs

HAZEL A. JONES

Imperial College London,
London, UK

I. Introduction

Gas exchange, the primary function of the lungs, requires close contact over a very large area, between the nonsterile external environment and the interior environment of the organism. As a consequence of this interface, the lungs have, out of necessity, developed extremely rapid and efficient mechanisms to control the potentially damaging substances to which they are exposed. The air we breathe is contaminated with infectious material including bacteria, viruses, and other respirable material, which may be toxic or merely mechanically irritating. Optimal gas exchange, achieved by minimizing gas to blood distance, requires that all inhaled particulate matter be cleared efficiently and that inflammatory responses to infection are resolved as soon as possible with no scarring. The gas-exchanging membrane can also become thickened after exposure to circulating drugs or external radiation. The responses to all these stimuli involve an inflammatory component.

The inflammatory response is thought to have evolved as a result of the requirement for a short, sharp response to repel attacks by invading organisms. The mechanisms that have developed involve the use of extremely potent bacteriocidal chemicals, which, if not subject to rigorous control, are also capable of tissue destruction.

The sequence of events that occurs involves the activation and mobilization of a variety of cell types and the production of numerous mediators. The prerequisite for any response is the detection of the threat. In the lungs, this function is largely undertaken by epithelial cells and the resident alveolar macrophages. These cells then signal the threat by releasing cytokines that stimulate the endothelium to express adhesion molecules, which link with surface molecules on neutrophils, causing them to marginate and then migrate through the vessel wall and interstitium into the region under attack. Further stimuli from bacteria present in the lungs initiate respiratory burst activity by the neutrophils, which release toxic contents, killing the invading organism with minimal collateral damage. Once the threat has been removed, the remaining neutrophils are inactivated by undergoing apoptosis, after which they are removed in a highly controlled manner by macrophages together with any cellular and bacterial debris.

In most cases of acute inflammation, these mechanisms work efficiently, and the infection resolves with little, if any, lasting damage. However, even when resolution ultimately occurs, the patient may require hospitalization and treatment when acute lung injury or bacterial pneumonia is present. Furthermore, in some circumstances the inflammatory response does not resolve and the inflammation persists. This persistence of inflammation is implicated in the pathogenesis of a number of lung diseases. These diseases often result in remodeling of the lung architecture, involving increases in lung matrix deposition and the consequent progressive loss of lung function. A number of these diseases are on the increase in the developed world, partly because of longer life spans and partly because of increasing levels of pollution, including cigarette smoke. Chronic obstructive pulmonary disease (COPD) leads to major morbidity and mortality as a consequence of loss of lung function (1). Asthma is an increasingly common disease responsible for loss of time from work and reduced quality of life (2). Both of these diseases have an inflammatory component (3,4).

Pulmonary inflammation is difficult to monitor in life. Difficulties in monitoring the pathogenic processes involved in the progression of lung disease *in vivo* have hampered the design and study of therapeutic interventions. Lung function tests can monitor progressive deterioration but provide no index of disease activity. Lung biopsy is invasive and difficult to repeat and may not be representative if disease distribution is heterogeneous. Chest X-ray films show changes in lung density but give no indication of disease activity. High-resolution computed tomography reveals lung architecture but does not allow monitoring of inflammatory cell behavior. Lavage of lung segments for inflammatory cells during bronchoscopy provides information about only the airspaces, when the disease process may be largely in the interstitium.

A number of imaging techniques routinely used in nuclear medicine departments are not very specific but are nevertheless clinically useful in the diagnosis and management of lung disease. However, external imaging of carefully validated intravenously injected radiolabeled markers of inflammatory processes has great potential for providing noninvasive and repeatable methods of monitoring the different components of the inflammatory process *in situ*. This will enable investigations of the factors that determine whether inflammation resolves or progresses to fibrosis and will also allow investigators to assess the efficacy of interventions targeted toward specific steps in the inflammatory process, thus potentially breaking the cycle of chronic inflammation.

II. Lung Water

Various stages of the pulmonary inflammatory process are associated with the development of lung edema, often with a concomitant protein leak. Increased lung water in the absence of a protein leak can be monitored by positron emission tomography (PET) with O-15-labeled water ($H_2{}^{15}O$) in tandem with a nondiffusible intravascular radiolabel (5,6). Damage to the epithelial and endothelial blood-gas barrier can be monitored by clearance of inhaled radioaerosol and/ or exudation of intravenously injected proteins, giving comparable results (7). These measurements are not widely used because they are relatively nonspecific, although sensitive. For instance, "healthy" smokers have rapid technetium-99m-labeled diethylenetriaminepentaacetic acid (^{99m}Tc-DTPA) clearance, despite a lack of clinically obvious disease associated with increased epithelial permeability. Kinetic modeling may help to reveal differences more specific to disease (8).

III. Amine Kinetics

Given the importance of the lungs in the control of circulating amines such as norepinephrine and serotonin, methods to study how the lungs handle amines in health and disease should prove to be both useful and informative. The kinetics of radiolabeled amines have been measured in a number of lung diseases, but the interpretation of the data so obtained still requires considerable development and validation (9).

IV. Components of the Pulmonary Inflammatory Process

There are several discrete components of inflammation that are susceptible to imaging with different techniques. Figure 9.1 shows a very simple linearized scheme of the major components of the archetypal neutrophilic inflammatory response.

A. Adhesion Molecule Expression

The vascular endothelium in an area of inflammation expresses adhesion molecules. These molecules interact with surface receptors on neutrophils, causing them to slow down and then marginate along the vessel walls. This musters

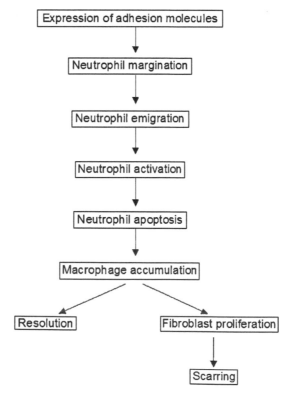

Figure 9.1 Components of the archetypal inflammatory response showing progression and resolution depicted as a linearized process.

the circulating inflammatory cells in the area of inflammation before emigration into the lungs. This component of lung inflammation has been studied only in animal models with an indium 111-labeled antibody to intercellular adhesion molecule 1 (ICAM-1). As predicted, this marker showed an increased uptake soon (1 h) after injury with oleic acid. The signal correlates with the time course of ICAM-1 expression of endothelial cells measured by immunofluorescence (10). In addition, studies have been carried out in patients with rheumatoid arthritis with an antibody fragment labeled with ^{111}In, which targets the adhesion molecule E-selectin. Both of these adhesion molecules are expressed by human endothelium during lung sepsis (11). The expression of adhesion molecules is an attractive target for imaging but has not yet been followed up, possibly because of significant uptake of the injected fragments by the liver and kidneys (12). There is evidence that different adhesion molecules are expressed in response to different stimuli, making the targeting almost too specific to be useful (13).

B. White Cell Trafficking

Chemotaxins caused by the presence of bacteria in the lungs, together with specific chemoattractants produced by resident cells, elicit trafficking of immune cells to the threatened region. This movement of white cells can be tracked by imaging the localization of radiolabeled leukocytes, and this technique is routinely used in nuclear medicine departments as a clinical tool to determine the location of pulmonary inflammation.

The technique involves the separation of white cells from the patient's blood and re-injection after labeling *in vitro* with an appropriate radiolabel (14). For the majority of clinical applications, mixed white cell preparations are labeled, but for research purposes in humans and animal models, it is feasible to separate the white cells further and to label only the granulocyte fraction or monocytes. The granulocyte fraction can itself be separated into neutrophils and eosinophils. The extreme radiosensitivity of lymphocytes renders them unsuitable for *ex vivo* labeling.

The manner in which the cells are handled is extremely important, principally to avoid any contamination, not only because the cells are to be re-injected into the patient, but also because neutrophils are very easily activated. Even with careful handling, cell separation techniques will cause priming of neutrophils; more vigorous handling or allowing the cells to settle out may cause the cells to degranulate and render them of little use for imaging studies. However, the clinical usefulness for localization of infection may well be enhanced by this increased activation because neutrophils require priming before they will respond to secondary stimuli to undergo respiratory burst activity. Furthermore, it is difficult to control for priming status because the cells will deprime and return to a quiescent state with time (15).

Radiolabeled leukocytes have also been widely used in clinical research of pulmonary inflammation and infection. Such investigations have advanced our understanding of the role of granulocytes in lung disease, particularly infection and chronic inflammation. The images from patients with bronchiectasis clearly show labeled cells in the airways and often also in the stomach because a proportion of sputum cells are swallowed after clearance through the respiratory tract. Because there is little loss of ^{111}In from the body other than by radioactive decay ($\sim$1%/day) (16), whole-body counting enables the loss of migrated cells from the body to be quantified, further elucidating the kinetics of granulocyte migration and providing a method for assessing the modulation of this aspect of the disease process by therapeutic intervention.

Patients with lobar pneumonia do not have a positive white cell scan (17) at a time when the lobe is known, from histologic measurement, to have undergone hepatization and be full of neutrophils. It appears that granulocyte migration is transient in this archetypal inflammatory response and that by the time the patient presents with the disease, cell migration has effectively stopped. The investigation of the initial stages of the acute inflammatory response occurs so rapidly that they can best be studied in animal models in which the exact timing of the challenge is controlled. Haslett (18) demonstrated in an animal model that migration in response to *Streptococcus pneumoniae* peaked at 2 h and had fallen to baseline values by 12 h after challenge. Thus, lack of a migration signal does not equate with absence of neutrophils in the lung.

The advent of positron emitters for cell labeling will render possible the quantification of the regional signal from sequestered and migrated cells (19). However, variability in the state of activation of cells that have been handled remains a concern regarding the interpretation of data obtained by using this or similar techniques.

C. *In Vivo* Cell Labeling

The possibility of using radiolabeled antibodies or antibody fragments to target cell surface antigens is very attractive, because this would enable the *in vivo* measurement of different cell types and phenotypes. Unfortunately, the development of these techniques is still in its infancy. A study of an antibody to NCA-90 surface antigen on granulocytes showed that clearance from the blood into inflamed areas appeared to be nonspecific (20).

D. Neutrophil Activation

Although *ex vivo*-labeled white cells give information regarding the destiny of intravenous cells, they provide no information regarding the distribution or the activation status of these immune cells within the body.

[^{18}F]-labelled fluorodeoxyglucose (^{18}FDG) is a positron-emitting glucose analog that is taken up into cells in proportion to their metabolic rate. It is taken into cells by facilitated transport through the same mechanism as glucose and is phosphorylated by the same hexokinase enzyme. At this point, it can be metabolized no further and accumulates in the cell in proportion to its glucose requirements.

Imaging of the fluorine-18 signal therefore reflects glucose requirements. [18]FDG-PET is widely used in nuclear medicine to monitor tumor glucose uptake. It also reflects the increased glucose requirements that accompany inflammation.

When the animal model of unilateral response to the instillation of *S. pneumoniae* developed by Haslett (18) is used, the rate of uptake of intravenously injected [18]FDG, measured by repeated PET scanning over 2 weeks (21), indicates that the [18]FDG-PET signal lags that of granulocyte migration by a number of hours, peaking at a time when a migration signal can no longer be detected (Fig. 9.2). The [18]FDG-PET signal reflects increased glucose metabolism in the inflamed area. Histologic examination of tissue obtained from this animal model [when tritiated deoxyglucose (^{3}H-DG) was co-injected with [18]FDG] indicates that signal is localized *in vivo* to neutrophil granulocytes in the airspaces (Fig. 9.3). Very few of the neutrophils in the alveolar walls (i.e., capillaries) show labeling. The implication of this is that, in response to this particular bacterial insult, neutrophils do not activate significantly until they reach the site of infection. This controlled response restricts tissue damage to a minimum. [18]FDG-PET scanning with corresponding tissue microautoradiography in a range of scarring and nonscarring challenges, instilled into animal models in the same manner, indicated in each case that neutrophil granulocytes were responsible for the majority of the deoxyglucose uptake (22). In models that resulted in scarring, labeled neutrophils were found in the thickened interstitium rather than in the airspaces (Fig. 9.4). This localization to neutrophils does not imply that glucose uptake by other cells makes no contribution to the signal, which will, in each case, be the product of the number of cells present and their individual glucose uptake. However, neutrophils, because they are able to upregulate their glucose metabolism to a much greater extent than other cells, make a major contribution to the signal.

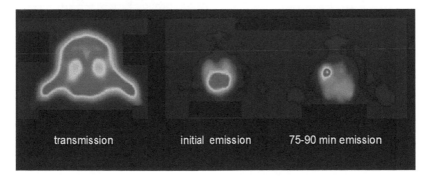

transmission   initial emission   75-90 min emission

Figure 9.2 **(See color insert)** Transthoracic PET images 15 h after instillation of *Streptococcus pneumoniae* into the right upper lobe of rabbit lung. Transmission image on the left shows distribution of lung density. Emission images show distribution of ^{18}F initially in the blood pool (middle) and localized to the challenged lung (right) 75–90 min after intravenous injection of [18]FDG. [Adapted from Jones et al. (21).]

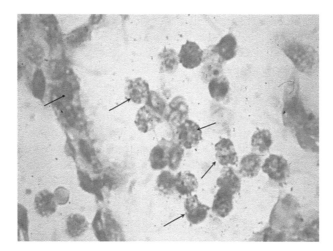

Figure 9.3 **(See color insert)** Microautoradiograph of lung tissue sample taken 1 h after injection of (^{3}H-DG) at a time of high ^{18}FDG uptake shown by PET (18 h after *Streptococcus pneumoniae* challenge to the rabbit lung). Silver grains developed by autoradiography show localization of ^{3}H-DG to neutrophils that have emigrated into the airspaces (arrowhead) but not in those in the capillaries (pinhead).

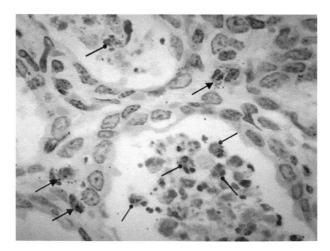

Figure 9.4 **(See color insert)** Microautoradiograph of lung tissue sample taken 1 h fter injection of ^{3}H-DG at a time of high ^{18}FDG uptake shown by PET in a scarring model of lung inflammation (2 weeks after bleomycin challenge to the rabbit lung). Silver grains developed by autoradiography show localization of ^{3}H-DG to neutrophils in the interstitium (arrowhead) but not in those in the airspaces (pinheads).

The findings from studies in animal models have been borne out in human lung disease. The [18]FDG-PET signal in patients with lobar pneumonia is high at a time when neutrophil migration measured by injection of radiolabeled white cells cannot be detected (Fig. 9.5, top). This demonstrates a clear dissociation between the migration and activation status of inflammatory cells in human lung disease (23). [18]F microautoradiography of bronchoalveolar lavage (BAL) fluid from a patient who underwent bronchoscopy immediately after a PET scan showed localization of radioactivity to neutrophils. This dissociation is also demonstrated in patients with bronchiectasis: chronic migration of white cells into the lungs is shown by radiolabeled white cell scanning, whereas [18]FDG-PET scans show very little increase in the lung signal (Fig. 9.5, bottom), indicating that although neutrophils are undoubtedly present, they are not highly activated. This low-grade activation of the cells may be due to a high throughput of cells, which could result in relatively immature neutrophils being sequestered (24), or may be due to factors in colonizing bacteria that suppress neutrophil activation. This might also explain the lack of an [18]FDG-PET signal in patients with cystic fibrosis (25).

A number of inflammatory lung diseases are diffuse and, because of the low density of the lungs, the emission images appear to the naked eye to show no increase in [18]FDG uptake relative to that observed in healthy subjects

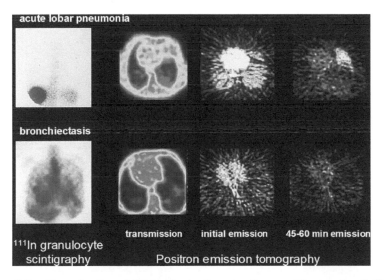

Figure 9.5 **(See color insert)** White blood cell scans of neutrophil migration (left) with PET images (right) in a patient 3 days after onset of symptoms of acute lobar pneumonia (top) and a patient with chronic bronchiectasis (bottom). White blood cell scans are clearly negative in pneumonia and positive in bronchiectasis. PET scans show transmission image, initial distribution after intravenous injection of [18]FDG and localization to affected lobe in the patient with pneumonia at 1 h. There is no apparent increase in [18]FDG uptake in the patient with bronchiectasis. [Adapted from Jones et al. (23).]

(Fig. 9.6). Quantification of the PET data, by using region-of-interest analysis and the construction of Patlak plots (26), however, can reveal significant differences between patient groups. Figure 9.7 shows an example of Patlak plots from a healthy subject and a patient with COPD.

Unlike the density of other organs, the density of the lung varies considerably with disease. The density of normal lung in the tidal breathing range is $\sim$0.3 g/cc. In the consolidated lung areas that occur with acute lobar pneumonia, this will approach 1 g/cc, and in emphysema, the density is dramatically reduced ($<$0.2 g/cc). [18]FDG can only be distributed into the tissue component of the lung and is therefore closely allied to density. The rate of uptake of [18]FDG is dependent on its initial volume of distribution, that is, the Patlak slope reflects the product of the number of cells in a ROI and the activity of these cells. For assessment of the activation status of the cells in the field, it must be taken into account that with no change in the metabolic activity of the cell population, doubling the lung density will double the slope purely as a result of doubling of volume of [18]FDG distribution per unit of thoracic volume. The activation status of the cells in the ROI can be measured by correcting the rate of uptake (Patlak slope) for the initial volume of distribution of the [18]FDG (the intercept of the Patlak slope at time zero) (23). Density, and hence, volume of [18]FDG distribution can also be increased

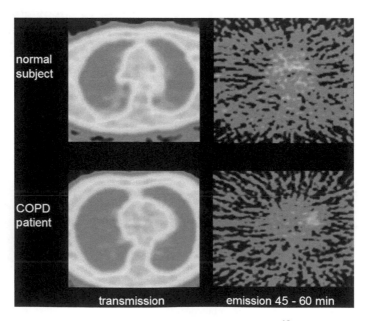

Figure 9.6 (See color insert) PET transmission images and [18]FDG emission images at 1 h after injection for a healthy subject (top) and a patient with COPD (bottom). No obvious difference is seen between the images. Differences can only be revealed by quantification of image data. [Adapted from Jones et al. (28).]

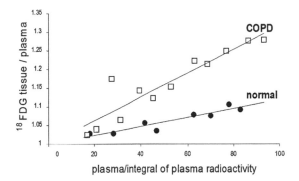

Figure 9.7 Quantification of image data. Patlak plots normalized to an intercept of 1.0 for the healthy subject and the patient with COPD whose images are shown in Fig. 9.6. [Adapted from Jones et al. (28).]

as a result of increased extracellular matrix (fibrosis) or edema. In these situations in which the increased volume of [18]FDG distribution is largely due to acellular components, this must be taken into consideration when data are interpreted. Under these circumstances, correction for the volume of distribution would be inappropriate as demonstrated by Chen et al. (27) in studies of acute lung injury.

Pulmonary [18]FDG-PET scanning in humans has shown high [18]FDG uptake in cases of infection (23), COPD (28), sarcoidosis (29), and acute lung injury (30) but not in stable asthma (28), cystic fibrosis (25), or rejection after transplantation (31). A very high signal is also found in patients with head injury, who are at risk for development of acute respiratory distress syndrome (ARDS) but who have no lung symptoms at the time of the scan (32). Figure 9.8 shows comparative [18]FDG-PET signals from a number of patient groups. The magnitude of the signal does not correlate closely with respiratory symptoms. These observations raise the question of which specific aspects of neutrophil function are responsible for the increase in deoxyglucose uptake.

The neutrophil granulocyte has a variety of functional responses, enabling it to respond to and effectively combat infection. These highly coordinated responses are dependent on an initial priming step, which enhances some steps and is a prerequisite for others (33). *In vitro* studies of neutrophils isolated from normal human peripheral blood demonstrate that the uptake of ^{3}H-DG is increased not only in cells that are primed and stimulated but also, and to the same extent, in cells that are only primed (34). Microautoradiography of the ^{3}H-DG distribution on cytospin preparations show the high level of labeling in all but the control samples (Fig. 9.9). This effect of priming could well explain the extremely high signals obtained in some patients with head injury, in whom respiratory symptoms never developed (32) (Fig. 9.8). Thus, a high pulmonary uptake of [18]FDG may reflect risk of damage, not necessarily actual

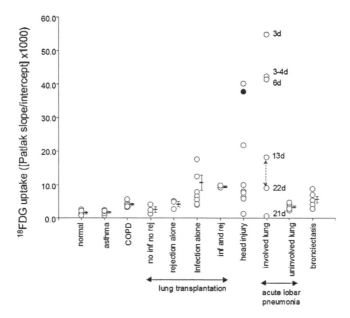

Figure 9.8 Individual values with standard error of the mean (SEM) bars, where appropriate, for [18]FDG uptake in healthy subjects and a number of patient groups. In the head injury series, the [18]FDG uptake in the only patient with lung symptoms is shown as a black dot. Although high, this was not the highest point. Individual points in showing [18]FDG uptake in the pneumonic lung are labeled with the number of days since the onset of symptoms. The double-headed arrow indicates repeat measurements made in an individual patient. [Composite illustration was constructed from results of several studies (23,28,31,32).]

damage. As the neutrophils remain in a primed state, any additional stimulus will precipitate actual tissue damage.

Activation may alter the uptake of [18]FDG through modulation of the number of glucose transporters on the cell membrane or changes in the phosphorylation enzyme such that they become limiting factors. However, *in vitro* studies performed by Burrows et al. (35) indicate that extracellular concentration of glucose has more impact on the rate of [18]FDG uptake than either transport or metabolism. The relevance of these findings to the *in vivo* situation remains to be evaluated.

E. Macrophage Kinetics

One of the key cells that orchestrate the inflammatory response is the macrophage. Resident macrophages comprise the majority of the cells inhabiting the alveolar spaces. These cells initiate the inflammatory response to bacterial or toxic insult by releasing mediators that coordinate the influx of neutrophils and monocytes from the blood. Once in the airspaces, the monocytes mature into inflammatory macrophages capable of phagocytosis and bacterial killing in

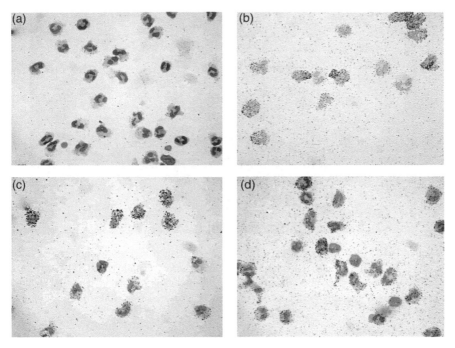

Figure 9.9 Microradiograph of neutrophils isolated from human peripheral blood and incubated with ^{3}H-DG for 1 h. (a) Control: unprimed cells; (b) tumor necrosis factor α (TNF-α)-primed and *N*-formyl-methionyl-leucyl-phenylalanine (fMLP)-stimulated cells; (c) unprimed cells stimulated with fMLP; (d) TNF-α-primed but unstimulated cells.

their own right, as well as disposal of tissue and cellular debris. The behavior of these cells, once they are in the inflammatory area, is the likely pivotal point that determines whether inflammation resolves or progresses to permanent lung damage. The interaction of macrophages with fibroblasts can lead to the production of extracellular matrix proteins and scarring.

A noninvasive measurement of macrophages in the lung should allow investigators to monitor the behavior of these key cells in a variety of diseases and help determine their relationship to the scarring process. The ligand PK11195 binds to receptors that are present in large numbers in macrophages (36). Labeled with carbon 11 for PET imaging, the R-isomer of this ligand localizes to the challenged regions of rabbit models after unilateral challenge with both scarring and nonscarring particulates (37). The initial signal correlates with macrophage influx. Changes in ^{11}C-*R*-PK11195 distribution with time can demonstrate the clearance from the lung of particle-bearing macrophages and has shown that clearance of nonscarring amorphous silica is efficient and rapid (Fig. 9.10), whereas clearance of microcrystalline silica by macrophages is delayed (Fig. 9.11). Histologic examination of lung tissue at different time points shows that amorphous silica particles are taken up into macrophages,

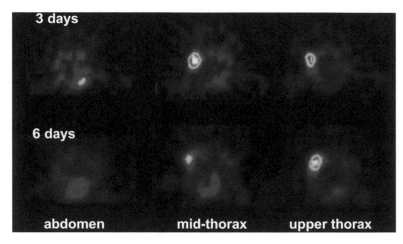

Figure 9.10 **(See color insert)** PET images of thorax after intravenous injection of [^{11}C]-*R*-PK11195 3 days (top) and 6 days (bottom) after challenge with 50 mg of 5 μm particles of microcrystalline silica into the right upper lobe of rabbit lung. Localization of radioactivity remains in the challenged region. [Adapted from Jones et al. (37).]

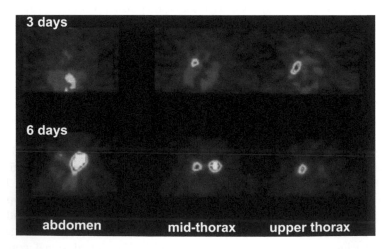

Figure 9.11 **(See color insert)** PET images of thorax after intravenous injection of [^{11}C]-*R*-PK11195 3 days (top) and 6 days (bottom) after challenge with 50 mg of 5 μm particles of amorphous (nonfibrogenic) silica into the right upper lobe of rabbit lung. Localization of radioactivity is to the challenged region at 3 days. By 6 days, there is a second signal, indicating clearance of particle-bearing macrophages through the lymphatics. [Adapted from Jones et al. (37).]

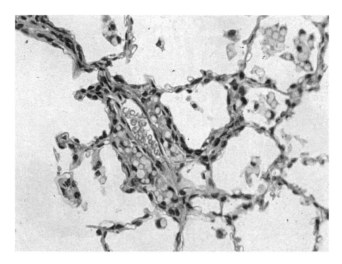

Figure 9.12 Photomicrograph of section of lung tissue 2 weeks after instillation of amorphous silica. Large numbers of particle-bearing macrophages are present in the perivascular sheath, most likely being cleared through the lymphatic system. The lung architecture is undamaged. [Adapted from Jones et al. (37).]

which are then cleared through the perivascular lymphatics, leaving the lung architecture undamaged (Fig. 9.12). Microcrystalline silica is also phagocytosed but not rapidly cleared from the lung undergoing extensive scarring. It may well be the compromised ability of the macrophage to clear particles efficiently from the lungs which results in lung scarring. The binding of PK11195 to macrophages has been confirmed by microautoradiography with the tritiated species in mixed inflammatory cells from animals (37) and humans (Fig. 9.13).

Imaging studies in patients with late fibrotic lung disease have shown that the PK11195 signal is low relative to that observed in healthy subjects and that early disease is associated with normal values (38). This was unexpected because histologic studies have shown that interstitial macrophages are a feature of lung fibrosis (39). The signal detected by ^{11}C-R-PK11195-PET scanning is, however, the product of cell numbers and receptor numbers per cell. Branley et al. (40) have subsequently demonstrated that the *in vitro* binding of PK11195 to cells in BAL samples is much lower than that in samples from healthy subjects. A single PK11195 scan obtained from a patient with lung fibrosis is therefore difficult to interpret, but repeat scans after therapeutic intervention would allow the effect of treatment to be assessed.

Pulmonary scanning of gallium 67 citrate is widely used in nuclear medicine departments for the detection of cancers and the active inflammation associated with interstitial lung disease and may also reflect macrophage activity. Tsuchiya et al. (41) demonstrated that the uptake measured by gamma-scintigraphy correlates with the expression of transferrin receptors (TFRs)

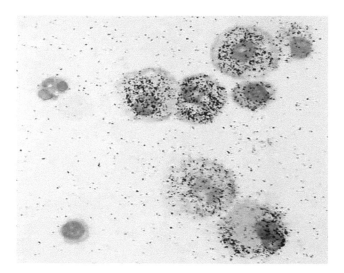

Figure 9.13 Microautoradiograph of BAL cells from a patient with interstitial lung disease. Cells were incubated with [^{3}H]-*R*-PK11195 for 10 min. Only the macrophages are labeled.

measured by immunohistochemistry. Biopsy samples from patients with interstitial lung disease show strong positive staining on the membranes of foamy or clustering macrophages in airspaces and on epithelioid cells in the granuloma present in sarcoidosis. No TFRs were demonstrated in other inflammatory cells, even fibroblasts. This is surprising because these cells are actively proliferating in lung fibroses (42). In lung cancer, TFR expression has been shown to be closely correlated with rate of proliferation (43,44).

F. Resolution of Inflammation

Ideally, an episode of inflammation will be followed by resolution with no permanent lung damage. The cessation of influx of inflammatory cells can be monitored by white cell scanning. The site of inflammation must be cleared of tissue debris and potentially damaging surplus inflammatory cells. The safe removal of these cells, predominantly neutrophil granulocytes, in a manner that prevents the release of their histotoxic contents, is critical to the resolution phase. In the absence of further production of inflammatory mediators, neutrophils undergo apoptosis and are then recognized and removed from the field by macrophages. This programmed cell death, which limits tissue damage and is antiinflammatory, contrasts strongly with necrosis that results in the toxic contents of the cell being released into the local environment, a process that causes potentiation of inflammation. Annexin V, used extensively *in vitro* to monitor apoptosis, has been radiolabeled with ^{18}F for PET imaging studies (45) and applied in inflammatory conditions. The information from these scans is difficult to interpret because annexin V links to phosphatidyl serine, which is exposed by both apoptotic and necrotic cells, not allowing discrimination between an antiinflammatory (apoptosis) and a proinflammatory (necrosis) process. Specific markers have been and are being developed that should allow specific identification of apoptosis *in vivo* (Chapter 13). This will greatly enhance the ability to monitor the critical balance point between resolution and progression to chronic inflammation. Interventions targeted to this process would be a major step forward in the control of pulmonary inflammatory disease.

V. Progression of Lung Disease

A. Fibroblast Proliferation

The interaction of macrophages with fibroblasts is thought to be a key step in the initiation of lung scarring. Fibroblasts are involved in remodeling processes in the lung and are capable of producing matrix proteins in large quantities. The proliferation of fibroblasts has been shown by histologic examination to be one of early signs of scarring. Inhaled particulates are particularly likely to elicit such a response. Proliferating fibroblasts express a number of receptors including AT1. Antagonists for these receptors have been labeled for imaging tumors. Pilot studies have shown increased uptake during fibroblast proliferation in animal models (unpublished data), but to date, this possibility has not yet been fully assessed or validated.

B. Control of the Extracellular Matrix

The complex balance between the synthesis of matrix proteins and their degradation is a very attractive target for therapeutic intervention. However, little is understood about the complex interactions that maintain the lung in a healthy condition or the processes that result in fibrotic lung disease as a consequence of chronic inflammation or other damage (46). The development of radiolabeled markers for discrete components of this system would greatly assist in the design of rational therapeutic strategies for these devastating diseases.

C. Synthesis of Matrix Proteins

Collagen is the major component responsible for increased extracellular matrix in lung fibrosis. The turnover of collagen in the lungs is very active, with $\sim$10% of total collagen normally being replaced every day (47). Thus, any minor imbalance such that synthesis exceeds degradation will lead to collagen accumulation, and hence, fibrosis (48). Collagen is unusually rich in proline residues; this distinguishes it from other proteins and has led to the use of proline incorporation into protein as a measure of active collagen synthesis (49,50).

The use of ^{18}F-labeled analogs of proline has enabled development of a method for monitoring collagen synthesis *in vivo* (51,52). The uptake of

[18]F-fluoroproline has been used to monitor scarring in rabbit models (53,54). After unilateral instillation with microcrystalline silica, ^{18}F-fluoroproline localizes in the challenged lung, and repeated measurements show a response that peaks at 6–8 weeks and is still detectable at 12 weeks after challenge (54). Microautoradiographs of lung tissue samples obtained 1 h after injection of tritiated proline show localization to fibroblasts in the actively scarring region. Acellular areas in scarred tissue show no radiolabeling. The scan time (90 min) is too short for the proline to be incorporated in the collagen itself, but the rate of proline uptake most likely reflects an active synthesis of collagen. The usefulness of the cis-isomer has been assessed in humans as a possible tumor marker (55) but has yet to be applied in human pulmonary fibrosis.

D. Extracellular Matrix Degradation

The other side of the extracellular matrix balance is the degradation of proteins by matrix metalloproteinases (MMPs) and their control by specific tissue inhibitors. The fibrosis that results from chronic inflammation is accompanied not only by increase in collagen synthesis but also by increase in the enzymes that control degradation (46). These enzymes are involved in the pathogenesis of tumors, and inhibitors to MMPs have been labeled with [18]F (56) and [11]C (57) for oncology imaging with PET. Unfortunately, the localization of markers developed so far in tumors appeared to be related to nonspecific binding (57).

The activity of MMPs is subject to complex regulation, involving both transcriptional and posttranslational mechanisms. The latter involves a group of endogenous protein inhibitors known as tissue inhibitors of metalloproteinases (TIMPs), of which there are several. The balance of these enzymes is a major determinant of extracellular matrix control (58). TIMPs have been radiolabeled for imaging studies but have not yet been validated *in vivo* (59).

There is a pressing need for validated markers for these processes to advance the development of treatment in various forms of lung fibrosis. At present, few treatments that make any significant impact on these debilitating diseases are available (60,61).

VI. Summary

Increasingly, imaging techniques are playing a major role in the diagnosis and treatment of patients with lung disease. A number of the scans offered routinely in nuclear medicine departments are nonspecific and not fully validated. There is still a considerable gap of knowledge between the clinical usefulness of such scans and the elucidation of mechanisms of disease.

PET scanning allows investigators to quantify radiolabel in tissues inaccessible by any other means. The challenge is in the interpretation of the signal. This requires rigorous validation of each newly developed marker to determine its specificity for the biologic target, its distribution kinetics, and its metabolic profile.

These studies usually involve a combination of *in vitro* studies and *in vivo* and *ex vivo* measurements in animal models before studies are performed with healthy human subjects and ultimately patients with well-characterized disease. The benefits of these major undertakings are that they should enable discrete cellular and biochemical mechanisms to be studied to evaluate their relative involvement in the pathogenesis of inflammatory lung disease. This in turn should allow us to devise strategies to target the pivotal stages with rationally designed therapeutic interventions and to monitor the efficacy of such treatments *in vivo*.

References

1. Lopez AD, Murray CC. The global burden of disease. 1990–2020. Nat Med 1998; 4:1241–1243.
2. National Institutes of Health. Global strategy for asthma management and prevention. *NHLBI/WHO Workshop Report*. National Heart Lung and Blood Institute, Publication number 95-3659, 1995.
3. Barnes PJ. Chronic obstructive pulmonary disease. N Engl J Med 2000; 343:269–280.
4. Vignola AM, Chanez P, Campbell AM, Souques F, Lebel B, Enander I, Bousquet J. Airway inflammation in mild intermittent and in persistent asthma. Am J Respir Crit Care Med 1998; 157:403–409.
5. Fazio F, Jones T, MacArthur CG, Rhodes CG, Steiner RE, Hughes JM. Measurement of regional pulmonary oedema in man using radioactive water (H215O). Br J Radiol 1976; 49:393–397.
6. Schuster DP. The evaluation of lung function with PET. Semin Nucl Med 1998; 28:341–351.
7. Braude S, Nolop KB, Hughes JM, Barnes PJ, Royston D. Comparison of lung vascular and epithelial permeability indices in the adult respiratory distress syndrome. Am Rev Respir Dis 1986; 133:1002–1005.
8. Bradvik I, Wollmer P, Evander E, Larusdottir H, Blom-Bulow B, Jonson B. Kinetics of lung clearance of 99mTc-DTPA in smoking patients with sarcoidosis compared to healthy smokers. Respir Med 2002; 96:317–321.
9. Peters AM. Radiolabelled amines and the lung. Nucl Med Commun 1998; 19:817–821.
10. Weiner RE, Sasso DE, Gionfriddo MA, Thrall RS, Syrbu S, Smilowitz HM, Vento J. Early detection of oleic acid-induced lung injury in rats using (111)In-labeled anti-rat intercellular adhesion molecule-1. J Nucl Med 2001; 42:1109–1115.
11. Tsokos M. Immunohistochemical detection of sepsis-induced lung injury in human autopsy material. Leg Med (Tokyo) 2003; 5:73–86.
12. Hnatowich DJ. Recent developments in the radiolabeling of antibodies with iodine, indium, and technetium. Semin Nucl Med 1990; 20:80–91.
13. Moreland JG, Bailey G, Nauseef WM, Weiss JP. Organism-specific neutrophil-endothelial cell interactions in response to *Escherichia coli, Streptococcus pneumoniae*, and *Staphylococcus aureus*. J Immunol 2004; 172:426–432.
14. Peters AM, Saverymuttu SH, Reavy HJ, Danpure HJ, Osman S, Lavender JP. Imaging of inflammation with indium-111 tropolonate labeled leukocytes. J Nucl Med 1983; 24:39–44.

256   *Jones*

15. Kitchen E, Rossi AG, Condliffe AM, Haslett C, Chilvers ER. Demonstration of reversible priming of human neutrophils using platelet-activating factor. Blood 1996; 88:4330–4337.
16. Currie DC, Saverymuttu SH, Peters AM, Needham SG, George P, Dhillon DP, Lavender JP, Cole PJ. Indium-111-labelled granulocyte accumulation in respiratory tract of patients with bronchiectasis. Lancet 1987; 1(8546):1335–1339.
17. Saverymuttu SH, Phillips G, Peters AM, Lavender JP. Indium-111 autologous leucocyte scanning in lobar pneumonia and lung abscesses. Thorax 1985; 40:925–930.
18. Haslett C. Resolution of acute inflammation and the role of apoptosis in the tissue fate of granulocytes. Clin Sci (Lond) 1992; 83:639–648.
19. Adonai N, Nguyen KN, Walsh J, Iyer M, Toyokuni T, Phelps ME, McCarthy T, McCarthy DW, Gambhir SS. *Ex vivo* cell labeling with 64Cu-pyruvaldehyde-*bis*(N4-methylthiosemicarbazone) for imaging cell trafficking in mice with positron-emission tomography. Proc Natl Acad Sci USA 2002; 99:3030–3035.
20. Skehan SJ, White JF, Evans JW, Parry-Jones DR, Solanki CK, Ballinger JR, Chilvers ER, Peters AM. Mechanism of accumulation of 99mTc-sulesomab in inflammation. J Nucl Med 2003; 44:11–18.
21. Jones HA, Clark RJ, Rhodes CG, Schofield JB, Krausz T, Haslett C. *In vivo* measurement of neutrophil activity in experimental lung inflammation. Am J Respir Crit Care Med 1994; 149:1635–1639.
22. Jones HA, Schofield JB, Krausz T, Boobis AR, Haslett C. Pulmonary fibrosis correlates with duration of tissue neutrophil activation. Am J Respir Crit Care Med 1998; 158:620–628.
23. Jones HA, Sriskandan S, Peters AM, Pride NB, Boobis AR, Haslett C. Dissociation of neutrophil emigration and metabolic activity in lobar pneumonia and bronchiectasis. Eur Respir J 1997; 10:795–803.
24. van Eeden SF, Kitagawa Y, Klut ME, Lawrence E, Hogg JC. Polymorphonuclear leukocytes released from the bone marrow preferentially sequester in lung microvessels. Microcirculation 1997; 4:369–380.
25. Labiris NR, Nahmias C, Freitag AP, Thompson ML, Dolovich MB. Uptake of 18fluorodeoxyglucose in the cystic fibrosis lung: a measure of lung inflammation? Eur Respir J 2003; 21:848–854.
26. Patlak CS, Blasberg RG, Fenstermacher JD. Graphical evaluation of blood-to-brain transfer constants from multiple time uptake data. J Cereb Blood Flow Metab 1983; 3:1–7.
27. Chen DL, Mintun MA, Schuster DP. A comparison of methods to quantitate 18F-fluorodeoxyglucose uptake with positron emission tomography during experimental acute lung injury. J Nucl Med 2004; 45:1583–1590.
28. Jones HA, Marino PS, Shakur BS, Morrell NW. *In vivo* assessment of lung inflammatory cell activity in patients with COPD and asthma. Eur Respir J 2003; 21:567–573.
29. Brudin LH, Valind SO, Rhodes CG, Pantin CF, Sweatman M, Jones T, Hughes JM. Fluorine-18 deoxyglucose uptake in sarcoidosis measured with positron emission tomography. Eur J Nucl Med 1994; 21:297–305.
30. Chen DL, Schuster DP. Positron emission tomography with 18F-fluorodeoxyglucose to evaluate neutrophil kinetics during acute lung injury. Am J Physiol Lung Cell Mol Physiol 2004; 286:L834–L840.

31. Jones HA, Donovan T, Goddard MJ, McNeil K, Atkinson C, Clark JC, White JF, Chilvers ER. Use of [18]FDG-PET to discriminate between infection and rejection in lung transplant recipients. Transplantation 2004; 77:2767–2777.

32. Jones HA, Clark JC, Minhas PS, Kendall IV, Downey SP, Menon DK. Pulmonary neutrophil activation following head trauma [abstract]. Am J Respir Crit Care Med 1998; 157:A349.

33. Condliffe AM, Kitchen E, Chilvers ER. Neutrophil priming: pathophysiological consequences and underlying mechanisms. Clin Sci (Lond) 1998; 94:461–471.

34. Jones HA, Cadwallader KA, White JF, Uddin M, Peters AM, Chilvers ER. Dissociation between respiratory burst activity and deoxyglucose uptake in human neutrophil granulocytes: implications for interpretation of ^{18}F-FDG-PET images. J Nucl Med 2002; 43:652–657.

35. Burrows RC, Freeman SD, Charlop AW, Wiseman RW, Adamsen TCH, Krohn KA, Spence AM. [^{18}F]-2-fluoro-2-deoxyglucose transport kinetics as a function of extracellular glucose concentration in malignant glioma, fibroblast and macrophage cells *in vitro*. Nucl Med Biol 2004; 31:1–9.

36. Zavala F, Lenfant M. Benzodiazepines and PK 11195 exert immunomodulating activities by binding on a specific receptor on macrophages. Ann N Y Acad Sci 1987; 496:240–249.

37. Jones HA, Valind SO, Clark IC, Bolden GE, Krausz T, Schofield JB, Boobis AR, Haslett C. Kinetics of lung macrophages monitored *in vivo* following particulate challenge in rabbits. Toxicol Appl Pharmacol 2002; 183:46–54.

38. Branley HM, du Bois RM, Black CM, Jones HA. Tissue uptake of the macrophage (mφ) radioligand ^{11}C-PK11195 measured by positron emission tomography (PET) in fibrosing alveolitis due to systemic sclerosis [abstract]. Am J Respir Crit Care Med 2003; 167:A474.

39. Katzenstein AL, Myers JL. Idiopathic pulmonary fibrosis: clinical relevance of pathologic classification. Am J Respir Crit Care Med 1998; 157:1301–1315.

40. Branley HM, Wells AU, du Bois RM, Jones HA. Quantification of the *in vitro* binding of 3H-PK11195 to bronchoalveolar lavage cells in patients with interstitial lung disease compared to normal non-smoking healthy individuals. Unpublished.

41. Tsuchiya Y, Nakao A, Komatsu T, Yamamoto M, Shimokata K. Relationship between gallium 67 citrate scanning and transferrin receptor expression in lung diseases. Chest 1992; 102:530–534.

42. Pardo A, Selman M. Molecular mechanisms of pulmonary fibrosis. Front Biosci 2002; 7:1743–1761.

43. Sutherland R, Delia D, Schneider C, Newman R, Kemshead J, Greaves M. Ubiquitous cell-surface glycoprotein on tumor cells is proliferation-associated receptor for transferrin. Proc Natl Acad Sci USA 1981; 78:4515–4519.

44. Inoue T, Cavanaugh PG, Steck PA, Brunner N, Nicolson GL. Differences in transferrin response and numbers of transferrin receptors in rat and human mammary carcinoma lines of different metastatic potentials. J Cell Physiol 1993; 156:212–217.

45. Murakami Y, Takamatsu H, Taki J, Tatsumi M, Noda A, Ichise R, Tait JF, Nishimura S. 18F-labelled annexin V: a PET tracer for apoptosis imaging. Eur J Nucl Med Mol Imaging 2004; 31:469–471.

46. Pardo A, Selman M. Idiopathic pulmonary fibrosis: new insights in its pathogenesis. Int J Biochem Cell Biol 2002; 34:1534–1538.

47. Laurent GJ, McAnulty RJ. Protein metabolism during bleomycin-induced pulmon-
     ary fibrosis in rabbits. Am Rev Respir Dis 1983; 128:82–88.
48. Selman M, Montano M, Ramos C, Chapela R. Concentration, biosynthesis and
     degradation of collagen in idiopathic pulmonary fibrosis. Thorax 1986; 41:355–359.
49. Laurent GJ. Rates of collagen synthesis in lung, skin and muscle obtained *in vivo* by a
     simplified method using [^{3}H]proline. Biochem J 1982; 206:535–544.
50. Gottlieb AA, Fujita Y, Udenfriend S, Witkop B. Incorporation of *cis*- and *trans*-4-
     fluoroprolines into proteins and hydroxylation of the trans-isomer during collagen
     biosynthesis. Biochemistry 1965; 4:2507–2513.
51. Bakerman S, Martin RL, Burgstahler AW, Hayden JW. *In vivo* studies with fluoro-
     prolines. Nature 1966; 212:849–850.
52. Wester HJ, Herz M, Senekowitsch-Schmidtke R, Hamacher K, Schwaiger,
     Stocklin G. Preclinical evaluation of 4-[18F]fluoroprolines: diastereomeric effects
     on metabolism and uptake in mice. Nucl Med Biol 1999; 26:259–265.
53. Wallace WE, Gupta NC, Hubbs AF, Mazza SM, Bishop HA, Keane MJ, Battelli LA,
     Ma J, Schleiff P. *Cis*-4-[^{18}F]Fluoro-L-Proline PET imaging of pulmonary fibrosis in a
     rabbit model. J Nucl Med 2002; 43:413–420.
54. Jones HA, Hamacher K, Hill AA, Clark JC, Krausz T, Boobis AR, Haslett C.
     ^{18}F-fluoroproline (^{18}FP) uptake monitored *in vivo* in a rabbit model of pulmonary
     fibrosis [abstract]. Am J Respir Crit Care Med 1997; 155:A185.
55. Langen KJ, Borner AR, Muller-Mattheis V, Hamacher K, Herzog H, Ackermann R,
     Coenen HH. Uptake of *cis*-4-[18F]fluoro-L-proline in urologic tumors. J Nucl Med
     2001; 42:752–754.
56. Furumoto S, Takashima K, Kubota K, Ido T, Iwata R, Fukuda H. Tumor detection
     using 18F-labeled matrix metalloproteinase-2 inhibitor. Nucl Med Biol 2003;
     30:119–125.
57. Zheng QH, Fei X, DeGrado TR, Wang JQ, Stone KL, Martinez TD, Gay DJ,
     Baity WL, Mock BH, Glick-Wilson BE, Sullivan ML, Miller KD, Sledge GW,
     Hutchins GD. Synthesis, biodistribution and micro-PET imaging of a potential
     cancer biomarker carbon-11 labeled MMP inhibitor (2R)-2-[[4-(6-fluorohex-1-
     ynyl)phenyl]sulfonylamino]-3-methylbutyric acid [11C]methyl ester. Nucl Med
     Biol 2003; 30:753–760.
58. Ruiz V, Ordonez RM, Berumen J, Ramirez R, Uhal B, Becerril C, Pardo A,
     Selman M. Unbalanced collagenases/TIMP-1 expression and epithelial apoptosis
     in experimental lung fibrosis. Am J Physiol Lung Cell Mol Physiol 2003;
     285:L1026–L1036.
59. Giersing BK, Rae MT, CarballidoBrea M, Williamson RA, Blower PJ. Synthesis and
     characterization of 111In-DTPA-N-TIMP-2: a radiopharmaceutical for imaging
     matrix metalloproteinase expression. Bioconjug Chem 2001; 12:964–971.
60. Hunninghake GW, Kalica AR. Approaches to the treatment of pulmonary fibrosis.
     Am J Respir Crit Care Med 1995; 151:915–918.
61. Davies HR, Richeldi L. Idiopathic pulmonary fibrosis: current and future treatment
     options. Am J Respir Med 2002; 1:211–224.

10

Bioluminescence Imaging of Transcription Factor Activity in the Lungs*

E. DUCO JANSEN and TIMOTHY S. BLACKWELL

Vanderbilt University School of Medicine,
Nashville, Tennessee

---

*Supported by NIH grants HL61419, HL66196, P20 CA86283 and the Whitaker Foundation.

I. Introduction

In vivo bioluminescence imaging (BLI) is a novel and powerful molecular imaging technique that enables one to study biological processes in their natural micro- and macroenvironment. This technology is based on the sensitive detection of light produced during the luciferase-mediated oxidation of a molecular substrate, where the luciferase enzyme is expressed *in vivo* as a molecular reporter. To date this technology has been applied in studies monitoring transgene expression (1–7), infectious disease progression (8–12), tumor growth and metastasis (13–19), transplantation (20,21), toxicology, viral infections, and gene therapy. Over the past few years, the number of studies applying this technology has grown exponentially. Here, we will describe methodology for quantitative *in vivo* measurement of a luciferase reporter construct expressed under the control of an important transcription factor, nuclear factor-kB (NF-κB). We will discuss utilization of this NF-κB driven promoter–reporter construct in transgenic mice to investigate the pathobiology of lung inflammation, injury, and host defense against bacterial pathogens.

II. Imaging Methodology

A. Bioluminescent Reaction

Bioluminescence refers to the process of emitting visible light from living organisms as a result of an enzyme-catalyzed reaction between a molecular oxygen and a suitable substrate. Bioluminescence manifests itself in nature in a variety of forms, ranging from the ubiquitous firefly to marine bacteria. Organisms exhibit bioluminescence for a variety of reasons: courtship and mating signaling, luring prey, defense, camouflage, and as a stress response (22). This natural phenomenon has now been harnessed for use in research as an optical reporter tool. Although a wide range of luciferase enzymes exist, each of which catalyzes the oxidation of a (luciferin) substrate with a corresponding release of photons of light (23), only a subset have been developed and used as reporter genes. Of these, the luciferase enzyme (*luc*) found in the North American firefly, *Photinus pyralis*, is the most commonly used optical reporter gene. The *luc* gene encodes a 550 amino acid protein luciferase that was first purified and characterized in 1978 by Gates et al. (24). The cDNA for firefly luciferase was then cloned in 1987 for use as an optical reporter (25). Since then, the *luc* gene has been modified to enhance expression in mammalian cells and to remove its peroxisome-targeting site to allow cytosolic accumulation of its product.

Firefly luciferase is a 62 kDa protein that catalyzes the oxidation of its molecular substrate in the presence of adenosine triphosphate (ATP) through the following reaction (26).

$$\text{Luciferase} + \text{Luciferin} + \text{ATP} + O_2 \xrightarrow{Mg^{2+}} \text{Luciferase--Luciferin}$$
$$+ \text{AMP} + PP_i \qquad (1)$$
$$\text{Luciferase--Luciferin} + \text{AMP} + O_2 \longrightarrow \text{Oxyluciferin}^*$$
$$+ CO_2 + \text{AMP} \qquad (2)$$
$$\text{Oxyluciferin}^* \longrightarrow \text{Oxyluciferin} + h\nu \qquad (3)$$

In the presence of oxygen, ATP, and Mg^{2+}, the reaction of luciferase enzyme with the substrate luciferin yields an electronically excited oxyluciferin. The return of oxyluciferin to its ground state is accompanied by the release of a single photon (27). Thus, in the presence of excess luciferin the number of photons emitted is proportional to the number of molecules of luciferase present (28).

Firefly luciferase emits a relatively broad spectrum of light (500–700 nm) with a peak wavelength of 563 nm in a reaction that requires a benzothiazolyl luciferin [D-(−)-2-(6′-hydroxy-2′-benzothiazolyl) thiazone-4-carboxylic acid]. Importantly, the peak emission is temperature dependent and is slightly red-shifted (~590 nm) at body temperature of 37°C (29). When using luciferase as a reporter *in vivo*, ATP is abundantly present and does not need to be provided exogenously. The required substrate, D-luciferin, is added exogenously [usually via intraperitoneal (IP) injection in mice] and distributes rapidly (within minutes) throughout the entire animal. Biodistribution of the substrate has been shown to peak by 15–20 min post administration (sooner if administered by tail vein injection) and crosses the blood–brain and placental barriers (3,14,30,31). As luciferase does not need to be optically excited in order to emit light and the light emitted is in the yellow–red part of the spectrum where mammalian tissue is semitransparent, the overall transmission of light is sufficient to enable detection *in vivo* from internal organs in small animals through several centimeters of tissue.

Various alternatives to *luc* have received attention recently. Notably Renilla luciferase (7,31–33) as well as a number of red-shifted mutants of *luc*. Although the use of Renilla luciferase, which emits at 480 nm and requires a different substrate, may have utility in two-color essays, strong absorption of the emission wavelength limits use for *in vivo* imaging. The development and use of red-shifted *luc* mutants is primarily aimed at reducing optical attenuation by tissue. However, given the bandpass filter effect of tissue chromophores (absorption of wavelengths <600 nm), the spectral components of even the native *luc*-mediate luminescence emitted *in vivo* are primarily in the red part of the spectrum (>600 nm) (34).

B. Tissue Optics

The propagation of light through biological tissue is governed by its tissue optical properties and geometry. The movement of photons through a turbid biological media is influenced by scattering and absorption events within the tissue and reflection and transmission events at tissue boundaries. An essential fact is that the tissue's optical properties are a direct function of the wavelength of light used or emitted. These phenomena have been studied in depth and can be mathematically analyzed and modeled (35,36). In the specific case of BLI, photons are generated inside the biological medium and emitted in all directions; however, only those photons that reach the surface of the animal and leave the animal in a direction such that they reach the aperture of the imaging camera contribute to the detected signal. After emission from their point of origin, photons can be absorbed or scattered by tissue components. Molecules that absorb light are known as chromophores; for visible light, (oxy)hemoglobin and melanin are the principle chromophores (Fig. 10.1). Hemoglobin absorbs blue light very strongly and has additional absorption peaks in the green/yellow part of the spectrum (577 nm). Absorption by melanin is strongest in the ultraviolet range and gradually reduces with increasing wavelength but is significant throughout the entire optical spectrum. Obviously, for BLI, the use of white (or albino) animals that lack melanin is preferable from a tissue optics point of view. Generally speaking, as far as tissue penetration by light is concerned, the rule of thumb is "the redder, the better." For methods of optical imaging, the ideal optical window lies in the red/near-infrared (NIR) light spectrum

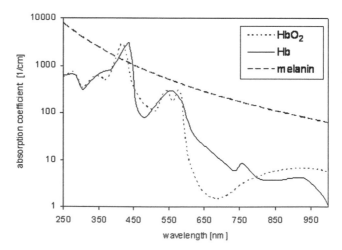

Figure 10.1 Illustration of the absorption coefficient of the main tissue chromophores as a function of wavelength. Shown are the spectra for (1) whole blood based on absorption characteristics of hemoglobin (solid line) and (2) whole blood based on the absorption characteristics of oxyhemoglobin (dotted gray line) and melanin (dashed line). Wavelengths <600 nm are strongly absorbed by blood and all wavelengths are strongly absorbed by melanin.

between 600 and 1350 nm (>1350 nm water, absorption becomes dominant). The net result is that for the spectrum emitted by *luc* (500–700 nm), it is primarily the wavelengths >600 nm that contribute to measured signal outside the animal. The shorter wavelengths are strongly absorbed and simply never penetrate the tissues unless the source is located very near the surface.

The likelihood of a photon being absorbed over some infinitesimal path distance is known as the wavelength dependent absorption coefficient, μ_a (cm^{-1}). The absorption coefficient is in essence a probabilistic term that lumps the molecular absorption coefficient and chromophore concentrations together in one parameter. For light at wavelengths of >600 nm, the absorption mean free path (the mean distance a photon can travel before it is absorbed) is $\sim$2 cm.

Light is not only absorbed but also strongly scattered in biological tissue. Unfortunately, even in the red/NIR window where absorption is minimal, scattering is still significant (scattering mean free path is $\sim$0.5 mm for wavelengths >600 nm). Spatial fluctuations in density and refractive index, n, result in changes in photon path direction. In biological tissue, discrete structures, such as cell membranes, nuclei, collagen bundles, or other cellular microstructure, can cause photon scattering. Elastic scatter simply causes the impinging photon to be redirected in a new path.

Scattering is treated much like absorption, that is, with a probabilistic approach using exponential decay. The scattering coefficient, μ_s, gives the probability of a photon being scattered per infinitesimal distance. Note that although the scattering coefficient provides information about the likelihood of scattering, it does not predict the direction in which the photon will be scattered. For this, an anisotropy factor, g, is introduced, where g is the average cosine of the scattering angle (and hence a number between -1 and 1). Although a detailed discussion of tissue optics is beyond the scope of this chapter [for a thorough review, see Ref. (37)], the combined parameter that describes scattering is known as the reduced scattering coefficient, $\mu'_s = (1 - g)\mu_s$. This reduced scatter coefficient, μ'_s, is combined with the absorption coefficient into the effective attenuation coefficient (μ_{eff}):

$$\mu_{eff} = \sqrt{3\mu_a(\mu_a + \mu'_s)}$$

This can then be used to calculate the effective penetration depth (δ_{eff}):

$$\delta_{eff} = \frac{1}{\mu_{eff}}$$

As scattering strongly affects light propagation in tissues, no simple method is available to estimate signal attenuation or spatial diffusion of light between its point of origin and the surface of a specific organ or tissue. Various solutions to the light transport equation have been developed, but many are computationally intensive (e.g., Monte Carlo simulation, diffusion approximation). Results of a diffusion approximation calculation estimating the signal attenuation and spatial spread as a function of the depth of a point source of light embedded in a tissue with a uniform set of optical properties is shown in Fig. 10.2. Although these results are illustrative, animal tissues do not have uniform optical properties. *In vivo* optical properties are difficult to measure (37) and *in vitro* measurements of optical properties are not necessarily valid for the same tissue *in vivo*. Biochemical and morphological changes accompanying tissue excision, temperature fluctuations, and changes in hydration can all affect the optical properties of

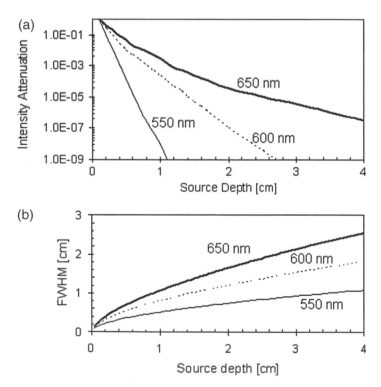

Figure 10.2 Calculated (diffusion approximation) signal attenuation (a) and spatial spread of light (b) as a function of depth of the light emitting point source. The source depth is plotted against intensity attenuation (a) or full width at half maximum (FWHM) (b), which represents the width of the spot at an intensity that is half of the value at its maximum point. Plots are shown for three different wavelengths with accompanying optical properties: 550 nm ($\mu_a = 5.0$ cm^{-1}, $\mu_s' = 20$ cm^{-1}), 600 nm ($\mu_a = 1.0$ cm^{-1}, $\mu_s' = 17$ cm^{-1}), and 650 nm ($\mu_a = 0.25$ cm^{-1}, $\mu_s' = 15$ cm^{-1}). Figure adapted from Ref. (34).

biological tissue (38,39). In addition to effects on sensitivity and resolution of planar imaging, these same issues make tomographic reconstruction of bioluminescence images a formidable task.

An experiment demonstrating the positional effects of a light emitting source on detected photon emission from the chest is shown in Fig. 10.3. A light emitting bead (1 mm diameter) with a spectrum similar to that of luciferase-induced luminescence and a constant emission intensity was implanted in the pleural space of a mouse posterior to the right lung (a), in the pleural space anterior to the right lung (b), or anterior to the rib cage (c). The difference in both light intensity and spatial spread of the light is striking. Measured photon emission, in this study, over the anterior thorax indicates that passage of light through the right lung attenuated signal by five fold. In addition, there was almost a seven fold reduction in signal by the chest wall. This study indicates that bioluminescent signals originating even in the posterior portions of mouse lungs can be detected externally; however, there is substantial attenuation and light scatter by tissue components, including lung parenchyma and chest wall.

C. Imaging System Design and Function

The enabling technology that has led to the breakthrough of optical molecular imaging is the highly sensitive detector (6,34,40,41). State-of-the-art charge couple device (CCD) cameras have seen significant improvements in sensitivity and noise characteristics in recent years. Only a few years ago, intensified CCD (ICCD) cameras were the instruments of choice for the imaging detection of

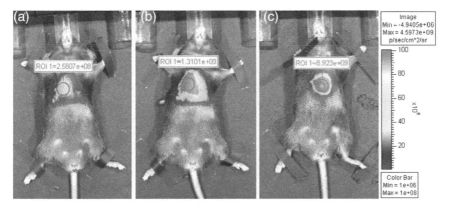

Figure 10.3 **(See color insert)** Bioluminescent imaging of a wild-type mouse after implantation of a light emitting bead (with a spectrum similar to that of firefly luciferase) in the pleural space posterior to the right lung (a), in the pleural space anterior to the right lung (b), or anterior to the rib cage (c). The pseudocolor scale is shown and the region of interest (ROI) for photon detection is indicated by a red circle. Detected photon counts are indicated for each ROI.

weak bioluminescence. These devices had relatively low quantum efficiencies (of ~15%) and did not detect light >600 nm particularly well (recall that this is exactly the light that emanates from the animal). Today back-thinned, back-illuminated, deep-depletion CCD cameras are available. In these devices, quantum wells on a semiconductor chip collect photons and build up charge in response. At the end of the image integration time, the chip is read out to a controller/computer. These instruments reach quantum efficiencies of >90% and are sensitive from 400 to 800 nm. Moreover, the main sources of noise, dark noise (generated by spontaneously generated electrons), and readout noise (generated when reading the signal from the CCD chip to the computer/controller) have been reduced significantly. Dark noise is dramatically decreased (resulting in improved signal/noise) by cooling the chip to below −90°C. Readout noise (random noise added to the signal during the transfer) can be effectively reduced by on-chip binning (a process whereby a block of pixels (e.g., 5×5 or 8 × 8) on the chip is grouped together and is read-out as one "superpixel"). Binning significantly increases the signal/noise of the signal at the expense of spatial resolution; however, because of light scattering in tissue, these larger superpixels are not the limiting factor in spatial resolution.

III. Applications

A. Transcription Factors and the Lungs

Protein transcription factors perform critical functions in biology by interacting with DNA and regulating RNA polymerase-mediated transcription of individual genes. These proteins influence the complement of proteins produced by the cell and, therefore, determine cellular phenotype. Although transcription factors are clearly important in development and homeostasis in the lungs, certain patterns of transcription factor activity in targeted cell populations may define particular disease processes. For example, pathogenesis of the acute respiratory distress syndrome (ARDS) is thought to be related to excessive production of pro-inflammatory molecules by the host in response to infection, trauma, or noxious stimuli (42–44). Production of these mediators is largely determined by new gene transcription and translation as most of the mediators implicated in this syndrome are not preformed and stored in cells in large amounts. Several key transcription factors have been identified that regulate generation of important mediators in ARDS including NF-κB.

The ubiquitous NF-κB transcription factor family plays an important role in innate (nonlymphocyte mediated) immunity in the lungs by regulating lung inflammation through transcriptional regulation of a variety of pro-inflammatory mediators including cytokines, chemokines, adhesion molecules, and enzymes (45). Signal transduction pathways initiated by ligand binding to toll-like receptors, interleukin (IL)-1 receptor, and tumor necrosis factor (TNF) type 1 receptor lead to activation of NF-κB, implicating this transcription factor family as a critical integrator of inflammatory signals. Although innate immune responses are necessary for effective lung host defense, dysfunctional or exaggerated inflammatory responses can lead to lung injury, as in ARDS. As NF-κB appears to be pivotal in determining immune/inflammatory responses in the lungs, we have investigated its role *in vivo* in the complex biological processes of lung inflammation, injury, and bacterial host defense.

B. Detection of NF-κB Activation in Reporter Mice

To quantitatively evaluate NF-κB dependent transcriptional activity over time and examine the consequences of NF-κB activation in multiple organs *in vivo*, we developed a transgenic reporter mouse model that was engineered to possess the following construct in each tissue—proximal 250 bases of the 5′ human immunodeficiency virus (HIV-1) long terminal repeat (LTR) driving the expression of *P. pyralis* luciferase cDNA [referred to as HLL mice (*HIV-LTR*/Luciferase)]. The proximal HIV-LTR is a NF-κB responsive promoter (46–48), containing a TATA box, an enhancer region between −82 and −103 with two NF-κB motifs, and three Sp1 boxes from −46 to −78. In primary cell culture, NF-κB activation is absolutely required for transcriptional activity of the HIV-LTR (49,50).

After generating HLL reporter mice, we validated the measurement of luciferase activity as a surrogate marker for NF-κB activation *in vivo* by comparing luciferase activation in lungs and other organs to NF-κB activation measured by electrophoretic mobility shift assays (EMSA) and production of NF-κB dependent mediators. Treatment of HLL mice with a single IP injection of *Escherichia coli* lipopolysaccharide (LPS) induced luciferase activity (measured in tissue homogenates by chemiluminescent luciferase activity assays) in lung and liver in a dose and time-dependent manner that correlated with NF-κB activation as measured by EMSA (51). As NF-κB dependent reporter gene transcription and translation must occur prior to accumulation of luciferase protein, peak NF-κB activation in lung and liver (as assayed by EMSA) preceded maximal detected luciferase activity. In these studies, lung luciferase activation was only found after LPS doses sufficient to induce neutrophilic lung inflammation. A close correlation was found between lung tissue luciferase activity and tissue concentration of the NF-κB dependent mouse neutrophil chemoattractant chemokine KC (51). In addition, targeting the liver by intravenous (IV) injection of adenoviral vectors expressing a dominant inhibitor of the NF-κB pathway resulted in significant inhibition of LPS-induced luciferase activity in this organ (51).

In addition to HLL mice, transgenic NF-κB reporter mice have been produced by other investigators and utilized to study lung and systemic NF-κB dependent inflammatory responses (13,52,53). We have made second generation NF-κB reporter mice containing a synthetic NF-κB responsive promoter with 8 κB binding sites and a minimal herpesvirus thymidine kinase promoter driving a green fluorescent protein (GFP)/luciferase fusion protein reporter. Studies with these different transgenic NF-κB reporter mouse lines yield similar patterns of luciferase activity in several inflammatory models, supporting the conclusion that luciferase activity in these mice reflects activation of NF-κB in cells and tissues.

An important limitation of previous animal model studies evaluating the role of NF-κB *in vivo* was that measurements of NF-κB activation were made by EMSA or western blots from nuclear protein extracts. EMSA and western blots are semiquantitative, evaluate NF-κB activation at only a single point in time, and do not address the functional effects of NF-κB activation in initiating gene transcription. In HLL mice, tissue luciferase activity measurements overcome some of these limitations by serving as an integrator of NF-κB transcriptional activity over time; however, to maximize the utility of this reporter we employed bioluminescent imaging technology. With this methodology, we can use each animal as its own control by obtaining baseline images prior to treatment. We can also perform multiple measurements after treatment in each mouse because luciferin is relatively nontoxic (17). In developing this technology for use in our transgenic reporter mice, we optimized luciferin dosing, defined the kinetics of a single injection of luciferin, and correlated photon emission with tissue luciferase activity (5,54–57). Following IP injection of D-luciferin in untreated HLL mice, we found that peak photon emission from the thorax occurred at 30–60 min and returned to baseline by 120 min (54). Maximal photon emission from both the head and thorax in these mice occurred after IP injection of 6 mg luciferin; however, the increment in photon emission (LPS-induced photon emission–baseline) was similar after 3 and 6 mg luciferin (57). Recently, the biodistribution of luciferin in mice has been reported. Lee et al. (58) showed that 3.8% of the injected dose could be found in lung tissue 45 min after IP injection. IV injection, however, produced the largest concentration of lung luciferase, 13.2% at 5 min. On the basis of this information and additional studies in our laboratory, we have found that IV injection of 1 mg luciferin followed by imaging at 5 min produces a similar bioluminescence pattern in HLL mice to 3–6 mg of luciferin given by IP injection and imaged at 30 min (unpublished observation).

In several different studies, we have shown an excellent correlation between tissue luciferase activity and bioluminescent detection of luciferase activity in HLL mice (5,54–57). Using models of lung inflammation induced by inhalation of aerosolized *E. coli* LPS or IP injection of *E. coli* LPS, we have shown that basal bioluminescence over the thorax of HLL mice derives primarily from skin and chest wall components, but LPS-inducible bioluminescence is primarily of lung origin. Figure 10.4 shows that untreated reporter mice have relatively high luciferase activity in the skin and chest wall compared with the lungs and heart. Treatment with aerosolized LPS or IP injection of LPS increased lung luciferase activity, but no significant changes in luciferase activity were found in skin, chest wall, or heart (57). In related studies, skin flap excisions were done over the right side of the thorax to examine the effect of skin bioluminescence on measured photon emission over the chest (57). Basal photon emission was substantially lower over the right chest after skin flap excision.

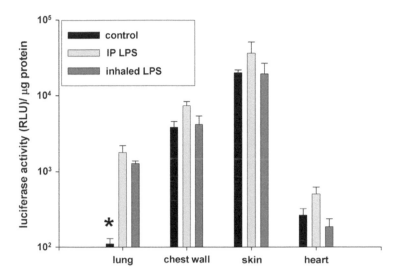

Figure 10.4 Luciferase activity measured as relative light units (RLU) per µg total protein from organs of HLL mice at baseline (control) and after intraperitoneal (IP) or aerosolized (inhaled) LPS. Mean $+/-$ SEM, *P < 0.05 compared with treatment groups. Reprinted with permission from Ref. (57).

Following treatment with LPS, bioluminescence increased 21.9-fold (mean) over the right chest following IP LPS and 15-fold after aerosolized LPS compared with 3.7-fold (IP LPS) and 3.9-fold (aerosolized LPS) increases over the left (intact) side of the chest. These studies demonstrate that basal photon emission over the thorax is due in large part to luciferase activity in the skin and chest wall; however, inducible bioluminescence in these models is predominantly due to increased lung luciferase activity. We have performed similar studies to evaluate the source of detected bioluminescence in the abdomen and head of HLL mice at baseline and after LPS treatment (57).

On the basis of these studies, it is clear that bioluminescence detection of luciferase activity in HLL mice is a powerful methodology for *in vivo* assessment of NF-κB dependent gene expression. There are, however, some limitations to this technique that must be considered. Background bioluminescence from basal luciferase activity can produce an unfavorable signal-to-noise ratio, making it difficult to identify low level induction of NF-κB activation. This issue is much more of a problem for the abdomen and head compared with the chest in HLL mice [Fig. 10.5(b)]. As previously discussed, photon emission from internal organs is detectable, but hemoglobin and other factors present in tissue attenuate the signal by photon absorption (8,59,60). This property implies that bioluminescence images are peripheral (surface) weighted because photons generated closer to the surface are more likely to escape than photons originating deeper in tissues. Lack of spatial resolution is an issue for bioluminescence imaging. Photon emission can be detected at the level of the organ (lung), but more specific localization is difficult at present and three dimensional localization of signals is currently not possible. Another limitation of bioluminescence detection of luciferase activity in transgenic reporter mice that

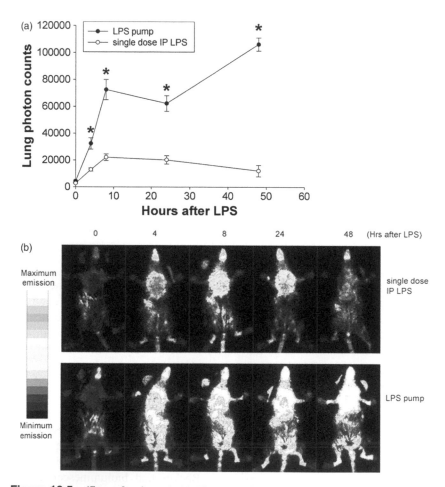

Figure 10.5 **(See color insert)** (a) Photon emission detected from the chest of HLL mice at 0–48 h after a single IP injection of LPS (2 µg/g) or LPS delivered to the peritoneal cavity by osmotic pump (LPS pump). (b) Bioluminescence of a representative HLL mouse treated with a single IP injection of LPS (upper panel) or LPS pump (lower panel). For detection of NF-κB dependent luciferase activity, luciferin (3 mg) was given by IP injection and photon emission was detected 30 min later. The scale for the pseudocolor images, indicative of relative pixel intensity, is shown at left (white is the highest emission). (c) Lung luciferase activity (relative light units, RLU) measured in lung homogenates from HLL mice 24 h after treatment with a single IP injection of LPS or LPS delivered by osmotic pump. Mean +/− SEM, *P < 0.05 compared with single dose IP LPS group.

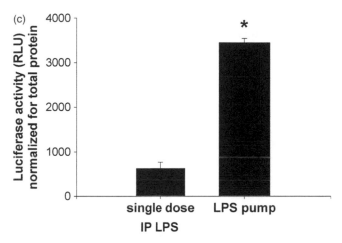

Figure 10.5 *Continued.*

have the ability to ubiquitously express the reporter construct is lack of cellular specificity. In HLL mice, it has been difficult to determine whether increased photon emission from the lungs following stimulation results from increased luciferase expression (on a per cell basis), induction of luciferase expression in a new population of resident cells, or recruitment of activated (inflammatory) cells expressing the reporter. In the future, utilization of multifunctional reporters, such as dual GFP-luciferase, offers opportunities to better address this important issue. For example, expression of GFP (along with luciferase) would allow specific identification of cells expressing the reporter on tissue sections by fluorescence (or confocal) microscopy or by immunohistochemistry. Using this approach, reliable identification of the distribution of cells expressing the transgene(s) would complement quantitative measurements of luciferase activity.

C. NF-κB Activation in Disease Models

By utilizing bioluminescent imaging of luciferase activity as an *in vivo* transcriptional reporter, we have measured timing, distribution, and intensity of NF-κB activation in a variety of disease models including lung inflammation induced by local and systemic stimuli. These models include treatment with Gram-negative bacterial LPS, direct hepatic injury, diet-induced pancreatitis, and *Pseudomonas* infection. In addition, these mice have been used to identify inflammation modulating effects of gene therapy targeted to the lungs.

Lung Inflammation Induced by Bacterial LPS

Gram-negative bacterial LPS is an integral component of the outer membrane of the cell wall, that is, responsible for much of the host inflammatory response to these organisms by interacting with cell surface toll-like receptor 4 (61). LPS-induced inflammatory signaling is an important paradigm for investigating the pathobiology of innate immunity. By utilizing models of LPS-induced inflammation in HLL mice, we have gained insight into the function of the NF-κB pathway in mediating lung inflammation and injury.

To investigate whether differences in NF-κB activation correlate with severity of lung inflammation and injury, we used two models of systemic inflammation induced by LPS. To create a transient lung inflammatory response without substantial lung injury, we injected mice with a single IP injection of *E. coli* LPS (2 μg/g). In contrast, delivering LPS by IP implantation of ALZET osmotic pumps (Alza Corporation, Palo Alto, CA) over 24 h causes a severe lung inflammatory response with neutrophilic influx, hemorrhage, and edema. In these studies, delivery of LPS by osmotic pump resulted in substantial mortality (50%) by 48 h (compared with no mortality in the single dose IP LPS group). Figure 10.5 shows the time course for bioluminescent detection of LPS-induced luciferase activity in HLL mice following single dose IP LPS or IP LPS delivered by osmotic pump. In these studies, mice were imaged for baseline bioluminescence 30 min after IP injection of luciferin (3 mg dissolved in 200 μL sterile phosphate buffered saline). Subsequently, osmotic pumps were loaded with 200 μL of LPS solution (1 mg/mL concentration to deliver 8 μg LPS/h). Both groups of mice ($n = 10$ per group) were imaged at 4, 8, 24, and 48 h following LPS injection, 30 min after repeated doses of IP luciferin (3 mg). Both groups had significantly increased bioluminescence over the chest by 4 h after LPS; however, the group treated with LPS pumps had significantly higher photon emission at every time point measured. In addition, the group treated with a single IP injection of LPS returned to near baseline bioluminescence values by 48 h, whereas the group treated with LPS pumps showed the greatest photon emission at 48 h. Mice treated with IP implantation of osmotic pumps alone (no LPS) showed only mild increases in bioluminescence at early time points (data not shown).

Representative bioluminescence pictures of mice treated with a single IP injection of LPS and LPS delivered by osmotic pump are shown in Fig. 10.5(b). The upper panel shows a mouse treated with single dose IP LPS. Compared with baseline, increased photon emission was identified by 4 h over the head, chest, and right upper quadrant of the abdomen. Photon emission peaked at 8 h and subsequently declined. The mouse treated with LPS delivered by osmotic pump (bottom panel) showed greater photon emission at each time point, with progressive increases in chest and head bioluminescence from 4 to 48 h. Interestingly, photon emission from the abdomen was initially high (at 4 and 8 h), but subsequently decreased (in distinct contrast to the chest and head). In a separate experiment, luciferase activity was measured in lung homogenates 24 h after single dose IP LPS or LPS delivered by osmotic pump [Fig. 10.5(c)]. Consistent with other findings, NF-κB dependent luciferase activity was significantly higher in lungs of mice treated with LPS delivered by osmotic pump compared with single dose IP LPS. These studies suggest that prolonged, high-level NF-κB activation in the lungs leads to protracted inflammation and lung injury (LPS pump), whereas less intense NF-κB activation is associated with mild, transient lung inflammation (single dose IP LPS).

Using another NF-κB luciferase reporter mouse model, Carlsen et al. (52) found that IV injection of LPS, TNFα, or IL-1β stimulated increased luciferase activity in the lungs and other organs as assessed by bioluminescence and tissue luciferase assays. Interestingly, they found that increased bioluminescence could be identified by imaging organs *ex vivo* and that this measurement correlated well with luciferase assays in most organs. We have performed analogous studies after IP or aerosolized LPS with similar findings (57).

BLI can be used to assess responses to anti-inflammatory therapies. In the study by Carlsen et al. (52), mice were pretreated with dexamethasone (4.5 mg/kg) 1 h prior to IV injection of LPS. These investigators found that this treatment suppressed LPS-induced whole mouse bioluminescence (52). In contrast, we pretreated mice with dexamethasone at 0.3, 1, or 10 mg/kg given in divided doses 24 h and 1 h prior to aerosolized LPS (54). We found that the lower doses of dexamethasone did not inhibit bioluminescence from the lungs of HLL mice in our model. In addition, there was no difference in lung neutrophil influx or expression of the chemokine macrophage inflammatory protein-2 (MIP-2). At the highest dose of dexamethasone, there was actually an increase of all of these parameters compared with LPS treatment alone. These findings show that bioluminescent detection of NF-κB activation correlates with important parameters of lung and systemic inflammation.

Lung Inflammation Following Direct Hepatic Injury and Pancreatitis

Injury to distal organs can lead to systemic inflammation and lung inflammation/ injury. Hepatic cryoablation, which is used to treat primary liver malignancies and metastases, has been associated with multiple organ failure and acute lung injury (5,62). In HLL mice, we showed that 35% hepatic cryoablation stimulated increased bioluminescence over the lungs, liver, and kidneys at 4 h after surgery (5). These findings correlated with increased concentrations of the chemokine MIP-2 and neutrophils in lung lavage. In addition, a close correlation was identified between detected bioluminescence and luciferase activity in each organ. These findings confirmed prior studies showing increased NF-κB activation in lung and liver (by EMSA) in a rat model of hepatic cryoablation compared with hepatic resection of similar amounts of tissue (62). In more recent studies, we have shown that IV delivery of adenoviral vectors expressing a dominant inhibitor of the NF-κB pathway blocked cryoablation-induced increases in NF-κB activation and decreased mortality in this model (unpublished data).

In a model of pancreatitis induced by a choline deficient, ethionine supplemented diet, we found that increased bioluminescence could be detected in the upper abdomen of HLL mice, reflecting increased luciferase activity in the liver and pancreas by 48 h after starting the diet (63). This increased bioluminescence in the abdomen was followed by increased luciferase activity in the lungs as determined by bioluminescence and tissue luciferase assays. These studies indicate that HLL reporter mice can be utilized to follow NF-κB activity in multiple organs. As shown in these studies and another recent article (64), NF-κB activation in one organ can signal downstream activation in other organs including the lungs.

Pseudomonas Pneumonia

The paradox of innate immunity is that this process is necessary for host defense against pathogens but is capable of host-derived tissue injury. To investigate the role of the NF-κB pathway in host defense, we established a model of *Pseudomonas aeruginosa* pneumonia in HLL mice. At 24 h after intratracheal administration of bacteria, we found a dose dependent increase in chest bioluminescence (Fig. 10.6) that correlated with tissue luciferase activity and neutrophilic alveolitis (56). We cross-bred HLL mice with mice deficient in the p47phox component of NADPH oxidase to investigate the role of reactive oxygen species in NF-κB activation. In the *Pseudomonas* model, p47phox$-/-$HLL mice showed deficient activation of luciferase as assessed by chest bioluminescence (56). This finding correlated with lower luciferase activity in lung tissue homogenates, decreased nuclear translocation of the RelA component of NF-κB as assessed by western blot, and lower lung TNFα levels. In contrast, *Pseudomonas* clearance was impaired in p47phox$-/-$HLL mice, indicating that suppression of NF-κB activation was not due to a diminished inflammatory stimulus. For these studies, *P. aeruginosa* expressing the lux operon from the bacterium *Photorhabdus luminescens* was obtained from Xenogen (Alemeda, CA). By bioluminescent detection of bacteria (which does not require luciferin injection), significantly more bacteria were present in the lungs of p47phox$-/-$ HLL mice compared with HLL mice at 24 h after administration. This finding was confirmed by colony counts from harvested lungs. From these studies, it is apparent that NADPH oxide derived reactive oxygen species are required for maximal NF-κB activation in this model and may impact host defense in ways other than direct effects on bacterial killing. In addition, these studies show that bioluminescence can be used to follow the host response to bacterial infection in the lungs. Future studies using bioluminescence to track both the bacterial burden and the host response to infection could lead to new insights into the pathogenesis of pneumonia or other infections.

Gene Therapy to Modulate NF-κB Activation

We postulated that epithelial cells play an important role in orchestrating NF-κB dependent inflammatory responses in the lungs. To investigate the NF-κB pathway in lung epithelium, we constructed replication deficient adenoviral vectors expressing NF-κB activators and inhibitors, including constitutively

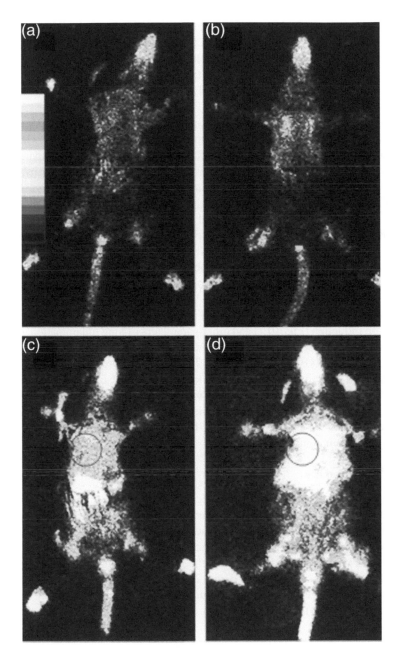

Figure 10.6 **(See color insert)** Bioluminescent images of HLL mice are shown at baseline (a) or 24 h after intratracheal injection of *Pseudomonas aeruginosa* at 10^5 (b), 10^6 (c), or 10^7 (d) colony forming units. The circle represents the region of interest used for quantization of photon emission. Reprinted with permission from Ref. (56).

active human IkappaB kinase 1 (cIKK1) and a trans-dominant inhibitor of NF-κB (IκBα-DN). In HLL mice, we intratracheally injected these adenoviral vectors alone or in combination to achieve selective, specific activation of NF-κB in lung epithelium (55). First, we titrated the dose of control adenoviral vectors to achieve transgene expression exclusively in lung epithelium without significant adenovirus associated inflammation at 72 and 96 h. We then administered this titer of adenoviral vectors expressing an activator of NF-κB (cIKK1) to HLL mice (Fig. 10.7). In these studies, we detected significantly increased NF-κB dependent luciferase activity in the lungs of Ad-cIKK1 treated mice compared with control mice treated with Ad-β-galactosidase (Ad-β-gal). Nuclear translocation of NF-κB in the lungs of Ad-cIKK1 treated mice was confirmed by immunoblots for RelA and EMSA from lung nuclear protein extracts. In addition to NF-κB activation, mice treated with intratracheal administration of Ad-cIKK1 showed: (1) induction of mRNA expression of several chemokines and cytokines in lung tissue, (2) elevated concentrations of NF-κB dependent chemokines MIP-2 and KC in lung lavage, (3) increased numbers of neutrophils in lung lavage, and (4) intra-alveolar accumulation of inflammatory cells, predominantly neutrophils, and mild alveolar septal thickening on lung sections (55). Co-administration of adenoviral vectors expressing IκB-αDN and Ad-cIKK1 resulted in abrogation of luciferase induction (Fig. 10.7) and other parameters of lung inflammation, demonstrating that the observed inflammatory effects of Ad-cIKK1 were dependent on activation of NF-κB by this kinase. These studies provide proof-of-concept evidence that selective activation of NF-κB in the absence of additional inflammatory stimuli induces lung inflammation *in vivo* that epithelial cells can produce a range of NF-κB linked cytokines that impact lung inflammation, and that BLI can be used to assess the impact of lung targeted gene therapy on NF-κB induced inflammation.

D. Summary

Studies using BLI in NF-κB reporter mice have added substantial insight into the regulation of lung inflammation, injury, and bacterial host defense by this transcription factor complex. These studies illustrate the utility of this imaging methodology in the lungs. As illustrated by these studies, bioluminescence offers several important advantages in the lungs including: (1) reduction of biological variation in the acquired data, (2) evaluation of biological effect within the context of the living animal, (3) reduction in the numbers of animals required for studies, and (4) high quality data with increased efficiency of time and resources.

IV. Challenges and Future Directions

The use of optically active reporter genes has been used successfully in a variety of applications to obtain quantitative information regarding biological processes.

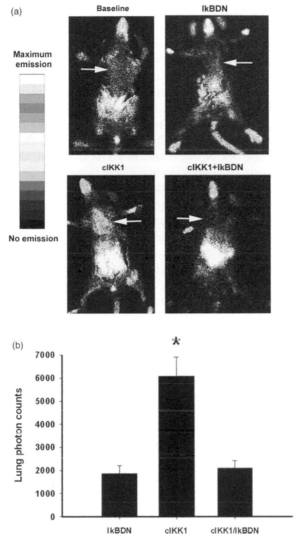

Figure 10.7 (**See color insert**) (a) Representative bioluminescent images from HLL mice prior to treatment (baseline) and 72 h after intratracheal treatment with adenoviral vectors expressing IκB-αDN, cIKK1, or cIKK1 + IκB-αDN. Photon emission from the area of the thorax overlying the lungs is identified by arrows and quantified (b). Mean $+/-$ SEM, $^{*}P < 0.05$ compared with other groups. Reprinted with permission from Ref. (55).

For the specific use of measuring transcriptional activity, the method provides several unique advantages; however, several issues must be treated with great care and simple quantification of light emission may not always provide a true representation of the biological effect studied. First, as luciferase expression is driven by a gene promoter of interest it can only be a surrogate marker for the activity of individual transcription factors. Second, the luciferase reaction is a complex interaction of a variety of molecules. As long as the enzyme (luciferase) is the rate limiting step, light emission can reasonably be expected to report on luciferase activity and thus on the transcriptional activity of the promoter used. If ATP, oxygen, or luciferin (substrate) is not abundantly present and become rate-limiting, light emission may not be a true representation of transcriptional activity. An additional complication is that light transmission from the point of origination to the surface of the animal is a function of both tissue geometry and the optical properties of the tissue. In some situations, dynamic changes may occur in geometry (e.g., growing tumor, scar tissue) and/or the optical properties (e.g., increase in perfusion due to inflammatory response causing a transient increase in the hemoglobin content of the tissue) that affect light emission. Collectively, although BLI is a unique and enabling molecular imaging method, quantitative analysis must be approached with care and validation for each specific application is necessary.

In recent years, technological advancements have enabled a range of molecular imaging methods. Modalities for human use as well as many modalities that are applicable to animal (mouse) models of human disease are now commonplace. Although vastly different in fundamental physical underpinnings, the overall goal of these methods is remarkably similar: the ability to image both structure and function in noninvasive fashion with exquisite sensitivity. Methods such as (functional) magnetic resonance imaging (MRI), (micro) positron emission tomography (PET), single photon emission computed tomography (SPECT), (micro) computed tomography (CT), and a variety of optical technologies have opened up many new possibilities of studying biological processes in live animals and humans in ways previously not possible. Clearly, each of these modalities has its own sets of advantages and disadvantages and no single modality can provide all the answers. For example, MRI and CT provide superior structural information but both are limited in elucidating function and neither is particularly sensitive. On the other hand, optical methods can provide superb sensitivity but suffers from limited probing depth or poor spatial resolution. However, compared with more traditional imaging modalities such as MRI or CT, BLI offers several advantages: (1) imaging systems are lower cost, (2) imaging time is shorter (typically <5 min), (3) systems can be operated by nonexperts, (4) multiple animals can be imaged simultaneously, and (5) sensitivity is orders of magnitude higher. For example, Lipshutz et al. (30) reported detection limits of as little as 35 pg luciferase/g tissue, similar to *ex vivo* luciferase and more sensitive than western blot.

Several challenges face the future development of BLI. First, the utility of BLI will be greatly enhanced if the spatial resolution of this method can be improved. Several approaches are currently being developed. Coquez et al. (65) reported an approach to use spectral information of light emission to estimate the depth of the luminescence source. Various investigators are working on approaches to use imaging from multiple angles to perform a tomographic reconstruction. The latter is a particularly challenging problem as neither the source location nor the transfer function is known (and the transfer function is spatially varying owing to the nonuniformity in distribution of optical properties) leaving one with a classic underdetermined problem that may not have a unique solution. The likelihood that constraining information from other imaging modalities (structure from MRI or CT) must be used to solve this problem is high. Rather than trying to reconstruct spatial distribution, another approach is to attempt to reduce the scattering properties of tissue. For example, by using hyperosmotic agents skin can be transiently rendered transparent allowing imaging with better spatial resolution (66,67). Other challenges include further development of luciferase mutants that will emit further into the infrared part of the spectrum and methodologies for labeling of multiple reporters with spectrally resolvable light emitting probes such that multiple processes can be imaged simultaneously.

Although BLI is a powerful imaging modality, it will never provide structural resolution equivalent to other modalities. Hence, the most exciting future developments will probably originate in multimodality imaging approaches where the strength of various imaging modalities can be combined.

References

1. Benaron DA, Contag PR, Contag CH. Imaging brain structure and function, infection and gene expression in the body using light. Philos Trans R Soc Lond B Biol Sci 1997; 352(1354):755–761.
2. Sadikot RT, Jansen ED, Blackwell TR, Zoia O, Yull F, Christman JW, Blackwell TS. High-dose dexamethasone accentuates nuclear factor-kappa B activation in endotoxin-treated mice. Am J Resp Crit Care Med 2001; 164(5):873–878.
3. Contag CH, Spilman SD, Contag PR, Oshiro M, Eames B, Dennery P, Stevenson DK, Benaron DA. Visualizing gene expression in living mammals using a bioluminescent reporter. Photochem Photobiol 997; 66(4):523–531.
4. Contag CH, Jenkins D, Contag FR, Negrin RS. Use of reporter genes for optical measurements of neoplastic disease in vivo. Neoplasia 2000; 2(1–2):41–52.
5. Sadikot RT, Wudel LJ, Jansen DE, Debelak JP, Yull FE, Christman JW, Blackwell TS, Chapman WC. Hepatic cryoablation-induced multisystem injury: bioluminescent detection of NF-kappa B activation in a transgenic mouse model. J Gastrointest Surg 2002; 6(2):264–270.
6. Contag CH, Bachmann MH. Advances *in vivo* bioluminescence imaging of gene expression. Ann Rev Biomed Eng 2002; 4:235–260.
7. Ray P, De A, Min JJ, Tsien RY, Gambhir SS. Imaging tri-fusion multimodality reporter gene expression in living subjects. Cancer Res 2004; 64(4):1323–1330.
8. Contag CH, Contag PR, Mullins JI, Spilman SD, Stevenson DK, Benaron DA. Photonic detection of bacterial pathogens in living hosts. Mol Microbiol 1995; 18(4):593–603.

9. Siragusa GR, Nawotka K, Spilman SD, Contag PR, Contag CH. Real-time monitoring of *Escherichia coli* O157:H7 adherence to beef carcass surface tissues with a bioluminescent reporter. Appl Environ Microbiol 1999; 65(4):1738–1745.

10. Rocchetta HL, Boylan CJ, Foley JW, Iversen PW, Letourneau DL, McMillian CL, Contag PR, Jenkins DE, Parr TR Jr. Validation of a noninvasive, real-time imaging technology using bioluminescent *Escherichia coli* in the neutropenic mouse thigh model of infection. Antimicrob Agents Chemother 2001; 45(1):129–137.

11. Francis KP, Joh D, Bellinger-Kawahara C, Hawkinson MJ, Purchio TF, Contag PR. Monitoring bioluminescent *Staphylococcus aureus* infections in living mice using a novel luxABCDE construct. Infect Immun 2000; 68(6):3594–3600.

12. Francis KP, Yu J, Bellinger-Kawahara C, Joh D, Hawkinson MJ, Xiao G, Purchio TF, Caparon MG, Lipsitch M, Contag PR. Visualizing pneumococcal infections in the lungs of live mice using bioluminescent *Streptococcus pneumoniae* transformed with a novel Gram-positive lux transposon. Infect Immun 2001; 69(5):3350–3358.

13. Contag PR, Olomu IN, Stevenson DK, Contag CH. Bioluminescent indicators in living mammals. Nat Med 1998; 4(2):245–247.

14. Rehemtulla A, Stegman LD, Cardozo SJ, Gupta S, Hall DE, Contag CH, Ross BD. Rapid and quantitative assessment of cancer treatment response using *in vivo* bioluminescence imaging. Neoplasia 2000; 2(6):491–495.

15. Edinger M, Sweeney TJ, Tucker AA, Olomu AB, Negrin RS, Contag CH. Noninvasive assessment of tumor cell proliferation in animal models. Neoplasia 1999; 1(4):303–310.

16. Edinger M, Cao YA, Hornig YS, Jenkins DE, Verneris MR, Bachmann MH, Negrin RS, Contag CH. Advancing animal models of neoplasia through *in vivo* bioluminescence imaging. Eur J Cancer 2002; 38(16):2128–2136.

17. Sweeney TJ, Mailander V, Tucker AA, Olomu AB, Zhang WS, Cao YA, Negrin RS, Contrag CH. Visualizing the kinetics of tumor-cell clearance in living animals. Proc Natl Acad Sci USA 1999; 96(21):12044–12049.

18. Vooijs M, Jonkers J, Lyons S, Berns A. Noninvasive imaging of spontaneous retinoblastoma pathway-dependent tumors in mice. Cancer Res 2002; 62(6):1862–1867.

19. Wetterwald A, van der Pluijm G, Que I, Sijmons B, Buijs J, Karperien M, Lowik CW, Gautschi E, Thalmann GN, Cecchini MG. Optical imaging of cancer metastasis to bone marrow: a mouse model of minimal residual disease. Am J Pathol 2002; 160(3):1143–1153.

20. Koransky ML, Ip TK, Wu S, Cao Y, Berry G, Contag C, Blau H, Robbins R. *In vivo* monitoring of myoblast transplantation into rat myocardium. J Heart Lung Transplant 2001; 20(2):188–189.

21. Tang Y, Shah K, Messerli SM, Snyder E, Breakefield X, Weissleder R. *In vivo* tracking of neural progenitor cell migration to glioblastomas. Hum Gene Ther 2003; 14(13):1247–1254.

22. Greer LF, Szalay AA. Imaging of light emission from the expression of luciferases in living cells and organisms: a review. Luminescence 2002; 17(1):43–74.

23. Hastings JW. Chemistries and colors of bioluminescent reactions: a review. Gene 1996; 173(1):5–11.

24. Gates BJ, Deluca M. Production of oxyluciferin during firefly luciferase light reaction. Arch Biochem Biophys 1975; 169(2):616–621.

25. de Wet JR, Wood KV, Deluca M, Helinski DR, Subramani S. Firefly luciferase gene: structure and expression in mammalian cells. Mol Cell Biol 1987; 7(2):725–737.

26. Gould SJ, Subramani S. Firefly luciferase as a tool in molecular and cell biology. Anal Biochem 1988; 175(1):5–13.

27. Nguyen VT, Morange M, Bensaude O. Firefly luciferase luminescence assays using scintillation counters for quantitation in transfected mammalian cells. Anal Biochem 1988; 171(2):404–408.

28. Brasier AR, Tate JE, Habener JF. Optimized use of the firefly luciferase assay as a reporter gene in mammalian cell lines. Biotechniques 1989; 7(10):1116–1122.

29. Rice BW. personal communication. 2004.

30. Lipshutz GS, Gruber CA, Cao YA, Hardy J, Contag CH, Gaensler KM. *In utero* delivery of adeno-associated viral vectors: intraperitoneal gene transfer produces long-term expression. Mol Ther 2001; 3(3):284–292.

31. Lorenz WW, Cormier MJ, Okane DJ, Hua D, Escher AA, Szalay AA. Expression of the *Renilla reniformis* luciferase gene in mammalian cells. J Biolumin Chemilumin 1996; 11(1):31–37.

32. Bhaumik S, Gambhir SS. Optical imaging of *Renilla* luciferase reporter gene expression in living mice. Proc Natl Acad Sci USA 2002; 99(1):377–382.

33. Ray P, Wu AM, Gambhir SS. Optical bioluminescence and positron emission tomography imaging of a novel fusion reporter gene in tumor xenografts of living mice. Cancer Res 2003; 63(6):1160–1165.

34. Rice BW, Cable MD, Nelson MB. In vivo imaging of light-emitting probes. J Biomed Opt 2001; 6(4):432–440.

35. Cheong WF, Prahl SA, Welch AJ. A review of the optical-properties of biological tissues. IEEE J Quantum Elect 1990; 26(12):2166–2185.

36. http://omlc.ogi.edu/spectra/hemoglobin/.

37. Welch AJ, Van Genert MJC. Optical–thermal Response of laser-irradiated tissue. In: Kogelnik H, ed. Lasers, Photonics, and Electro-Optics. New York: Plenum Press, 1995.

38. Zhu D, Luo Q, Cen J. Effects of dehydration on the optical properties of *in vitro* porcine liver. Lasers Surg Med 2003; 33(4):226–231.

39. Kitamoto Y, Tokunaga H, Tomita K. Vascular endothelial growth factor is an essential molecule for mouse kidney development: glomerulogenesis and nephrogenesis. J Clin Invest 1997; 99(10):2351–2357.

40. Oshiro M. Cooled CCD versus intensified cameras for low-light video—applications and relative advantages. Methods Cell Biol 1998; 56:45–62.

41. http://www.princetoninstruments.com/library.shtml.

42. Ware LB, Matthay MA. The acute respiratory distress syndrome. N Engl J Med 2000; 342(18):1334–1349.

43. Bhatia M, Moochhala S. Role of inflammatory mediators in the pathophysiology of acute respiratory distress syndrome. J Pathol 2004; 202(2):145–156.

44. Fan J, Ye RD, Malik AB. Transcriptional mechanisms of acute lung injury. Am J Physiol Lung Cell Mol Physiol 2001; 281(5):L1037–L1050.

45. Blackwell TS, Christman JW. The role of nuclear factor-kappa B in cytokine gene regulation. Am J Respir Cell Mol Biol 1997; 17(1):3–9.

46. Nabel G, Baltimore D. An inducible transcription factor activates expression of human immunodeficiency virus in T cells. Nature 1987; 326(6114):711–713.

47. Kretzschmar M, Meisterernst M, Scheidereit C, Li G, Roeder RG. Transcriptional regulation of the HIV-1 promoter by Nf-kappa B *in vitro*. Genes Dev 1992; 6(5):761–774.

48. Kingsman SM, Kingsman AJ. The regulation of human immunodeficiency virus type-1 gene expression. Eur J Biochem 1996; 240(3):491–507.

49. Moses AV, Ibanez C, Gaynor R, Ghazal P, Nelson JA. Differential role of long terminal repeat control elements for the regulation of basal and Tat-mediated transcription of the human immunodeficiency virus in stimulated and unstimulated primary human macrophages. J Virol 1994; 68(1):298–307.

50. Alcami J, de Lera T, Folgueira L, Pedraza MA, Jacque JM, Bachelerie F, Noriega AR, Hay RT, Harrich D, Gaynor RB et al. Absolute dependence on kappa B responsive elements for initiation and Tat-mediated amplification of HIV transcription in blood CD4 T lymphocytes. EMBO J 1995; 14(7):1552–1560.

51. Blackwell TS, Yull FE, Chen CL, Venkatakrishnan A, Blackwell TR, Hicks DJ, Lancaster LH, Christman JW, Kerr LD. Multiorgan nuclear factor kappa B activation in a transgenic mouse model of systemic inflammation. Am J Respir Crit Care Med 2000; 162(3):1095–1101.

52. Carlsen H, Moskaug JO, Fromm SH, Blomhoff R. *In vivo* imaging of NF-kappa B activity. J Immunol 2002; 168(3):1441–1446.

53. Hubbard AK, Timblin CR, Shukla A, Rincon M, Mossman BT. Activation of NF-kappa B-dependent gene expression by silica in lungs of luciferase reporter mice. Am J Physiol Lung Cell Mol Physiol 2002; 282(5):L968–L975.

54. Sadikot RT, Jansen ED, Blackwell TR, Zoia O, Yull F, Christman JW, Blackwell TS. High-dose dexamethasone accentuates nuclear factor-kappa B activation in endotoxin-treated mice. Am J Respir Crit Care Med 2001; 164(5):873–878.

55. Sadikot RT, Han W, Everhart MB, Zoia O, Peebles RS, Jansen ED, Yull FE, Christman JW, Blackwell TS. Selective I kappa B kinase expression in airway epithelium generates neutrophilic lung inflammation. J Immunol 2003; 170(2):1091–1098.

56. Sadikot RT, Zeng H, Yull FE, Li B, Cheng DS, Kernodle DS, Jansen ED, Contag CH, Segal BH, Holland SM, Blackwell TS, Christman JW. p47(phox) deficiency impairs NF-kappa B activation and host defense in *Pseudomonas* pneumonia. J Immunol 2004; 172(3):1801–1808.

57. Yull FE, Han W, Jansen ED, Everhart MB, Sadikot RT, Christman JW, Blackwell TS. Bioluminescent detection of endotoxin effects on HIV-1 LTR-driven transcription *in vivo*. J Histochem Cytochem 2003; 51(6):741–749.

58. Lee KH, Byun SS, Paik JY, Lee SY, Song SH, Choe YS, Kim BT. Cell uptake and tissue distribution of radioiodine labelled D-luciferin: implications for luciferase based gene imaging. Nucl Med Commun 2003; 24(9):1003–1009.

59. Colin M, Moritz S, Schneider H, Capeau J, Coutelle C, Brahimi-Horn MC. Haemoglobin interferes with the *ex vivo* luciferase luminescence assay: consequence for detection of luciferase reporter gene expression *in vivo*. Gene Ther 2000; 7(15):1333–1336.

60. Weissleder R. A clearer vision for *in vivo* imaging. Nat Biotechnol 2001; 19(4):316–317.

61. Beutler B, Rietschel ET. Innate immune sensing and its roots: the story of endotoxin. Nat Rev Immunol 2003; 3(2):169–176.

62. Blackwell TS, Debelak JP, Venkatakrishnan A, Schot DJ, Harley DH, Pinson CW, Williams P, Washington K, Christman JW, Chapman WC. Acute lung injury after hepatic cryoablation: correlation with NF-kappa B activation and cytokine production. Surgery 1999; 126(3):518–526.

63. Gray KD, Simovic MO, Chapman WC, Blackwell TS, Christman JW, Washington MK, Yull FE, Jaffal N, Jansen ED, Gautman S, Stain SC. Systemic NF-kappa B activation in a transgenic mouse model of acute pancreatitis. J Surg Res 2003; 110(1):310–314.

64. Chen LW, Egan L, Li ZW, Greten FR, Kagnoff MF, Karin M. The two faces of IKK and NF-kappa B inhibition: prevention of systemic inflammation but increased local injury following intestinal ischemia–reperfusion. Nat Med 2003; 9(5):575–581.

65. Coquez O, Troy TL, Rice BW. Quantification and depth localization of *in vivo* bioluminescent signals in small animals using spectral imaging techniques. Soc Mol Imaging, Annual Meeting, San Francisco, CA, 2003 (Abstract 174).

66. Pickett PM, Izfar S, MacKanos MA, Virostko J, Jansen ED. Use of hyperosmotic agent to increase spatial resolution of optical imaging of photoactive reporter genes. Laser Surg Med Unpublished data.

67. Vargas G, Chan KF, Thomsen SL, Welch AJ. Use of osmotically active agents to alter optical properties of tissue: effects on the detected fluorescence signal measured through skin. Lasers Surg Med 2001; 29(3):213–220.

11

Molecular Imaging of Lung Cancer

PHILIPP MAYER-KUCKUK, MICHAEL DOUBROVIN, INNA SERGANOVA, and RONALD G. BLASBERG

Memorial Sloan-Kettering Cancer Center,
New York, New York, USA

Medical imaging has undergone a remarkable revolution and expansion in the past two decades. This is largely due to improved imaging technology involving all the major imaging modalities: magnetic resonance (MR), computed tomography (CT), positron emission tomography (PET), ultrasound and optical imaging. These advances and improvements in technology are being rapidly translated into the clinic and have established new standards of medical practice. For example, "Cancer imaging" was identified as one of six "extraordinary scientific opportunities" by the National Cancer Institute (NCI) in 1997–1998, and subsequent funding initiatives from NCI have provided a major stimulus for further developments. A major component of this imaging initiative included the development and support for molecular imaging.

Molecular imaging provides visualization in space and time of normal as well as abnormal cellular processes at a molecular-genetic or cellular level. Molecular imaging has its roots in molecular biology and cell biology as well as in imaging technology and chemistry. Three different noninvasive, *in vivo* imaging technologies have developed more or less in parallel: (i) MR imaging (1), (ii) nuclear imaging [quantitative autoradiography (QAR), gamma camera, and PET] (2), (iii) optical imaging of small animals (3,4), as well as 2-photon fluorescent imaging of viable cells, small organisms, and embryos (5). It is the convergence of the imaging and molecular/cell biology disciplines that is at the heart of this success story and is the wellspring for further advances in this new field. The development of versatile and sensitive noninvasive assays that do not require tissue samples will be of considerable value for monitoring molecular-genetic and cellular processes in animal models of human disease, as well as for studies in human subjects in the future. Imaging molecular-genetic and cellular processes will compliment established molecular-biological assays that are invasive and require tissue sampling, and imaging can provide a spatial as well as temporal dimension to our understanding of various diseases.

I. Molecular Imaging Strategies

Before discussing specific issues related to imaging oncogenesis and lung cancer, it would be helpful to briefly outline three previously described and currently used molecular imaging strategies to noninvasively monitor and measure molecular events. They have been broadly defined as "direct," "indirect," and "biomarker" imaging. These strategies have been discussed previously in several recent reviews (6–13) and in other perspectives on molecular imaging (14–20).

A. Direct Imaging

Direct imaging strategies are usually described in terms of a specific target and a target-specific probe. This strategy has been established using nuclear, optical, and MR imaging technology. The resultant image of probe localization and concentration (signal intensity) is directly related to its interaction with the target. Imaging cell surface-specific antigens with radiolabeled antibodies and genetically engineered antibody fragments, such as minibodies, are examples of direct molecular imaging that has evolved over the past 30 years. In addition, *in vivo* imaging of receptor density/occupancy using small radiolabeled ligands has also been widely used, particularly in neuroscience research, over the past two decades. These examples represent some of the first molecular imaging applications used in clinical nuclear medicine research. More recent research has focused on chemistry and the synthesis of small radiolabeled or fluorescent molecules that target specific receptors (e.g., the estrogen or androgen receptors) (21,22) and florescent probes that are activated by endogenous proteases (23). For example, the alpha(v)beta3 integrin is highly expressed on tumor vasculature and plays an important role in metastasis and tumor-induced angiogenesis; initial studies of targeting and imaging of the alpha(v)beta3 integrin with radio-labeled glycosylated Arg-Gly-Asp (RGD)-containing peptides are very encouraging (Fig. 11.1) (24). Another example is direct imaging of the cell surface receptor-tyrosine kinase HER2. Imaging was used to sequentially monitor the pharmacodynamics of HER2 degradation in response to treatment with an HER2-chaperone protein (HSP90) inhibitor [17-allylamino-17-demethoxy-geldanamycin (17-AAG)] (25). This study demonstrates that a highly specific, small F(ab')$_2$ antibody fragment can be radiolabeled with a short-lived nuclide and used for repetitive noninvasive imaging of HER2 degradation and recovery (Fig. 11.2).

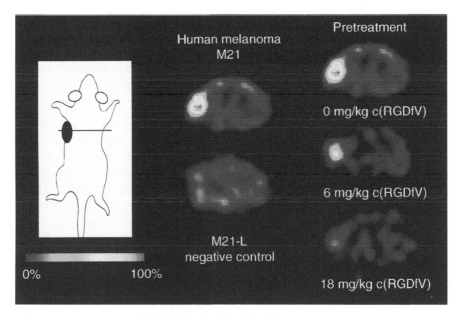

Figure 11.1 (**See color insert**) Noninvasive imaging of $\alpha v \beta 3$ expression. Transaxial PET images of nude mice bearing human melanoma xenografts. Images were acquired 90 min after injection of $\sim$5.5 MBq of [^{18}F]Galacto-RGD. (Top left image) Selective accumulation of the tracer in the $\alpha v \beta 3$-positve (M21) tumor on the left flank. No focal tracer accumulation is visible in the $\alpha v \beta 3$-negative (*M21-L*) control tumor (bottom left image). The three images on the right were obtained from serial [^{18}F]Galacto-RGD PET studies in one mouse. These images illustrate the dose-dependent blockade of tracer uptake by the $\alpha v \beta 3$-selective cyclic pentapeptide cyclo ($-$Arg$-$Gly$-$Asp$-$D$-$he$-$Val$-$). [Figure adapted from Haubner et al. (24)]

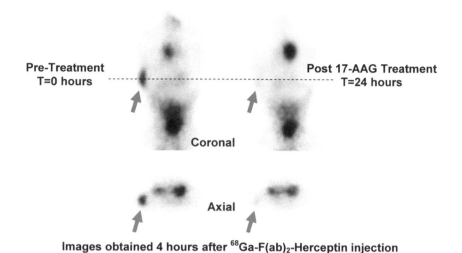

Pre-Treatment
T=0 hours

Post 17-AAG Treatment
T=24 hours

Coronal

Axial

Images obtained 4 hours after ^{68}Ga-F(ab)$_2$-Herceptin injection

Figure 11.2 Noninvasive imaging of HER2 expression. Coronal and transaxial micro-PET images of [^{68}Ga]-F(ab)$_2$-Herceptin in a nude mouse bearing single BT 474 xenograft. Both image sets were acquired 3 h after i.v. injection of ~5 MBq of [^{68}Ga]-F(ab)$_2$-Herceptin. The pretreatment images are shown on the left; the post-treatment images are shown on the right. Treatment involved 17-AAG administered 3 × 50 mg/kg, followed by imaging 24 h later. [Figure adapted from Smith-Jones et al. (25)]

Other direct imaging strategies involve the development of labeled antisense and aptomer oligonucleotide probes [respirable antisense oligonucleotides (RASONs)] that specifically hybridize to target mRNA. Some efficacy for gamma camera and PET imaging of endogenous gene expression using RASONs has been reported (26–29). Nevertheless, RASON imaging has several serious limitations including (i) low number of target mRNA/DNA molecules per cell, (ii) limited tracer delivery (poor cell membrane, vascular, and blood-brain barrier permeability), (iii) poor stability, (iv) slow clearance of nonbound oligonucleotides), (v) comparatively high background activity and low specificity of localization (low target/background ratios).

A further constraint limiting direct imaging strategies is the necessity to develop a specific probe for each molecular target, and then to validate the sensitivity, specificity, and safety of each probe for specific applications. This can be very time consuming and costly. For example, the development, validation, and regulatory approval for [fluorine18]-fluorodeoxyglucose ([^{18}F]-FDG) PET imaging of glucose utilization in tumors has taken over 20 years.

B. Indirect Imaging

Indirect imaging strategies are a little more complex. One example of indirect imaging that is now being widely used is reporter gene imaging. It requires "pre-targeting" (delivery) of the reporter gene to the target tissue (by transfection/transduction), and it usually includes transcriptional control components that can function as "molecular-genetic sensors" and initiate reporter gene expression. This strategy has been widely applied in optical- (30–32) and radionuclide-based imaging (33–37), and to a lesser degree for MR (38,39) imaging. Early reporter gene imaging approaches required postmortem tissue sampling and processing (e.g., beta-galactosidase assay), but more recent studies have emphasized noninvasive imaging techniques involving live animals and human subjects (40).

A general paradigm for noninvasive reporter gene imaging using radiolabeled probes was initially described in 1995 (32) and is diagrammatically shown in Fig. 11.3. A simplified description and cartoon of a reporter gene is shown in Fig. 11.3(a), and a representation of different reporter genes for imaging transduced cells is shown in Fig. 11.3(b). This paradigm requires the appropriate combination of a reporter/marker transgene and a reporter/marker probe. The reporter transgene usually encodes for an enzyme, receptor, or transporter that selectively interacts with the radiolabeled probe and results in its accumulation in the transduced cell. It may be helpful to consider this reporter imaging paradigm as an example of an *in vivo* radiotracer assay that reflects reporter gene expression. Enzymatic amplification of the signal (e.g., level of radioactivity) facilitates imaging the location and magnitude of reporter gene expression. Viewed from this perspective, reporter gene imaging is similar to imaging hexokinase activity with FDG. It is important to note that imaging transgene expression is largely independent of the vector used to shuttle the reporter gene into the cells of the target tissue; that is, any of several currently available vectors can be used (e.g., retrovirus, adenovirus, adeno-associated virus, lentivirus, liposomes, etc.). The reporter transgene can encode for an enzyme [e.g., *HSV1-tk* (32) or *luciferase* (41)], a receptor [e.g., *hD2R* (42) or *hSSTR2* (43)], or a transporter [e.g., *hNIS* (44)], or it can encode for a fluorescent protein [e.g., *eGFP* (45)] [Fig. 11.3(b)].

A common feature of all reporter constructs (and their vectors) is the cDNA expression cassette containing the reporter transgene(s) of interest (e.g., HSV1-tk) which can be placed under the control of specific promoter–enhancer elements. The up-stream promoter–enhancer elements can be used to regulate transcription of the reporter cDNA. The versatility of reporter constructs (and their vectors) is due in part to their modular design, as arrangements in the expression cassette can be varied to some extent. For example, reporter genes can be "always turned on" by constitutive promoters [such as long terminal repeat (LTR), Rous sarcoma virus (RSV), cytomegalovirus (CMV), phosphoglycerate kinase (PGK), elongation factor 1 (EF1), etc.] and used to monitor cell trafficking by identifying the location, migration, targeting, and proliferation of stably transduced cells or vectors. Reporter gene labeling provides the opportunity for repetitive imaging and sequential monitoring of tumor growth rate and response to treatment (32), as well as imaging metastases (45). Alternatively,

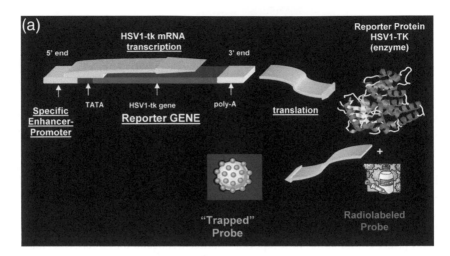

Figure 11.3 HSV1-*tk* reporter construct and the indirect reporter imaging paradigm (a). The basic structure of a reporter gene complex is shown, in this case Herpes simplex virus type 1 thymidine kinase (HSV1-*tk*). The control and regulation of gene expression is performed through promoter and enhancer regions that are located at the 5′ end ("up-stream") of the reporter gene. These promoter/enhancer elements can be "constitutive" and result in continuous gene expression ("always on"), or they can be "inducible" and sensitive to activation by endogenous transcription factors and promoters. Following the initiation of transcription and translation, the gene product—a protein—accumulates. In this case the reporter gene product is an enzyme (HSV1-TK). HSV1-TK will phosphorylate selected thymidine analogs (e.g., FIAU or FHBG), whereas these probes are not phosphorylated by endogenous mammalian TK1. The phosphorylated probe does not cross the cell membrane readily; it is "trapped" and accumulates within transduced cells. Thus, the magnitude of probe accumulation in the cell (level of radioactivity) reflects the level of HSV1-TK enzyme activity and level of HSV1-*tk* gene expression. Different reporter systems (b). The reporter gene complex is transfected into target cells by a vector. Inside the transfected cell, the reporter gene may or may not be integrated into the host-cell genome; transcription of the reporter gene to mRNA is initiated by "constitutive" or "inducible" promoters, and translation of the mRNA to a protein occurs in the ribosomes. The reporter gene product can be a cytoplasmic or nuclear enzyme, a transporter in the cell membrane, a receptor at the cell surface or part of cytoplasmic or nuclear complex, an artificial cell surface antigen, or a fluorescent protein. Often, a complimentary reporter probe (e.g., a radiolabeled, magnetic or bioluminescent molecule) is given and the probe concentrates (or emits light) at the site of reporter gene expression. The level of probe concentration (or intensity of light) is usually proportional to the level reporter gene product and can reflect several processes, including the level of transcription, the modulation and regulation of translation, protein–protein interactions, and posttranslational regulation of protein conformation and degradation.

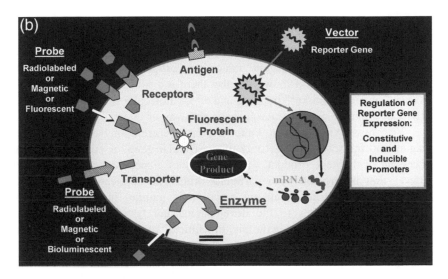

Figure 11.3 *Continued.*

the promoter–enhancer elements can be constructed to be "inducible" and "sensitive" to activation and regulation by specific endogenous transcription factors and promoters (factors that bind to and activate specific enhancer elements in the promoter region of the reporter vector construct leading to the initiation of reporter gene transcription).

Considerable progress in reporter gene imaging has been achieved during the past 5 years. Important proof-of-principle experiments in small animals include the imaging of endogenous regulation of transcription (46–48), posttranscriptional modulation of translation (49), protein–protein interactions (50–52), protein degradation and activity of the proteosomal ubiquination pathway (53), apoptosis (54), and so on. Noninvasive imaging of viral (55,56), bacterial (57) and cell trafficking (58), plus tissue-specific reporter gene imaging in prostate cancer (59), hepatocytes (60), and colorectal cancer cells (61) have also been reported.

C. Biomarker Imaging

Biomarker imaging or surrogate marker imaging can be used to assess downstream effects of one or more endogenous molecular-genetic processes. This approach is particularly attractive for potential translation into clinical studies in the near-term, because existing radiopharmaceuticals and imaging paradigms may be useful for monitoring down-stream effects of changes in specific molecular-genetic pathways in diseases such as cancer. The biomarker imaging approach is very likely to be less specific and more limited with respect to the number of molecular-genetic processes that can be imaged. Nevertheless, it benefits from the use of radiolabeled probes that have already been developed and studied in human subjects. Thus, the translation of biomarker imaging paradigms into patients will be far easier than either the direct imaging paradigms outlined earlier or the reporter transgene imaging paradigms outlined subsequently. However, it remains to be shown whether there is a sufficiently high correlation between "surrogate marker" imaging and direct molecular assays that reflect the activity of a particular molecular/genetic pathway of interest.

Very few studies have attempted a rigorous correlation between biomarker imaging and transcriptional activity of a particular gene, or posttranscriptional processing of the gene product, or the activity of a specific signal transduction pathway that is targeted by a particular drug. The application of biomarker imaging for monitoring treatment response is gaining increasing attention, particularly as it relates to the development and testing of new pathway-specific drugs. One recent example of clinically useful biomarker imaging is the early (1–7 days) assessment of treatment response with FDG-PET imaging, as applied to gastrointestinal stromal tumors (GIST) pre- and post-STI571 (Gleevec) treatment (62,63) (Fig. 11.4). This is significant because STI571 (Gleevec) treatment specifically targets the cKIT receptor tyrosine kinase (RTK) that is mutated and constitutively over-expressed in GIST, and the metabolic response to treatment is observed within hours.

Although glucose uptake and glycolytic enzyme activity are homeo-statically regulated, glucose metabolism has also been shown to be regulated

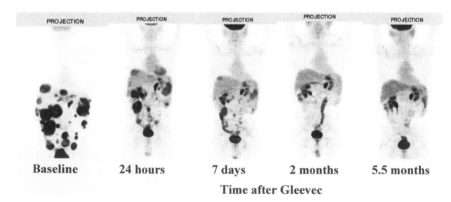

Baseline   24 hours   7 days   2 months   5.5 months

Time after Gleevec

Figure 11.4   FDG-PET imaging of GIST before and after treatment. In patients with GIST, tumor glucose utilization is very high and these tumors can be readily visualized by [^{18}F]-FDG-PET. A striking observation in patients with GIST who are treated with STI571 (Gleevec) was the rapid and sustained decrease in FDG uptake determined by PET scan as early as 24 h following one dose of STI571, and this was sustained over many months. The high FDG levels seen in the kidney, ureter, and bladder are normal in both the pre- and post-Gleevec images. [Figure adapted from Van den Abbeele et al. (63)]

by extracellular signals mediated by cell surface receptors such as cKIT. Receptor mediated regulation of glucose uptake is thought to involve activation of phosphoinositide 3-kinsase (PI3K), Akt, mammalian target of rapamycin (mTOR), and S6 kinase (S6K). Examples of this include the CD28 signaling pathway in T-cells and insulin receptor signaling (64). A likely explanation for the dramatic effect of STI571 (Gleevec) on glucose uptake in GIST is that Kit receptor signaling regulates/mediates glucose uptake as well as glucose metabolism. Interestingly, in yeast and a lymphocyte cell line, mTOR depletion or rapamycin treatment and glucose deprivation trigger a stress response similar to a starvation phenotype (65). Whether imaging "surrogate markers" will be of value for assessing treatment directed at other molecular-genetic abnormalities in tumors [epidermal growth factor receptor (EGFR), p53, c-Met, hypoxia-inducile-factor-1 (HIF-1), etc.] remains to be demonstrated.

Selective use of FDG-PET imaging in nonsmall cell lung cancer (NSCLC) has also been shown to be of value. FDG-PET has been repeatedly shown to improve staging accuracy compared to CT scanning alone, and it provides a cost-effective adjunct to the preoperative staging of NSCLC and lung metastases (66). However, in patients with adenocarcinoma and mediastinal lymph nodes of <1 cm, FDG-PET scanning cannot yet replace mediastinoscopy (67). FDG-PET is also having an impact on radiation therapy volume delineation in NSCLC. Radiation targeting based on fused FDG-PET and CT images resulted in alterations in radiation therapy planning in >50% of patients when compared with CT targeting (68). FDG-PET is also being used to assess response to chemotherapy and may have predictive value. A reduction in metabolic activity after one cycle of chemotherapy has been shown to be correlated with final outcome of therapy (69). The use of metabolic markers to determine response (Fig. 11.5) may shorten the duration of phase II studies evaluating new cytotoxic drugs, and may decrease the morbidity and costs of therapy in nonresponding patients.

II. Oncogenic Cell Transformation

Oncogenesis means "creation of cancer." A considerable amount of recent research has focused on experiments designed to better understand the complex processes that underlies and leads to cancer formation. Nevertheless, our understanding of oncogenic cell transformation remains incomplete. A widely accepted basic model of how a normal body cell transforms into a cancer cell describes oncogenesis as a step-wise accumulation of genetic alterations including gene amplification, insertional mutagenesis, and translocation. As a result, cancer cells acquire significant genetic instability. The genes that are affected by the genetic alterations may vary among different types of cancer and are also highly specific for the cancer of an individual. However, in essence, the activation of oncogenes and the inactivation of tumor suppressor genes triggers oncogenesis. Prior and

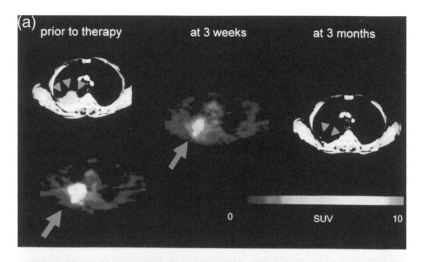

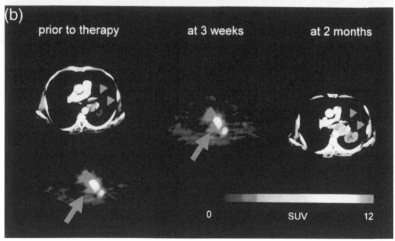

Figure 11.5 (**See color insert**) FDG-PET imaging lung tumors before and after treatment. [^{18}F]-FDG-PET and CT scans of a responding (a) and nonresponding (b) lung tumor. In the responding tumor, there is a 61% decrease in FDG uptake 3 weeks after initiation of chemotherapy. In contrast, tumor FDG uptake is essentially unchanged in the nonresponding tumor. [Adapted from Weber et al. (69)]

recent research has identified critical gene alterations in several cancers. For example, in most lung cancers, K-Ras, H-Ras, ErbB1, and Myc are affected (70,71). The majority of genetic alterations translate into dysregulation of cellular signal transduction and gene expression. In this way, cancer cells escape their growth control systems; for example, through modification and activation of cell cycle genes and the inactivation or elimination of cell death pathways.

Continuous cell proliferation then results in tumor formation. In addition, tumor growth beyond a millimeter size is dependent on tumor blood vessel formation, and changes resulting in enhanced cell mobility and migration allow tumor cells to metastasize to distant body sites (72).

Tumorigenesis is a complex, yet highly regulated process. It is clearly dependent on the cellular microenvironment, as illustrated by the angiogenic switch. Thus, *in vitro* studies of tumorigenesis are significantly limited. For example, *in vitro* models cannot accurately replicate the cascade of interacting signaling molecules and interactions between adjacent cells that will govern the cancer cell development and progression. To overcome these limitations, *in vivo* models of tumor formation have been developed in the past.

A. The Study of Lung Cancer in Experimental Mouse Models

Initially, mouse models of lung cancer utilized either human cancer cells as xenografts or syngeneic models of mouse lung cancer (73). Xenograft models use immunodeficient animals and provide the opportunity to study lung cancer formation at ectopic sites, as well as directly in the lungs. Xenotransplants usually maintain histology of the parent tumor; more importantly they can retain similar growth characteristics and may display the anticancer drug responsiveness of the original tumor. However, lung xenografts in immunocompromised animals generally do not metastasize, and it is likely that xenograft models select for cells which acquire a phenotype different from the original tumor (74). In contrast, transplantation of mouse lung cancer cells provides a model to observe tumorigenesis of pulmonary lesions. To circumvent the need for transplantation of exogenous cancer cells, lung tumors can be induced through exposure to chemical carcinogens.

Chemical induction of lung tumors provides a method for studying lung tumorigenesis in mice. Although induction of pulmonary lesions by agents such as ethyl carbamate is a reliable way of generating lung cancer, it can be difficult to analyze the underlying genetic alterations. Nevertheless, induction studies have indicated some correlations; for example, the relationship between systemic vinyl carbamate treatment and abnormal activation of K-Ras (75). K-Ras is an oncogene that is expected to play a critical role in lung cancer formation. To redefine the role of specific genes in lung tumorigenesis, attempts have been made to generate genetically defined alterations in the mouse genome. This approach will be outlined in the following section.

B. Genetic Mouse Models of Lung Cancer

Transgenic and gene ablation mouse models for lung cancer provide a genetic approach to dissect lung cancer tumorigenesis in living mice. Conventional transgenic models have been used to determine the effect of forced expression of proto-oncogenes, such as the kinases RON (76) and c-Raf-1 (77), on the

formation of lung lesions. Further examples include overexpression of a dominant negative variant of the tumor suppressor p53 gene (78), as well as enforced
expression of the transcription factor c-myc (79). To achieve lung cancer cell
restricted gene expression, the promoters for Clara cell secretory protein and
surfactant protein C have been most widely used. However, these promoters
do not allow the expression of genes in all of the highly diverse cell types that
are present in the lung. Hence, improved models may require the identification
and cloning of promoters suitable for defined gene expression in a larger
number of specific lung cell types. A further restriction in the use of uncontrolled
overexpression of genes that may alter cell proliferation and differentiation is
the potential for lethal lung damage during mouse development. This has been
recently emphasized by Kwak et al., who provide an excellent review on genetically engineered lung cancer mouse models (80).

An alternative to conventional transgenic mouse models, is the use of
conditional transgenic mouse models that have been generated. In this section,
we will first briefly summarize the application of drug-dependent protein overexpression in the lungs. We will focus on the tet regulatory system as the most
successfully used method to study the role of specific genes in lung cancer
formation. Then, we will discuss conditional gain of function approaches;
particularly, the Cre recombinase-based approach because of its potential for
molecular imaging of tumorigenesis.

The tet repressor was originally derived from Tn10 tetracycline (Tc)
resistance operon in *Escherichia coli*. Fusion of the tet repressor to a C-terminal
fragment of activator VP16 generated the Tc transactivator (tTA). To control
expression of a gene of interest, tTA is placed under control of a specific promoter,
while expression of the gene of interest is regulated by a promoter harboring the tet
operator sequence. Tet regulatory systems have been studied and used extensively
and excellent reviews, which give detailed information about function and applications, are available (81). In particular, tet on systems provide an elegant and
robust method to induce the expression of a cancer-related gene following the systemic administration of a drug such as doxycycline. Gene products that were overexpressed in lung tissue via the tet on system include fibroblast growth factor
(FGF) and K-Ras. The study by Clark et al. (82) indicates the potential of FGF-
10 to induce lung adenomas. A higher degree of tumorigenesis was observed by
Fisher et al. (83) following forced expression of K-Ras in lung tissue. In both
studies, withdrawal of doxycycline resulted in rapid tumor regression. Interestingly, this regression was also observed when K-Ras was overexpressed in
tumors that were deficient in either p53 or Ink4A/Arf. This finding emphasizes
the critical role of mutant K-Ras in lung cancer.

Site-specific recombinases of the α-integrase family have been developed as
a tool to artificially induce genetic changes in selected genes at a specific point in
time. For example, the bacteriophage P1 derived Cre recombinase catalyzes the
genetic recombination to sequences flanked by locus of crossover P1 (loxP)
sites. Utilizing this unique enzymatic activity, gene excision, insertion, inversion,

and translocation can be initiated in a controlled fashion. Meuwissen et al. (84) have employed Cre (loxP) recombinase facilitated activation of K-Ras to generate a mouse model of lung cancer. Mice transgenic for an exogenous gene comprising the oncogene K-Ras^{v12} and a human alkaline phosphatase were generated. The β-actin promoter driven expression of the transgene was activated by Cre mediated recombination of the loxP sites. An adenovirus was used to deliver Cre activity following intra-tracheal administration. This method generated sporadic pulmonary adenocarcinoma with an NSCLC phenotype.

III. Imaging Oncogenesis in Genetic Mouse Models

Genetic mouse models take advantage of the fact that cancer results from mutations in proto-oncogenes and tumor suppressor genes. They allow examination of the consequence of a specific gene alteration on the formation of tumors in their physiological environment. Important for the interpretation of data obtained from mouse models is the ability to accurately detect the consequences that arise from the generated genetic alteration. In most circumstances, onset and temporal dynamics of tumor growth will be a critical assessment. As the discussed mouse models require gene manipulation, it is rational to use reporter genes for the noninvasive detection and assessment of tumor growth.

A proof-of-principle study that utilizes bioluminescence imaging to detect and measure K-Ras dependent lung tumorigenesis has been recently reported by Lyons et al. (85). Mice engineered to induce lung tumors following Cre recombinase mediated activation of K-Ras overexpression were crossed with animals which provide Cre controlled luciferase expression. Following adenoviral delivery of Cre to the lungs, the formation of multiple lung tumors was observed. Optical bioluminescence imaging using the luciferase reporter gene was capable of monitoring the temporal dynamics of tumor development and progression in the lung of an individual animal (Fig. 11.6).

An important aspect of the report by Lyons et al. (85) is their methodological approach. Imaging oncogenesis was accomplished by combining a conditional transgenic mouse model of tumorigenesis with a conditional transgenic reporter gene mouse. This approach is highly versatile and easily translatable to other mouse models of cancer. However, reporter gene imaging was restricted to monitor tumor development and therefore, activation of the reporter was only indirectly related to the activation of oncogenic pathways. Furthermore, all noninvasive *in vivo* imaging systems have defined limits with respect to image resolution and sensitivity. Hence, it can be anticipated that only established tumors of a minimum size and with an established blood supply can be efficiently monitored by our molecular imaging techniques (e.g., micro-PET, bioluminescence, fluorescence). It is therefore unlikely that the very early events which lead to the formation of cancer can be imaged using some of our currently available molecular imaging techniques, and that further developments in imaging technology will

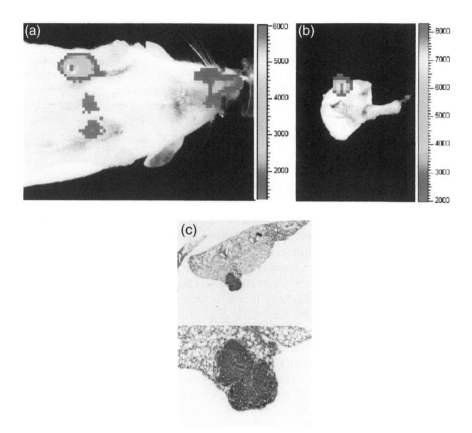

Figure 11.6 (**See color insert**) Bioluminescence imaging of spontaneous lung tumorigenesis. Tumors arising from LucRep/conditional $Kras2^{v12}$ mice were visualized noninvasively. (a) image of a compound LucRep/conditional $Kras2^{v12}$ mouse 13 weeks after AdCre intubation shows a bright focal region of luminescence originating from the thorax. (b) image of the lungs dissected from the mouse depicted in (a) also shows a single origin of light. (c) The same lungs after H&E processing (at 2.5× and 10× magnification) showing that the light detected in (a) and (b) originated from a single lesion measuring between 1 and 2 mm in diameter. [Adapted from Lyons et al. (85)]

be required to image very small populations of cells. Nevertheless, as described in the next section, reporter gene imaging has a great potential to directly assess the molecular changes that occur during oncogenesis.

IV. Imaging Oncogenesis Pathways

Despite the issues related to image resolution and sensitivity or the limitations of optical imaging deep tissue due to light absorption and scatter, reporter gene imaging can be used to visualize and measure oncogenic gene expression. For example, during tumorigenesis the activation of a specific oncogene may be monitored through an oncogene promoter that controls the expression of a reporter gene. The feasibility of imaging activation of cancer-related endogenous genes was demonstrated by Doubrovin et al. (46). It was shown that p53-dependent gene expression can be imaged *in vivo* with PET and by *in situ* fluorescence. A retroviral vector generated by placing the Herpes simplex virus type 1 thymidine kinase and enhanced green fluorescent protein fusion gene under control of a p53-specific response element. DNA damage-induced upregulation of p53 transcriptional activity was demonstrated and correlated with the expression of p53-dependent down-stream genes, including p21. These findings were observed in U87 (p53$^{+/+}$) cells and xenografts, but not in SaOS (p53$^{-/-}$) cells. This was the first demonstration that a *cis*-reporter system [*cis*-p53/thymidine kinase green fluorescent protein (TKGFP)] was sufficiently sensitive to image endogenous gene expression using noninvasive nuclear PET imaging. The PET images corresponded with upregulation of genes in the p53 signal transduction pathway (p53-dependent genes) in response to DNA damage induced by 1,3-bis-[2-chlororethyl]-1-nitrosourea (BCNU) chemotherapy. PET imaging of p53 transcriptional activity in tumors using the *Cis*-p53TKGFP reporter system lays the foundation to develop imaging of, for example, signal transduction pathways during oncogenesis (Fig. 11.7).

Platelet-derived growth factor (PDGF) and epidermal growth factor (EGF) signaling as well as Ras/Raf/MEK/Erk and protein kinase B (PKB)/Akt/mTOR mediated pathways have been shown to be important for oncogenesis and tumor development. PDGF, EGF, and HER2 receptors are frequently mutated, amplified, or overexpressed in tumors (86–88). This suggests that these RTK signaling pathways are critical targets in oncogenesis. RTKs signal through several effector arms, including Ras/MAPK (mitogen-activated protein kinase), PI3K, PLC-γ (phospholipase C), and JAK-STAT (Janus kinase-signal transducers and activators of transcription), which regulate cellular proliferation, migration and invasion, and cytokine stimulation. Given the scope of biological effects from RTK stimulation, it is reasonable to investigate how the dysregulation of these pathways drives malignant transformation, progression, and maintenance of these tumors.

Furthermore, the PI3K-PKB/Akt signaling pathway plays a critical role in mediating survival signals in a wide range of cell types. The binding of growth factors to specific RTKs activates the PI3K and the serine–threonine kinase Akt (also called PKB). Akt promotes cell survival and proliferation in part by directly phosphorylating and inhibiting members of the FOXO subfamily of forkhead transcription factors. Akt has been shown to be activated in many tumors and upregulation of Akt activity is consistently observed in PTEN (phosphatase and tensin homolog on chromosome 10)-mutant gliomas, which correlates with elevated activity of signaling components down-stream of

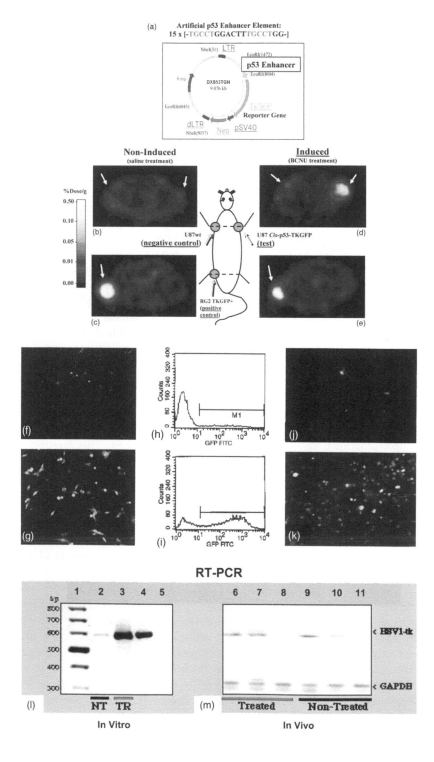

(a) **Artificial p53 Enhancer Element:**
15 x [-TGCCTGGACTTTGCCTGG-]

Non-Induced
(saline treatment)

Induced
(BCNU treatment)

%Dose/g

U87wt
(negative control)

U87 *Cis*-p53-TKGFP
(test)

RG2 TKGFP+
(positive
control)

RT-PCR

In Vitro   In Vivo

Table 11.1 Target-Specific Drugs, Signaling Pathways and Reporter Imaging

Drug	Target	Pathway	Reporter system
PTK 787[a]	PDGFR	Growth factor (RTK)	STAT3 and/or E2F1
OSI 774[a]	EGFR	Growth factor (RTK)	STAT3 (SRE, E2F1)
PD 98059[a]	MEK	Ras/Raf/MEK/Erk	SRE (E2F1)
Ly 294002[b]	PI3K	PI3K/PKB/Akt/mTOR	FLKHRL1 (SRE)
CCI-779[a]	mTor	mTOR (S6K/4E-PBI)	FLKHRL1 (SRE)

[a]Drugs in Phase I/II clinical trials; [b]a less toxic analog of Wortmannin.
Note: Reporter systems: STAT3 (cell surface receptor tyrosine kinase activation); SRE (Ras pathway activation); E2F1 (cell cycle activation); FLKHRL1 (PI3K-mTor activation).

mTOR, such as S6K and 4E-binding protein 1 (4E-BP1). Expression of activated Akt inhibits apoptosis and G1 arrest induced by growth factor withdrawal. The biological effects of Akt have also been linked to the induction of c-myc and Bcl-2 (89). Activated forms of Akt substitute for interleukin 2 (IL-2)

Figure 11.7 (**See color insert**) PET imaging of endogenous p53 activation and validation of *Cis*-p53/TKGFP reporter system in cell cultures and sampled tumor tissue. The p53-sensitive reporter vector (a) contains an artificial p53 specific enhancer that activates expression of the TKeGFP reporter gene. Transaxial PET images (GE Advance tomograph) through the shoulder (b, d) and pelvis (c, e) of two rats are shown (upper panel); the images are color-coded to the same radioactivity scale (%dose/g). An untreated animal is shown on the left, and a BCNU-treated animal is shown on the right. Both animals have three s.c. tumor xenografts: U87p53TKGFP (test) in the right shoulder, U87 wild-type (negative control) in the left shoulder, and RG2TKGFP (positive control) in the left thigh. The nontreated animal on the left shows localization of radioactivity only in the positive control tumor (RG2TKGFP); the test (U87p53TKGFP) and negative control (U87 wt) tumors are at background levels. The BCNU-treated animal on the right shows significant radioactivity localization in the test tumor (right shoulder) and in the positive control (left thigh), but no radioactivity above background in the negative control (left shoulder). Fluorescence microscopy and FACS analysis of a transduced U87p53/TKGFP cell population in the noninduced (control) state (f, h), and 24 h after a 2 h treatment with BCNU 40 mg/mL (g, i). Fluorescence microscopic images of U87p53/ TKGFP s.c. tumor samples obtained from nontreated rats (j) and rats treated with 40 mg/kg BCNU i.p. (k). The RT-PCR blots from *in vitro* (l) and *in vivo* (m) experiments show very low HSV1-*tk* expression in nontreated U87p53TKGFP transduced cells and xenografts-bearing animals, respectively, and no HSV1-*tk* expression in wild-type U87 cells and tumor tissue, respectively. When U87p53TKGFP transduced cells and xenografts-bearing animals are treated with BCNU, there is a marked increase in HSV1-*tk* expression comparable to that in constitutively HSV1-*tk* expressing RG2TK+ cells and xenografts. The numbered blots are: 1: ladder; 2: U87p53TKGFP non-treated, 3: U87p53TKGFP treated, 4: RG2TKGFP, and 5: wild-type U87 cells; 6: RG2TKGFP, 7: U87p53TKGFP, and 8: U87 treated animal xenografts; 9: RG2TKGFP, 10: U87p53TKGFP, 11: wild-type U87 non-treated animal xenografts. [Figure adapted from Doubrovin et al. (46)]

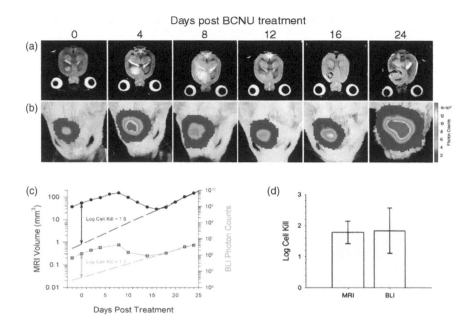

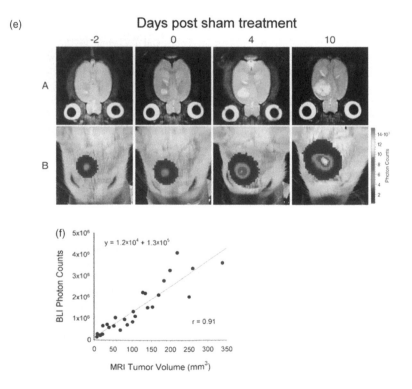

signals that phosphorylate Rb and activate E2 factor (E2F) during G1 progression (90). Because E2F can upregulate the expression of c-myc (91–93), c-myc induction by Akt may be mediated, at least in part, via E2F. In addition, recent experiments suggest that Akt may also use metabolic pathways to regulate cell survival.

There is a strong rationale to assess the effects of drugs that target PDGF/ EGFR signaling or Ras/Raf/MEK/Erk and PKB/Akt/mTOR mediated pathways by noninvasive imaging in transgenic animals. Specific drugs which are known (or thought) to target specific signaling pathways and down-stream effectors can be assessed in the transgenic oncogenic/reporter animals (Table 11.1).

V. Imaging Tumor Treatment

Imaging the effects of treatment targeted to a particular signaling pathway is described earlier, and it can be applied to tumors or xenografts that have been transduced with the appropriate reporter construct or to transgenic reporter animal models of cancer. A more widely used variant of this application, particularly in the pharmaceutical industry, is the monitoring of tumor or

---

Figure 11.8 (**See color insert**) Temporal analysis of the response of 9L ^{Luc} tumor to BCNU chemotherapy (panels a–d). Tumor cells were implanted 16 days before treatment. Tumor volume was monitored with T2-weighted MRI (a) and intratumoral luciferase activity was monitored with BLI (b). The days post BCNU therapy on which the images were obtained are indicated at the top. The scale to the right of the BL images describes the color map for the photo count. Quantitative analysis of tumor progression and response to BCNU treatment (c). Tumor volumes and total tumor photon emission obtained by T2-weighted MRI and BLI, respectively, are plotted vs. days post BCNU treatment. The dashed lines are the regression fits of exponential tumor repopulation following therapy. The solid vertical lines denote the apparent tumor-volume and photon-production losses elicited by BCNU on the day of treatment from which log cell kill values were calculated as previously described (9). Comparison of log cell kill values determined from MRI and BLI measurements (d). Log cell kill elicited by BCNU chemotherapy was calculated using MRI (1.78 ± 0.36) and BLI (1.84 ± 0.73). Data are represented as mean ± SEM for each animal ($n = 5$). There was no statistically significant difference between the log kills calculated using the MRI abd BLI data ($P = 0.951$). [Figure adapted from Rehemtulla et al. (32)] Kinetics of intracranial glioma growth (panels e and f). 9L^{Luc} cells were implanted intracerebrally and tumor progression was monitored with MRI (A) and BLI (B). The days, after sham treatment, on which the images were obtained are indicated at the top. The MR images are T2-weighted and are of a representative slice from the multislice dataset. The scale to the right of the BL images describes the color map for luminescent signal. Correlation of tumor volume with *in vivo* photon emission is shown where tumor volume was measured from T2-weighted MR images and plotted against total measured photon counts (f). The relationship between the two measurements was defined by regression analysis ($r = 0.91$). [Figure adapted from Rehemtulla et al. (32)]

xenograft growth using bioluminescence imaging. The popularity of bioluminescence imaging is due to its relative simplicity, low cost, and high throughput, and
because orthotopic xenograft growth and response to treatment can be monitored
effectively in mice (32). In this system, the desired cell lines are stably transduced
with a luciferase reporter gene, the transduced cells are selected and used to
produce subcutaneous (sc) or orthotopic xenografts. Monitoring tumor growth
and response to treatment is performed by bioluminescence imaging, sequentially
over time (Fig. 11.8).

An alternative to reporter imaging, is to image the target of drug treatment
directly. For example, the cell surface RTK HER2 is overexpressed in many

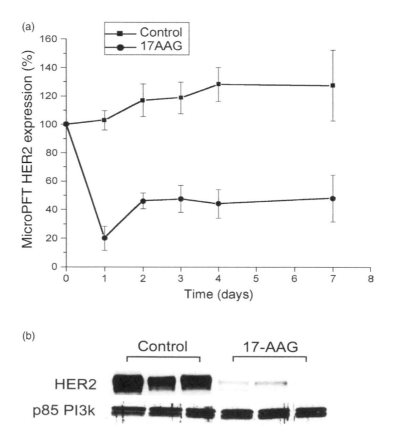

Figure 11.9 Monitoring the effect of 17-AAG on tumor HER2 expression. (a) MicroPET
determination of average HER2 expression in two groups of mice ($n = 5$) over a 1-week
period. One group of mice were treated with 3×50 mg/kg 17-AAG after the initial micro-
PET scan; the control group was treated with vehicle only. The data normalized to the initial
pretreatment uptake value. (b) Western blot analysis of HER2 and the 85 kDa regulatory
subunit of P13 kinase expression in BT-474 tumors from control mice and from mice
24 h after treatment with 17-AAG. [Figure adapted from Smith-Jones et al. (25)]

breast tumors and the level of expression can be imaged with radiolabeled (94–96) or gadolinium-chelated (97) antibodies specific for HER2. In a recent study, the pharmacodynamics of HER2 degradation and recovery in response to treatment was determined in a noninvasive imaging study (25). What was novel in this study was the ability to image the target of therapy, HER2, through the effects of the drug on the HER2 chaperone protein (HSP90) rather than through an inhibition of HER2 function. The ansamycin class of antibiotics, including geldanamycin and its derivative 17-AAG, bind to the adenosine triphosphate (ATP)-binding pocket of HSP90 and inhibit HSP90 chaperone function. The HSP90 chaperone is required for conformational maturation and stability of a number of key signaling molecules including HER2, AKT, RAF, cdk4 serine kinases (98). HER2 is dependent on HSP90 and is particularly sensitive to 17-AAG treatment, which results in rapid proteosomal degradation of this RTK. Smith-Jones et al. (25) exploited the mechanism of action of 17-AAG to image the pharmacodynamic effects of 17-AAG on HER2, through its effect on the chaperone protein (Figs. 11.2 and 11.9). This approach could be extended to other targets of drug therapy, such as MET, insulin-like growth factor-I (IGF-I) and other RTKs that are HSP90 chaperone-dependent.

This approach could be easily adapted to human studies and would provide the opportunity to noninvasively image the pharmacodynamics of drug action by repetitive imaging over time using short-lived radionuclides such as 68-Ga ($t_{1/2} = 68$ min). The ability to image drug pharmacodynamic effects addresses a major impediment to the development of rational therapeutic strategies, namely, the determination of whether the drug treatment protocol (dose and schedule) is actually inhibiting the target and whether the level of inhibition is sufficient. Furthermore, it is not inconceivable that noninvasive imaging of drug pharmacodynamic effects could be applied to individual patients in order to optimize dose and administration schedule.

Acknowledgments

A special acknowledgment is given to our friend and colleague, Juri Gelovani-Tjuvajev, who joined our group in 1991. He has recently accepted a well-deserved appointment as Chairman, Department of Experimental Diagnostic Imaging at MD Anderson Cancer Center in Houston in 2003. He was a leading investigator in our group and initiated many of the projects in our laboratory, including the development of noninvasive multi-modality reporter transgene imaging.

References

1. Ichikawa T, Hogemann D, Saeki Y, Tyminski E, Terada K, Weissleder R, Chiocca EA, Basilion JP. MRI of transgene expression: correlation to therapeutic gene expression. Neoplasia 2002; 4:523–530.

2. Blasberg RG, Gelovani J. Molecular-based imaging: a nuclear based perspective. (Review) Mol Imaging 2002; 1:280–300.
3. Edinger M, Cao YA, Hornig YS, Jenkins DE, Verneris MR, Bachmann MH, Negrin RS, Contag CH. Advancing animal models of neoplasia through *in vivo* bioluminescence imaging. Eur J Cancer 2002; 38:2128–2136.
4. Weissleder R. Scaling down imaging: molecular mapping of cancer in mice. Nat Rev Cancer 2002; 2:11–18.
5. Hadjantonakis AK, Macmaster S, Nagy A. Embryonic stem cells and mice expressing different GFP variants for multiple non-invasive reporter usage within a single animal. BMC Biotechnol 2002; 2:11.
6. Blasberg R, Tjuvajev J. *In vivo* monitoring of gene therapy by radiotracer imaging. In: Ernst Shering Research Foundation Workshop 22. Impact of Molecular Biology and New Technical Developments on Diagnostic Imaging. Berlin-Heidelberg: Springer Verlag, 1997.
7. Gambhir SS, Herschman HR, Cherry SR, Barrio JR, Satyamurthy N, Toyokuni T, Phelps ME, Larson SM, Balatoni J, Finn R, Sadelain M, Tjuvajev J, Blasberg R. Imaging transgene expression with radionuclide imaging technologies. Neoplasia 2000; 2:118–138.
8. Tavitian B. *In vivo* antisense imaging. Q J Nucl Med 2000; 44:236–255.
9. Ray P, Bauer E, Iyer M, Barrio JR, Satyamurthy N, Phelps ME, Herschman HR, Gambhir SS. Monitoring gene therapy with reporter gene imaging. Semin Nucl Med 2001; 31:312–320.
10. Blasberg RG, Gelovani J. Molecular-genetic imaging: a nuclear medicine-based perspective. Mol Imaging 2002; 1:280–300.
11. Luker GD, Sharma V, Piwnica Worms D. Visualizing protein–protein interactions in living animals. Methods 2003; 29:110–122.
12. Weissleder R, Ntziachristos V. Shedding light onto live molecular targets. Nat Med 2003; 9:123–128.
13. Gelovani Tjuvajev J, Blasberg RG. *In vivo* imaging of molecular-genetic targets for cancer therapy. Cancer Cell 2003; 3:327–332.
14. Berger F, Gambhir SS. Recent advances in imaging endogenous or transferred gene expression utilizing radionuclide technologies in living subjects: applications to breast cancer. Breast Cancer Res 2001; 3:28–35.
15. Contag CH, Ross BD. It's not just about anatomy: *in vivo* bioluminescence imaging as an eyepiece into biology. J Magn Reson Imaging 2002; 16:378–387.
16. Gambhir SS. Molecular imaging of cancer with positron emission tomography. Nat Rev Cancer 2002; 2:683–693.
17. Blasberg RG, Tjuvajev JG. Molecular-genetic imaging: current and future perspectives. J Clin Invest 2003; 111:1620–1629.
18. Weissleder R, Ntziachristos V. Shedding light onto live molecular targets. Nat Med 2003; 9:123–128.
19. Min JJ, Gambhir SS. Gene therapy progress and prospects: noninvasive imaging of gene therapy in living subjects. Gene Ther 2004; 11:115–125.
20. Shah K, Jacobs A, Breakefield XO, Weissleder R. Molecular imaging of gene therapy for cancer. Gene Ther 2004; 11:1175–1187.
21. Dehdashti F, Mortimer JE, Siegel BA, Griffeth LK, Bonasera TJ, Fusselman MJ, Detert DD, Cutler PD, Katzenellenbogen JA, Welch MJ. Positron tomographic

assessment of estrogen receptors in breast cancer: comparison with FDG-PET and *in vitro* receptor assays. J Nucl Med 1995; 36:1766–1774.

22. Larson SM, Morris M, Gunther I, Beattie B, Humm JL, Akhurst TA, Finn RD, Erdi Y, Pentlow K, Dyke J, Squire O, Bornmann W, McCarthy T, Welch M, Scher H. Tumor localization of 16beta-18F-fluoro-5alpha-dihydrotestosterone versus 18F-FDG in patients with progressive, metastatic prostate cancer. J Nucl Med 2004; 45:366–373.

23. Jaffer FA, Tung CH, Gerszten RE, Weissleder R. *In vivo* imaging of thrombin activity in experimental thrombi with thrombin-sensitive near-infrared molecular probe. Arterioscler Thromb Vasc Biol 2002; 22:1929–1935.

24. Haubner R, Wester HJ, Weber WA, Mang C, Ziegler SI, Goodman SL, Senekowitsch-Schmidtke R, Kessler H, Schwaiger M. Noninvasive imaging of alpha(v)beta3 integrin expression using 18F-labeled RGD-containing glycopeptide and positron emission tomography. Cancer Res 2001; 61:1781–1785.

25. Smith-Jones PM, Solit DB, Akhurst T, Afroze F, Rosen N, Larson SM. Imaging the pharmacodynamics of HER2 degradation in response to Hsp90 inhibitors. Nat Biotechnol 2004; 22:701–706.

26. Dewanjee MK, Ghafouripour AK, Kapadvanjwala M, Dewanjee S, Serafini AN, Lopez DM, Sfakianakis GN. Noninvasive imaging of c-myc oncogene messenger RNA with indium-111-antisense probes in a mammary tumor-bearing mouse model. J Nucl Med 1994; 35:1054–1063.

27. Cammilleri S, Sangrajrang S, Perdereau B, Brixy F, Calvo F, Bazin H, Magdelenat H. Biodistribution of iodine-125 tyramine transforming growth factor alpha antisense oligonucleotide in athymic mice with a human mammary tumour xenograft following intratumoral injection. Eur J Nucl Med 1996; 23:448–452.

28. Phillips JA, Craig SJ, Bayley D, Christian RA, Geary R, Nicklin PL. Pharmacokinetics, metabolism, and elimination of a 20-mer phosphorothioate oligodeoxynucleotide (CGP 69846A) after intravenous and subcutaneous administration. Biochem Pharmacol 1997; 54:657–668.

29. Tavitian B, Terrazzino S, Kuhnast B, Marzabal S, Stettler O, Dolle F, Deverre JR, Jobert A, Hinnen F, Bendriem B, Crouzel C, Di Giamberadio L. *In vivo* imaging of oligonucleotides with positron emission tomography. Nat Med 1998; 4:467–471.

30. Contag CH, Spilman SD, Contag PR, Oshiro M, Eames B, Dennery P, Stevenson DK, Benaron DA. Visualizing gene expression in living mammals using a bioluminescent reporter. Photochem Photobiol 1997; 66:523–531.

31. Contag PR, Olomu IN, Stevenson DK, Contag CH. Bioluminescent indicators in living mammals. Nat Med 1998; 4:245–247.

32. Rehemtulla A, Stegman LD, Cardozo SJ, Gupta S, Hall DE, Contag CH, Ross BD. Rapid and quantitative assessment of cancer treatment response using *in vivo* bioluminescence imaging. Neoplasia 2000; 2:491–495.

33. Tjuvajev JG, Stockhammer G, Desai R, Uehara H, Watanabe H, Gansbacher B, Blasberg RG. Imaging the expression of transfected genes *in vivo*. Cancer Res 1995; 55:6126–6132.

34. Tjuvajev JG, Finn R, Watanabe K, Joshi R, Oku T, Kennedy J, Beattie B, Koutcher J, Larson S, Blasberg RG. Noninvasive imaging of herpes virus thymidine kinase gene transfer and expression: a potential method for monitoring clinical gene therapy. Cancer Res 1996; 15:4087–4095.

35. Tjuvajev JG, Avril N, Oku T, Sasajima T, Miyagawa T, Joshi R, Safer M, Beattie B, DiResta G, Daghighian F, Augensen F, Koutcher J, Zweit J, Humm J, Larson SM, Finn R, Blasberg R. Imaging herpes virus thymidine kinase gene transfer and expression by positron emission tomography. Cancer Res 1998; 58:4333–4341.

36. Gambhir SS, Barrio JR, Wu L, Iyer M, Namavari M, Satyamurthy N, Bauer E, Parrish C, MacLaren DC, Borghei AR, Green LA, Sharfstein S, Berk AJ, Cherry SR, Phelps ME, Herschman HR. Imaging of adenoviral-directed herpes simplex virus type 1 thymidine kinase reporter gene expression in mice with radiolabeled ganciclovir. J Nucl Med 1998; 39:2003–2011.

37. Gambhir SS, Barrio JR, Phelps ME, Iyer M, Namavari M, Satyamurthy N, Wu L, Green LA, Bauer E, MacLaren DC, Nguyen K, Berk AJ, Cherry SR, Herschman HR. Imaging adenoviral-directed reporter gene expression in living animals with positron emission tomography. Proc Natl Acad Sci USA 1999; 96:2333–2338.

38. Weissleder R, Simonova M, Bogdanova A, Bredow S, Enochs WS, Bogdanov A Jr. MR imaging and scintigraphy of gene expression through melanin induction. Radiology 1997; 204:425–429.

39. Louie AY, Huber MM, Ahrens ET, Rothbacher U, Moats R, Jacobs RE, Fraser SE, Meade TJ. *In vivo* visualization of gene expression using magnetic resonance imaging. Nat Biotechnol 2000; 18:321–325.

40. Halbhuber KJ, Konig K. Modern laser scanning microscopy in biology, biotechnology and medicine (review). Ann Anat 2003; 185:1–20.

41. Contag CH, Spilman SD, Contag PR, Oshiro M, Eames B, Dennery P, Stevenson DK, Benaron DA. Visualizing gene expression in living mammals using a bioluminescent reporter. Photochem Photobiol 1997; 66:523–531.

42. Liang Q, Satyamurthy N, Barrio JR, Toyokuni T, Phelps MP, Gambhir SS, Herschman HR. Noninvasive, quantitative imaging in living animals of a mutant dopamine D2 receptor reporter gene in which ligand binding is uncoupled from signal transduction. Gene Ther 2001; 8:1490–1498.

43. Rogers BE, Zinn KR, Buchsbaum DJ. Gene transfer strategies for improving radiolabeled peptide imaging and therapy. Q J Nucl Med 2000; 44:208–223.

44. Haberkorn U. Gene therapy with sodium/iodide symporter in hepatocarcinoma. Exp Clin Endocrinol Diabetes 2001; 109:60–62.

45. Chishima T, Miyagi Y, Wang X, Yamaoka H, Shimada H, Moossa AR, Hoffman RM. Cancer invasion and micrometastasis visualized in live tissue by green fluorescent protein expression. Cancer Res 1997; 57:2042–2047.

46. Doubrovin M, Ponomarev V, Beresten T, Balatoni J, Bornmann W, Finn R, Humm J, Larson S, Sadelain M, Blasberg R, Gelovani Tjuvajev. Imaging transcriptional regulation of p53-dependent genes with positron emission tomography *in vivo*. Proc Natl Acad Sci USA 2001; 98:9300–9305.

47. Ponomarev V, Doubrovin M, Lyddane C, Beresten T, Balatoni J, Bornmann W, Finn R, Akhurst T, Larson S, Blasberg R, Sadelian M, Tjuvajev JG. Imaging TCR-dependent NFAT-mediated T-cell activation with positron emission tomography *in vivo*. Neoplasia 2001; 3:480–488.

48. Iyer M, Wu L, Carey M, Wang Y, Smallwood A, Gambhir SS. Two-step transcriptional amplification as a method for imaging reporter gene expression using weak promoters. Proc Natl Acad Sci USA 2001; 98:14595–14600.

49. Mayer-Kuckuk P, Banerjee D, Malhotra S, Doubrovin M, Iwamoto M, Akhurst T, Balatoni J, Bornmann W, Finn R, Larson S, Fong Y, Gelovani Tjuvajev J,

Blasberg R, Bertino JR. Cells exposed to antifolates show increased cellular levels of proteins fused to dihydrofolate reductase: a method to modulate gene expression. Proc Natl Acad Sci USA 2002; 99:3400–3405.

50. Ray P, Pimenta H, Paulmurugan R, Berger F, Phelps ME, Iyer M, Gambhir SS. Noninvasive quantitative imaging of protein–protein interactions in living subjects. Proc Natl Acad Sci USA 2002; 99:3105–3110.

51. Luker GD, Sharma V, Pica CM, Dahlheimer JL, Li W, Ochesky J, Ryan CE, Piwnica-Worms H, Piwnica-Worms D. Noninvasive imaging of protein–protein interactions in living animals. Proc Natl Acad Sci USA 2002; 99:6961–6966.

52. Luker GD, Sharma V, Pica CM, Prior JL, Li W, Piwnica-Worms D. Molecular imaging of protein–protein interactions: controlled expression of p53 and large T-antigen fusion proteins *in vivo*. Cancer Res 2003; 63:1780–1788.

53. Luker GD, Pica CM, Song J, Luker KE, Piwnica-Worms D. Imaging 26S proteasome activity and inhibition in living mice. Nat Med 2003; 9:969–973.

54. Laxman B, Hall DE, Bhojani MS, Hamstra DA, Chenevert TL, Ross BD, Rehemtulla A. Noninvasive real-time imaging of apoptosis. Proc Natl Acad Sci USA 2002; 99:16551–16555.

55. Gambhir SS, Barrio JR, Phelps ME, Iyer M, Namavari M, Satyamurthy N, Wu L, Green LA, Bauer E, MacLaren DC, Nguyen K, Berk AJ, Cherry SR, Herschman HR. Imaging adenoviral-directed reporter gene expression in living animals with positron emission tomography. Proc Natl Acad Sci USA 1999; 96:2333–2338.

56. Tjuvajev JG, Chen SH, Joshi A, Joshi R, Guo ZS, Balatoni J, Ballon D, Koutcher J, Finn R, Woo SL, Blasberg RG. Imaging adenoviral-mediated herpes virus thymidine kinase gene transfer and expression *in vivo*. Cancer Res 1999; 59:5186–5193.

57. Tjuvajev J, Blasberg R, Luo X, Zheng LM, King I, Bermudes D. Salmonella-based tumor-targeted cancer therapy: tumor amplified protein expression therapy (TAPET) for diagnostic imaging. J Control Release 2001; 74:313–315.

58. Koehne G, Doubrovin M, Doubrovina E, Zanzonico P, Gallardo HF, Ivanova A, Balatoni J, Teruya-Feldstein J, Heller G, May C, Ponomarev V, Ruan S, Finn R, Blasberg RG, Bornmann W, Riviere I, Sadelain M, O'Reilly RJ, Larson SM, Tjuvajev JG. Serial *in vivo* imaging of the targeted migration of human HSV-TK-transduced antigen-specific lymphocytes. Nat Biotechnol 2003; 21:405–413.

59. Zhang L, Adams JY, Billick E, Ilagan R, Iyer M, Le K, Smallwood A, Gambhir SS, Carey M, Wu L. Molecular engineering of a two-step transcription amplification (TSTA) system for transgene delivery in prostate cancer. Mol Ther 2002; 5:223–232.

60. Green LA, Nguyen K, Bauer E, Barrio JR, Namavari M, Satyamurthy N, Tokokuni T, Phelps ME, Sandgren EP, Herchmann HR, Gambhir SS. Indirect monitoring of endogenous gene expression by imaging PET reporter gene expression in transgenic mice. J Nucl Med 2000; 5:81S.

61. Qiao J, Doubrovin M, Sauter MV, Huang Y, Guo ZS, Balatoni J, Akhurst T, Blasberg R, Tjuvajev JG, Chen SH, Woo SL. Tumor-specific transcriptional targeting of suicide gene therapy. Gene Ther 2002; 9:168–175.

62. Demetri GD, von Mehren M, Blanke CD, Van den Abbeele AD, Eisenberg B, Roberts PJ, Heinrich MC, Tuveson DA, Singer S, Janicek M, Fletcher JA, Silverman SG, Silberman SL, Capdeville R, Kiese B, Peng B, Dimitrijevic S, Druker BJ, Corless C, Fletcher CD, Joensuu H. Efficacy and safety of imatinib mesylate in advanced gastrointestinal stromal tumors. N Engl J Med 2002; 347:472–480.

63. Van den Abbeele AD, for the GIST Collaborative PET Study Group (Dana-Farber Cancer Institute, Boston, Massachusetts, USA, OSU, Portland, Oregon, Helsinki University Central Hospital, Turku University Central Hospital, Finland, Novartis Oncology). F18-FDG-PET provides early evidence of biological response to ST1571 patients with malignant gastrointestinal stromal tumors (GIST). Proc Am Soc Clin Oncol 2001; 20:362a.

64. Frauwirth KA, Riley JL, Harris MH, Parry RV, Rathmell JC, Plas DR, Elstrom RL, June CH, Thompson CB. The CD28 signaling pathway regulates glucose metabolism. Immunity 2002; 16:769–777.

65. Peng T, Golub TR, Sabatini DM. The immunosuppressant rapamycin mimics a starvation-like signal distinct from amino acid and glucose deprivation. Mol Cell Biol 2002; 22:5575–5584.

66. Hoekstra CJ, Stroobants SG, Hoekstra OS, Vansteenkiste J, Biesma B, Schramel FJ, van Zandwijk N, van Tinteren H, Smit EF. The value of [18F]fluoro-2-deoxy-D-glucose positron emission tomography in the selection of patients with stage IIIA-N2 non-small cell lung cancer for combined modality treatment. Lung Cancer 2003; 39:151–157.

67. Kelly RF, Tran T, Holmstrom A, Murar J, Segurola RJ Jr. Accuracy and cost-effectiveness of [18F]-2-fluoro-deoxy-D-glucose-positron emission tomography scan in potentially resectable non-small cell lung cancer. Chest 2004; 125:1413–1423.

68. Bradley J, Thorstad WL, Mutic S, Miller TR, Dehdashti F, Siegel BA, Bosch W, Bertrand RJ. Impact of FDG-PET on radiation therapy volume delineation in non-small-cell lung cancer. Int J Radiat Oncol Biol Phys 2004; 59:78–86.

69. Weber WA, Petersen V, Schmidt B, Tyndale Hines L, Link T, Peschel C, Schwaiger M. Positron emission tomography in non-small-cell lung cancer: prediction of response to chemotherapy by quantitative assessment of glucose use. J Clin Oncol 2003; 21:2651–2657.

70. Rodenhuis S, van de Wetering ML, Mooi WJ, Evers SG, van Zandwijk N, Bos JL. Mutational activation of the K-ras oncogene: a possible pathogenetic factor in adenocarcinoma of the lung. N Engl J Med 1987; 317:929–935.

71. Zajac-Kaye M. Myc oncogene: a key component in cell cycle regulation and its implication for lung cancer. Lung Cancer 2001; 34(suppl 2):S43–S46.

72. Chambers AF, Groom AC, MacDonald IC. Dissemination and growth of cancer cells in metastatic sites. Nat Rev Can 2002; 2:563–572.

73. Malkinson AM. Primary lung tumors in mice as an aid for understanding, preventing, and treating human adenocarcinoma of the lung. Lung Cancer 2001; 32:265–279.

74. Kang Y, Siegel PM, Shu W, Drobnjak M, Kakonen SM, Cordon-Cardo C, Guise TA, Massague J. A multigenic program mediating breast cancer metastasis to bone. Cancer Cell 2003; 3:537–549.

75. You M, Wang Y, Lineen AM, Gunning WT, Stoner GD, Anderson MW. Mutagenesis of the K-ras protooncogene in mouse lung tumors induced by N-ethyl-N-nitrosourea or N-nitrosodiethylamine. Carcinogenesis 1992; 13:1583–1586.

76. Chen YQ, Zhou YQ, Fu LH, Wang D, Wang MH. Multiple pulmonary adenomas in the lung of transgenic mice overexpressing the RON receptor tyrosine kinase. Recepteur d'origine nantais. Carcinogenesis 2002; 23:1811–1819.

77. Kerkhoff E, Fedorov LM, Siefken R, Walter AO, Papadopoulos T, Rapp UR. Lung-targeted expression of the c-Raf-1 kinase in transgenic mice exposes a novel oncogenic character of the wild-type protein. Cell Growth Differ 2000; 11:185–190.

78. Tchou-Wong KM, Jiang Y, Yee H, LaRosa J, Lee TC, Pellicer A, Jagirdar J, Gordon T, Goldberg JD, Rom WN. Lung-specific expression of dominant-negative mutant p53 in transgenic mice increases spontaneous and benzo(a)pyrene-induced lung cancer. Am J Respir Cell Mol Biol 2002; 27:186–193.

79. Geick A, Redecker P, Ehrhardt A, Klocke R, Paul D, Halter R. Uteroglobin promoter-targeted c-MYC expression in transgenic mice cause hyperplasia of Clara cells and malignant transformation of T-lymphoblasts and tubular epithelial cells. Transgenic Res 2001; 10:501–511.

80. Kwak I, Tsai SY, DeMayo FJ. Genetically engineered mouse models for lung cancer. Annu Rev Physiol 2004; 66:647–663.

81. Baron U, Bujard H. Tet repressor-based system for regulated gene expression in eukaryotic cells: principles and advances. Methods Enzymol 2000; 327:401–421.

82. Clark JC, Tichelaar JW, Wert SE, Itoh N, Perl AK, Stahlman MT, Whitsett JA. FGF-10 disrupts lung morphogenesis and causes pulmonary adenomas *in vivo*. Am J Physiol Lung Cell Mol Physiol 2001; 280:L705–L715.

83. Fisher GH, Wellen SL, Klimstra D, Lenczowski JM, Tichelaar JW, Lizak MJ, Whitsett JA, Koretsky A, Varmus HE. Induction and apoptotic regression of lung adenocarcinomas by regulation of a K-Ras transgene in the presence and absence of tumor suppressor genes. Genes Dev 2001; 24:3249–3262.

84. Meuwissen R, Linn SC, van der Valk M, Mooi WJ, Berns A. Mouse model for lung tumorigenesis through Cre/lox controlled sporadic activation of the K-Ras oncogene. Oncogene 2001; 20:6551–6558.

85. Lyons SK, Meuwissen R, Krimpenfort P, Berns A. The generation of a conditional reporter that enables bioluminescence imaging of Cre/loxP-dependent tumorigenesis in mice. Cancer Res 2003; 63:7042–7046.

86. Lazar-Molnar E, Hegyesi H, Toth S, Falus A. Autocrine and paracrine regulation by cytokines and growth factors in melanoma. Cytokine 2000; 12:547–554.

87. Dai C, Celestino JC, Okada Y, Louis DN, Fuller GN, Holland EC. PDGF autocrine stimulation dedifferentiates cultured astrocytes and induces oligodendrogliomas and oligoastrocytomas from neural progenitors and astrocytes *in vivo*. Genes Dev 2001; 15:1913–1925.

88. Holland EC. Gliomagenesis: genetic alterations and mouse models. Nat Rev Genet 2001; 2:120–129.

89. Ahmed NN, Grimes HL, Bellacosa A, Chan TO, Tsichlis PN. Transduction of interleukin-2 antiapoptotic and proliferative signals via Akt protein kinase. Proc Natl Acad Sci USA 1997; 94:3627–3632.

90. Brennan P, Babbage JW, Burgering BM, Groner B, Reif K, Cantrell DA. Phosphatidylinositol 3-kinase couples the interleukin-2 receptor to the cell cycle regulator E2F. Immunity 1997; 7:679–689.

91. Wong KK, Zou X, Merrell KT, Patel AJ, Marcu KB, Chellappan S, Calame K. v-Abl activates c-myc transcription through the E2F site. Mol Cell Biol 1995; 15:6535–6544.

92. Oswald F, Lovec H, Moroy T, Lipp M. E2F-dependent regulation of human MYC: trans-activation by cyclins D1 and A overrides tumour suppressor protein functions. Oncogene 1994; 9:2029–2036.

93. Moberg KH, Logan TJ, Tyndall WA, Hall DJ. Three distinct elements within the murine c-myc promoter are required for transcription. Oncogene 1992; 7:411–421.

94. Funovics MA, Kapeller B, Hoeller C, Su HS, Kunstfeld R, Puig S, Macfelda K. MR imaging of the her2/neu and 9.2.27 tumor antigens using immunospecific contrast agents. Magn Reson Imaging 2004; 22:843–850.

95. Blend MJ, Stastny JJ, Swanson SM, Brechbiel MW. Labeling anti-HER2/neu monoclonal antibodies with 111In and 90Y using a bifunctional DTPA chelating agent. Cancer Biother Radiopharm 2003; 3:355–363.

96. Palm S, Enmon RM Jr, Matei C, Kolbert KS, Xu S, Zanzonico PB, Finn RL, Koutcher JA, Larson SM, Sgouros G. Pharmacokinetics and Biodistribution of (86)Y-Trastuzumab for (90)Y dosimetry in an ovarian carcinoma model: correlative MicroPET and MRI. J Nucl Med 2003; 44:1148–1155.

97. Artemov D, Mori N, Ravi R, Bhujwalla ZM. Magnetic resonance molecular imaging of the HER-2/neu receptor. Cancer Res 2003; 63:2723–2727.

98. Neckers L. Hsp90 inhibitors as novel cancer chemotherapeutic agents. Trends Mol Med 2002; 8(suppl 4):S55–S61.

12

Molecular Imaging of Protein–Protein Interactions in Living Animals

**DAVID PIWNICA-WORMS, KATHRYN E. LUKER, and
VICTOR M. VILLALOBOS**

Washington University Medical School,
St. Louis, Missouri, USA

I. Introduction

Refinement of the human genome is expected to facilitate investigations into normal physiology and disease processes, leading to discovery of targets for new medical therapies and drugs (1). However, regulation of gene expression, posttranslational modifications of proteins (e.g., phosphorylation or myristoylation), or interactions between proteins cannot be deduced or inferred from DNA sequences (2). Thus, a biological function has been assigned to only a small portion of the genome. The vast amount of available sequence data has produced a demand for tools to integrate these data into the complex physiology of whole organisms (3). To determine the function of a particular protein within its cellular context, researchers are developing and applying several different techniques for identifying and characterizing protein function and interactions *in vivo*.

Regulated protein–protein interactions are fundamental to living systems, mediating many cellular functions including cell cycle progression, signal transduction, and metabolic pathways (4,5). On a whole organism scale, protein–protein interactions regulate signals that affect overall homeostasis, patterns of development, normal physiology, and disease in living animals (5–7). In addition, protein–protein interactions have considerable potential as therapeutic targets (8,9).

Furthermore, complexes of transcription factors, co-repressors, and chromatin-binding proteins maintain normal cell homeostasis, and disruption of these protein interactions may be significant in permitting unregulated growth of cancer cells (5). In cancers including lung cancer, aberrant patterns of protein interactions arise from dysregulated phosphorylation of receptor tyrosine kinases [e.g., epidermal growth factor receptor (EGFR), Erb2/HER2], tumor suppressors [e.g., p53, phosphatase and tensin homologue on chromosome 10 (PTEN)], and targets that mediate downstream signaling in cell proliferation, survival, and growth [e.g., signal transducers and activators of transcription (STATs), mammalian target of rapamycin (mTOR), phosphoinositide 3-kinase (PI3K)–Akt] (10). Thus, protein kinases and mediated protein–protein interactions comprising the kinome have emerged as important therapeutic targets in cancer and other human diseases (8–11). However, evidence is accumulating that pathways of protein interactions in specific tissues produce regional effects that cannot be investigated fully with *in vitro* systems. Many protein interactions and signaling cascades arise from a dialog between cells and their matrix in a tissue-specific manner and, thus, there is considerable interest in imaging protein–protein interactions noninvasively in their normal physiological context within living animals with positron emission tomography (PET) (12,13) or bioluminescence imaging (14,15).

Fundamentally, the detection of physical interaction among two or more proteins can be assisted if association between the interactive partners leads to production of a readily observed biological or physical readout (16). Current strategies for detecting protein–protein interactions include activation of transcription, repression of transcription, activation of signal transduction pathways, or reconstitution of a disrupted enzymatic activity (13,16,17). Most strategies for detecting protein–protein interactions in intact cells are based on fusion of the pair of interacting molecules to defined protein elements to reconstitute a biological or biochemical function. Compared with studies of protein interactions in cultured cells, strategies to interrogate protein–protein interactions in living organisms impose even further constraints on reporter systems and mechanisms of detection. Briefly summarized subsequently are various strategies for detecting protein-binding partners with the intent of identifying properties that might be exploited for molecular imaging applications *in vivo*.

II. Detecting Protein Interactions in Intact Cells and Animals

A variety of techniques have been developed to investigate protein–protein inter-actions in cultured cells, including the two-hybrid system and protein-fragment complementation (PFC). The two-hybrid system is the most widely applied method to identify and characterize protein interactions. However, several fea-tures of PFC make it attractive as an approach for *in vivo* imaging of protein inter-actions in cells, and particularly, in live animals. Subsequently, we describe major features of these two methods and other strategies with potential utility for *in vivo* imaging.

A. Two-Hybrid

Two-hybrid systems exploit the modular nature of transcription factors, many of which can be separated into discrete DNA-binding and activation domains (18). Proteins of interest are expressed as fusions with either a DNA-binding domain or an activation domain, creating hybrid proteins. If the hybrid proteins bind to each other as a result of interaction between the proteins of interest, then the separate DNA-binding domain and activation domain of the transcription factor are brought together within the cell nucleus to drive expression of a reporter gene. In the absence of specific interaction between the hybrid proteins, the reporter gene is not expressed because the DNA-binding domain and activation domain do not associate independently. Two-hybrid assays can detect transient and/or unstable interactions between proteins, and the technique is reported to be inde-pendent of expression of endogenous proteins (19). Although the two-hybrid assay originally was developed in yeast, commercial systems (BD Biosciences Clontech) are now available for studies in bacteria and mammalian cells. We and other investigators have shown that two-hybrid systems can be used to image protein interactions in living mice with PET (12,13,20,21) or biolumines-cence imaging (14). For example, to enable noninvasive molecular imaging of protein–protein interactions *in vivo* by PET and fluorescence imaging, we engin-eered a fusion reporter gene comprising a mutant herpes simplex virus 1 thymi-dine kinase (*mNLS-sr39-HSV1-tk*) fused in frame to enhance green fluorescent protein (*eGFP*) for readout of a two-hybrid system *in vivo* (Fig. 12.1). Using microPET and the *HSV1-tk* substrate 9-(4-[^{18}F]-fluoro-3 hydroxymethylbutyl) guanine (^{18}F-FHBG), interactions between p53 tumor suppressor and the large T antigen (TAg) of simian virus 40 (SV40) were visualized in mice engrafted with tumor xenografts of HeLa cells stably transfected with the imaging con-structs (12). Further control of the system could be imposed by use of a bidirec-tional tetracycline-inducible promoter driving expression of the hybrid proteins. Thus, the PET reporter signals induced by tetracycline analogs *in vivo* could be shown to be both time- and concentration-dependent (20), directly demonstrating the ability to image regulated protein–protein interactions *in vivo* with PET.

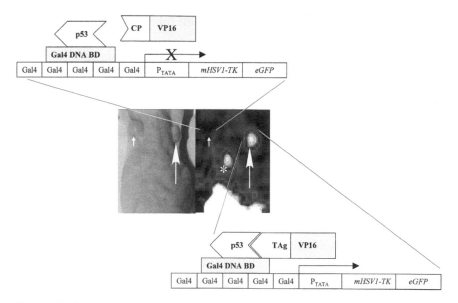

Figure 12.1 **(See color insert)** Two-hybrid strategy for molecular imaging of protein–protein interactions *in vivo* using microPET and dual reporter genes. *Lower right*: The p53 tumor suppressor and the transforming SV40 large T antigen (TAg), two known interacting proteins, are each fused to different domains of a hybrid transcription factor. Both portions of the transcription factor are required to activate the dual PET-fluorescence reporter gene (*mHSV1-tk-egfp*), but only the DNA binding domain (Gal4BD) can bind on its own to specific DNA sequences that regulate activation of the reporter. However, when p53 and TAg proteins interact, the activation domain (VP16) is now properly assembled, thereby switching on the dual reporter. The activated reporter can be detected by microPET imaging of living mice using the positron-emitting radiopharmaceutical ^{18}F-FHBG, a substrate phosphorylated and trapped within cells by mHSV1-TK, and detected independently by fluorescence microscopy of eGFP. *Upper left*: In contrast, when the VP16 activation domain is fused to a nonintereacting protein (in this case, polyoma virus coat protein, CP), the reporter gene cannot be activated. *Middle left:* Photograph of the anterior thorax of a mouse with axillary xenograft tumors of HeLa cells containing noninteracting p53-CP proteins (small arrow) and interacting p53-TAg proteins (large arrow). *Middle right*: coronal microPET image (10 min acquisition time) of the same mouse showing accumulation of ^{18}F-FHBG only in the tumor expressing the interacting p53-TAg proteins (large arrow). Asterisk denotes radiotracer in the gallbladder. Intestinal activity from normal hepatobiliary clearance of the radiotracer is observed in the lower portion of the image. [Reproduced from Ref. (57).]

However, the two-hybrid method has limitations. Some types of proteins do not lend themselves to study by the two-hybrid method. For example, because production of signal in the two-hybrid method requires nuclear localization of the hybrid proteins, integral membrane proteins cannot be studied in their intact state. In addition, the time delay associated with transcriptional activation of the reporter, and degradation of the reporter protein, and mRNA lifetime limits kinetic analysis of protein interactions (22).

B. Protein-Fragment Complementation

PFC assays depend on division of a monomeric reporter enzyme into two separate inactive components that can reconstitute function upon association [Fig. 12.2(a)]. When these reporter fragments are fused to interacting proteins, reporter activity is reconstituted upon association of the interacting proteins. PFC strategies based on several enzymes including β-galactosidase,

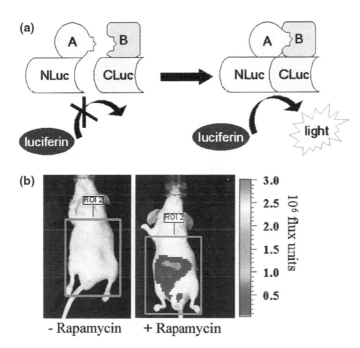

Figure 12.2 **(See color insert)** Protein complementation strategy for molecular imaging of protein–protein interactions *in vivo* using bioluminescence. (a) Schematic of luciferase complementation imaging. Rapamycin-induced association of the proteins FRB (A) and FKBP (B) bring fused, but inactive N-terminal-Luc (NLuc) and C-terminal-Luc (CLuc) fragments of luciferase into close proximity to reconstitute bioluminescence activity. (b) Luciferase complementation imaging of representative nu/nu mice implanted intraperitoneally with HEK-293 cells co-expressing FRB-N-terminal-Luc and C-terminal-Luc-FKBP fusion proteins. Bioluminescence images were taken 10 h after administration of a single dose of rapamycin (4.5 μg/g, intraperitoneal) (right panel) or vehicle control (left panel). Mice were anesthetized with isoflurane, injected i.p. with D-luciferin (150 μg/g in PBS) and then imaged 10 min later with a CCD camera (1 min exposure, binning 8, f-stop 1, FOV 15 cm). Regions of interest (ROI) used for analysis are shown. Flux units are photons/sec/cm^2/sr.

dihydrofolate reductase (DHFR), β-lactamase, and luciferase have been used to monitor protein–protein interactions in mammalian cells (23–30).

Of the available strategies, complementation of firefly and *Renilla* luciferases are potentially amenable to near real-time applications in living animals (28,29). A complementation strategy based on two random fragments of *Renilla* luciferase has been applied to evaluate constitutive MyoD-Id interaction (29), and rapamycin-mediated heterodimerization of FKBP-rapamycin-binding domain (FRB) and FK506 binding protein 12 (FKBP-12) (31) and homodimerization of HSV-TK (32). However, these studies showed low overall bioluminescence output relative to intact luciferase, as well as considerable constitutive activity of the N-terminal complementation fragment, necessitating expression control for that fragment to minimize background. Similar residual bioluminescence was also reported for the N-terminal complementation fragment of firefly luciferase in a MyoD-Id complementation scheme (15) on the basis of a previously developed split-intein strategy (28). These technical considerations of residual background and low signal constrain the user to evaluation of strong protein interactions and highly expressed interacting pairs, thereby precluding general use. In addition, *Renilla* luciferase has several biochemical and optical characteristics (discussed subsequently) that significantly detract from its utility for molecular imaging applications *in vivo*. Thus, until recently, no enzyme fragment pair had been found that satisfied all criteria for noninvasive analysis of protein–protein interactions, while enabling interrogation in cell lysates, intact cells, and living animals.

To develop an optimized PFC imaging system for broad use in living cells and animals, we screened a combinatorial incremental truncation library for reconstitution of the enzymatic activity of a heterodimeric firefly (*Photinus pyralis*) luciferase (Luc) (30,33). This library employed a well-characterized protein interaction system: rapamycin-mediated association of the FRB domain of human mTOR (residues 2024–2113) with FKBP-12 (25,27,34). Initial fusions of FRB and FKBP with N- and C-terminal fragments of luciferase, respectively, were designed such that the enzymatic activities of the individual overlapping fragments were weak or absent. From these constructs, N- and C-terminal incremental truncation libraries were generated by unidirectional exonuclease digestion and validated (35). The libraries were co-expressed in *Escherichia coli* and screened in the presence of rapamycin for bioluminescence. From this screen, one could identify an optimal pair of overlapping amino acid sequences for the N-terminal and C-terminal Luc fragments. The optimized combination of fragments produced no signal in the absence of rapamycin and strong bioluminescence in the presence of the dimerizing agent rapamycin (Fig. 12.2A).

In live cells and in cell lysates, our optimized complementation system successfully reproduced published apparent K_d values for rapamycin (25,27,30,33,34). To test the specificity of the complementation system, we mutated the FRB fragment in the FRB-N-terminal Luc construct to a form FRB(S2035I) (34), rendering it insensitive to rapamycin. We showed that this mutation, even in the presence of rapamycin, produced low bioluminescence signal, similar to the optimal pair in the absence of rapamycin (33). In addition, expression of single constructs produced no detectable signal relative to untransfected cells. Thus, our optimized complementation pair eliminated the substantial bioluminescence activity of the N-terminal luciferase fragment that was problematic with previous split-luciferase systems based on simple bisection of luciferase (15).

Furthermore, bioluminescence imaging of animals using charge-couple device (CCD) cameras such as the IVIS (Xenogen) enabled us to quantify relative expression of the luciferase reporter activity *in vivo*. In mice bearing implants of cells expressing our FRB-N-terminal Luc/C-terminal Luc-FKBP fusion pair, rapamycin-induced luciferase activity could be readily observed *in vivo* [Fig. 12.2(b)]. Repetitive bioluminescence imaging showed dose- and time-dependent luciferase activity induced by rapamycin with a maximal *in vivo* signal-to-background ratio of over 20:1, 10 times greater than prior attempts (33).

A fundamental advantage of PFC is that the expressed hybrid proteins form a complete assay system independent of activation of cell-specific processes such as transcription. In principle, therefore, protein interactions may be detected in any subcellular compartment, and assembly of protein complexes may be monitored in real-time. Because many PFC strategies are based on reconstituting active enzymes, these systems also offer the potential benefits of signal amplification to enhance sensitivity for detecting interacting proteins. A disadvantage of complementation approaches is that re-assembly of an enzyme may be susceptible to steric constraints imposed by the interacting proteins. Another potential limitation of PFC for application in living animals is that transient interactions between proteins may produce insufficient amounts of active enzyme to allow noninvasive detection. Nonetheless, because most PFC strategies are based on reconstituting active enzymes, the potential benefits of signal amplification enhance sensitivity for detecting interacting proteins in living animals.

C. Other Strategies

The split-ubiquitin system enables signal amplification from a transcription factor-mediated reporter readout (36,37). In one application, the interaction of two membrane proteins forces reconstitution of two halves of ubiquitin, leading to a cleavage event mediated by ubiquitin-specific proteases that release an artificial transcription factor to activate a reporter gene. As discussed, indirect readout of the reporter limits kinetic analysis, and the released transcription factor must translocate to the nucleus.

Several variations of recruitment systems have been developed for use in whole cells, including the Ras-recruitment system (38,39) and interaction traps (40). Cells that co-express a test protein fused to a membrane localization signal, such as a myristoylation sequence, and a protein binding partner fused to a cytoplasmic protein, such as activated Ras devoid of its membrane targeting signal, will localize mammalian Ras to the membrane only in the presence of interacting proteins. However, Ras-recruitment systems, as originally configured, cannot be applied to mammalian cells, and, while readout is not directly dependent on transcriptional activation, indirect readout by colony growth nonetheless limits kinetic analysis and interrogation of subcellular compartmentation of the interactions.

An interesting variation of the recruitment approach applicable to living mammalian cells is the cytokine-receptor-based interaction trap. Here, a signaling-deficient receptor provides a scaffold for recruitment of interacting fusion proteins that phosphorylate endogenous STAT3. Activated STAT complexes then drive a nuclear reporter (40). This system permits detection of both modification-independent and phosphorylation-dependent interactions in intact mammalian cells, but the transcriptional readout again limits kinetic analysis. In addition, the impact of endogenous STATs on the strength of readout in a variety of cells remains to be characterized.

Other approaches to detect protein–protein interactions in live mammalian cells include fluorescence resonance energy transfer (FRET) and bioluminescence resonance energy transfer (BRET) (41–44). For FRET, fluorescently labeled proteins, one coupled to a donor fluorophore and the other coupled to an acceptor fluorophore, produce a characteristic shift in the emission spectra of the system when protein binding partners interact. Thus, in the absence of target protein interactions, excitation of the donor fluorophore will produce emissions characteristic of the donor fluorophore. However, upon close approximation of interacting proteins and excitation of the donor fluorophore, resonance energy transfer will excite the acceptor flourophore, which in turn, will emit at a longer (red-shifted) wavelength. A limitation of FRET is inter- and intra-molecular spatial constraints and sensitivity of detection, because there is no amplification of the signal. For BRET, the donor molecule is luciferase or a related bioluminescent protein, whereas the acceptor is green fluorescent protein or a color variant. Although intermolecular spatial constraints are thought to be less restrictive with BRET, similar limitations related to sensitivity may apply. However, as the photon donor in BRET is produced by an enzymatic activity (luciferase), the potential for signal amplification exists.

BRET as a tool for monitoring protein–protein interaction *in vivo* may be advantageous over FRET due to several factors (42,43,45). Most importantly is that no incident light is required to activate BRET probes. Because tissue absorption increases exponentially for wavelengths below <600 nm, excitation of fluorescent proteins for FRET requires monochromatic light of high intensity, thereby introducing problems such as autofluorescence and photobleaching (46). For example, at the maximal excitation wavelength (490 nm) of the most red-shifted currently available FRET pair, EGFP-mRFP1, tissue absorption is >100 times that produced at 600 nm, limiting the utility of the pair *in vivo* (47). Nonetheless, both BRET and FRET suffer from issues related to spectral overlap that can render quantitative analysis of the two interacting fragments difficult in whole cells when expression levels of the two components are not exactly matched. This arises when using resonance energy transfer due to factors involving the actual and effective ratios of the donor and acceptor proteins in a cellular environment. The actual ratio of donor-to-acceptor depends upon expression levels of each separate construct. The effective ratio is further modulated by the differential localization of either fluorophore or the two proteins that are being measured. Thus, both spectral overlap and subcellular compartmentalization can adversely impact results with interacting FRET pairs or BRET pairs. One solution to this is use of a single chain multidomain biosensor, thereby assuring co-localization and a 1:1 ratio of donor and acceptor proteins. Thus, use of single chain biosensors for measuring protein–protein interactions may have advantages for selected applications. Measurements of inducible protein conformational changes, inducible protein–protein interactions, and cleavable events have been demonstrated using single chain biosensor folding strategies (48–51).

III. Applications *In Vivo*

When adapting any of these strategies for detection of protein–protein interactions in whole animals *in vivo*, several points must be considered. First, because whole animal reporters must be detected noninvasively with remote imaging devices [PET, single photon emission tomography (SPECT), magnetic resonance imaging (MRI), fluorescence or bioluminescence optical imaging], signal strength and signal-to-noise of the reporter are of primary concern. As a general rule, any signal detected by biochemical or cell culture-based assays will be attenuated *in vivo*. This arises from pharmacokinetic considerations of substrate delivery, substrate metabolism, and excretion pathways, as well as signal loss by absorption, attenuation, or dilution of substrate, and its emitted photon. Thus, any system possessing signal amplification strategies will more likely produce a signal detectable in a whole animal. For example, substrate binding strategies inherent to reporters involving one-to-one correlation of a labeled ligand and its cognate receptor lack an amplification mechanism. These would be inferior to transcriptional activation or enzyme reconstitution strategies, such as two-hybrid assays or enzyme complementation, for applications *in vivo*.

Detection and spatial localization of the reporter are other important considerations for *in vivo* imaging. For example, reporter substrates that are radiopharmaceuticals formulated with either PET or SPECT radionuclides can be detected readily deep within the body, and well-developed technologies already exist to tomographically map the location of the signal source (the radiotracer) within cross-sections of body tissue. The emitted radiation particles are for all practical purposes minimally attenuated by overlying tissues in mice and other small animals, and can be detected and directly mapped to specific deep body parts using standard back-projection and deconvolution software schemes well established in the field. The physical properties of radionuclide detection enable spatial resolution of ~ 1 mm for second-generation microPET instruments (52) and approaching 3–4 mm for small animal SPECT instruments (53). By comparison, tissue diffusion and nonlinearities inherent to optical emissions within the body can severely attenuate and delocalize optical signals *in vivo*. In addition, optical detection technologies are for the most part planar and, thus, the signal source can only be mapped as a projection over the surface of the animal. Depth resolution is a problem in current optical instruments. However, technologies enabling tomographic localization of optical signals in intact animals are under active development (54). Furthermore, for reasons related to attenuation and detection, radionuclide approaches are quantitative and, thus, absolute molar masses of reporter substrate can be calculated and related to the underlying reporter or biochemical pathway. In contrast, optical technologies are generally qualitative, but can approach semiquantitative readout when each animal serves as its own control under an established geometry.

Another consideration for whole animal reporters is duration of the reporter signal. For example, *Renilla* luciferase, a reporter commonly used in cell biology assays, is characterized by a burst of bioluminescence followed by rapid decay of light. Thus, the kinetics of the *Renilla* luciferase reaction is much more rapid than the prolonged signals generated by firefly luciferase variants or even radioactive decay by standard isotopes. Although bioluminescence from *Renilla* luciferase has been imaged in living mice (29,55,56), practical issues include animal anesthesia, delivery of substrate *in vivo*, positioning of the animal within the instrument, and detection time. These issues place temporal constraints on rapid enzyme-based readouts of biological processes characterized by slow rate constants. In addition, the spectral output of *Renilla* luciferase is generally more blue-shifted ($\lambda_{max} = 475$ nm) than that of green–yellow firefly luciferase ($\lambda_{max} = 570$ nm), thereby increasing tissue absorption of the photons emitted by *Renilla* luciferase and limiting sensitivity when the reporter is expressed in tissues or cells deep within the animal (47). In addition, coelenterazine, the chromophoric substrate for *Renilla* luciferase, is avidly transported by P-glycoprotein (ABCB1; Pgp), a 170 kDa transmembrane protein encoded by the *MDR1* gene (56). Thus, although enabling molecular imaging and high throughput screening of drug resistance pathways, these data raise concern for the indiscriminate use of *Renilla* luciferase as a reporter in intact cells or transgenic animals, wherein P-glycoprotein-mediated alterations in coelenterazine permeability may impact results.

IV. Concluding Comments

In summary, availability of gene sequences provide an essential framework for studying signaling pathways in pulmonary disease, but these data typically are insufficient to understand the full range of biological functions of proteins. A key step in characterizing any protein is determining its interactions with other proteins in signal transduction pathways and biochemical processes. Identifying binding partners for a protein can suggest possible functions and potentially identify targets for therapeutic intervention. Although *in vitro* assays can provide important data about interacting proteins, these studies do not reproduce the complex regulatory, transport and localization pathways that exist in living animals. Recent advances in imaging technology have enabled *in vivo* studies of cellular and molecular signaling processes. Thus, investigations of protein—protein interactions in living animals require researchers to integrate knowledge about the biological hypothesis with molecular imaging reporters and pharmacokinetics of contrast agents or tracers. These studies demonstrate that noninvasive molecular imaging of protein—protein interactions may enable investigators to determine how intrinsic binding specificities of proteins are regulated in a wide variety of normal and pathophysiologic conditions.

Further research is necessary to increase the sensitivity of imaging systems for monitoring protein-interactions in real-time, therefore expanding the biological questions that can be studied *in vivo*. Development and application of technologies for molecular imaging of protein—protein interactions *in vivo* will allow researchers to determine how intrinsic binding specificities of proteins are regulated during normal development and pulmonary disease progression. In addition, evaluation of the pharmacokinetics and targeting of drugs that promote or disrupt these interactions will enable novel aspects of drug action to be studied directly within the living organism.

Acknowledgments

We thank colleagues of the Molecular Imaging Center for insightful discussions and excellent technical assistance. Work reviewed herein was supported by grants from the National Institutes of Health (P50 CA94056) and Department of Energy (DE FG02 94ER61885).

References

1. Pennisi E. Human genome: finally, the book of life and instructions for navigating it. Science 2000; 288:2304–2307.
2. Rudert F, Ge L, Ilag L. Functional genomics with protein—protein interactions. Biotechnol Annu Rev 2000; 5:45–86.
3. Kitano H. Looking beyond the details: a rise in system-oriented approaches in genetics and molecular biology. Curr Genet 2002; 41:1–10.
4. Newton A. Regulation of the ABC kinases by phosphorylation: protein kinase C as a paradigm. Biochem J 2003; 370:361–371.

5. Ogawa H, Ishiguro S, Gaubatz S, Livingston D, Nakatani Y. A complex with chromatin modifiers that occupies E2F- and Myc-responsive genes in G0 cells. Science 2002; 296:1132–1136.

6. Zhang H, Hu G, Wang H et al. Heterodimerization of Msx and Dlx homeoproteins results in functional antagonism. Mol Cell Biol 1997; 17(5):2920–2932.

7. Stark G, Kerr I, Williams B, Silverman R, Schreiber R. How cells respond to interferons. Annu Rev Biochem 1998; 67:227–264.

8. Heldin C. Signal transduction: multiple pathways, multiple options for therapy. Stem Cells 2001; 19(4):295–303.

9. Darnell JE Jr. Transcription factors as targets for cancer therapy. Nat Rev Cancer 2002; 2:740–749.

10. Luo J, Manning B, Cantley L. Targeting the PI3K-Akt pathway in human cancer: rationale and promise. Cancer Cell 2003; 4:257–262.

11. Manning G, Whyte D, Martinez R, Hunter T, Sudarsanam S. The protein kinase complement of the human genome. Science 2002; 298:1912–1934.

12. Luker G, Sharma V, Pica C et al. Noninvasive imaging of protein–protein interactions in living animals. Proc Natl Acad Sci USA 2002; 99:6961–6966.

13. Luker G, Sharma V, Piwnica-Worms D. Visualizing protein–protein interactions in living animals. Methods 2003; 29:110–122.

14. Ray P, Pimenta H, Paulmurugan R et al. Noninvasive quantitative imaging of protein–protein interactions in living subjects. Proc Natl Acad Sci USA 2002; 99:2105–3110.

15. Paulmurugan R, Umezawa Y, Gambhir SS. Noninvasive imaging of protein–protein interactions in living subjects by using reporter protein complementation and reconstitution strategies. Proc Natl Acad Sci USA 2002; 99(24):15608–15613.

16. Toby G, Golemis E. Using the yeast interaction trap and other two-hybrid-based approaches to study protein–protein interactions. Methods 2001; 24:201–217.

17. Lievens S, Heyden J, Vertenten E, Plum J, Vandekerckhove J, Tavernier J. Design of a fluorescence-activated cell sorting-based mammalian protein–protein interaction trap. Methods Mol Biol 2004; 263:293–310.

18. Fields S, Song O. A novel genetic system to detect protein–protein interaction. Nature 1989; 340:245–246.

19. von Mering C, Krause R, Snel B et al. Comparative assessment of large-scale sets of protein–protein interactions. Nature 2002; 471:399–403.

20. Luker G, Sharma V, Pica C, Prior J, Li W, Piwnica-Worms D. Molecular imaging of protein–protein interactions: controlled expression of p53 and large T antigen fusion proteins *in vivo*. Cancer Res 2003; 63:1780–1788.

21. Luker G, Sharma V, Piwnica-Worms D. Noninvasive imaging of protein–protein interactions in living animals. In: Conn PM, ed. Handbook of Proteomic Methods. Totowa, NJ: Humana Press, Inc, 2003:283–298.

22. Rossi F, Blakely B, Blau H. Interaction blues: protein interactions monitored in live mammalian cells by beta-galactosidase complementation. Trends Cell Biol 2000; 10(3):119–122.

23. Rossi F, Charlton C, Blau H. Monitoring protein–protein interactions in intact eukaryotic cells by beta-galactosidase complementation. Proc Natl Acad Sci USA 1997; 94(16):8405–8410.

24. Wehrman T, Kleaveland B, Her JH, Balint RF, Blau HM. Protein–protein interactions monitored in mammalian cells via complementation of beta-lactamase enzyme fragments. Proc Natl Acad Sci USA 2002; 99(6):3469–3474.
25. Remy I, Michnick S. Clonal selection and *in vivo* quantitation of protein interactions with protein-fragment complementation assays. Proc Natl Acad Sci USA 1999; 96:5394–5399.
26. Remy I, Wilson I, Michnick S. Erythropoietin receptor activation by a ligand-induced conformation change. Science 1999; 283:990–993.
27. Galarneau A, Primeau M, Trudeau L-E, Michnick S. β-Lactamase protein fragment complementation assays as *in vivo* and *in vitro* sensors of protein–protein interactions. Nat Biotechnol 2002; 20:619–622.
28. Ozawa T, Kaihara A, Sato M, Tachihara K, Umezawa. Split luciferase as an optical probe for detecting protein–protein interactions in mammalian cells based on protein splicing. Anal Chem 2001; 73:2516–2521.
29. Paulmurugan R, Gambhir S. Monitoring protein–protein interactions using split synthetic *Renilla* luciferase protein-fragment-assisted complementation. Anal Chem 2003; 75:1584–1589.
30. Luker K, Piwnica-Worms D. Optimizing luciferase protein fragment complementation for bioluminescent imaging of protein–protein interactions in live cells and animals. Methods Enzymol 2004; 385:349–360.
31. Paulmurugan R, Massoud T, Huang J, Gambhir S. Molecular imaging of drug-modulated protein–protein interactions in living subjects. Cancer Res 2004; 64:2113–2119.
32. Massoud T, Paulmurugan R, Gambhir S. Molecular imaging of homodimeric protein–protein interactions in living subjects. FASEB J 2004; 18:1105–1107.
33. Luker K, Smith M, Luker G, Gammon S, Piwnica-Worms H, Piwnica-Worms D. Kinetics of regulated protein–protein interactions revealed with firefly luciferase complementation imaging in cells and living animals. Proc Natl Acad Sci USA 2004; 101:12288–12293.
34. Chen J, Zheng X, Brown E, Schreiber S. Identification of an 11-kDa FKBP12-rapamycin-binding domain within the 289-kDa FKBP12-rapamycin-associated protein and characterization of a critical serine residue. Proc Natl Acad Sci USA 1995; 92(11):4947–4951.
35. Ostermeier M, Nixon A, Shim J, Benkovic S. Combinatorial protein engineering by incremental truncation. Proc Natl Acad Sci USA 1999; 96:3562–3567.
36. Johnsson N, Varshavsky A. Split ubiquitin as a sensor of protein interactions *in vivo*. Proc Natl Acad Sci USA 1994; 91:10340–10344.
37. Stagljar I, Korostensky C, Johnsson N, te Heesen S. A genetic system based on split - ubiquitin for the analysis of interactions between membrane proteins *in vivo*. Proc Natl Acad Sci USA 1998; 95:5187–5192.
38. Aronheim A, Zandi E, Hennemann H, Elledge S, Karin M. Isolation of an AP-1 repressor by a novel method for detecting protein–protein interactions. Mol Cell Biol 1997; 17:3094–3102.
39. Broder Y, Katz S, Aronheim A. The Ras recruitment system, a novel approach to the study of protein–protein interactions. Curr Biol 1998; 8:1121–1124.
40. Eyckerman S, Verhee A, Van der Heyden J et al. Design and application of a cyto-kine-receptor-based interaction trap. Nat Cell Biol 2001; 3:1114–1119.

41. Gautier I, Tranier M, Durieux C et al. Homo-FRET microscopy in living cells to measure monomer–dimer transition of GFP-tagged proteins. Biophys J 2001; 80:3000–3008.

42. Boute N, Jockers R, Issad T. The use of resonance energy transfer in high-throughput screening: BRET versus FRET. Trends Pharmacol Sci 2002; 23(8):351–354.

43. Zhang J, Campbell R, Ting A, Tsien R. Creating new fluorescent probes for cell biology. Nat Rev Mol Cell Biol 2002; 3:906–918.

44. Xu Y, Kanauchi A, von Arnim A, Piston D, Johnson C. Bioluminescence resonance energy transfer: monitoring protein–protein interactions in living cells. Methods Enzymol 2003; 360:289–301.

45. Kenworthy A. Imaging protein–protein interactions using fluorescence resonance energy transfer microscopy. Methods 2001; 24:289–296.

46. Tsien R. The green fluorescent protein. Annu Rev Biochem 1998; 67:509–544.

47. Strangmann G, Boas D, Sutton J. Non-invasive neuroimaging using near-infrared light. Biol Psychiatry 2002; 52:679–693.

48. Mochizuki N, Yamashita S, Kurokawa K et al. Spatio-temporal images of growth-factor-induced activation of Ras and Rap1. Nature 2001; 411:1065–1068.

49. Miyawaki A, Tsien R. Monitoring protein conformations and interactions by fluorescence resonance energy transfer between mutants of green fluorescent protein. Methods Enzymol 2000; 327:472–500.

50. Kurokawa K, Mochizuki N, Ohba Y, Mizuno H, Miyawaki A, Matsuda M. A pair of fluorescent resonance energy transfer-based probes for tyrosine phosphorylation of the CrkII adaptor protein *in vivo*. J Biol Chem 2001; 276:31305–31310.

51. Chan FK-M, Siegel R, Zacharias D et al. Fluorescence resonance energy transfer analysis of cell surface receptor interactions and signaling using spectral variants of the green fluorescent protein. Cytometry 2001;44:361–368.

52. Tai Y, Chatziioannou A, Yang Y et al. MicroPET II: design, development and initial performance of an improved microPET scanner for small-animal imaging. Phys Med Biol 2003; 48:1519–1537.

53. Cherry S. *In vivo* molecular and genomic imaging: new challenges for imaging physics. Phys Med Biol 2004; 49:R13–R48.

54. Ntziachristos V, Tung C, Bremer C, Weissleder R. Fluorescence molecular tomography resolves protease activity *in vivo*. Nat Med 2002; 8:757–761.

55. Bhaumik S, Gambhir S. Optical imaging of *Renilla* luciferase reporter gene expression in living mice. Proc Natl Acad Sci USA 2001; 99(1):377–382.

56. Pichler A, Prior J, Piwnica-Worms D. Imaging reversal of multidrug resistance in living mice with bioluminescence: MDR1 P-glycoprotein transports coelenterazine. Proc Natl Acad Sci USA 2004; 101:1702–1707.

57. Piwnica-Worms D, Schuster D, Garbow J. Molecular imaging of host–pathogen interactions in intact small animals. Cell Microbiol 2004; 6:319–331.

13

Functional Imaging of Cellular Death

ROBERT H. MACH

Washington University School of Medicine,
St. Louis, Missouri

I. Introduction

Apoptosis is a tightly regulated mode of cellular death that does not result in injury to neighboring cells or elicit an inflammatory response. On the other hand, necrosis is a catastrophic, unregulated mode of cell death that is followed by the invasion of inflammatory cells (1). Although apoptosis and necrosis are caused by distinct biochemical pathways, there is a great deal of experimental evidence to suggest that both processes are observed in diseases characterized by abnormal cellular death. Although there are a number of factors that can induce cell death, both apoptosis and necrosis are often the end result of the exposure of normal tissue to oxidative stress. When this occurs, the balance between the amount of tissue undergoing apoptosis and necrosis is dependent on a variety of factors including the severity of the oxidative stress. The development of non-invasive imaging procedures for measuring apoptosis and necrosis could provide valuable information regarding the relative contribution of each in tissues undergoing abnormal cellular death. This chapter will provide a review of noninvasive imaging procedures for imaging cellular death *in vivo*. Procedures that are currently being used in human imaging studies as well as newer strategies currently under development will be presented. A description of the use of the imaging agents, ^{99m}Tc-pyrophophate and ^{111}In-antimyosin, for imaging necrosis in myocardial infarction will not be presented but can be found in the recent review by Flotats and Carrio (2).

II. Apoptosis vs. Necrosis

Apoptosis, or programmed cell death, has received a great deal of attention over the past 10 years. It has been estimated that the human body eliminates about 10^{11} cells daily, mostly by apoptosis (3). This level of cellular death represents a mass of cells equivalent to an entire body weight on an annual basis. Therefore, apoptosis is critical for the normal development and function of multicellular organisms, and the fundamental process of apoptosis has been highly conserved throughout evolution. The abnormal regulation of cellular death via apoptosis is believed to play a key role in a variety of human diseases.

There are two separate pathways by which cells can undergo apoptosis, extrinsic, and intrinsic pathways. The extrinsic pathway is initiated by the activation of extracellular receptors, termed death receptors. A classification of the various death receptors, and the ligands known to activate these receptors, is given in Table 13.1. The binding of the death receptor ligand to its receptor results in the initiation of a sequence of cellular signaling events leading to the activation of a series of enzymes termed caspases. A detailed description of the cascade of molecular events leading to apoptosis is beyond the scope of this chapter but can be found in a number of excellent reviews (1–5).

The term caspase is a contraction of name, cysteine-dependent aspartate-specific proteases (3). The enzymatic properties of the caspases are determined by their specificity for substrates containing an aspartic acid residue and the utilization of a cysteine side chain for catalyzing peptide bond cleavage. Caspases exist in the cytosol as inactive zymogens termed procaspases. Caspase activation occurs when the cell receives an apoptotic signal, a process that involves cleavage of the inactive zymogen into large ($\sim$20 kDa) and small ($\sim$10 kDa)

Table 13.1 Death Receptors and Death Receptor Ligands Associated with the Extrinsic Pathway of Apoptosis

Receptors	Ligand
Death receptors[a]	
CD95 (a.k.a. Fas, Apo1)	CD95L
TNFR1 (a.k.a. p55, CD120a)	TNF
TNFR2	TNF
Death Receptor 2 (DR2)	TRAIL
DR3 (a.k.a. Apo3, WSL-1, TRAMP, or LARD)	Apo3L (a.k.a. TWEAK)
NGFR	NGF, BDNF, NT-3, NT-4
LTβR	LT$\alpha2\beta1$, LT$\alpha1\beta2$
Decoy receptor[b]	
DCR1	TRAIL
DCR2	TRAIL
DR4	TRAIL
DR5	TRAIL
DR6	?

[a]Binding of death receptor ligand to death receptor induces apoptosis.
[b]Binding of death receptor ligand to decoy receptor protects cell against apoptosis.

subunits, and dimerization to form the catalytically active form of the enzyme. There are two different classes of caspases involved in apoptosis, the initiator caspases and the executioner caspases. The initiator caspases (caspase-6, -8, -9, and -10) are located at the top of the signaling cascade; their primary function is to activate the executioner caspases (caspase-2, -3, and -7). The executioner caspases are responsible for the physiological (e.g., cleavage of the DNA repair enzyme PARP-1, nuclear laminins and cytoskeleton proteins) and morphological changes (DNA strand breaks, nuclear membrane damage, membrane blebbing) that occur in apoptosis (1). A third class of caspases, caspases-1, -4, -5, and -13, are involved in the processing of proinflammatory cytokines and are not believed to play an active role in apoptosis.

A second signaling pathway leading to apoptosis is the intrinsic pathway. The death receptors are responsible for initiating the extrinsic pathway of apoptosis, whereas the mitochondria are responsible for initiating the intrinsic pathway of apoptosis (1). The intrinsic pathway of apoptosis occurs in response to intracellular events such as increased reactive oxygen and nitrogen species (ROS/RNS) such as peroxynitrite, peroxynitrous acid, and alkyl peroxynitrites. The intrinsic pathway is triggered by senescence and environmental insults and involves the release of cytochrome c from the mitochondrial membrane. Cytochrome c binds with the protein, Apaf-1, resulting in the formation in the apoptosome complex. The apoptosome complex activates caspase-9, which in turn activates caspase-3. The regulation of the intrinsic pathway of apoptosis is also determined by the interaction and relative abundance of the Bcl-2 family of proteins. The proteins of the Bcl-2 family can be divided into two groups, the proapoptotic (Bax, Bak, and Bod) and antiapoptotic (Bcl-2, Bcl-Xl, Bfl-1, and Bcl-W) proteins. The cascade of events regulating the intrinsic pathway of apoptosis is a rapidly evolving area of research. A detailed discussion of the complex interactions between pro- and antiapoptotic proteins is beyond the scope of this chapter, but several excellent reviews of this subject have been recently published (3–5).

Apoptosis represents a tightly regulated, conserved mode of cell death that does not injure neighboring cells, whereas necrosis represents a more severe form of cell demise compared with apoptosis. Necrosis consists of a catastrophic, unregulated mode of cell death that is followed by an invasion of inflammatory cells (1). In addition to the numerous biochemical and morphological differences between apoptosis and necrosis, perhaps the most distinctive feature of necrosis is the disintegration of the plasma membrane, as opposed to the compaction of cells undergoing apoptosis (6). The loss of the plasma membrane results in the leakage of cell content from necrotic cells into the surrounding tissue, which induces an inflammatory response and secondary tissue damage. Cells undergoing apoptosis are rapidly cleared by macrophages, resulting in little or no secondary tissue damage.

The key molecular event characterizing necrosis is the activation of the enzyme poly(ADP-ribose) polymerase-1 (PARP-1). PARP-1 is a chromatin-associated enzyme that detects and repairs single strand breaks in DNA that are induced by a variety of toxic insults (6). Although the degradation of PARP-1 is a key initial step in the induction of apoptosis, the functional activation of this enzyme plays a critical role in necrosis. Exposure of the cell to a variety of toxic stimuli such as ROS/RNS, ionizing radiation, and genotoxic chemicals results in the formation of nicks and breaks in the DNA strand. In response to this DNA damage, PARP-1 becomes activated and catalyzes the formation of poly-ADP on acceptor proteins such as topoisomerases I and II, DNA polymerase, DNA ligase 2, and histones (7). As NAD^+ is a substrate for the formation of poly-ADP ribosylation reactions, the activation of PARP-1 under genotoxic stimuli results in a depletion of cellular NAD^+ levels and a disruption cellular energetics (i.e., glycolysis, β-oxidation of fatty acids and the TCA cycle require NAD^+ and are disrupted following PARP-1 activation). Therefore, the difference in level of PARP-1 activity represents a major feature in discriminating between cell death caused by apoptosis and that caused by necrosis. Apoptosis is characterized by a *reduction* in PARP-1 levels through the enzymatic action of caspase-3 and caspase-7, which results in an increase in DNA strand breaks and DNA fragmentation. As necrosis does not involve the activation of caspases, genotoxic stimuli resulting in DNA nicks and strand breaks results in an *activation* of PARP-1 to the extent where NAD^+ levels are depleted, resulting in cell death due to a disruption in cellular energetics (6,7).

III. The Need to Discriminate Between Apoptosis and Necrosis

On the basis of the earlier discussion, it is clear that apoptosis and necrosis represent two ends of a continuum: apoptosis is a highly regulated form of cellular death, that is, triggered by the exposure of a cell to mild oxidative stress, whereas necrosis is a severe form of cell death, that is, triggered by the exposure of a cell to severe oxidative stress (Fig. 13.1). It is currently believed that cellular death under a variety of pathological conditions represents a balance between apoptosis and necrosis. Although it was initially thought that apoptosis and necrosis could not be stopped once the process was initiated, recent studies suggest that pharmacological intervention can minimize cell death and tissue damage resulting from via these pathways. For example, inhibitors of both caspase-3 (apoptosis) and PARP-1 (necrosis) have been shown to reduce the amount of cellular and tissue damage in cell culture and animal models of disease (8–10). Although these data are encouraging, it must be emphasized that these studies were conducted under experimental conditions that favored one form of cell death over the other. It is more likely that cell death under pathological conditions consists of a mixture of both apoptosis and necrosis, with the relative balance between the two different pathways determined by the severity and the duration of the

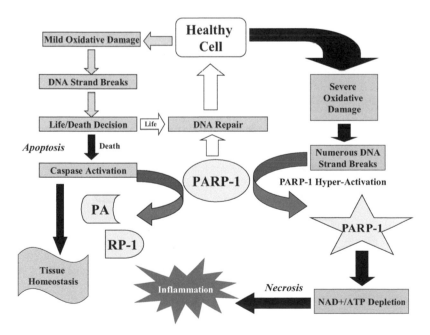

Figure 13.1 Cartoon showing the two different pathways of cellular death following exposure of a cell to oxidative stress.

toxic insult. Therefore, methods that could be used to determine the level of apoptosis vs. necrosis under a variety of pathological conditions would be of tremendous value in identifying a pharmacological treatment aimed at minimizing the extent of cellular death.

Figure 13.2 represents two hypothetical situations illustrating this point. The picture on the left consists of a large area of necrosis surrounded by a penumbra of apoptosis. The picture on the right consists of a large region of apoptosis containing a small necrotic core. Treatment of the condition on the left with a pancaspase inhibitor or a selective caspase-3, caspase-7 inhibitor would result in only a marginal effect because most of the tissue is undergoing cellular death via necrosis, which does not involve caspase activation (Fig. 13.1). In this case, an inhibitor of PARP-1 would be more effective in minimizing cell death. Similarly, treatment of the condition on the right with a PARP-1 inhibitor would be relatively ineffective as PARP-1 is cleaved by caspase-3 and caspase-7 in the large region undergoing apoptosis and only the small necrotic core would be spared. In this case, treatment with either a pancaspase inhibitor or a selective inhibitor of caspase-3, caspase-7 would result in a greater sparing of tissue. Unfortunately, the factors determining the balance between apoptosis and necrosis in tissue undergoing abnormal cellular death are not clear at this time.

Although Fig. 13.2 describes a hypothetical situation, there is ample experimental evidence to suggest that both apoptosis and necrosis occur in a wide variety of disease conditions. A prominent example of this is the condition of ischemia–reperfusion injury in cardiovascular disease. Prolonged regional myocardial ischemia without reperfusion causes myocyte cell death. However, reperfusion after even a brief period of ischemia can also lead to cellular death even though restoration of blood flow is necessary to salvage the myocardium.

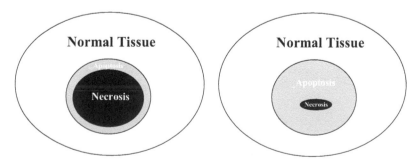

Figure 13.2 Representation of two hypothetical conditions of abnormal cellular death (Apoptosis: Caspase-3 active, PARP-1; Necrosis: Caspase-3 inactive, PARP-1 hyperactivated). The example on the left consists of a large area of necrosis surrounded by a small penumbra of apoptosis. This condition would benefit greater from treatment with a PARP-1 inhibitor. The condition on the right consists of a large area of apoptosis surrounding a small necrotic core. This condition would benefit more from treatment with either a pancaspase inhibitor or a selective inhibitor of caspase-3.

This condition is referred to as ischemia–reperfusion injury. Several studies in animal models of ischemia–reperfusion injury have shown that the principal cause of cellular death is necrosis (11–13). However, other studies have shown that cellular death consisted of a necrotic core surrounded by a perinecrotic area that displayed properties consistent with apoptosis (11,14–18). Therefore, it is likely that cellular death resulting from ischemia–reperfusion injury can consist of a mixture of apoptosis and necrosis, depending on the extent and duration of the ischemia prior to reperfusion. Other disease conditions where evidence demonstrating both apoptosis and necrosis occur includes diabetic cardiomyopathy, sepsis, stroke, and the neurodegenerative disorders Alzheimer's disease and Parkinson's disease. The development of a noninvasive imaging technique capable of measuring apoptosis and necrosis independently could provide valuable information on the balance between apoptosis and necrosis, and if there is a temporal shift in the balance of these mechanisms of cellular death, in a wide variety of pathological conditions.

IV. Measurement of Apoptosis and Necrosis *In Vitro*

There are a number of *in vitro* methods for determining whether cells are undergoing apoptosis. One method involves the use of the anticoagulant annexin V. Annexin V is a member of a family of Ca-dependent phospholipid binding proteins that binds with high affinity to phosphatidyl serine (PS). One of the early events occurring in apoptosis is the "PS shift" (Fig. 13.2). The outer leaflet of the plasma membrane contains mainly neutral phospholipids or cationic phospholipids such as phosphatidylcholine and sphingomyelin. The inner membrane contains aminophospholipids such as PS and phosphatidylethanolamine. Cationic phospholipids are pumped to the outer leaflet by the enzyme floppase, whereas the enzyme translocase is responsible for recruiting PS and phosphatidylethanolamine to the inner leaflet of the plasma membrane. Therefore, PS is generally absent from the extracellular space in healthy cells. During apoptosis, there is an increase in intracellular calcium levels that deactivates translocase and floppase [for a review, see Ref. (2)]. The calcium increase also activates the enzyme scramblase, which facilitates the bidirectional movement of phospholipids within the lipid bilayer and a translocation of PS from the cytoplasmic surface of the plasma membrane to the external cell surface (PS shift). *In vitro* detection of externalized PS can be measured with either flow cytometry or fluorescence microscopy by using annexin V that has been derivatized with a fluorescent tag. However, as the PS shift occurs in both necrosis and apoptosis, the discrimination between apoptosis and necrosis using either flow cytometry or fluorescence microscopy requires a second step, the propidium iodide (PI) exclusion test (1). PI is an intercalating agent that forms a fluorescent complex with DNA. As PI is a charged molecule, it is unable to cross the cell membrane and intercalate the DNA of cells undergoing apoptosis because apoptotic cells have an intact cell membrane (Fig. 13.3). In contrast, necrosis is characterized by the loss of integrity of the plasma and nuclear membranes, which enables the PI to enter the cell and label DNA. Therefore, cells having a positive fluorescent signal from the annexin V study and a negative fluorescent signal from the PI labeling study are undergoing apoptosis, whereas cells giving a positive fluorescent signal under both conditions (i.e., annexin V and PI labeling) are undergoing necrosis.

Another common method for measuring apoptosis is the DNA labeling technique, terminal deoxytransferase-mediated dUTP nick-end labeling (TUNEL). In this method, labeling of DNA strand breaks at the 3′ end is achieved by using the enzyme, terminal deoxynucleotidyl transferase (TdT) and either a radioactive or a fluorescently-labeled deoxynucleotide. This method provides a very sensitive measurement of DNA strands breaks. However, as DNA strand

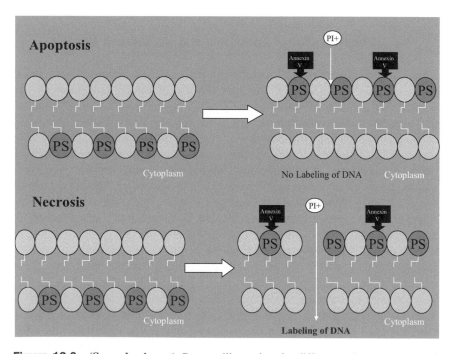

Figure 13.3 **(See color insert)** Cartoon illustrating the differences between apoptosis and necrosis. Membrane inversion resulting in the exposure of phosphatidyl serine (PS) to the extracellular space occurs in both apoptosis and necrosis. Since the cell membrane remains intact during apoptosis, the charged molecule propidium iodide (PI) cannot enter the cell and label DNA, whereas the disruption of the cell and nuclear membrane that occurs in necrosis allows PI to enter the cell and label DNA. Therefore, cells that are annexin V (+)/PI (−) are undergoing apoptosis, whereas cells that are annexin V (+)/ PI (+) are undergoing necrosis.

breaks occur in apoptosis and necrosis, this method can not be used to discriminate between the two different mechanisms of cellular death.

An alternative strategy for measuring apoptosis is the use of antibodies directed toward the enzymes involved in apoptosis. As caspase-3 activation occurs in both extrinsic and intrinsic pathways, the use of caspase-3 immunohistochemical staining is a common method used in measuring apoptosis. Because caspase-3 is not activated in necrosis, the immunohistochemical measurement of activated caspase-3 provides a sensitive method for measuring apoptosis.

As stated earlier, one of the primary functions of caspase-3 and caspase-7 in the induction of apoptosis is to degrade the DNA repair enzyme, PARP-1. Caspase-3 and caspase-7 recognize a DEVD motif and cleavage at this site separates the DNA binding domain from the catalytic domain. This degradation of PARP-1 is critical for the ensuing DNA fragmentation that is characteristic of apoptosis. Therefore, the immunohistochemical measurement of the two PARP-1 *cleavage products* is another sensitive method for measuring apoptosis vs. necrosis (1).

There are two methods for measuring PARP-1 function in tissues. The first method involves using immunohistochemistry techniques using antibodies raised against PARP-1 itself. However, many of the antibodies for PARP-1 recognize both the full length 116 kDa protein as well as the large (89 kDa) and small (24 kDa) fragments resulting from cleavage by caspase-3 and caspase-7 during apoptosis. PARP-1 is also one of the most abundant nuclear proteins, with one molecule of PARP-1 present per 1000 bp of DNA. Therefore, the depletion of NAD and ATP that results in cellular death by necrosis is thought to occur via a hyperactivation of PARP-1 and not an increase in synthesis of PARP-1 protein. A second method for measuring PARP-1 function is the use of antibodies raised for the product of PARP-1, poly-ADP ribose. PARP-1 catalyzes the ADP ribosylation of a number of proteins involved in the DNA repair process, including histones, DNA topoisomerases I and II, DNA polymerases, and DNA ligase 2. Therefore, the significant signal amplification obtained by using antibodies raised against poly-ADP ribose provides a sensitive method for measuring the hyperactivation of PARP-1 that occurs in necrosis.

V. Measurement of Apoptosis and Necrosis *In Vivo* Using Functional Imaging Techniques

Although there are numerous methods for measuring apoptosis and necrosis *in vitro* utilizing commercially-available reagents, the development of radiotracers or contrast agents that can make similar measurements *in vivo* with noninvasive imaging techniques such as positron emission tomography (PET), single photon emission computed tomography (SPECT), magnetic resonance imaging (MRI) and spectroscopy (MRS), and optical imaging has occurred at a much slower pace.

A. Radiolabeled Annexin V Analogs

Annexin V is an endogenous intracellular human protein with a molecular weight of 35 kDa. It has a high affinity for anionic phospholipids such as PS that are exposed to the extracellular space during PS inversion that occurs early in the process of apoptosis. Binding of annexin V to PS is a reversible, calcium-dependent process. The affinity of annexin V for PS is ~7 nM (2) and is comparable to many small molecule radiotracers used for imaging receptors systems. The success of fluorescein-tagged annexin V for the *in vitro* measurement of apoptosis has lead to annexin V analogs labeled with a radionuclide compatible with noninvasive imaging techniques such as SPECT and PET.

The first group to report the use of a radiolabeled annexin V analog in non-invasive imaging studies of apoptosis was Blankenberg et al. (19). In this study, ^{99m}Tc-HYNIC annexin V was used and a series of studies were conducted in three different animal models of apoptosis: (1) Fas antibody-mediated fulminant hepatic apoptosis, (2) cardiac allograft rejection model in Sprague-Dawley rats, and (3) a murine model of lymphoma following treatment with cyclophosphamide (100 mg/kg, i.p.). In mice treated with Fas antibody, there was a progressive increase in ^{99m}Tc-HYNIC annexin V uptake in liver and spleen which was confirmed with annexin V immunohistochemical staining. Similar results were reported in the cardiac allograft and cyclosphamide-treated tumor models. However, as noted by the authors, ^{99m}Tc-HYNIC annexin V does not discriminate between apoptosis and necrosis as PS is located on the outer membrane leaflet in both forms of cellular death. Annexin V has also been labeled with ^{99m}Tc using the N_2S_2 chelation systems, 4,5-*bis*(thioacetamido)pentanoyl annexin V (BTAP annexin V) (20,21) and ethylenedicysteine (^{99m}Tc-EC annexin V) (22). The ^{99m}Tc-complex of *N*-1-immino-4-mercaptobutyl-annexin V (^{99m}Tc-I annexin V) has also been reported (23).

Although all forms of annexin V labeled with ^{99m}Tc are capable of imaging cellular death, there are some subtle differences in the *in vivo* characteristics of each radiotracer. For example, Boersma et al. (21) conducted a study directly comparing ^{99m}Tc-I annexin V and ^{99m}Tc-BTAP annexin V in humans. They found that the radiochemical yield of ^{99m}Tc-I annexin V was lower than that of ^{99m}Tc-BTAP annexin V, with unlabeled ^{99m}Tc-pertechnetate being the main radiolabeled impurity. Both complexes displayed biphasic clearance kinetics from plasma, consisting of a fast compartment ($t_{1/2} = 4 - 40$ min) and a slow compartment ($t_{1/2} = 1.2 - 7.4$ h). Both ^{99m}Tc-I annexin V and ^{99m}Tc-BTAP annexin V displayed a high uptake in the kidney and liver, which correspond to the routes of excretion of the radiotracers. In contrast to the plasma clearance kinetics, there was also a significant difference between the biological half-life of the two different complexes; ^{99m}Tc-I annexin V had a biological half-life of 62 ± 13 h, whereas ^{99m}Tc-BTAP annexin V had a half-life of 16 ± 7 h. SPECT studies also revealed that the best time for imaging myocardial infarction ranged between 15 and 20 h after administration of the radiotracer, whereas imaging of tumors is best performed between 5 and 15 h after tracer administration, depending on the location of the tumor (21). The difference in biological half-life between the two agents indicates that ^{99m}Tc-I annexin V is suitable for imaging myocardial infarction, whereas ^{99m}Tc-BTAP annexin V is better suited for imaging the response to therapy in tumor imaging protocols.

A number of clinical research studies using ^{99m}Tc-labeled annexin V complexes have been reported over the past 5 years (Table 13.2) (20,22–30). Both ^{99m}Tc-I annexin V and ^{99m}Tc-BTAP annexin V have been used to measure cell death occurring in myocardial infarction. For example, Thimister et al. (26)

Table 13.2 Clinical Imaging Studies Using Radiolabeled Annexin V Analogs

Agent	Study	Reference
Human studies		
^{99m}Tc-HYNIC annexin V	Acute heart- or lung-transplant rejection	Blankenberg and Strauss (24)
^{99m}Tc-HYNIC annexin V	Lung transplant rejection	Blankenberg et al. (25)
^{99m}Tc-HYNIC annexin V	Heart transplant rejection	Narula et al. (27)
^{99m}Tc-HYNIC annexin V	Head and neck cancer	Van der Wiele et al. (28)
^{99m}Tc-BTAP annexin V	Acute myocardial infarction	Thimister et al. (26)
^{99m}Tc-BTAP annexin V	Pharmacokinetic studies	Kemerink et al. (29)
^{99m}Tc-BTAP annexin V	Lung cancer, lymphoma, breast cancer	Belhocine et al. (30)
[99m]Tc-i-annexin V	Acute myocardial infarction	Hofstra et al. (23)
[99m]Tc-i-annexin V	Pharmacokinetic studies	Kemerink et al. (30)
[99m]Tc BTAP annexin V and ^{99m}Tc-i-annexin V	Pharmacokinetic studies	Kemerink et al. (21)
Animal studies		
^{99m}Tc-HYNIC annexin V	Allograft rejection, FAS-antibody, cyclophosphamide treatment in tumor bearing rodents	Blankenberg et al. (19)
^{99m}Tc-EC annexin V	Paclitaxel treatment in tumor bearing rodents	Yang et al. (22)
^{99m}Tc-HYNIC annexin V	Cyclophosphamide induced apoptosis in rodents	Blankenberg et al. (31)
^{99m}Tc-HYNIC annexin V	Thymic apoptosis	Ohtsuki et al. (32)
[124]I-annexin V and [124]I-SIB annexin	Biodistribution studies	Collingridge et al. (33)
[124]I-SIB annexin	5-HU treatment in tumor bearing mice	Glazer et al. (39)

recently demonstrated that the high uptake of [99mTc]-BTAP annexin V following percutaneous transluminal coronary angioplasty corresponded to the region of perfusion deficit identified with the myocardial blood flow [99mTc]MIBI prior to intervention (Fig. 13.4). The authors also suggested that it is possible to differentiate reversible myocardial cell damage from necrosis by conducting repeat [99mTc]MIBI perfusion/[99mTc]-BTAP annexin V imaging studies days to weeks after revascularization (24). Another important clinical application of [99mTc]-labeled annexin V imaging is the prediction of the response of tumors to chemotherapy. Many functionally-diverse anticancer agents, such as topoisomerase inhibitors, alkylating agents, antimetabolites, and hormone antagonists, generate apoptosis in sensitive cells (34–36). The ability of a tumor to respond to chemotherapy and enter apoptosis can vary significantly from patient to patient. Therefore, a high uptake of [99mTc]-labeled annexin V should be indicative to a positive response to chemotherapy. A recent study demonstrating this concept was reported by Belhocine et al. (20). Using [99mTc]-BTAP annexin V, these investigators reported that it was possible to detect a positive response to chemotherapy as early as 1 day after the first course of chemotherapy. Furthermore, the investigators reported a positive correlation between [99mTc]-BTAP annexin V and overall patient survival in a mixed-patient population of lung cancer and lymphoma patients (Fig. 13.5). This study clearly demonstrates the utility of SPECT imaging with [99mTc]-labeled annexin V complexes in monitoring the response to treatment in cancer patients.

A recent study presented data indicating that it is possible to improve the plasma clearance kinetics of radiolabeled annexin V analogs by treatment of the protein with polyethylene glycol (PEG) (37). Previous studies have shown that PEG-modified proteins exhibit a reduced liver uptake, increased blood circulating half-lives, and an improved signal-to-noise ratio for imaging purposes. In this study, which used [111In]-DTPA-PEG-annexin V, the fast component of plasma clearance ($t_{1/2}$, α) in nude mice was 4.9 h compared with 4.2 min for the nonPEGylated annexin V. The [111In]-DTPA-PEG-annexin V had a much

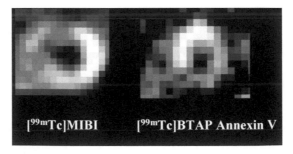

Figure 13.4 (**See color insert**) SPECT study of myocardial infarction. Notice that the increase in uptake of [99mTc]BTAP annexin V corresponds to the perfusion deficit identified in the [99mTc]MIBI scan. This data is reproduced with permission from Ref. (16).

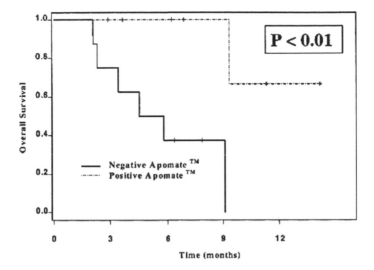

Figure 13.5 Difference in patient outcome in cancer patients showing an increased uptake of [^{99m}Tc]BTAP annexin V (Apomate™), indicating a positive response to chemotherapy-induced apoptosis, vs. those demonstrating a low uptake of the radiotracer. This data is reproduced with permission from Ref. (12).

higher uptake than ^{111}In-DTPA-annexin V in breast tumor-bearing mice treated with poly(L-glutamic acid)-paclitaxel (Xyotax). Furthermore, there was a high correlation between the tumoral uptake of ^{111}In-DTPA-PEG-annexin V and apoptotic index and TUNEL staining (Fig. 13.6) (37). This modification is likely to lead to a dramatic improvement in the signal-to-noise ratio in SPECT studies in cancer patients.

The relatively long biological half-life of radiolabeled annexin V analogs and prolonged time between i.v. administration of the radiotracer and imaging

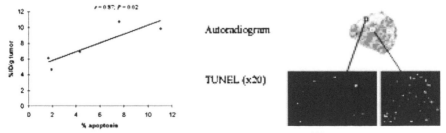

Figure 13.6 (See color insert) Increased tumor uptake of [^{111}In]DTPA-PEG-annexin V. Note the high correlation of tumor uptake of the radiotracer with the apoptotic index (left) and TUNEL staining. This data is reproduced with permission from Ref. (29).

has placed limits on the development of radiotracers for PET imaging studies of apoptosis. Therefore, the PET-based radiotracers for imaging apoptosis using annexin V to label PS have relied on positron-emitting radionuclides having a relatively long half-life such as ^{18}F ($t_{1/2} = 110$ min), ^{124}I ($t_{1/2} = 4.2$ days), and ^{64}Cu ($t_{1/2} = 16.4$ h). The preparation of [^{18}F]-fluorobenzoyl annexin V was accomplished using the four-step procedure outlined in Fig. 13.7 (38). *In vitro* studies indicate that this radiotracer displays a high uptake in Jurkat T-cells undergoing apoptosis induced by UV irradiation. ^{124}I-labeled annexin has been prepared by direct labeling using oxidative radioiodination techniques or by coupling with the reagent *N*-succinimidyl 3-[^{124}I]*m*-iodobenzoate ([^{124}I]SIB annexin V; Fig. 13.7) (39). *In vivo* studies in rodents revealed that [^{124}I]annxein V (prepared via direct labeling of annexin V) undergoes rapid *in vivo* deiodination and accumulation of radioactivity in the thyroid. However, [^{124}I]SIB annexin V was found to have a higher stability with respect to deiodination *in vivo*. The authors also reported that the uptake of [^{124}I]SIB annexin V was higher in human leukemia (HL60) cells undergoing apoptosis induced by the DNA topoisomerase I inhibitor, camphothecin (39). The uptake of [^{124}I]SIB annexin V in apoptotic HL60 cells was blocked by incubation with 100-fold excess annexin V, which is consistent with the labeling of PS residues exposed to the extracellular leaflet during camphothecin-induced apoptosis. Similar results have been reported with [^{124}I]SIB annexin V imaging studies in RIF-I tumor-bearing mice receiving treatment with 5-fluorouracil (33).

B. Imaging Agents Based on Caspase-3

The activation of caspase-3 represents a key event in both pathways of apoptosis, the extrinsic pathway resulting from the activation of death receptors and the intrinsic pathway caused by the release of cytochrome *c* and the formation of the apoptosome complex. Therefore, one method for imaging apoptosis would be to develop radiotracers having a high affinity for activated caspase-3 vs. the inactive zymogen, procaspase-3. Unfortunately, progress in this area of research has been hampered by the limited availability of lead compounds that can be used for radiotracer development. Although a number of potent, peptide-based inhibitors of the caspases have been reported, many of these compounds lack selectivity for caspase-3 (effector caspase) vs. the initiator caspases. An example of this is the pancaspase inhibitor, benzyloxycarbonyl-Val-Ala-DL-Asp(*O*-methyl)-flyoromethyl ketone (Z-FAD-fmk), which has been radiolabeled with ^{131}I and shown to have a high uptake in hepatoma cells in which apoptosis has been induced by exposure to 25 μM ganciclovir (40).

An interesting variation on imaging caspase-3 activity in cells undergoing apoptosis was recently reported by Laxman et al. (41). In this chapter, the authors created a construct in which the firefly luciferase gene (Luc) was inserted between two estrogen receptor-DEVD sequences (i.e., ER-DEVD-Luc-DEVD-ER), which is the peptide sequence recognized and cleaved by caspase-3.

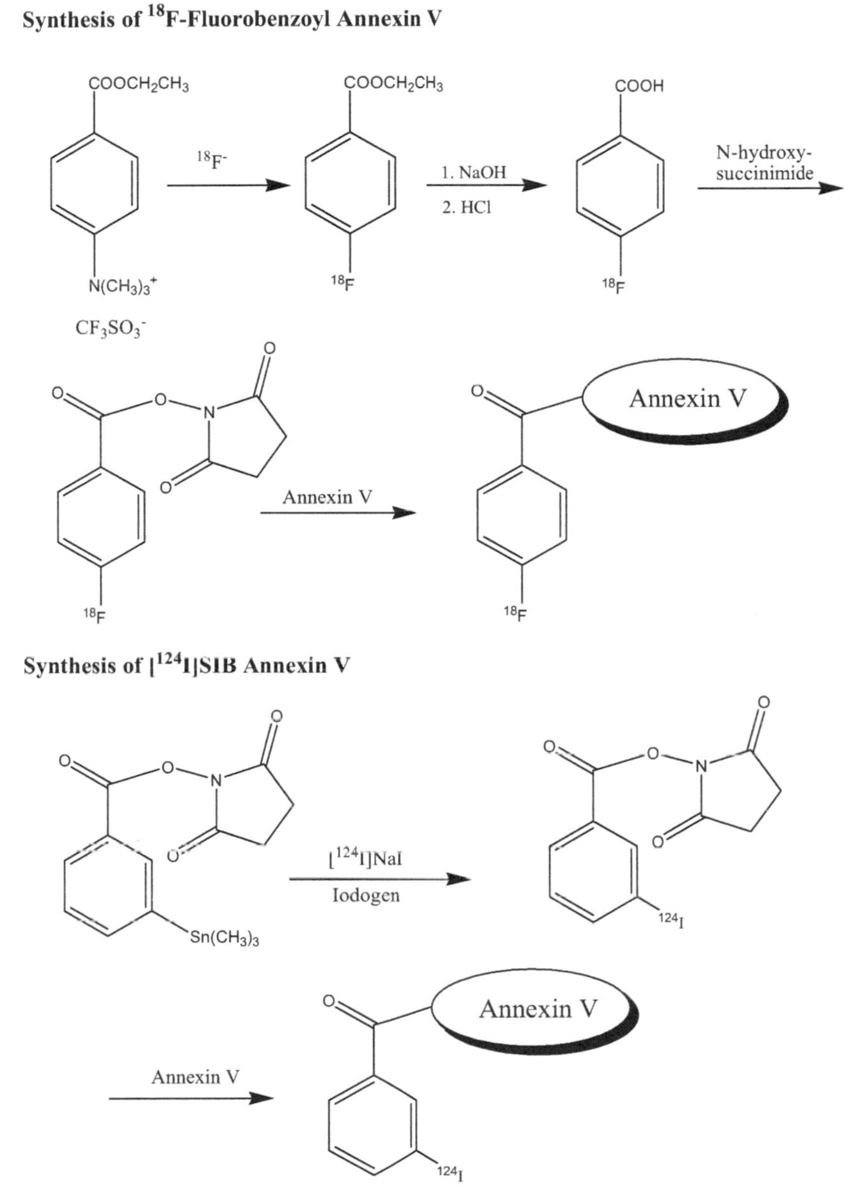

Synthesis of ^{18}F-Fluorobenzoyl Annexin V

Synthesis of [^{124}I]SIB Annexin V

Figure 13.7 Synthesis of ^{18}F- and ^{124}I-labeled annexin V analogs.

The function of the ER domains is to silence the enzymatic activity of the luciferase. The construct was then stably transfected into human glioma (D54) cells and the cells constitutively expressing ER-DEVD-Luc-DEVD-ER were grown in cell culture and subcutaneous tumors were implanted in athymic mice. The animals were then anesthetized with 2% isoflurane and given a single i.p. dose of 150 mg/kg luciferin in normal saline. Bioluminescent imaging studies were conducted under baseline conditions and following induction of apoptosis via intratumoral administration of tumor necrosis factor α-related apoptosis-inducing ligand (TRAIL). The results of this study are shown in Fig. 13.8 and clearly reveal an apoptosis-induced increase in signal. Although this imaging protocol cannot be applied to cancer patients, it demonstrates the ability to image activated caspase-3 in solid tumors undergoing apoptosis. This procedure is currently being used to assess the ability of anticancer drugs to induce apoptosis in animal models.

C. Imaging PARP-1 Activity in Cells Undergoing Necrosis

As stated earlier, the overactivation of PARP-1 levels and depletion of NAD^+ pools is currently believed to be the principal pathway responsible for cellular death via necrosis. Therefore, PARP-1 is thought to play a major role in a variety of pathological conditions including ischemia–reperfusion injury (i.e., myocardial infarction and stroke), septic shock, diabetic cardiomyopathy, and neurodegeneration (Table 13.2). The measurement of PARP-1 levels is currently limited to the use of immunohistochemistry techniques in tissue slices. The development of a radiotracer that could image PARP-1 levels with PET and SPECT would provide a useful tool in studying the role of this enzyme in a variety of pathological conditions.

Previous studies have shown that the phenanthridinone derivative, PJ 34, has a high affinity for PARP-1 (42). PJ 34 inhibits PARP-1 by competing for the NAD^+ binding site in the activated form of the enzyme. Therefore, a radio-labeled version of PJ 34 should be able to measure the hyperactivation of PARP-1 that occurs in the early stages of necrosis.

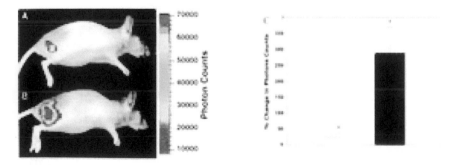

Figure 13.8   (**See color insert**) Bioluminescent imaging study showing TNF-α-induced activation of caspase-3. This data is reproduced with permission from Ref. (33).

Recently, [^{11}C]PJ 34 was synthesized by Mach et al. (43). This was accomplished by N-alkylation of the des-methyl precursor, **1**, with [^{11}C]methyl iodide (Fig. 13.9). Preliminary studies indicate that it is possible to measure PARP-1 activation in animal models of disease. For example, an increase in uptake of [^{11}C]PJ 34 was observed in a rat model of myocardial infarction. In this study, the left anterior descending coronary artery was ligated for 1 h, followed by release of the ligature and reperfusion for 2 h. [^{11}C]PJ 34 was then injected via intravenous administration and a dynamic acquisition microPET imaging study was conducted. The results of this study indicated a dramatic increase in [^{11}C]PJ 34 accumulation in the area distal to the ligation (Fig. 13.10), which is consistent with the activation of PARP-1 activity using immunohistochemical measurements of poly-ADP-ribose formation (44). These data indicate that [^{11}C]PJ 34 may be useful in measuring PARP-1 activation occurring in the early stages of necrosis in a variety of disease states.

VI. Imaging Cell Death During Lung Health and Disease

The various mechanisms of cell death reviewed in this chapter are important to the pathogenesis of lung disease. Of course, both apoptosis and necrosis are important in lung cancer, as they are in virtually all forms of malignancy. However, apoptosis is also important for normal lung development and as part of the normally regulated inflammatory response. Indeed, dysregulation of normal apoptosis may underlie a variety of lung diseases.

For instance, the histopathologic counterpart of acute lung injury is known as "diffuse alveolar damage," a significant component of which is type I alveolar cell necrosis. During the reparative phase of acute lung injury, type II alveolar cells proliferate and differentiate into type I cells as part of a hyperplastic response that is designed to repopulate the alveolar wall, thereby restoring normal lung architecture. As the number of proliferating type II cells is far greater than the number needed to reconstitute the alveolar wall, apoptosis provides a mechanism to clear unnecessary cells without eliciting any additional injurious inflammatory response (45).

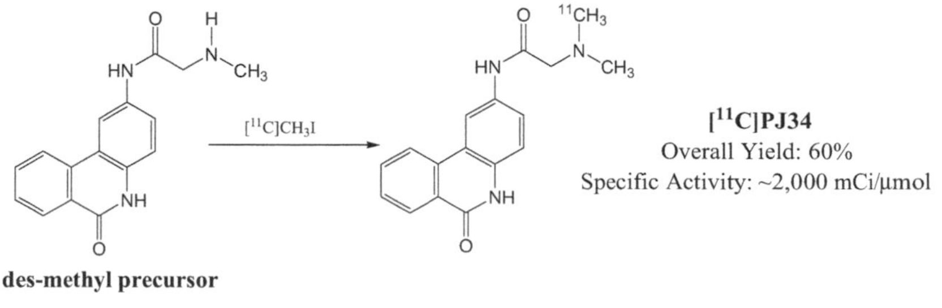

Figure 13.9 Synthesis of [^{11}C]PJ 34.

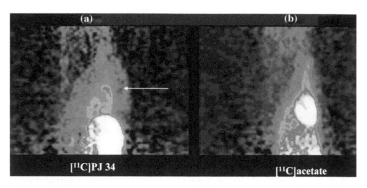

Figure 13.10 (**See color insert**) MicroPET imaging study in a rodent model of ischemia–reperfusion injury. The high uptake of [^{11}C]PJ 34 was distal to the site of the coronary artery ligation (arrow) and is consistent with PARP-1 mediated necrosis. This is in contrast to uniform uptake of the metabolic radiotracer, [^{11}C]acetate, in normal heart.

Not all patients with acute lung injury, however, repair their lungs normally, but instead develop significant tissue fibrosis, impairing normal lung function. Interestingly, increased apoptosis of lung epithelial cells is characteristic of experimental models that result in pulmonary fibrosis (45,46), despite the conventional view that apoptosis provides a mechanism for cell elimination without associated tissue scarring. Furthermore, the blockade of apoptosis in these experimental models reduces collagen deposition that is associated with scar formation (46). Similar observations have been made in diseases of chronic lung fibrosis (46).

Neutrophilic inflammation is characteristic of many lung diseases including acute lung injury, pneumonia, idiopathic pulmonary fibrosis, and asthma. Normally, neutrophils are cleared from the lungs by macrophages and other phagocytic cells after they become apoptotic. However, in the early stages of acute lung injury, neutrophil apoptosis appears to be delayed, prolonging neutrophil life-span, and potentially providing a mechanism for neutrophil-induced tissue injury (45).

Evidence for PARP-1 activation during lung disease also exists. For instance, shear forces associated with mechanical ventilation may result in alveolar epithelial cell necrosis, that is, mediated in part by PARP-1 activation (45). Likewise, PARP-1 activation has been implicated in the pathogenesis of septic shock, an important cause of acute lung injury (47).

It is clear from these observations that more information about mechanisms of cell death during lung health and disease is needed. Most studies of apoptosis in the lungs, however, have been conducted in animal models. Evidence in humans is largely limited to tissue biopsy material and/or biochemical analysis of bronchoalveolar lavage fluid. Such studies are imperfect because of sampling limitations, both temporally (over time) and spatially (selection of sites for tissue biopsy or lavage). Noninvasive imaging methods of monitoring both necrotic and apoptotic forms of cell death should add considerably to our knowledge about the importance of these processes in human lung disease. Furthermore, imaging studies should be useful as markers of treatment effect as strategies are developed that target modification of apoptosis. The interpretation of such studies in humans will have to take into account (after careful validation studies in animal models) that the imaging signal may be affected by increases in apoptosis in some cell populations (e.g., type II cells) and decreases in others (e.g., neutrophils).

VII. Conclusion

The past 5 years have witnessed tremendous progress in the development of non-invasive imaging strategies for measuring programmed cell death in a variety of disease conditions. The most successful strategy examined to date involves the use of radiolabeled annexin V, which measures PS exposed to the extracellular membrane leaflet during the early stages of programmed cell death. However, PS inversion occurs in both apoptosis and necrosis, and this imaging strategy is not able to differentiate between these two functionally different forms of cellular death. The next stage of radiotracer development is expected to focus on targeting specific enzymatic pathways intrinsic to apoptosis or necrosis. The two enzymatic pathways that are likely targets for radiotracer development are the caspase system for apoptosis and PARP-1 for necrosis. Within the caspase system, caspase-3 and/or caspase-7 are the best targets because they are executioner caspases, which are activated once the cell has made the commitment to undergo apoptosis. The most likely molecular target for necrosis in PARP-1, and preliminary studies with [^{11}C]PJ 34 indicate that it is possible to measure PARP-1 hyperactivation occurring in animal models of disease. The development of imaging agents targeting caspase-3 and PARP-1 is likely to be an active area of research over the next few years.

Acknowledgments

The author would like to thank Ms. Terry Sharp for doing the surgery for the rat myocardial ischemia–reperfusion injury model and Dr. Michael Welch for providing the [^{11}C]acetate image. The editorial suggestions of Dr. Dan Schuster were also greatly appreciated. The PARP-1 study described in this chapter was funded by the NIH grant HL13851.

References

1. Neuss M, Crow MT, Chesley A, Lakatta EG. Symposium: programmed cell death-clinical reality and therapeutic strategies. Cardiovasc Drug and Ther 2001; 15:507–523.

2. Flotats A, Carrio I. Non-invasive *in vivo* imaging of myocardial apoptosis and necrosis. Eur J Nucl Med Biol 2003; 30:615–630.
3. Troy CM, Salvessen GS. Caspases on the brain. J Neurosci Res 2002; 69:145–150.
4. Reed JC. Apoptosis-based therapies. Nat Rev Drug Discov 2002; 1:111–121.
5. Leist M, Jaattela M. Four deaths and a funeral: from caspases to alternative mechanisms. Nat Rev Mol Cell Biol 2001; 2:1–10.
6. Virag L, Szabo C. The therapeutic potential of poly(ADP-ribose)polymerase inhibitors. Pharmacol Rev 2002; 54:375–429.
7. Szabo C, Dawson VL. Role of poly(ADP-ribose) synthetase in inflammation and ischaemia–reperfusion. Trends Pharm Sci 1998; 19:287–298.
8. Uchiyama T, Otani H, Okada T, Ninomiya H, Kido M, Imamura H, Nogi S, Kobayashi Y. Nitric oxide induces caspase-dependent apoptosis and necrosis in neonatal rat cardiomyocytes. J Mol Cell Cardiol 2002; 34:1049–1061.
9. Pacher P, Liaudet L, Garcia Soriano F, Mabley JG, Szabo E, Szabo C. The role of poly(ADP-ribose) polymerase activation in the development of myocardial and endothelial dysfunction in diabetes. Diabetes 2002; 51:514–521.
10. McDonald MC, Mota-Filipe H, Wright JA, Abdelrahman M, Threadgill MD, Thompson AS, Thiermermann C. Effects of 5-aminoisoquinoline, a water soluble, potent inhibitor of the activity of poly(ADP-ribose) polymerase on the organ injury and dysfunction caused by haemorrhagic shock. Brit J Pharmacol 2000; 130:843–850.
11. Zhao Z-Q, Vinten-Johansen J. Myocardial apoptosis and ischemic preconditioning. Cardiovascular Res 2002; 55:438–455.
12. Rochitte CE, Lima JAC, Bluemke DA, Reeder SB, McVeigh ER, Furuta T, Becker LC, Melin JA. Magnitude and time course of microvascular obstruction and tissue injury after acute myocardial infarction. Circulation 1998; 98:1006–1014.
13. Matsumura K, Jeremy RW, Schaper J, Becker LC. Progression of myocardial necrosis during reperfusion of ischemic myocardium. Circulation 1998; 97:795–804.
14. Krijnen PAJ, Nijmeijer R, Meijer, CJLM, Visser CA, Hack CE, Niessen HWM. Apoptosis in myocardial ischaemia and infarction. J Clin Pathol 2002; 55:801–811.
15. Saraste A, Pulkki KI, Kallajoki M, Henriksen K, Parvinen M, Liisa-Maria Voipio-Pulkki L-M. Apoptosis in human acute myocardial infarction. Circulation 1997; 95:320–323.
16. Freude B, Masters TN, Kostin S, Robicsek F, Schaper J. Cardiomyocyte apoptosis in acute and chronic conditions. Basic Res Cardiol 1998; 93:85–89.
17. Freude B, Masters TN, Kostin S, Robicsek F, Schaper J. Apoptosis is initiated by myocardial ischemia and executed during reperfusion. J Am Coll Cardiol 2000; 32:197–208.
18. Veinot JP, Gattinger DA, Fliss H. Early apoptosis in human myocardial infarcts. Hum Pathol 1997; 28:485–492.
19. Blankenberg FG, Katsikis PD, Tait JF, Davis RE, Naumovski L, Ohtsuki K, Kopiwoda S, Abrams MJ, Darkes M, Robbins RC, Maecker HT, Strauss HW. *In vivo* detection and imaging of phosphatidylserine expression during programmed cell death. PNAS 1998; 95:6349–6354.

20. Belhocine T, Steinmetx N, Hustinx R, Bartsch P, Jerusalem G, Seidel L, Rigo P, Green A. Increased uptake of the apoptosis-imaging agent ^{99m}Tc recombinant human annexin V in human tumors after one course of chemotherapy as a predictor of tumor response and patient prognosis. Clin Cancer Res 2002; 8:2766–2774.

21. Boersma HH, Liem IH, Kemerink GJ, Thimister PWL, Hofstra L, Stolk LML, van Heerde WL, Pakbiers M-TW, Janssen D, Beysens AJ, Reutelingsperger CPM, Heidendal GAK. Comparison between human pharmacokinetics and imaging properties of two conjugation methods for ^{99m}Tc-Annexin A5. Brit J Radiol 2003; 76:553–560.

22. Yang DJ, Azhdarinia A, Wu P, Yu DF, Tansey W, Kalimi SK, Kim EE, Podoloff DA. *In vivo* and *in vitro* measurement of apoptosis in breast cancer cells using ^{99m}Tc-EC-annexin V. Cancer Biother Radio 2001; 16:73–83.

23. Hofstra L, Liem IH, Dumont EA, Boersma HH, van Heerde WL, Doevendans PA, DeMuinck E, Wellens HJJ, Kemerink GJ, Reutelingsperger CPM, Heidendal GA. Visualization of cell death in patients with acute myocardial infarction. Lancet 2000; 356:209–212.

24. Blankenberg FG, Strauss HW. Non-invasive diagnosis of acute heart- or lung-transplant rejection using radiolabeled annexin V. Pediatr Radiol. 1999; 29:299–305.

25. Blankenberg FG, Robbins RC, Stoot JH, Vriens PW, Berry GJ, Tait JF, Strauss HW. Radionuclide imaging of acute lung transplant rejection with annexin V. Chest 2000; 117:834–840.

26. Thimister PWL, Hofstra L, Liem IH, Boersma HH, Kemerink G, Reutelingsperger CPM, Heidendal GAK. *In vivo* detection of cell death in the area at risk in acute myocardial infarction. J Nucl Med 2003; 44:391–396.

27. Narula J, Acio ER, Narula N, Samuels LE, Fyfe B, Wood D, Fitzpatrick JM, Raghunath PN, Tomaszewski JE, Kelly C, Steinmeitz N, Green A, Tait JF, Leppo J, Blankenberg FG, Jain D, Strauss HW. Annexin-V imaging for noninvasive detection of cardiac allograft rejection. Nat Med 2001; 7:1347–1352.

28. van der Wiele C, Lahorte C, Vermeersch H, Loose D, Merville K, Steinmetz ND, Vanderheyden J-L, Cuvelier CA, Slegers G, Dierck RA. Quantitative tumor apoptosis imaging using Technetium-99m HYNIC annexin V single photon emission computed tomography. J Clin Oncol 2003; 21:3483–3487.

29. Kemerink GJ, Boersma HH, Thimister PW, Hofstra L, Liem IH, Pakbiers MT, Janssen D, Reutelingsperger CP, Heidendal GA. Biodistribution and dosimetry of ^{99m}Tc BTAP-annexin-V in humans. Eur J Nucl Med 2001; 28:1373–1378.

30. Kemerink GJ, Liem IH, Hofstra L, Boersma HH, Buijs CAMW, Reutelingsperger CP, Heidendal GAK. Patient dosimetry of intravenously administered ^{99m}Tc-annexin-V. J Nucl Med 2001; 28:1373–1378.

31. Blankenberg FG, Naumovski L, Tait JF, Post AM, Strauss HW. Imaging cyclophosphamide-induced intramedullary apoptosis in rats using ^{99m}Tc-radiolabelled annexin V. J Nucl Med 2001; 42:309–316.

32. Ohtsuki K, Akashi K, Aoka Y, Blankenberg FG, Kopiwoda S, Tait JF, Strauss HW. Technetium-99m HYNIC-annexin V: a potential radiopharmaceutical for the *in vivo* detection of apoptosis. Eur J Nucl Med 1999; 26:1251–1258.

33. Collingridge DR, Glaser M, Osman S, Barthel H, Hutchinson OC, Luthra SK, Brady F, Bouchier-Hayes L, Martin SJ, Workman P, Price P, Aboagye EO.

In vitro selectivity, *in vivo* biodistribution and tumour uptake of annexin V radio-labelled with a positron emitting radioisotope. Brit J Cancer 2003; 89:1327–1333.

34. Hickman JA. Apoptosis induced by anticancer agents. Cancer Metast Rev 1992; 11:121–139.

35. Dive C, Evans CA, Whetton AD. Induction of apoptosis: new targets for cancer chemotherapy. Semin Cancer Biol 1992; 3:417–427.

36. Lowe SW, Lin AW. Apoptosis in cancer. Carcinogenesis (Lond.) 2000; 21:485–495.

37. Ke S, Wen X, Wu Q-P, Wallace S, Charnsangevi C, Stachowiak AM, Stephens CL, Abbruzzese JL, Podoloff DA, Li C. Imaging taxane-induced tumor apoptosis using PEGylated, ^{111}In-labeled annexin V. J Nucl Med 2004; 45:108–115.

38. Zijlstra S, Gunawan J, Burchert W. Synthesis and evaluation of a ^{18}F-labelled recombinant annexin V derivative, for identification and quantification of apoptotic cells with PET. Appl Radiat Isot 2003; 58:201–207.

39. Glaser M, Collingridge DR, Aboagye EO, Bouchier-Hayes L, Hutchinson OC, Martin SJ, Price P, Brady F, Luthra SK. Iodine-124 labelled annexin V as a potential radiotracer to study apoptosis using positron emission tomography. Appl Radiat Isop 2003; 58:55–62.

40. Haberkorn U, Klinscherf R, Krammer PH, Mier W, Eisenhut M. Investigation of a potential scintigraphic marker of apoptosis: radioiodinated Z-Val-Ala-DL-Asp(O-methyl)-fluoromethyl ketone. Nucl Med Biol 2001; 28:793–798.

41. Laxman B, Hall DE, Bhojani MS, Hamstra DA, Chenevert TL, Ross BD, Rehemtulla A. Noninvasive real-time imaging of apoptosis. PNAS 2002; 99:16551–16555.

42. Soriano FG, Virag L, Jagtap P, Szabo E, Mabley JG, Liaudet L, Marton A, Hoyt DG, Murthy KGK, Salzman AL, Southman GJ, Szabo C. Nature Med 2001; 7:108–113.

43. Mach RH, Chu W, Tu Z, Dence CS, Welch MJ. [^{11}C]PJ34: a PET radiotracer for imaging the role of PARP-1 in necrosis. J Label Compd Radiopharm 2003; 46:S98.

44. Liaudet L, Szabo E, Timashpolsky L, Virag L, Cziraki A, Szabo C. Supression of poly (ADP-ribose) polymerase activation by 3-aminobenzamide in a rat model of myocardial infarction: long-term morphological and functional consequences. Brit J Pharmacol 2001; 133:1424–1430.

45. Martin TR, Nakamura M, Mastute-Bello G. The role of apoptosis in acute lung injury. Crit Care Med 2003; 31(suppl):S184–S188.

46. Uhal BD. Apoptosis in lung fibrosis and repair. Chest 2002; 122 (suppl):293S–298S.

47. Liaudet L. Role of poly(ADP-ribose) polymerase activation in the pathophysiology of septic shock. Adv Sepsis 2002; 2:86–93.

14

Imaging Cell Trafficking

NAOTO OKU and TOMOHIRO ASAI

School of Pharmaceutical Sciences, University of Shizuoka,
Shizuoka, Japan

I. Introduction

Cancer metastasis occurs through a complex cascade of events including the dissociation of malignant cells from the primary site, intravasation, adhesion and invasion to target organs, and growth at the sites of cell disposition (1–3) (Fig. 14.1). A number of molecules are important to this sequential process. Cell adhesion molecules, such as selectins (4) and integrins (5), are involved in the tumor cells' adhesion and invasion to the target organ. Matrix

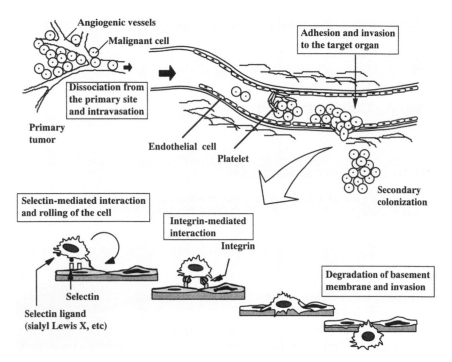

Figure 14.1 Diagram illustrating possible mechanisms involved in producing cancer metastases.

metalloproteinases (6) help to trigger degradation of the basement membrane and are involved in both intravasation and extravasation. Finally, chemokines (7,8) derived from target tissues are thought to be important for determining target tissues.

There are two major theories regarding the determination of metastatic organs. One is the "seed and soil theory" initially introduced by Paget. This theory claims that metastasis is a nonrandom phenomenon, occurring at specific sites which are appropriate for each type of metastatic tumor cell. The second theory is the "anatomical–mechanical theory," which claims that metastasis simply occurs at those sites where enough tumor cells accumulate above some critical level. It may well be that both theories are true.

The adhesion and invasion relationships of metastatic cancer cells to target organs are thought to be similar to those of leukocytes to inflammatory sites in which various cell adhesion molecules are involved (9,10). However, studies of tumor cell trafficking during metastasis have been hampered by the lack of noninvasive techniques to determine real-time trafficking *in vivo*. New and emerging imaging methods may allow an analysis of cell trafficking, thereby helping to clarify the early events of metastasis. We recently reported that posi-tron emission tomography (PET) could be used to monitor cell trafficking of metastasis *in vivo* (11). In this chapter, we review our experience with this method to illustrate how imaging can be used to study cell trafficking in intact animals and humans.

II. Relationship Between Tumor Cell Trafficking and Metastatic Potential

PET with [2-^{18}F]2-fluoro-2-deoxy-D-glucose ([2-^{18}F]FDG) is widely used for the diagnosis of cancer and metastasis because of it's ability to functionally image metabolically active cells. A cancer diagnosis using [2-^{18}F]FDG is based on the higher metabolic demand of tumor cells over normal cells. Once [2-^{18}F]FDG is taken up by a cell, it is phosphorylated and retained inside the cell ("metabolic trapping") (Chapter 9). This feature is also useful for labeling cancerous cells *in vitro*. Therefore, we used [2-^{18}F]FDG as a method for labeling tumor cells. Tumor cells were incubated with [2-^{18}F]FDG for 15–30 min *in vitro*, and highly positron-labeled cells were easily obtained. After washing, the positron-labeled cells were injected into the bloodstream of experimental animals such as rats and mice [Fig. 14.2(a)]. Then, cell trafficking was determined with a PET scanner (SHR-2400 or SHR-7700, Hamamatsu Photonics K.K. Japan) (11). The resolution of this scanner (2.7 mm) is sufficient to discriminate each organ in which the tumor cells accumulate in these small animals.

As an experimental model of animal metastasis, we first used sub-lines of rat 13762NF mammary adenocarcinoma: MTLn3 cells from spontaneous lung metastasis and MTC cells established from a locally growing tumor (12). The [2-^{18}F]FDG-labeled cells were injected into female Fisher 344 rats via a tail vein. The PET emission scan was started immediately after injection and was continued for 1 h. Tissue radioactivity in the form of coincidence gamma photons was measured and then converted to Bq/cm^3 of tissue volume after calibration. Highly metastatic MTLn3 cells accumulated in lungs more than MTC cells which have lower metastatic potential [Fig. 14.2(b)]. Free (noncell associated) [2-^{18}F]FDG accumulated in the heart, liver, and kidneys; however, the radioactivity of the [2-^{18}F]FDG-labeled cells localized to the lungs, suggesting specific disposition of these cells. The data also indicate that accumulation of cells in the target organ correlates strongly with actual metastatic potential; that is, highly metastatic cells tended to accumulate more in target organs than did those with low metastatic potential. Furthermore, sialidase treatment of MTLn3 cells reduced the accumulation of MTLn3 cells in lungs, suggesting that cell surface sialyl conjugates are important for the recognition of metastatic tumor cells by the endothelium of the target organ (11). These findings indicate that PET imaging could detect real-time cell trafficking *in vivo*, thus showing the disposition of specific cells. Actual disposition may be dependent on cell surface properties such as types of adhesion molecules or their ligands including sialyl conjugates.

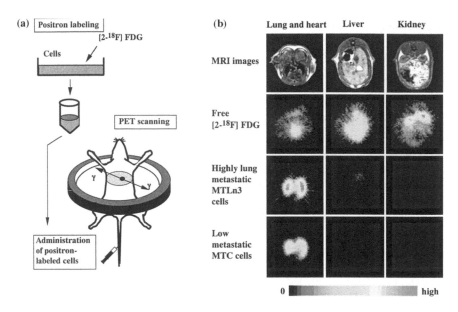

Figure 14.2 (**See color insert**) Experimental scheme of PET analysis for studying cell trafficking and accumulation of lung metastatic cells having differential metastatic potential in lungs. (a) First, cells are incubated with [2-^{18}F]FDG for 15–30 min at 37°C. Cells are washed to remove any free [2-^{18}F]FDG and are then injected into appropriate animals. PET imaging was started immediately after injection and performed for 60–120 min. Tissue radioactivity in the form of coincidence gamma photons was measured and converted to Bq/cm^3 of tissue volume by calibration. (b) Trafficking of [2-^{18}F]FDG-labeled highly lung metastatic MTLn3 cells and low metastatic MTC cells during the first 10 min after iv administration, as imaged by PET [reprinted with permission from Ref. (11)]. Images are in the coronal plane with a slice size of 3 mm. Scaling was corrected to be comparable in each organ. For reference to the PET images, magnetic resonance (MR) images of lungs, heart, liver, and kidneys are presented in the top panel. Lower three panels show PET images of free [2-^{18}F]FDG (upper), [2-^{18}F]FDG-labeled MTLn3 cells (middle), and [2-^{18}F]FDG-labeled MTC cells (lower).

Next, we examined the trafficking of tumor cells having different metastatic organ-specificity, using a highly lung metastatic sub-line of murine B16 melanoma (B16BL6 cells) and a highly liver metastatic sub-line of mouse RAW117 large cell lymphoma (RAW117-H10). The metastatic potential of B16BL6 cells was determined as follows: B16BL6 cells (1×10^6 cells per mouse) were injected intravenously into 7-week-old female C57BL/c mice, and deposition in lungs and other tissues was determined on day 14 after injection. As a result, 137 ± 42 colonies were detected on the surface of the lungs, and no deposition was observed on the surface of the liver or the spleen. The metastatic potential of RAW117-H10 cells was determined in a similar fashion, except that organ weights rather than colony counting were used for this group because discrete colonies of RAW117-H10 cells were difficult to determine. The liver, spleen, and lung weights of RAW117-H10-injected mice were, respectively, 1.60-, 2.39-, and 1.38-fold greater than those of control mice, suggesting that the cells metastasized to these organs.

After injecting B16BL6 and RAW117-H10 cells pre-labeled with [2-^{18}F]FDG into the tail veins of mice, the trafficking of these cells was examined using PET (13). Figure 14.3(a) shows typical images after injection of B16BL6 melanoma cells into a mouse. Specific accumulation of cells was observed only in the lungs. Both types of cells accumulated in the lungs immediately after injection, presumably because the lung was the first organ to be reached [Fig. 14.3(b)]. Elimination of RAW117-H10 cells from the lungs was fast when compared with elimination of B16BL6 cells. No accumulation of B16BL6 cells occurred in the liver; however, gradual accumulation of RAW117-H10 cells did occur in the liver. The time–activity curves of ^{18}F in the lungs and in the liver shown in Fig. 14.3(c) reflect the relatively rapid removal of RAW117-H10 from the lungs. At 60 min after injection, the liver/ lung accumulation per volume ratios of B16BL6 or RAW117-H10 cells were 0.097 and 0.326, respectively. These data indicate that lung metastatic cells tend to interact with lungs, and liver metastatic cells tend to accumulate in livers. This suggests that the accumulation of tumor cells *in vivo* is strongly influenced by tumor cell adhesion to the microvascular endothelium, not just organ location.

Further evidence was found for the importance of adhesion for accumulation. Treatment of RAW117-H10 cells with the protein kinase C inhibitor, H-7, decreased adhesion to murine hepatic sinusoidal endothelial (HSE) cells *in vitro* and suppressed accumulation in the livers analyzed by PET (14). In contrast, treatment of RAW117-P cells (which are from a low liver metastatic parental line of RAW117), with an activator of protein kinase C, TPA, resulted in increased adhesiveness to HSE and enhanced specific accumulation in livers. These data strongly suggest that the adhesiveness of cancerous cells *in vitro* reflects actual interaction with the endothelial cells of the target organ *in vivo*. Therefore, we can conclude that the accumulation of tumor cells in their target organs, and possibly the resulting metastasis, is related to the specific interaction of the cells with a target organ, and that the interaction is mediated by some specific cell adhesion molecule(s).

III. Involvement of Cell Adhesion Molecules in Metastatic Cell Trafficking

As described earlier, early trafficking (or accumulation of metastatic cells) correlates with metastatic potential to some extent and is dependent on cell adhesion molecule(s). Therefore, we examined the involvement of cell adhesion molecules, such as integrins and selectins, to the accumulation of metastatic cells

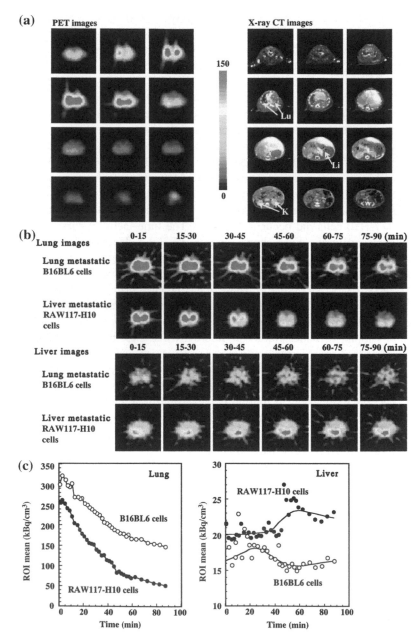

Figure 14.3 (**See color insert**) *In vivo* trafficking of lung metastatic B16BL6 melanoma cells and liver metastatic RAW117-H10 cells as determined by PET. (a) [2-^{18}F]FDG-labeled B16BL6 cells were injected via the tail vein of a C57BL/6 mouse.

(continued)

in their target organs. These adhesion molecules are important for adhesion and invasion of leukocytes at inflammatory sites. These, or similar molecules, are thought to be also involved in determining sites of metastatic cell accumulation. A first step is thought to involve the interaction of selectins such as E-selectin expressed on cytokine-activated endothelial cells and their ligands such as sialyl Lewis X (sLe^x) and sialyl Lewis A, or other sialyl conjugates expressed on the metastatic cell surface (15,16). In fact, a correlation between expression of these sialyl conjugates on cancerous cells and their metastatic potential has been reported (17,18). This selectin-mediated interaction is not strong but is enough to anchor the metastatic cells onto the endothelium of target organs. During this interaction, the endothelial cells are activated to express integrin receptors, causing a stronger interaction of cancerous cells with the endothelium. The cancerous cells then extravasate and invade the secondary colonizing site. If this scheme is correct, selectin-mediated interactions appear to occur at an early stage of metastatic cell adhesion and invasion of target organs followed by integrin-mediated interactions. Thus, we have used imaging to examine the trafficking of metastatic cells in the presence of inhibitors for selectin-mediated interaction or integrin-mediated interaction (19).

First, B16BL6 cells were co-injected into a tail vein of mice with either sLe^x-incorporated liposomes, which may bind to selectins, or with an Arg-Gly-Asp RGD-related peptide, DGRGDS conjugated with trimesic acid [Ar(GRGDS)$_3$], which is known to suppress interaction with certain integrins. Both sLe^x-liposome and RGD-related peptide suppressed actual metastasis of B16BL6 cells to the lungs.

We then examined the trafficking of B16BL6 cells in the presence of these inhibitors. As shown in Fig. 14.4(a), accumulation of [2-^{18}F]FDG-labeled B16BL6 cells in the lungs was suppressed in the presence of sLe^x-liposome, but was not affected by the liposome modified with methylated sLe^x (Me-sLe^x), which lacked the ability to bind to selectins. Neither the Me-sLe^x-liposome nor the nonmodified liposome suppressed B16BL6 metastasis to the lungs. Interestingly, the RGD-related peptide did not reduce the accumulation

---

Biodistribution during 30 min after administration of the cells was imaged by PET, and corresponding X-ray CT images are shown with a slice aperture of 3.25 mm [reprinted with permission from Ref. (28)]. Twelve slices from the head (upper left) to the tail (lower right) are shown. Scaling was corrected to be comparable between all images. Li, liver; Lu, lung; and K, kidney. (b) PET analysis of [2-^{18}F]FDG-labeled B16BL6 and RAW117-H10 cells was performed over 90 min, and 15 min frames show cell accumulation in lungs and liver [reprinted with permission from Ref. (13)]. (c) Time–activity curves of ^{18}F in lungs and liver after injection of [2-^{18}F]FDG-labeled B16BL6 and RAW117-H10 cells were obtained from mean pixel radioactivity in the region-of-interest (ROI) of the PET images, where the injected dose was calibrated as 740 kBq.

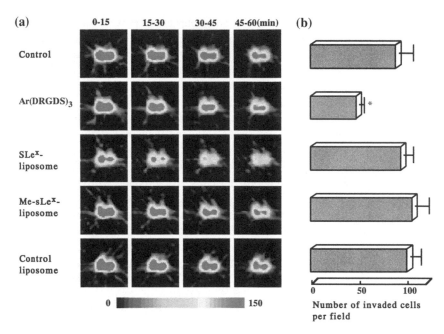

Figure 14.4 **(See color insert)** Effect of sLe^x-liposome or RGD-related peptide on the trafficking and invasion activity of B16BL6 melanoma cells. (a) C57BL6 mice were injected with [2-^{18}F]FDG-labeled B16BL6 cells (5 × 10^5 cells) with or without sLex-liposome, Me-sLex-liposome, empty liposome (3 nmol as egg yolk phosphatidylcholine), or Ar(DRGDS)$_3$. PET imaging of the lungs was started immediately after tumor cell injection and performed over 90 min and divided into every 15 min frames [reprinted with permission from Ref. (19)]. (b) B16BL6 cells (2 × 10^5 cells/well) were seeded with or without sLex-liposome, Me-sLex-liposome, empty liposome, or Ar(DRGDS)$_3$ into the upper compartment of a Transwell cell-culture chamber, the filters of which had been precoated with fibronectin on their lower surfaces and with Matrigel on their upper surfaces. After a 4 h incubation, cells per field which had invaded to the lower surfaces were counted [reprinted with permission from Ref. (13)]. *$P < 0.001$ vs. control.

of B16BL6 cells in the lungs, although it suppressed metastasis of these cells. To understand the reason for metastasis suppression by RGD-related peptide, we examined the effect of the peptide on the invasion of B16BL6 to Matrigel *in vitro* [Fig. 14.4(b)]. As shown in the figure, RGD-related peptide suppressed the invasion of B16BL6 cells, but sLe^x-liposome did not.

These data suggest that the binding of metastatic cells to the target organ occurs in the early stages of metastasis and is mediated by selectins or selectin-like molecules; integrin-mediated interaction may follow selectin-mediated interaction. This is the first evidence of selectin-mediated interaction during the early stages of metastasis, followed by integrin-related interaction. This study of interactions between cancer cells within the bloodstream and the endothelium of target organs in living animals was only possible because of noninvasive imaging methods with PET.

In the case of RAW117 cells, highly liver metastatic RAW117-H10 cells accumulated more in the liver than the low metastatic parental line, RAW117-P, again as determined by PET image analysis. Therefore, we examined differences in selectin ligands expressed on these cells. RAW117-H10 cells expressed more sialyl Lewis A than RAW117-P cells as determined by FACS analysis; the two cell lines expressed sLe^x equally (20). However, integrin $\alpha v\beta3$ is also reported to play an important role in the initial stages of liver metastasis in RAW117-H10 cells (21). It is possible, then, that the expression of some integrin species affects the early stages of trafficking of certain metastatic cells. In fact, integrin $\alpha v\beta3$ overexpressed in Chinese hamster ovary (CHO)-K1 cells, accumulated more in the liver than did untransfected CHO-K1 cells (22). Integrin $\alpha v\beta3$ expression actually affected the trafficking of metastatic cells. Interestingly, the accumulation pattern of both $\alpha v\beta3$ transfectants and control CHO-K1 cells in lung was almost the same.

The results of these studies suggest that integrin-mediated interactions may affect adhesion of cancerous cells to the target organ or the invasion process itself, depending on the specific integrin species and the target organ.

IV. Determination of Intraorgan Trafficking of Metastatic Cells

During the first stage of blood-borne metastasis, metastatic tumor cells that have intravasated from the primary site adhere to and extravasate through the vascular endothelium of the target organ. PET image analyses show that the metastatic potential of various intravenously injected tumor cells correlates well with the early accumulation of these cells in the target organ, suggesting that the target organ is initially engaged by metastatic tumor cells through specific interactions between adhesion molecules on the tumor cells and their ligands on the target endothelium. PET analysis is useful for understanding bulk trafficking of metastatic cells *in vivo*; however, it cannot detect the precise location of each metastatic cell within an organ. However, the movement of individual cells can be tracked using intravital fluorescence microscopy (IVM), although, this method is invasive in nature. With this technique, fluorescently labeled cells are injected into the bloodstream and the target organ is examined under a fluorescence microscope (23).

As mentioned earlier, the liver accumulation of integrin $\alpha v\beta3$ transfectants of CHO-K1 cells ($\alpha v\beta3$-CHO-K1 cells) was significantly higher than that of CHO-K1 cells after injection via the portal vein. On the other hand, lung accumulation of transfected and nontransfected cells was not significantly different (22). To determine the precise location of each cell in the liver (i.e., to determine whether individual cells were sequestered intravascularly or had extravasated), we performed IVM on the liver. We used stable transfectants bearing the green fluorescent protein (GFP) gene: GFP-CHO-K1 and GFP-$\alpha v \beta 3$-CHO-K1 cells (22). In both cases, 1×10^6 cells were injected via the portal vein of Balb/c nu/nu mice, and an IVM analysis was performed. The anesthetized mouse was placed on the viewing platform of the fluorescent microscope with the liver protruding through an abdominal incision. Fluorescence images were monitored directly on a computer display through the CCD camera. Cells remaining in the bloodstream and those which had extravasated into the surrounding tissue were recorded [Fig. 14.5(a)]. Invasion percent was determined from the average number of cells that had migrated into the parenchyma.

Both types of cells remained in the hepatic blood vessels 1 h after injection [Fig. 14.5(b)]. On the other hand, cells expressing the integrin $\alpha v \beta 3$ had moved extravascularly more than control CHO-K1 cells within 24 h. These results suggest the possibility that the specific accumulation of $\alpha v \beta 3$-CHO-K1 cells in the liver is followed by migration of the cells into the extravascular region.

As the adhesion of the two types of cells to HSE cells *in vitro* did not correspond to accumulation of these cells *in vivo*, the integrin $\alpha v \beta 3$ may function to promote extravasation of $\alpha v \beta 3$ integrin-expressing tumor cells in the liver. It is possible that this extravasation is mediated by vitronectin. Vitronectin, a classical integrin $\alpha v \beta 3$ ligand, is produced in the liver along with other serum components (24,25); mouse vitronectin mRNA has been detected mainly in hepatocytes (26). Thus, in this study, PET analysis showed an enhanced cellular accumulation of $\alpha v \beta 3$ integrin-expressing cells in the liver, whereas IVM analysis indicated that the expression of the integrin $\alpha v \beta 3$ promotes invasion of the target organ.

V. Topological Distribution of Metastatic Cells as Analyzed by Whole-Body Autoradiography

PET analysis of cell trafficking is noninvasive and is useful for investigating bulk cell behavior in the body. However, it is difficult to determine the intraorgan distribution of infiltrating cells with this method. As an alternative, we have used another invasive technique, whole-body autoradiography, to examine the precise intraorgan distribution of metastatic tumor cells. Specifically, we used a bioimaging analyzer system (BAS) to determine the distribution of lung metastatic B16BL6 cells and liver metastatic RAW117-H10 cells after injection of 5-[^{125}I]iodo-2'-deoxyuridine ([^{125}I]IUDR)-labeled metastatic cells.

B16BL6 cells were incubated in the presence of 3.7 MBq of [^{125}I]IUDR for 4 h. The cells were washed and harvested with EDTA–phosphate-buffered saline (PBS), and suspended in medium. [^{125}I]IUDR-labeled B16BL6 cells (1×10^6 cells) were intravenously injected into C57BL/6 mice via a tail vein. Animals were sacrificed at 15 and 120 min after injection, and frozen immediately with

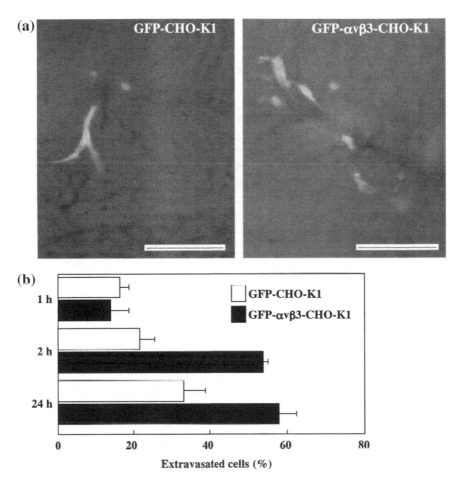

Figure 14.5 (**See color insert**) IVM observation of GFP-CHO-K1 and GFP-αvβ3-CHO-K1 cells in liver after portal vein injection. (a) Invasion of GFP-CHO-K1 (left) and GFP-αvβ3-CHO-K1 (right) cells; 1×10^6 cells were injected into Balb/c nu/nu mice via a portal vein. At 24 h after the injection, liver was examined under a fluorescence microscope [reprinted with permission from Ref. (22)]. Bars represent 100 μm. (b) IVM analysis was performed as described in (a), at 1, 2, and 24 h after the injection of GFP-expressing CHO-K1 cells; the number of fluorescent cells sequestered in blood vessels or extravasated into surrounding tissue were counted under a fluorescence microscope. The data indicate the percentage of cells that had invaded into tissue vs. total cells counted.

acetone-dry ice. Frozen mice were embedded in 8% carboxymethylcellulose and sagittal slices of 30 μm thickness were prepared in every 1 mm aperture with an autocryotome. Imaging plates were exposed to the whole-body slice specimens taken from labeled cell-inoculated mice: 60 min (for lung analysis) and 6 days (for other tissues). Then, the BAS (BAS2000, Fuji Photo Film Co. Ltd) was used for whole-body autoradiography; $[^{125}I]$IUDR-labeled RAW117-H10 cells were similarly prepared and analyzed.

Figure 14.6(a) shows the whole-body autoradiogram of a specimen slice of a mouse and injection of RAW117-H10 cells (13), reflecting accumulation of these cells in the lungs and in the liver. As shown in Fig. 14.6(b), at 15 min after injection, accumulation of B16BL6 cells was greater in the lungs than that of RAW117-H10 cells. The intralung distribution of these cells was rather homogeneous, although the cells were distributed as colonies throughout the lung tissue. Accumulation of cells in the liver is also shown in Fig. 14.6(b). The data from BAS analysis are consistent with the data from PET analysis: lung metastatic B16BL6 cells tended to accumulate in the lungs, and liver metastatic RAW117-H10 cells tended to accumulate in the liver. Accumulation of the cells seemed to be rather homogeneous throughout the liver [dark area shown in Fig. 14.6(b)]. At 120 min post-injection, colony distribution also occurred in the liver with both B16BL6 and RAW117 cells. Figure 14.6(c) shows typical B16BL6 accumulation in lung tissue and typical RAW117-H10 accumulation in liver tissue. The colony distribution of the cells is obvious, although the precise number of cells in each colony is unknown due to halation during exposure.

With regard to the accumulation of cells in "colonies" in their target organ, we believe trafficking of metastatic cells may occur in the following manner. At first, each cell is trapped in the capillary vessel because the vessel opening is smaller than the cells. The cell does manage though, to flowout gradually from the capillary vessel if there are no specific interactions with endothelial cells. This may be the case for RAW117 cells in the lungs. On the other hand, the cell is sequestered in the tissue if there are specific interactions between the metastatic cell and the endothelium. This may occur for B16BL6 cells in the lungs and for RAW117 cells (which pass through the lungs) in the liver. Populations of B16BL6 cells that fail to interact with the lungs flow through the bloodstream, but some of these cells may be trapped in the lungs during subsequent passes through the lung capillaries. If a cell becomes sequestered in the lungs, cells coming after it, or cells in the second passage, may interact more easily with the lung endothelium, due to slower blood flow. This would account for the creation of "colonies" of cells in target organs, detected by BAS analysis.

VI. Influence of the Immune Surveillance System on Metastasis Cell Trafficking

Host resistance factors may also be important in metastatic cell trafficking. For instance, immune surveillance may reduce the number of metastatic cells in the bloodstream, resulting in a reduced accumulation of cells in a target organ. Likewise, even after surgical removal of the primary tumor, a substantial number of viable tumor cells can be detected in the circulation. However, this

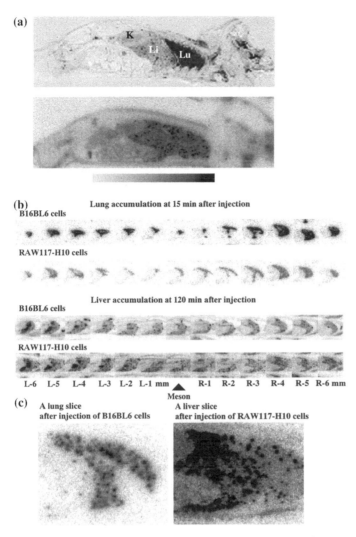

Figure 14.6 Whole-body autoradiography of a mouse injected with [^{125}I]IUDR-labeled metastatic cells. (a) [^{125}I]IUDR-labeled metastatic cells were injected intravenously into syngeneic mice. The mouse specimen was prepared, and the distribution of radiolabeled cells was detected by a BAS [reprinted with permission from Ref. (13)]. A specimen for whole-body autoradiography is shown (upper) along with a BAS image at 120 min after injection of RAW117-H10 cells (lower). The imaging plate was exposed for 6 days. Lu, lung; Li, liver; K, kidney. (b) BAS analysis of [^{125}I]IUDR-labeled B16BL6 and RAW117 cells was performed. Images represent accumulation in lung 15 min post-injection, and in liver 120 min post-injection. The arrowhead indicates the meson, and labels under frames represent left (L) or right (R) distance from the meson. (c) Typical images represent accumulation of B16BL6 cells in lung (left) and RAW117-H10 cells in liver (right) 120 min post-injection.

phenomenon does not correlate well with the subsequent development of detectable metastases. It is also empirically known that a certain number of metastatic tumor cells are required to establish metastatic foci, and metastasis is not observed if a smaller number of cells are inoculated in experimental metastasis models. This evidence indicates that metastasis may develop only if the metastatic cells can circumvent the immune surveillance of the host. Macrophages and natural killer cells are thought to be the first line of defense in target organs (the lung and the liver) against invading metastatic tumor cells (27).

Once again, we have used imaging with PET and [2-^{18}F]FDG, this time to investigate the importance of immune surveillance in allowing metastases to become established in target organs. We investigated the trafficking of lung-metastatic B16BL6 cells in relation to the number of injected cells, because the immune defense system may work more effectively when fewer tumor cells are injected (28). B16BL6 cells (1×10^6 cells including [2-^{18}F]FDG-labeled 1×10^4 cells, 1×10^5 cells including [2-^{18}F]FDG-labeled 1×10^4 cells, and [2-^{18}F]FDG-labeled 1×10^4 cells) were injected into the tail vein of each mouse. A PET emission scan was started immediately after injection of the cells and lasted 90 min. Cells accumulated in the lungs at a similar rate when 1×10^6 or 1×10^5 B16BL6 cells were injected into the mice [Fig. 14.7(a)]. There was an approximate 10-fold difference in the number of accumulated cells between the two doses. Figure 14.7(b) indicates the elimination of both labeled cells and calculated total cells from the lungs. Elimination from the lungs was not dependent on cell number, but on the proportion of accumulated cells.

The injection of 1×10^4 cells resulted in lung accumulation less than one-tenth of that obtained with 1×10^5 cell-injection. Metastasis was observed when 1×10^5 or 1×10^6 B16BL6 cells were injected (colony number on the surface of each mouse lungs was 174, 173, 170, 165, and 148 for 1×10^5 cells injected, and >300 in all five mice tested for 1×10^6 cells injected). Metastasis was not observed after injection of 1×10^4 cells (no colony was observed in five mice tested).

To clarify the role of immune surveillance in preventing metastasis, we challenged macrophage-depleted mice with 1×10^4 tumor cells. Mice were treated with 2-chloroadenosine (2ClAd) (which is known to deplete macrophages) (29), 2 days prior to the tumor cell challenge. This canceled the suppression of not only metastasis (colony number on the surface of each mouse lungs was 37, 11, 3, 3, and 1), but also of lung accumulation [Fig. 14.7(c)]. 2ClAd is known to increase lung metastasis of M109 tumor cells after intraperitoneal injection (30). In our study, administration of this compound following the tumor cell challenge had little effect on metastatic potential (colony number on the surface of each mouse lungs was 1, 0, 0, 0, and 0).

Similar results were obtained with liver metastatic RAW117-H10 cells (31): when 1×10^6 or 1×10^5 RAW117-H10 cells were injected into mice via a portal vein, both numbers of cells caused liver metastasis and cells accumulated

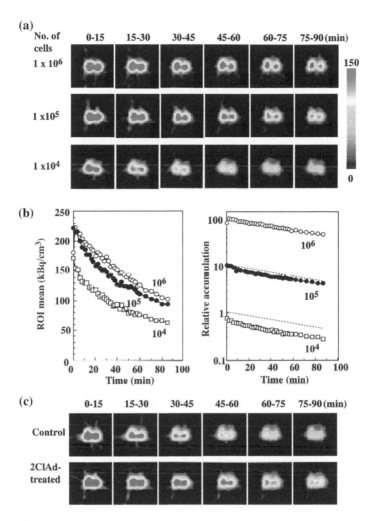

Figure 14.7 (**See color insert**) Trafficking of B16BL6 cells after injection of various numbers of cells. (a) [2-^{18}F]FDG-labeled B16BL6 cells (1×10^6 cells including [2-^{18}F]FDG-labeled 1×10^4 cells, 1×10^5 cells including [2-^{18}F]FDG-labeled 1×10^4 cells, and [2-^{18}F]FDG-labeled 1×10^4 cells) were injected into C57BL6 mice via the tail vein. PET imaging was started immediately after injection of the cells and was performed for 90 min in 15 min frames. The accumulation of B16BL6 cells in the lungs is shown [reprinted with permission from Ref. (28)]. (b) Time–activity curves of ^{18}F accumulation in the lungs were determined by analysis of the PET images (left panel). Relative cell accumulation is shown in the right panel where the highest accumulation after injection of 1×10^6 cells is 100. Dashed line shows 1/10 and 1/100 amount of the relative accumulation of cells after injection of 1×10^6 cells. (c) Mice were intraperitoneally pre-treated with 25 mg/kg of 2ClAd or PBS. Two days later, the mice were injected with [2-^{18}F]FDG-labeled B16BL6 cells (1×10^4 cells) via the tail vein. PET imaging, representing the accumulation of B16BL6 cells in the lungs, was performed as just described.

in the liver at similar rates. However, injection of 1×10^4 cells did not produce metastasis, and the accumulation rate in liver was less than one-tenth of that after injection of the 1×10^5 cells. Treatment of mice with 2ClAd to deplete macrophages 2 days prior to the injection of 1×10^4 cells resulted in suppression of the fast elimination component of cells from the liver. Corresponding to this change, metastasis was observed after injection of the 1×10^4 cells into 2ClAd pre-treated mice.

These data allow us to conclude that immune surveillance is a strong factor preventing metastasis during the first phase of the metastatic process, but not at later stages. Further, macrophages appear to play an important role in this immune surveillance, as revealed obvious when a small number of tumor cells is used for the challenge.

VII. Conclusions and Future Prospects

PET imaging can be used for both qualitative and quantitative studies of the trafficking of metastatic cells *in vivo*. In the PET studies described in this chapter, we found that specific interactions between metastatic cells and passing organs were important determinants of which organs were affected. Highly metastatic cells accumulated more than low metastatic cells. Metastasis organ specificity correlated with an early accumulation of cells to the target organ. Anatomical–mechanical trapping of metastatic cells may also be determined partly by which organ the tumor cells reach first, especially when the cell has the potential to interact with the endothelia of various organs. PET studies appear to be especially useful for studying lung metastasis, because the lung has a narrow capillary bed and is the first organ affected after intravenous injection. Such studies can be supplemented with IVM analyses, and BAS analyses to study the intraorgan distribution of metastatic cells. PET studies can also be used to clarify the role of cell adhesion molecules or their ligands in the metastatic process after specific inhibitors are used to affect the adhesion of cells to endothelium, causing a reduction of metastatic cell accumulation in the target organ. Thus, PET studies would also be useful for screening of new metastasis inhibitors or for elucidating the mode of action of these inhibitors.

Although the utility of PET imaging to study cell trafficking in this chapter has focused on tumor metastasis as an illustration of the relevant principles involved, similar approaches might be useable with other cell types, especially those with elevated glucose metabolism. Hematopoietic cells or some precursor (stem) cells are also possible candidates.

References

1. Nicolson GL. Molecular mechanisms of cancer metastasis: tumor and host properties and the role of oncogenes and suppressor genes. Curr Opin Oncol 1991; 3:75–92.

2. Liotta LA, Steeg PS, Steiler-Stevenson WG. Cancer metastasis and angiogenesis: an imbalance of positive and negative regulation. Cell 1991; 64:327–336.

3. Fidler IJ. The pathogenesis of cancer metastasis: the "seed and soil" hypothesis revisited. Nat Rev Cancer 2003; 3:453–458.

4. Kannagi R. Transcriptional regulation of expression of carbohydrate ligands for cell adhesion molecules in the selectin family. Adv Exp Med Biol 2001; 491:267–278.

5. Hood JD, Cheresh DA. Role of integrins in cell invasion and migration. Nat Rev Cancer 2002; 2:91–100.

6. Egeblad M, Werb Z. New functions for the matrix metalloproteinases in cancer progression. Nat Rev Cancer 2002; 2:161–174.

7. Liotta LA. An attractive force in metastasis. Nature 2001; 410:24–25.

8. Muller A, Homey B, Soto H, Ge N, Cartron D, Buchanan ME, McClanahan T, Murphy E, Yuan W, Wagner SN, Barrera JL, Mohar A, Verastegui E, Zlotnik A. Involvement of chemokine receptors in breast cancer metastasis. Nature 2001; 410:50–56.

9. Muller WA. Leukocyte-endothelial-cell interactions in leukocyte transmigration and the inflammatory response. Trends Immunol 2003; 24:327–334.

10. Lafrenie R, Shaughnessy SG, Orr FW. Cancer cell interactions with injured or activated endothelium. Cancer Metastasis Rev 1992, 11.377–388.

11. Oku N, Koike C, Sugawara M, Tsukada H, Okada S. Positron emission tomography analysis of metastatic tumor cell trafficking. Cancer Res 1994; 54:2573–2576.

12. Neri A, Welch D, Kawaguchi T, Nicolson GL. Development and biologic properties of malignant cell sublines and clones of a spontaneously metastasizing rat mammary adenocarcinoma. J Natl Cancer Inst 1982; 68:507–517.

13. Koike C, Watanabe M, Oku N, Tsukada H, Irimura T, Okada S. Cancer Res 1997; 37:3612–3619.

14. Koike C, Oku N, Watanabe M, Tsukada H, Kakiuchi T, Irimura T, Okada S. Real-time PET analysis of metastatic tumor cell trafficking *in vivo* and its relation to adhesion properties. Biochim Biophys Acta 1995; 1238:99–106.

15. Ugorski M, Laskowska A. Sialyl Lewis(a): a tumor-associated carbohydrate antigen involved in adhesion and metastatic potential of cancer cells. Acta Biochim Pol 2002; 49:303–311.

16. Zhang J, Nakayama J, Ohyama C, Suzuki M, Suzuki A, Fukuda M, Fukuda MN. Sialyl Lewis X-dependent lung colonization of B16 melanoma cells through a selectin-like endothelial receptor distinct from E- or P-selectin. Cancer Res 2002; 62:4194–4198.

17. Yamada N, Chung YS, Takatsuka S, Arimoto Y, Sawada T, Dohi T, Sowa M. Increased sialyl Lewis A expression and fucosyltransferase activity with acquisition of a high metastatic capacity in a colon cancer cell line. Br J Cancer 1994; 76:582–587.

18. Nakamori S, Kameyama M, Furukawa H, Takeda O, Sugai S, Imaoka S, Nakamura Y. Genetic detection of colorectal cancer cells in circulation and lymph nodes. Dis Colon Rectum 1997; 40:S29–S36.

19. Saiki I, Kioke C, Obata A, Fujii H, Murata J, Kiso M, Hasegawa A, Komazawa H, Tsukada H, Azuma I, Okada S, Oku N. Int J Cancer 1996; 65:833–839.

20. Kikkawa H, Miyamoto D, Imafuku H, Koike C, Suzuki Y, Okada S, Tsukada H, Irimura T, Oku N. Jpn J Cancer Res 1998; 89:1296–1305.

21. Yun Z, Smith TW, Menter DG, McIntire LV, Nicolson GL. Differential adhesion of metastatic RAW117 large-cell lymphoma cells under static or hydrodynamic conditions: role of integrin $\alpha v \beta 3$. Clin Exp Metastasis 1997; 15:3–11.

22. Kikkawa H, Kaihou M, Horaguchi, N, Uchida T, Imafuku H, Takiguchi A, Yamazaki Y, Koike C, Kuruto R, Kakiuchi T, Tsukada H, Takada Y, Matsuura N, Oku N. Role of integrin $\alpha v \beta 3$ in the early phase of liver metastasis: PET and IVM analyses. Clin Exp Metastasis 2002; 19:717–725.

23. Chambers AF, MacDonald IC, Schmidt EE, Koop S, Morris VL, Khokha R, Groom AC. Steps in tumor metastasis: new concepts from intravital videomicroscopy. Cancer Metastasis Rev 1995; 14:279–301.

24. Weerasinghe D, McHugh KP, Ross FP, Brown EJ, Gisler RH, Imhof BA. A role for the alphavbeta3 integrin in the transmigration of monocytes. J Cell Biol 1998; 142:595–607.

25. Salcedo R, Patarroyo M. Constitutive $\alpha v \beta 3$ integrin-mediated adhesion of human lymphoid B cells to vitronectin substrate. Cell Immunol 1995; 160:165–172.

26. Seiffert D, Crain K, Wagner NV, Loskutoff DJ. Vitronectin gene expression *in vivo*. Evidence for extrahepatic synthesis and acute phase regulation. J Biol Chem 1994; 269:19836–19842.

27. Griffini P, Smorenburg SM, Vogels IMC, Tigchelaar VW, Van Noorden CJF. Clin Exp Metastasis 1996; 14:367–380.

28. Kikkawa H, Imafuku H, Tsukada H, Oku N. Possible role of immune surveillance at the initial phase of metastasis produced by B16BL6 melanoma cells. FEBS Lett 2000; 467:211–216.

29. Kubota Y, Iwasaki Y, Harada H, Yokomura I, Ueda M, Hashimoto S et al. Depletion of alveolar macrophages by treatment with 2-chloroadenosine aerosol. Clin Diagn Immunol 1999; 6:452–456.

30. Schultz RM, Tang JC, DeLong DC, Ades EW, Altom MG. Cancer Res 1986; 46:5624–5628.

31. Kikkawa H, Tsukada H, Oku N. Usefulness of positron emission tomographic visualization for examination of *in vivo* susceptibility to metastasis. Cancer 2000; 89:1628–1633.

15

Imaging Angiogenesis in the Lung

WAYNE MITZNER

Johns Hopkins Bloomberg School of
Public Health,
Baltimore, Maryland, USA

ELIZABETH WAGNER

Johns Hopkins Asthma and Allergy Center,
Baltimore, Maryland, USA

I. Imaging Neovascularization in the Lung: Challenges for Measurement

Angiogenesis refers to the process by which new blood vessels form to meet new needs demanded by ischemic tissue. In several pathologic processes, angiogenesis arises as a response to specific insults. For instance, when lung tumors grow beyond the point at which they can be nourished by the existing pulmonary circulation, the cancerous tissue becomes ischemic and starts signaling a need for increased perfusion. Without such increased perfusion, tumor growth could not continue, and this is the motivation for the intensive search for inhibitors of angiogenesis as a therapy for cancer. In chronic asthma, there is often a slight thickening of the airway wall, accompanied by increased smooth muscle and vascularization. These new blood vessels may contribute to the warming or humidification of inspired air, but their precise role in this disease remains somewhat controversial (1). Angiogenesis in the lung also occurs where there is pathologic obstruction of the pulmonary vasculature. In such cases, the bronchial circulation expands to meet the needs of the ischemic tissue. Although this process is clearly beneficial in keeping the lung tissue alive, the gas exchange function of the lung is not corrected. Although hypoxia is often listed as a stimulus for angiogenesis, the fact that angiogenesis readily occurs in the ventilated lung with obstruction of deoxygenated pulmonary blood flow proves that ischemia is the more relevant stimulus. Because these new vessels to ischemic tissue always originate from the microcirculation, attempts to visualize such vessels will clearly stress the limits of all imaging modalities. In a recent excellent review article, the applications and limitations of many of these techniques in systemic organs are described (2). However, the lung poses unique challenges because efforts to visualize angiogenesis in this organ are hampered by several physiological factors. Most significant is the fact that new vessel growth predominantly arises from the systemic circulation that normally perfuses the airways and thorax. Although changes in pulmonary vessels occasionally appear in metastases (3), nearly all observations of lung angiogenesis can trace the origin of new vessels to their arterial sources from either the tracheobronchial vasculature or intercostal arteries surrounding the lungs. Although in animal models this neovascularization can develop to as much as 30% of the cardiac output (4), under normal conditions the bronchial circulation represents <3% of cardiac output (5). Because of the two distinct vascular systems within the lungs, the larger and recruitable pulmonary vasculature obscure small angiogenic alterations of the bronchial vasculature. *In vivo* imaging of the lungs with bronchial arteriograms can provide qualitative information about neovascularization. However, to confirm new vessel proliferation, investigators have resorted to histologic evaluation of tissue biopsy specimens with quantification of vascular density. Even this approach has been difficult because unique endothelial markers distinguishing new angiogenic vessels relative to pulmonary vessels are not currently apparent, although a few studies have focused on defining endothelial heterogeneity within normal lungs (6,7). Thus, *in vivo* imaging of neovascularization within the lungs represents a significant challenge requiring further characterization of vascular phenotype. This chapter is organized around three different but well-characterized pathophysiologic conditions, for which different imaging modalities are being used to assess vascular function and angiogenesis: asthma, pulmonary artery obstruction, and lung cancer.

II. Imaging Neovascularization in Asthma

Much of our current knowledge regarding neovascularization of the airways during conditions of airway inflammation depends on histologic examination of postmortem tissue and biopsy specimens. However, each of these sources for tissue sampling presents problems for an accurate assessment of changes in airway vascularity. Neither airway specimens obtained at autopsy nor biopsy samples obtained during bronchoscopy are acquired while normal airway vascular volumes and pressures are maintained. Because vascular area is also a function of distending pressure of the lungs, tissue obtained without a fixed lung distending pressure will also be subject to error. Thus, vascular area measurements, although frequently reported, are likely to be unreliable.

This sampling and analytic problem is akin to the question of whether there are more or larger smooth muscle cells in patients with asthma. Although this issue can be addressed in human biopsy tissue with careful and proper sampling technique (8), it does not resolve the problems associated with the appearance of unpressurized small blood vessels in biopsy tissue. Nonetheless, the number of vessels can be counted and correlated with length of basement membrane or other fixed markers. For instance, Li and Wilson (9) found a significantly greater number of vessels in biopsy specimens of subjects with mild asthma than in biopsy specimens from healthy control volunteers (739 $\pm$ 150 mm^2 vs. 539 $\pm$ 276 mm^2). In contrast, Chu et al. (10) found no difference in the number of blood vessels counted in biopsy specimens from healthy subjects and patients with mild to moderate asthma. Only biopsy specimens from patients with asthma and concurrent *Mycoplasma pneumoniae* infections demonstrated significantly increased numbers of vessels (10). Finally, Kuwano et al. (11) demonstrated that increased numbers of vessels in patients with asthma were proportional to the overall increase in airway wall area (11). Thus, accurate histologic assessment of airway neovascularization requires complete and controlled tissue sampling, which may not always be possible.

However, an exciting, recently published study, in which a new imaging technique was applied, holds promise for visualization of new vessel growth in the airways of human subjects. Using bronchovideomicroscopy, Tanaka et al. (12) demonstrated increased vascularity of the submucosa of the distal trachea in-patients with asthma compared with healthy control subjects. In their study a conventional fiberoptic bronchoscope was used to guide and position an additional side-viewing high-magnification (65–105-fold image magnification) bronchovideoscope positioned with a 1 mm focal distance from the side lens to the tracheal wall. Signals obtained through this bronchovideoscope were reconstructed by a video processor and projected onto a monitor. Figure 15.1 shows representative images obtained from control subjects and subjects with chronic obstructive pulmonary disease (COPD) compared with images obtained from patients with asthma. Images were quantified offline for total vascular area density. Patients with COPD showed no difference in airway vascularity when compared with healthy control subjects, despite significant loss of pulmonary function. Patients with a new diagnosis of asthma, as well as patients with asthma who had been taking inhaled corticosteroids for ≥ 5 years, showed significantly increased vascularity when compared with control subjects and patients

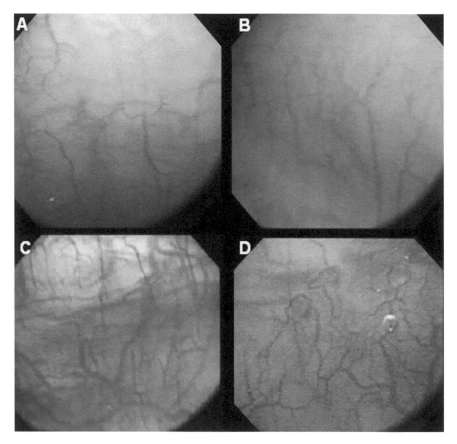

Figure 15.1 **(See color insert)** Side view and high-magnification bronchovideoscopic images of lower trachea of control subject (A), subject with COPD (B), steroid-naïve patient with newly diagnosed, stable asthma (C), and patient who has had stable asthma for >5 years, treated with inhaled corticosteroids (D). Fine vessel networks are prominently increased in the patients with asthma when compared with the control subject and the patient with COPD [From Tanaka et al. (12), by permission].

with COPD. Furthermore, within the group of patients with asthma, the degree of vascularity was not correlated with pulmonary function. This technique offers the only means of *in vivo* estimation of neovascularization in airways of human subjects. However, limitations acknowledged by the authors include the difficulty in discerning whether the increased vascular density could be explained by vasodilation or vascular engorgement of existing vessels, as well as the detection threshold limit of 20 μm. Histologic assessments of neovascularization in animal models of chronic airway inflammation and remodeling are subject to similar criticisms, although perhaps with fewer limitations. Using rodent models of airway remodeling after *Mycoplasma pulmonis* infection, McDonald and coworkers (13) have demonstrated increased airway vascularity by examining tracheal whole mounts (13). Figure 15.2 shows *Lycopersicon esculentum* lectin staining of tracheal vessels in control and *M. pulmonis*-infected mice. Obvious differences in vascular phenotype are apparent in the two mice strains studied; C57Bl/6 mice showed increased numbers of tracheal vessels, whereas C3H mice showed increased vessel diameters. Careful morphometric analysis confirmed these visual assessments. Although a comparison of control mice with infected mice demonstrates increased numbers overall, lectin staining does not distinguish existing vessels from new vessels. *In vivo* imaging of airway vessels within the trachea after remodeling could be used to assess vascular function.

A new application of the technique of intravital microscopy to tracheal vessels has been demonstrated in rats (14,15). Shown in Fig. 15.3 is a still image taken from the videotaping of a postcapillary venule of a rat. Several adherent leukocytes are evident. Recruitment in real time can be evaluated, as can alterations in the permeability of different-sized fluorescent dextrans. Vasomotion as assessed by vessel diameters and red blood cell velocity can also be measured. This *in vivo* imaging approach can be used for a functional assessment of angiogenic vessels of large airways.

III. Imaging Neovascularization after Pulmonary Artery Obstruction

Perhaps the most extensively studied form of new systemic vessel growth in the lung is that which occurs after pulmonary artery embolization. Virchow (16), in 1847, recognized that the bronchial circulation could proliferate and sustain lung tissue distal to a pulmonary embolism. Since that time, neovascularization of the systemic circulation into the lung after pulmonary artery obstruction has been confirmed and studied in humans (17), sheep (18), dogs (4), pigs (19), and rats (20). In these models the importance of the bronchial circulation in supporting the ischemic parenchymal tissue has been confirmed and both the structure and physiology of the new vasculature have been studied. Bronchial arteriograms in patients with chronic thromboembolic disease demonstrate the unique capacity of systemic vessels to proliferate and to invade the ischemic lung parenchyma. Figure 15.4 shows both a dilated bronchial artery and a fine meshwork of vessels distal to the pulmonary occlusion (21). Systemic blood flow to the lung has been shown to increase to as much as 30% of the original pulmonary blood flow after pulmonary artery occlusion (4). In addition to bronchial neovascularization, several intercostal arteries have been shown to participate in the neovascularization of the ischemic lung (22). Arteriograms of several thoracic arteries in a patient with Takayasu arteritis with pulmonary artery involvement demonstrate the proliferative nature of these vessels supplying the ischemic

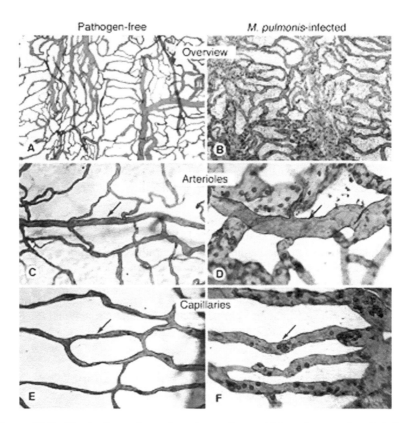

Figure 15.2   Tracheal vasculature in pathogen-free and *Mycoplasma pulmonis*-infected C57BL/6 and C3H mice. The vasculature was perfusion-stained with biotinylated *Lycopersicon esculentum* lectin and ABC/DAB peroxidase reaction and visualized by light microscopy in tracheal whole mounts. (A) Organized pattern of mucosal vessels in trachea of pathogen-free C57BL/6 mouse, showing capillaries across a cartilaginous ring (cartilage), fed from arterioles (arrows) and drained by venules (arrowheads) in inter-cartilaginous regions. (B) Enlarged vessels in trachea of C57BL/6 mouse at 2 weeks after infection. (C) Enlarged vessels and regions with increased numbers of capillary-sized vessels (arrow) in trachea of C57BL/6 mouse at 4 weeks after infection. (D) Numerous capillary-sized vessels and enlarged vessels in trachea of C57BL/6 mouse at 8 weeks after infection. Many capillary-sized vessels are out of focus, as vessels are no longer confined to plane of epithelium. (E) Trachea of pathogen-free C3H mouse, showing organized pattern of mucosal vessels. (F) Enlarged vessels in trachea of C3H mouse at 8 weeks after infection. All segments of the vasculature appear enlarged. Similar enlarged vessels were seen at 1, 2, and 4 weeks after inoculation of C3H mice. Scale bar (A–F), 100 mm. [From Thurston et al. (13), by permission].

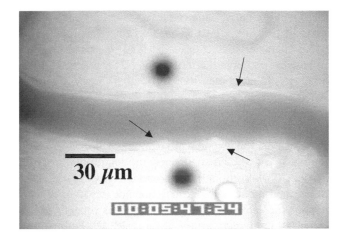

Figure 15.3 Still image of rat postcapillary venule with few adherent leukocytes (arrows).

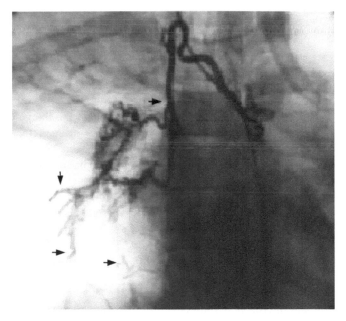

Figure 15.4 Bronchial arteriogram in-patient with thromboembolic pulmonary hypertension. The dilated bronchial artery is clearly seen, as well as a mesh of small bronchial vessels connected to the pulmonary arterial branches downstream from the embolic occlusion. Large arrowhead points to bronchial artery, and small arrows point to branches of pulmonary artery distal to the occlusion [From Endrys et al. (21), by permission].

lung (Fig. 15.5). Additionally, each of these systemic vessels demonstrates significant hypertrophy at the point of aortic origin. Thus, both proliferation and hypertrophy are characteristic features that can be visualized by conventional angiography and by computed tomography (CT), respectively. In additional studies, investigators have measured bronchial artery diameters from CT images in patients with chronic pulmonary embolism vs. acute pulmonary embolism and demonstrated that only in patients with chronic pulmonary embolism is there an increase in bronchial artery diameter (23).

To further explore the mechanisms responsible for neovascularization after pulmonary embolism, we established a new model of pulmonary artery obstruction in the mouse (24). Although the bronchial vasculature extends from the carina to the terminal bronchioles in most species (5), in mice there is no functional bronchial vasculature beyond the mainstem bronchi (24,25). We have shown that after left pulmonary artery ligation (LPAL) in the mouse, intercostal arteries provide the source for new vascularization of the lung (24). Casting the new vasculature demonstrated that intercostal arteries in proximity to the ischemic lung developed a dense vascular plexus that bridged the pleural space and invaded the lung parenchyma. Further imaging of the cast with micro-CT revealed the extent of neovascularization 3 months after LPAL. Figure 15.6 (right) is a dorsal view of the new vasculature in the left lung observed through the thorax. The CT density window was set to show bone and methacrylate cast material. The casting material filled the aorta where the methacrylate was injected and the extensive new systemic vasculature invading the left lung (Fig. 15.6, arrow). In the lung, this new plexus establishes connections to the existing pulmonary vascular tree that then fills with the casting material. No cast material entered the normal right lung. Figure 15.6 (left) shows a vascular cast of new blood vessels from another animal in which the thoracic cage was removed. A dense vascular plexus of new vessels is seen in the upper left lung, which was fed by vascular connections from the chest wall. These images provide confirmation of the new systemic vasculature invading the substance of the left lung after LPAL.

Additional imaging of the lung vasculature with fluorescent microspheres is based on findings of Glenny and coworkers (26) established for the pulmonary circulation. Fluorescent microspheres (15 μm) were injected into the jugular vein (grey) and left ventricle (white) 14 days after LPAL in mice. After histologic sectioning of the lungs and three-dimensional reconstruction of fluorescent images, a composite image was produced (Fig. 15.7). The composite image shows that microspheres injected into only the jugular vein appeared in the right lung and microspheres injected into only the left ventricle appeared in the upper left lung. No spheres were apparent in the lower left lung.

Single photon emission computed tomography (SPECT) imaging of technetium 99m-labeled albumen aggregates can provide new insights into the distribution of blood flow in this model of pulmonary artery obstruction. Recently, Clough et al. (27) and Wietholt et al. (28) used micro-CT coupled

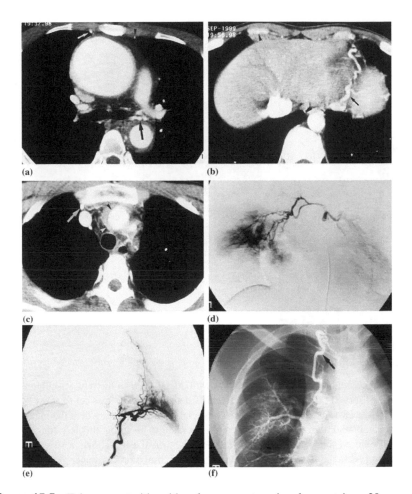

Figure 15.5 Takayasu arteritis with pulmonary artery involvement in a 20-year-old man. (a) CT scan obtained at the level of the tracheal carina shows a hypertrophied right bronchial artery in the retrobronchial area (black arrow). The right internal mammary artery (white arrow) is also enlarged when compared with the left internal mammary artery (arrowhead). The aortic wall is thickened, and the pulmonary arteries are relatively small. The dilated ascending aorta suggests aortic involvement by Takayasu arteritis. (b) CT scan obtained at the level of the dome of the liver shows a hypertrophied left inferior phrenic artery (arrow). The right internal mammary artery is also demonstrated in the anterior chest wall (arrowhead). (c) CT scan obtained at the level of the aortic arch vessels shows the hypertrophied right internal mammary artery (arrow). Note the thickening of the arch vessels (arrowheads). (d) Bronchial angiogram shows hypervascular staining in the right lung. (e) Selective left inferior phrenic arteriogram shows the hypertrophied left inferior phrenic artery supplying the left lower lung. (f) Selective right internal mammary arteriogram shows the hypertrophied right internal mammary artery (arrow) and pulmonary vessels opacified by the systemic-to-pulmonary artery shunt [From Do et al. (22), by permission].

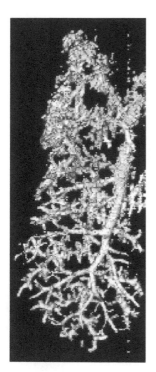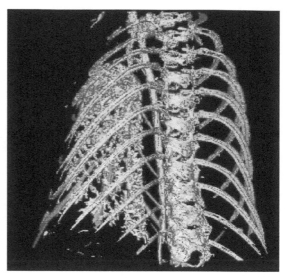

Figure 15.6   The image on the right shows a dorsal view of the new vasculature in the left lung observed through the thorax. The CT density window was set to show bone and methacrylate cast material. Note the cast material filling the aorta where the methacrylate was injected and the extensive systemic vasculature invading the left lung. No cast material entered the normal right lung. The image on the left shows a vascular cast of new blood vessels from another animal without the thoracic cage. Note the dense plexus of new vessels in the upper left lung, fed by vascular connections from the chest wall. In the lung, this new plexus establishes connections to the existing pulmonary vascular tree, which also fills with the casting material. These images provide confirmation of the new systemic vasculature invading the substance of the left lung after LPAL (Image done in collaboration with Chris Dawson at the Medical College of Wisconsin).

with SPECT to visualize this distribution in a rat model. Figure 15.8 shows a nominal image obtained after aortic injection of aggregates in a rat 40 days after LPAL. Images were obtained by using a gamma camera equipped with a 5 mm pinhole after a 2 mCu aortic injection of aggregates (1 mL). SPECT reconstruction of 128 views at 20 s per view was performed by using ordered-subset expectation maximization. Subsequently, without repositioning the animal, micro-CT imaging was performed by using 360 projection images acquired over 360°. The SPECT and micro-CT image volumes were co-registered, the lung fields within the SPECT images were identified from the micro-CT

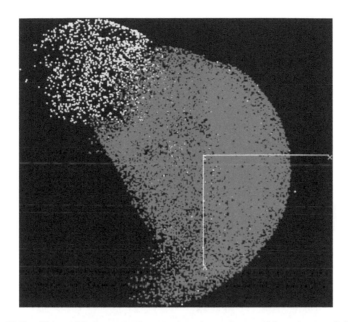

Figure 15.7 (**See color insert**) Fluorescent microspheres (15 μm) were injected into the jugular vein (grey) and left ventricle (white) 14 days after LPAL in mice. After histologic sectioning of the lungs and three-dimensional reconstruction of fluorescent images, the composite image shows that only spheres injected into the jugular vein appeared in the right lung and only spheres injected into the left side of the heart appeared in the upper left lung. In this experiment, no spheres were seen in the lower left lung (Image done in collaboration with Susan Bernard and Robb Glenny at the University of Washington).

images, and the activity within the left lung was quantified and used as a measure of perfusion through the bronchial circulation. A time course sequence of such images can provide important information about the functional development of angiogenesis. This should help provide new insights into the mechanisms responsible for angiogenesis. For instance, this model has been used to show that both lung ischemia and systemic wound healing (thoracotomy) in immediate proximity to the ischemic lung are essential for neovascularization. Additional studies demonstrated that the C-X-C chemokines play a prominent role in the generation of new vessels to the lung (29).

IV. Imaging Neovascularization in Lung Cancer

The role of angiogenesis in cancer has received an enormous amount of attention in recent years, with the hope that by blocking angiogenesis, the spread and growth of cancer might be controlled. The ability to visualize new vessels in patients with cancer provides an opportunity not only to follow the growth of

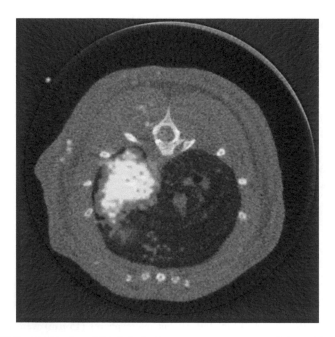

Figure 15.8 Technetium 99-labeled albumen aggregates were injected into the aorta 40 days after LAPL in rats. Micro-CT/SPECT image shows restoration of left lung perfusion, independently measured to be 20% of cardiac output (Unpublished image provided by Anne Clough at Marquette University).

the tumor but also to assess functional changes in the vasculature. Such imaging technology is critically important in the evaluation of new therapies that involve inhibition or destruction of tumor vasculature. In the thorax, at least three approaches have been applied to this objective. Using a method related to that described previously for imaging airway walls through a bronchoscope, Shibuya et al. (30) have been able to follow the growth of the vasculature in bronchial tumors. Their approach was to use high-magnification bronchovideoscopy with a narrow-band imaging (NBI) filter that included the Blue-1 wavelength range of 400–430 nm. This range covers the 410 nm absorption wavelengths for hemoglobin and allows more accurate detection of vasculature structure. This method provides sufficient resolution to enable quantification of capillary diameters in visualized regions. Figure 15.9 shows one example from this work. The figure compares four different bronchoscopic images obtained by using different optical approaches. The increased diagnostic ability of the NBI Blue-1 approach is apparent.

Visualization of blood vessels in the lung by CT can be enhanced by addition of contrast media to the blood. This approach, known as contrast-enhanced dynamic CT, was shown by Tateishi et al. (31) to be able to predict

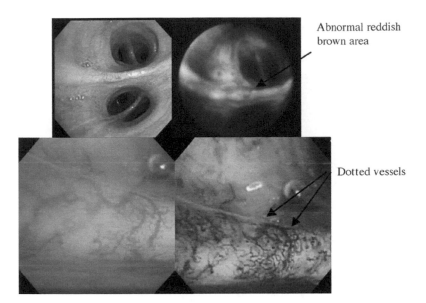

Abnormal reddish
brown area

Dotted vessels

Figure 15.9 **(See color insert)** High-magnification bronchovideoscopy combined with
NBI of the bronchial mucosa at sites of abnormal fluorescence. Shown are four different
bronchoscopic findings (white light bronchoscopy, fluorescence bronchoscopy, high-
magnification bronchovideoscopy, and high-magnification bronchovideoscopy with NBI)
at the right basal bronchus of a patient with sputum cytologic findings suggestive of malignancy. Redness and swelling at the bifurcation were observed under white light examination,
and an abnormal reddish-brown area was identified by fluorescence examination. Increased
vessel growth and complex networks of tortuous vessels were observed at sites of abnormal
fluorescence by high-magnification bronchovideoscopy with conventional RGB broadband
filter. In the NBI images, the vessels were seen to be clearly dotted among the complex
networks of tortuous vessels. The pathologic diagnosis, as determined by biopsy, was angiogenic squamous dysplasia [From Shibuya et al. (30), by permission].

tumor angiogenesis in patients with lung cancer. In particular, the maximum
attenuation values in selected regions of interest during the dynamic CT scans
were correlated with vascular endothelial growth factor-positive tumor biopsy
specimens. Figure 15.10 shows one result from their study, including an image
from the dynamic CT and the findings from histologic examination of tissue
biopsy specimens. This approach has great promise for the ability to monitor
the growth of vascular intense tumors in the lung.

Green fluorescent protein (GFP) has been used to visualize tumor growth in
many organs. By transfecting tumor cells with the pLEIN expression vector,
enhanced expression of GFP can be induced (32,33). Chishima et al. (32) were
able to follow the progressive growth of human lung tumors in the mouse lung
and pleural space. Although this approach does not provide direct images of
the blood vessels, by identifying the leading growth edge of the tumor, it is

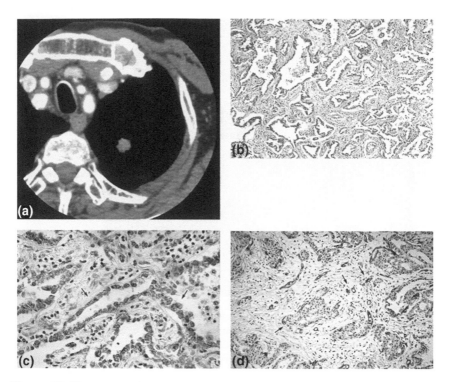

Figure 15.10   Images of stage IA lung adenocarcinoma from a 67-year-old male patient. (a) This contrast-enhanced, dynamic CT image, which was taken 50 s after the administration of contrast material, reveals the maximum attenuation value of the time-attenuation curve of 48 Hounsfield units. (b) This photomicrograph shows papillary growth of tumor cells consistent with (hematoxylin and eosin stain; original magnification, 100×). (c) Immunohistochemical staining of anti-vascular endothelial growth factor (anti-VEGF) antibody is shown (original magnification, 200×). There are positive findings for VEGF in the cytoplasm of tumor cells (arrows). (d) Immunohistochemical staining of anti-CD34 antibody is shown (original magnification, 200×). Delineated CD34-positive cells were counted as microvessels (arrows) [From Ref. (31) by permission].

possible to visualize the new vessel growth that accompanies the growing tumor. One of the problems with using such intravital microscopy to visualize tumors with a GFP label is that the resolution of the image is limited by light scattering through the skin. Yang et al. (33) have recently described a method in which a reversible skin-flap is used to reduce light attenuation and scattering. Using this method, they were able to follow the growth of Lewis lung tumors that expressed GFP. Figure 15.11 shows results from their recent study of lung visualization. This method has increased the detection sensitivity and observable depth of tissue, allowing visualization of tumor growth with its concomitant new vasculature.

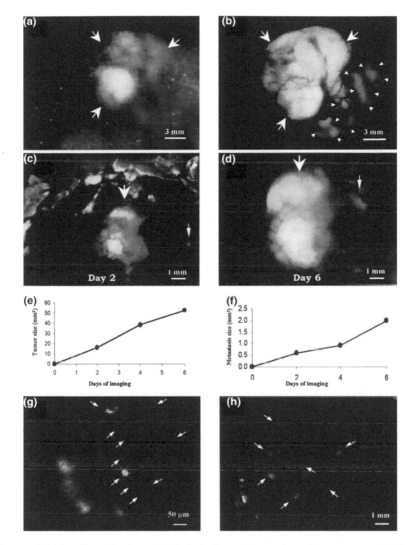

Figure 15.11 (See color insert) Whole-body and direct view of lung cancer. (a) Whole-body transcutaneous image of orthotopically growing Lewis lung tumor (arrows) in an intact live mouse on day 14 after surgical orthotopic implantation (SOI) (Bar = 3 mm). (b) Direct view of orthotopically growing Lewis lung tumor through skin-flap window also imaged in a (arrows). The primary tumor (large arrows) and invading tumor cells (small arrows) are visible. Vessels can also be visualized in the primary tumor (Bar = 3 mm). (c) Direct view of microfoci (arrows) on the ipsilateral lung on day 5 after SOI (Bar = 1 mm). (d) Same as c, day 9 after SOI (Bar = 1 mm). (e) Growth curve of large tumor determined by direct-view images (c and d, indicated by thick arrows). (f) Growth curve of microfocal tumor determined by direct-view images (c and d, indicated by fine arrows). (g) Two three-cell microfoci in the ipsilateral lung on day 5 after SOI visualized by direct-view imaging (Bar = 50 μm). (h) Micrometastases (arrows) in the contralateral lung on day 7 after SOI visualized by direct-view imaging (Bar = 1 mm) [From Yang et al. (33), by permission].

V. Concluding Comments and Future Expectations

Although the focus of this book is on molecular imaging, this chapter deals primarily with structural imaging. The reasons for this altered focus are related to the unique aspects of lung structure and its dual circulations. However, with the accelerated development and improvement of new technologies, we expect that the ability to obtain molecular images from the lungs may soon become routine. One potential approach is to incorporate reporter probes in the genome that can be detected with optical detectors (Chapters 4 and 10). Several systems exist (e.g., xenogen, is available http://www.xenogen.com/prodimag1.html or are being developed to visualize a luciferase reporter in intact mice. With three-dimensional detectors in a darkened enclosure, it is now possible to detect low levels of molecular signaling even within the lungs. The probes needed to detect angiogenesis in the lungs are currently being evaluated in gene array experiments by several groups (29,34).

Along these lines, the research with selective light band filtering shown in Fig. 15.9 may lead to the detection of other tagged molecules by means of bronchoscopy. For example, it may be possible to visualize the GFP tag used by Yang et al. (33) from within the airway lumen. It may also be possible to apply colored tags to other molecular markers of angiogenesis that could then be visualized by means of bronchoscopy from the airway lumen. Given that angiogenesis normally arises from the bronchial circulation, this approach may actually allow better access to imaging changes in the vasculature, even in longitudinal studies in humans. Of course, questions about sensitivity of detection and signal/noise ratio remain to be answered, but this multifaceted approach may eventually make the lungs more accessible than other organs to molecular imaging of angiogenesis.

References

1. Anderson SD, Daviskas E. The mechanism of exercise-induced asthma is ... J Allergy Clin Immunol 2000; 106:453–459.
2. McDonald DM, Choyke PL. Imaging of angiogenesis: from microscope to clinic. Nat Med 2003; 9:713–725.
3. Milne EN, Zerhouni EA. Blood supply of pulmonary metastases. J Thorac Imaging 1987; 2:15–23.
4. Michel RP, Hakim TS, Petsikas D. Segmental vascular resistance in postobstructive pulmonary vasculopathy. J Appl Physiol 1990; 69:1022–1032.
5. Deffebach ME, Charan NB, Lakshminarayan S, Butler J. The bronchial circulation-small, but vital attribute of the lung. Am Rev Respir Dis 1987; 135:463–481.
6. Moldobaeva A, Wagner EM. Heterogeneity of bronchial endothelial cell permeability. Am J Physiol Lung Cell Mol Physiol 2002; 283:L520–L527.
7. Moldobaeva A, Wagner EM. Angiotensin-converting enzyme activity in ovine bronchial vasculature. J Appl Physiol 2003; 95:2278–2284.

8. Woodruff PG, Dolganov GM, Ferrando RE, Donnelly S, Hays SR, Solberg OD, Carter R, Wong HH, Cadbury PS, Fahy JV. Hyperplasia of smooth muscle in mild/moderate asthma without changes in cell size or gene expression. Am J Respir Crit Care Med 2004; 169(9):1001–1006.

9. Li X, Wilson JW. Increased vascularity of the bronchial mucosa in mild asthma. Am J Respir Crit Care Med 1997; 156:229–233.

10. Chu HW, Kraft M, Rex MD, Martin RJ. Evaluation of blood vessels and edema in the airways of asthma patients: regulation with clarithromycin treatment. Chest 2001; 120:416–422.

11. Kuwano K, Bosken CH, Pare PD, Bai TR, Wiggs BR, Hogg JC. Small airways dimensions in asthma and in chronic obstructive pulmonary disease. Am Rev Respir Dis 1993; 148:1220–1225.

12. Tanaka H, Yamada G, Saikai T et al. Increased airway vascularity in newly diagnosed asthma using a high-magnification bronchovideoscope. Am J Respir Crit Care Med 2003; 168:1495–1499.

13. Thurston G, Murphy TJ, Baluk P, Lindsey JR, McDonald DM. Angiogenesis in mice with chronic airway inflammation: strain-dependent differences. Am J Pathol 1998; 153:1099–1112.

14. Lim LH, Bochner BS, Wagner EM. Leukocyte recruitment in the airways. an intravital microscopic study of rat tracheal microcirculation. Am J Physiol Lung Cell Mol Physiol 2002; 282:L959–L967.

15. Lim LH, Wagner EM. Airway distension promotes leukocyte recruitment in rat tracheal circulation. Am J Respir Crit Care Med 2003; 168:1068–1074.

16. Virchow R. Uber die standpunkte in den wissenschaftlichen medizin. Virchow Archiv 1847; 1:1–19.

17. Karsner H, Ghoreyeb A. Studies in infarction: the circulation in experimental pulmonary embolism. J Exp Med 1913; 18:507–522.

18. Charan NB, Carvalho P. Angiogenesis in bronchial circulatory system after unilateral pulmonary artery obstruction. J Appl Physiol 1997; 82:284–291.

19. Fadel E, Riou JY, Mazmanian M et al. Pulmonary thromboendarterectomy for chronic thromboembolic obstruction of the pulmonary artery in piglets. J Thorac Cardiovasc Surg 1999; 117:787–793.

20. Weibel ER. Early stages in the development of collateral circulation to the lung in the rat. Circ Res 1960; 8:353–376.

21. Endrys J, Hayat N, Cherian G. Comparison of bronchopulmonary collaterals and collateral blood flow in patients with chronic thromboembolic and primary pulmonary hypertension. Heart 1997; 78:171–176.

22. Do KH, Goo JM, Im JG, Kim KW, Chung JW, Park JH. Systemic arterial supply to the lungs in adults: spiral CT findings. Radiographics 2001; 21:387–402.

23. Hasegawa I, Boiselle PM, Hatabu H. Bronchial artery dilatation on MDCT scans of patients with acute pulmonary embolism: comparison with chronic or recurrent pulmonary embolism. AJR Am J Roentgenol 2004; 182:67–72.

24. Mitzner W, Lee W, Georgakopoulos D, Wagner E. Angiogenesis in the mouse lung. Am J Pathol 2000; 157:93–101.

25. Verloop MC. On the arteriae bronchiales and their anastomosing with the arteria pulmonalis in some rodents; a micro-anatomical study. Acta Anat 1949; 7:1–32.

26. Bernard SL, Ewen JR, Barlow CH, Kelly JJ, McKinney S, Frazer DA, Glenny RW. High spatial resolution measurements of organ blood flow in small laboratory animals. Am J Physiol Heart Circ Physiol 2000; 279:H2043–H2052.
27. Clough AV, Weitholt C, Molthen RC, Gordon JC, Roerig DL. SPECT/micro-CT imaging of bronchial angiogenesis in a rat. In: Barrett HH, Kupinski M, eds. Small Animal SPECT Imaging. Kluwer, 2004.
28. Wietholt C, Molthen RC, Haworth ST, Dawson CA, Roerig DL, Clough AV. Quantification of bronchial circulation perfusion in rats. In: Amani AA, Manduca A, eds. Physiology, Function, and Structure from Medical Images. Vol. 5370. SPIE Proceedings, 2004.
29. Srisuma S, Biswal SS, Mitzner WA, Gallagher SJ, Mai KH, Wagner EM. Identification of genes promoting angiogenesis in mouse lung by transcriptional profiling. Am J Respir Cell Mol Biol 2003; 29:172–179.
30. Shibuya K, Hoshino H, Chiyo M et al. High magnification bronchovideoscopy combined with narrow band imaging could detect capillary loops of angiogenic squamous dysplasia in heavy smokers at high risk for lung cancer. Thorax 2003; 58:989–995.
31. Tateishi U, Kusumoto M, Akiyama Y, Kishi F, Nishimura M, Moriyama N. Role of contrast-enhanced dynamic CT in the diagnosis of active tuberculoma. Chest 2002; 122:1280–1284.
32. Chishima T, Miyagi Y, Wang X et al. Metastatic patterns of lung cancer visualized live and in process by green fluorescence protein expression. Clin Exp Metastasis 1997; 15:547–552.
33. Yang M, Baranov E, Wang JW et al. Direct external imaging of nascent cancer, tumor progression, angiogenesis, and metastasis on internal organs in the fluorescent orthotopic model. Proc Natl Acad Sci USA 2002; 99:3824–3829.
34. McDonald SL, Edington HD, Kirkwood JM, Becker D. Expression analysis of genes identified by molecular profiling of VGP melanomas and MGP melanoma-positive lymph nodes. Cancer Biol Ther 2004; 3.

16

New Methods for Visualizing the Airways

WILLIAM LUNN and ARMIN ERNST

Harvard Medical School,
Boston, Massachusetts, USA

I. Introduction

Lung cancer is the leading cause of cancer related deaths in the United States. The American Cancer Society estimates that there will be 173,770 new cases of lung cancer diagnosed in 2004 and that 160,440 people will die of lung cancer in the same year (1). According to these estimates, lung cancer will represent ~13% of all new cases of cancer diagnosed when compared with 17% for prostate cancer, 16% for breast cancer, 8% for colon cancer, and 4% for skin cancer. However, more people will die of lung cancer in 2004 than of the earlier listed cancers combined. In fact, deaths due to lung cancer are estimated to account for 28% of all the cancer related deaths in the United States in 2004.

Despite enormous research efforts and recent advances in multimodality therapy, the mortality rate for lung cancer is significant. The American Cancer Society reports a 5 year survival rate for lung cancer in the United States, combining all cell types, of 15%. This compares to a rate of 13% for the interval from 1974 to 1976. Although patients with early stage nonsmall cell carcinoma have the best prognosis, $\sim$50% of these patients will eventually die of their cancer despite surgical resection.

Given the lack of significant improvement in survival in patients with lung cancer over the last 30 years, investigators have begun to explore other options to combat this disease. Primary prevention, halting the appearance of disease by avoiding tobacco use, has been part of the strategy to combat lung cancer since the Surgeon General's 1964 report on the health consequences of tobacco habituation. Although it is noteworthy that the number of adult smokers has declined, it is disappointing that the number of adolescent smokers, particularly women, is on the rise. The lack of success of abstention from tobacco has led to an interest in chemoprevention strategies. The concept is that if patients cannot be convinced to quit smoking, they can be given medications designed to prevent carcinogenesis. The National Cancer Institute's Specialized Program of Research Excellence has launched parallel studies of such agents in the prevention of lung cancer. The primary objective of these investigations is to prevent the appearance or halt the progression of premalignant lesions as assessed by sputum cytology or tissue histology. The final results of these studies are pending, but are being anticipated with much enthusiasm.

Other efforts to improve survival in patients with lung cancer have centered on the concept of early detection of premalignant lesions. As it is known that patients diagnosed and treated in early stage disease have a better survival, it seems logical that improving detection techniques would lead to improvement in survival statistics. Indeed, identifying and treating premalignant lesions in the colon and cervix have resulted in a decreased incidence of malignancies in these organs. Unfortunately, all of the studies to date looking at early detection techniques for lung cancer have not led to improvements in cancer related mortality. It should be noted that the majority of these studies are dated over 15 years old, rely on plain chest radiographs and sputum cytology, and thus may not be applicable in the age of ultrafast computed tomography (CT) scanning. Investigators are currently studying the role of CT in lung cancer screening. Despite much debate in the literature on the preliminary results of these studies, final conclusions are pending. As a result, the American Cancer Society does not recommend sputum cytology, bronchoscopy, or chest roentgens for lung cancer screening at this time. This is in contrast to Japan, which employs a screening program on the basis of CT and sputum cytology that has proven effective in their population. Other screening tools, such as ultrafast CT, sputum DNA, and serum biomarkers, are under development and their use is investigational.

Among the most promising technologies to screen for lung abnormalities are imaging modalities. Physicians have been fascinated with the ability to image the living airways ever since Gustav Killian, a German otolaryngologist, performed the first bronchoscopy on a living person via the translaryngeal route with a modified rigid esophagoscope in 1897. Bronchoscopy was further advanced by Shigeto Ikeda, who developed the first flexible bronchoscope in Japan in 1966 and popularized its use worldwide (2). The purpose of this discussion is to review current airway imaging modalities that are, or may become, of clinical use to the thoracic endoscopist in detection and/or treatment of airway diseases.

II. Cellular Evolution of Lung Cancer

Auerbach et al. (3,4) were the first to describe premalignant changes in the airways of smokers and former smokers. In autopsy studies of 1522 adult smokers, former smokers, and nonsmokers, multiple bronchial cross-sectional biopsies were analyzed, nearly 42,000 in total. Abnormal airway histology was reported in >90% of the smokers, whereas only ~1% of the patients who had never been smokers had biopsy sections with cellular atypia. Though the histology of the lesions had been described in detail, a formal classification system was not developed until later. In 1999, the World Health Organization published the most recent classification system detailing seven types of airway histology: 1) normal, 2) reserve cell hyperplasia, 3) squamous metaplasia, 4) mild dysplasia, 5)moderate dysplasia, 6) severe dysplasia, and 7) carcinoma *in situ* (CIS). Current opinion holds that there is a stepwise progression from normal tissue through each of these stages before cancer develops. Additionally, other changes in the airway wall have been noted to correlate with the development of malignancy. Angiogenic squamous dysplasia (ASD), for example, develops from the growth of new capillaries into dysplastic airway epithelium. This is thought to occur in response to tumor growth factors that facilitate neoangiogenesis. The earlier mentioned molecular changes are exploited by imaging technologies that allow physicians to visualize these changes in the living human lung.

III. Imaging Modalities

A. Autoflourescence Bronchoscopy

Light reflecting on living airway tissue interacts with electrons in chromophores, such as collagen and elastin, causing them to become excited and then return to ground level. It is the return of electrons to ground level that results in emission of fluorescence—light energy. When light wavelength 400–450 nm is directed in the normal airway, the resultant fluorescence is green. This property of the airway to fluoresce has been called "autoflourescence" (AF) by investigators as

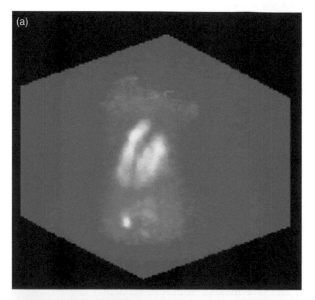

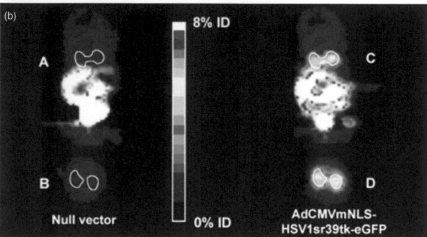

Figure 8.2 (a) Three-dimensional views of the lungs in a rat infected with 1×10^{11} viral particles (VP) of AdCMV-mNLS-HSV1sr39*tk-egfp*. A movie version of this figure is available at: http://ccs.wustl.edu/schuster_avifile/avi.htm. Reproduced with permission from Ref. (43). (b) Reporter gene expression imaging with PET in a control mouse infected with a null vector (a and b) and a mouse expressing the mutant HSV1-*tk* gene (C and D). Panels A and C are coronal views of the mice, whereas B and D are corresponding transverse slices obtained at the mid-lung level. In both mice, regions-of-interest (ROIs) are drawn to indicate lung boundaries (white lines) and tracer uptake was expressed as a percentage of injected dose (ID). There was significant pulmonary uptake of the tracer in the mouse expressing the viral TK when compared with the control mouse. High levels of activity in the abdomen are due to a combination of urinary excretion and of biliary excretion into the gastrointestinal tract.

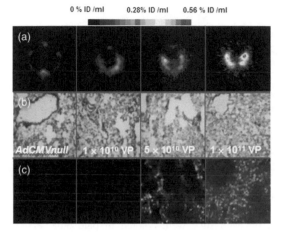

Figure 8.3 PET images (a), light microscopic micrographs (b), and corresponding fluorescence micrographs (c) obtained in one rat infected with AdCMVnull (left panel) and three rats, respectively, infected with 1×10^{10}, 5×10^{10}, and 1×10^{11} viral particles (VP) of AdCMV-mNLS-sr39tk-$egfp$ (panel 2, 3, and 4 from left to right). The PET images are transverse slices obtained at the mid-chest level. Light and fluorescent micrographs ($10\times$ magnification) represent identical lung areas in the left lung from adjacent sections. Exposure time for each fluorescent micrograph was the same (960 ms). Fluorescence was mainly seen in distal parenchymal (alveolar) cells rather than in airway epithelium or microvessel endothelium. [Reproduced with permission from Richard et al. (43).]

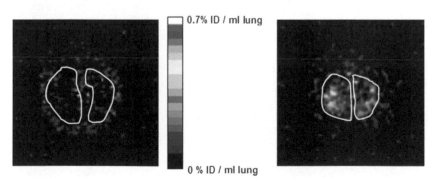

Figure 8.4 (Left) Transverse image taken 1 h after IV administration of [^{64}Cu]-TETA-OC from a rat after null vector administration. (Right) Three days after intratracheal administration of adenovectors containing $hSSTr2$. The image is at the mid-thoracic level. The white lines on each figure depict lung ROIs. The color bar shows units of percentage of injected dose (ID) per gram.

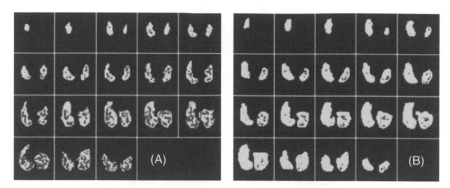

Figure 8.7 Parametric images of lung [^{18}F]-FHBG distribution in a rat administered adenovectors in a surfactant vehicle (A) or a saline vehicle (B). The pixels within each ROI drawn on each slice were colored in pale blue. Pixels with radioactivity values greater than 0.3% of [^{18}F]-FHBG ID/mL were colored in red. [^{18}F]-FHBG = 9-(4-[^{18}F]-fluoro-3-hydroxymethylbutyl)guanine. Note that higher levels of expression with the surfactant vehicle are apparent, without any specific spatial dependence. [Reproduced with permission from Richard et al. (41).]

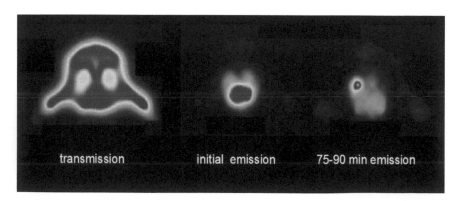

transmission   initial emission   75-90 min emission

Figure 9.2 Transthoracic PET images 15 h after instillation of *Streptococcus pneumoniae* into the right upper lobe of rabbit lung. Transmission image on the left shows distribution of lung density. Emission images show distribution of ^{18}F initially in the blood pool (middle) and localized to the challenged lung (right) 75–90 min after intravenous injection of ^{18}FDG. [Adapted from Jones et al. (21).]

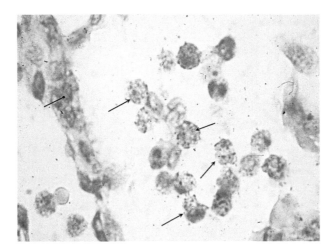

Figure 9.3 Microautoradiograph of lung tissue sample taken 1 h after injection of (^{3}H-DG) at a time of high ^{18}FDG uptake shown by PET (18 h after *Streptococcus pneumoniae* challenge to the rabbit lung). Silver grains developed by autoradiography show localization of ^{3}H-DG to neutrophils that have emigrated into the airspaces (arrowhead) but not in those in the capillaries (pinhead).

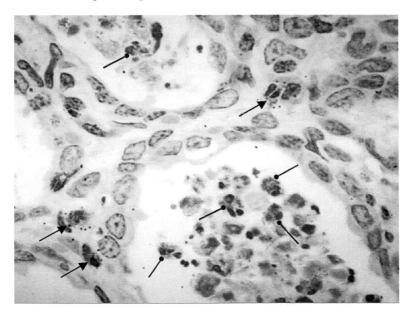

Figure 9.4 Microautoradiograph of lung tissue sample taken 1 h fter injection of ^{3}H-DG at a time of high ^{18}FDG uptake shown by PET in a scarring model of lung inflammation (2 weeks after bleomycin challenge to the rabbit lung). Silver grains developed by autoradiography show localization of ^{3}H-DG to neutrophils in the interstitium (arrowhead) but not in those in the airspaces (pinheads).

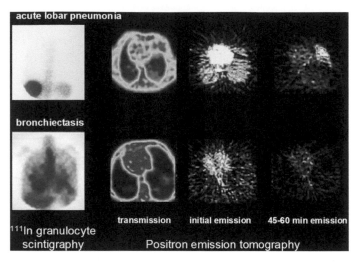

Figure 9.5 White blood cell scans of neutrophil migration (left) with PET images (right) in a patient 3 days after onset of symptoms of acute lobar pneumonia (top) and a patient with chronic bronchiectasis (bottom). White blood cell scans are clearly negative in pneumonia and positive in bronchiectasis. PET scans show transmission image, initial distribution after intravenous injection of ^{18}FDG and localization to affected lobe in the patient with pneumonia at 1 h. There is no apparent increase in ^{18}FDG uptake in the patient with bronchiectasis. [Adapted from Jones et al. (23).]

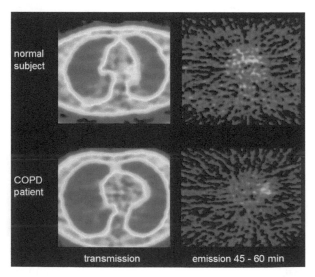

Figure 9.6 PET transmission images and ^{18}FDG emission images at 1 h after injection for a healthy subject (top) and a patient with COPD (bottom). No obvious difference is seen between the images. Differences can only be revealed by quantification of image data. [Adapted from Jones et al. (28).]

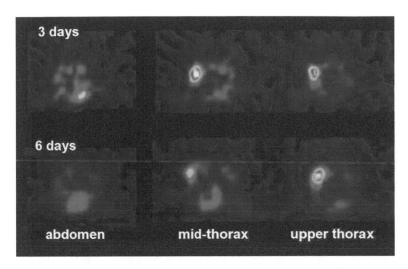

Figure 9.10 PET images of thorax after intravenous injection of [^{11}C]-*R*-PK11195 3 days (top) and 6 days (bottom) after challenge with 50 mg of 5 μm particles of microcrystalline silica into the right upper lobe of rabbit lung. Localization of radioactivity remains in the challenged region. [Adapted from Jones et al. (37).]

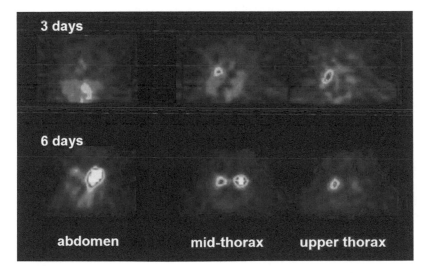

Figure 9.11 PET images of thorax after intravenous injection of [^{11}C]-*R*-PK11195 3 days (top) and 6 days (bottom) after challenge with 50 mg of 5 μm particles of amorphous (nonfibrogenic) silica into the right upper lobe of rabbit lung. Localization of radioactivity is to the challenged region at 3 days. By 6 days, there is a second signal, indicating clearance of particle-bearing macrophages through the lymphatics. [Adapted from Jones et al. (37).]

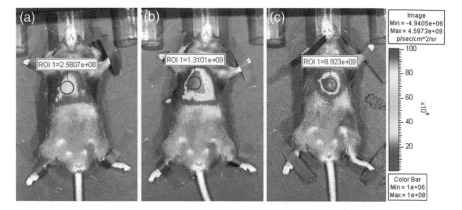

Figure 10.3 Bioluminescent imaging of a wild-type mouse after implantation of a light emitting bead (with a spectrum similar to that of firefly luciferase) in the pleural space posterior to the right lung (a), in the pleural space anterior to the right lung (b), or anterior to the rib cage (c). The pseudocolor scale is shown and the region of interest (ROI) for photon detection is indicated by a red circle. Detected photon counts are indicated for each ROI.

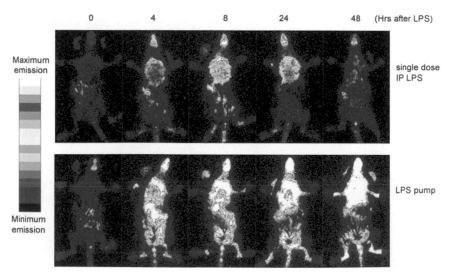

Figure 10.5 Bioluminescence of a representative HLL mouse treated with a single IP injection of LPS (upper panel) or LPS pump (lower panel). For detection of NF-κB dependent luciferase activity, luciferin (3 mg) was given by IP injection and photon emission was detected 30 min later. The scale for the pseudocolor images, indicative of relative pixel intensity, is shown at left (white is the highest emission). Mean $+/-$ SEM, *P $<$ 0.05 compared with single dose IP LPS group.

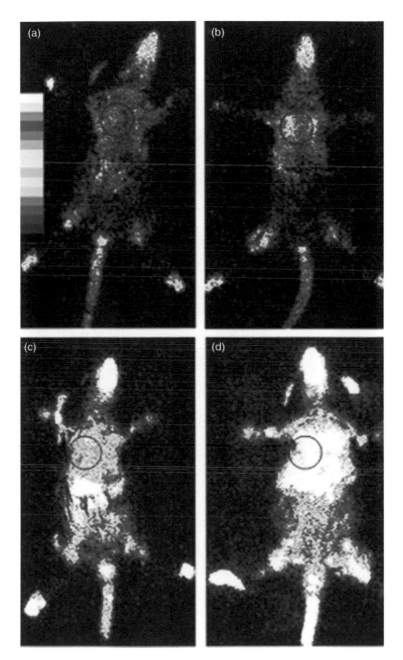

Figure 10.6 Bioluminescent images of HLL mice are shown at baseline (a) or 24 h after intratracheal injection of *Pseudomonas aeruginosa* at 10^5 (b), 10^6 (c), or 10^7 (d) colony forming units. The circle represents the region of interest used for quantization of photon emission. Reprinted with permission from Ref. (56).

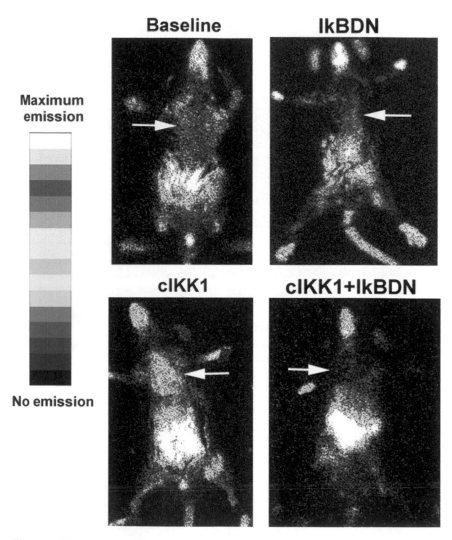

Figure 10.7 Representative bioluminescent images from HLL mice prior to treatment (baseline) and 72 h after intratracheal treatment with adenoviral vectors expressing IκB-αDN, cIKK1, or cIKK1 + IκB-αDN. Photon emission from the area of the thorax overlying the lungs is identified by arrows and quantified. Reprinted with permission from Ref. (55).

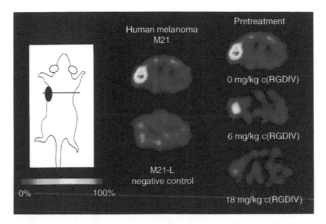

Figure 11.1 Noninvasive imaging of $\alpha v\beta 3$ expression. Transaxial PET images of nude mice bearing human melanoma xenografts. Images were acquired 90 min after injection of ~5.5 MBq of [^{18}F]Galacto-RGD. (Top left image) Selective accumulation of the tracer in the $\alpha v\beta 3$-positve (M21) tumor on the left flank. No focal tracer accumulation is visible in the $\alpha v\beta 3$-negative (*M21-L*) control tumor (bottom left image). The three images on the right were obtained from serial [^{18}F]Galacto-RGD PET studies in one mouse. These images illustrate the dose-dependent blockade of tracer uptake by the $\alpha v\beta 3$-selective cyclic pentapeptide cyclo (−Arg−Gly−Asp−D−he−Val−). [Figure adapted from Haubner et al. (24)]

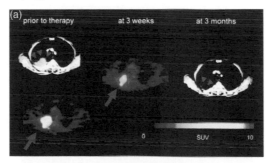

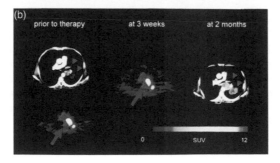

Figure 11.5 FDG-PET imaging lung tumors before and after treatment. [^{18}F]-FDG-PET and CT scans of a responding (a) and nonresponding (b) lung tumor. In the responding tumor, there is a 61% decrease in FDG uptake 3 weeks after initiation of chemotherapy. In contrast, tumor FDG uptake is essentially unchanged in the nonresponding tumor. [Adapted from Weber et al. (69)]

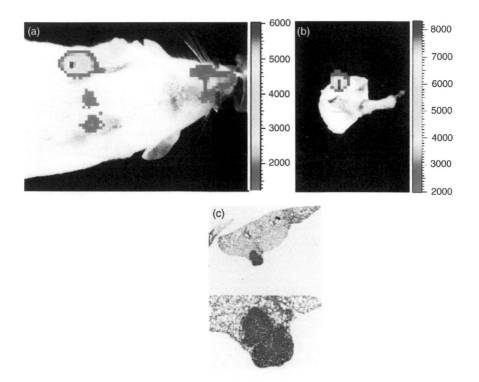

Figure 11.6 Bioluminescence imaging of spontaneous lung tumorigenesis. Tumors arising from LucRep/conditional $Kras2^{v12}$ mice were visualized noninvasively. (a) image of a compound LucRep/conditional $Kras2^{v12}$ mouse 13 weeks after AdCre intubation shows a bright focal region of luminescence originating from the thorax. (b) image of the lungs dissected from the mouse depicted in (a) also shows a single origin of light. (c) The same lungs after H&E processing (at 2.5× and 10× magnification) showing that the light detected in (a) and (b) originated from a single lesion measuring between 1 and 2 mm in diameter. [Adapted from Lyons et al. (85)]

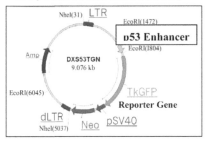

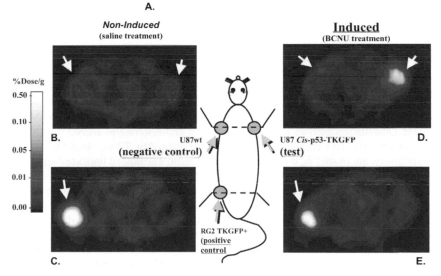

Figure 11.7 PET imaging of endogenous p53 activation and validation of *Cis*-p53/ TKGFP reporter system in cell cultures and sampled tumor tissue. The p53-sensitive reporter vector contains an artificial p53 specific enhancer that activates expression of the TKeGFP reporter gene. [Figure adapted from Doubrovin et al. (46)]

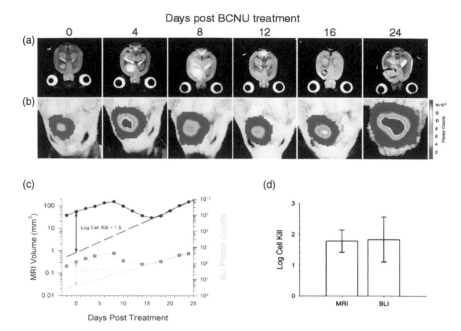

Figure 11.8 Temporal analysis of the response of 9L ^{Luc} tumor to BCNU chemotherapy (panels a–d). Tumor cells were implanted 16 days before treatment. Tumor volume was monitored with T2-weighted MRI (a) and intratumoral luciferase activity was monitored with BLI (b). The days post BCNU therapy on which the images were obtained are indicated at the top. The scale to the right of the BL images describes the color map for the photo count. Quantitative analysis of tumor progression and response to BCNU treatment (c). Tumor volumes and total tumor photon emission obtained by T2-weighted MRI and BLI, respectively, are plotted vs. days post BCNU treatment. The dashed lines are the regression fits of exponential tumor repopulation following therapy. The solid vertical lines denote the apparent tumor-volume and photon-production losses elicited by BCNU on the day of treatment from which log cell kill values were calculated as previously described (9). Comparison of log cell kill values determined from MRI and BLI measurements (d). Log cell kill elicited by BCNU chemotherapy was calculated using MRI (1.78 ± 0.36) and BLI (1.84 ± 0.73). Data are represented as mean ± SEM for each animal ($n = 5$). There was no statistically significant difference between the log kills calculated using the MRI abd BLI data ($P = 0.951$). [Figure adapted from Rehemtulla et al. (32)] Kinetics of intracranial glioma growth (panels e and f). 9L^{Luc} cells were implanted intracerebrally and tumor progression was monitored with MRI (A) and BLI (B). The days, after sham treatment, on which the images were obtained are indicated at the top. The MR images are T2-weighted and are of a representative slice from the multislice dataset. The scale to the right of the BL images describes the color map for luminescent signal. Correlation of tumor volume with *in vivo* photon emission is shown where tumor volume was measured from T2-weighted MR images and plotted against total measured photon counts (f). The relationship between the two measurements was defined by regression analysis ($r = 0.91$). [Figure adapted from Rehemtulla et al. (32)]

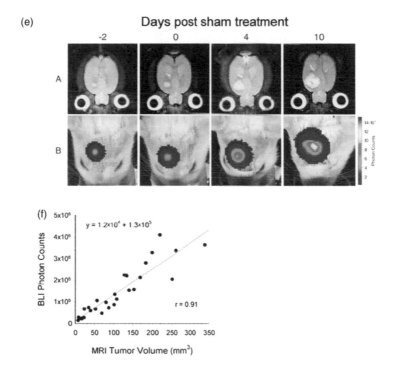

Figure 11.8 *Continued*

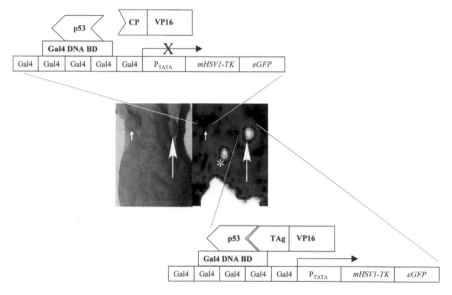

Figure 12.1 Two-hybrid strategy for molecular imaging of protein–protein interactions *in vivo* using microPET and dual reporter genes. *Lower right*: The p53 tumor suppressor and the transforming SV40 large T antigen (TAg), two known interacting proteins,
are each fused to different domains of a hybrid transcription factor. Both portions of the
transcription factor are required to activate the dual PET-fluorescence reporter gene
(*mHSV1-tk-egfp*), but only the DNA binding domain (Gal4BD) can bind on its own to
specific DNA sequences that regulate activation of the reporter. However, when p53
and TAg proteins interact, the activation domain (VP16) is now properly assembled,
thereby switching on the dual reporter. The activated reporter can be detected by
microPET imaging of living mice using the positron-emitting radiopharmaceutical
^{18}F-FHBG, a substrate phosphorylated and trapped within cells by mHSV1-TK, and
detected independently by fluorescence microscopy of eGFP. *Upper left*: In contrast,
when the VP16 activation domain is fused to a nonintereacting protein (in this case,
polyoma virus coat protein, CP), the reporter gene cannot be activated. *Middle left:*
Photograph of the anterior thorax of a mouse with axillary xenograft tumors of HeLa
cells containing noninteracting p53-CP proteins (small arrow) and interacting p53-TAg
proteins (large arrow). *Middle right*: coronal microPET image (10 min acquisition time)
of the same mouse showing accumulation of ^{18}F-FHBG only in the tumor expressing
the interacting p53-TAg proteins (large arrow). Asterisk denotes radiotracer in the gallbladder. Intestinal activity from normal hepatobiliary clearance of the radiotracer is
observed in the lower portion of the image. [Reproduced from Ref. (57).]

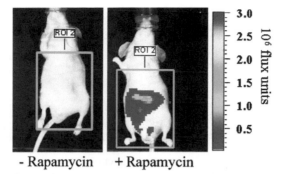

- Rapamycin   + Rapamycin

Figure 12.2 Bioluminescence images were taken 10 h after administration of a single dose of rapamycin (4.5 μg/g, intraperitoneal) (right panel) or vehicle control (left panel). Mice were anesthetized with isoflurane, injected i.p. with D-luciferin (150 μg/g in PBS) and then imaged 10 min later with a CCD camera (1 min exposure, binning 8, f-stop 1, FOV 15 cm). Regions of interest (ROI) used for analysis are shown. Flux units are photons/sec/cm^2/sr.

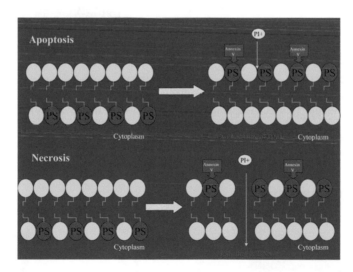

Figure 13.3 Cartoon illustrating the differences between apoptosis and necrosis. Membrane inversion resulting in the exposure of phosphatidyl serine (PS) to the extracellular space occurs in both apoptosis and necrosis. Since the cell membrane remains intact during apoptosis, the charged molecule propidium iodide (PI) cannot enter the cell and label DNA, whereas the disruption of the cell and nuclear membrane that occurs in necrosis allows PI to enter the cell and label DNA. Therefore, cells that are annexin V (+)/PI (−) are undergoing apoptosis, whereas cells that are annexin V (+)/PI (+) are undergoing necrosis.

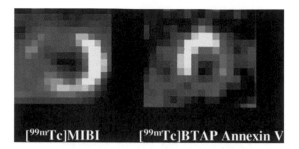

Figure 13.4 SPECT study of myocardial infarction. Notice that the increase in uptake of [99mTc]BTAP annexin V corresponds to the perfusion deficit identified in the [99mTc]MIBI scan. This data is reproduced with permission from Ref. (16).

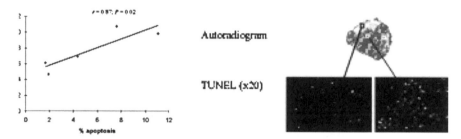

Figure 13.6 Increased tumor uptake of [111In]DTPA-PEG-annexin V. Note the high correlation of tumor uptake of the radiotracer with the apoptotic index (left) and TUNEL staining. This data is reproduced with permission from Ref. (29).

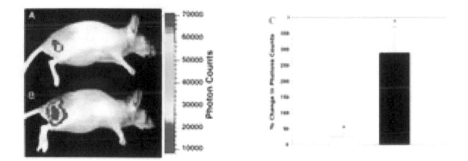

Figure 13.8 Bioluminescent imaging study showing TNF-α-induced activation of caspase-3. This data is reproduced with permission from Ref. (33).

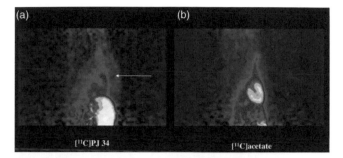

Figure 13.10 MicroPET imaging study in a rodent model of ischemia–reperfusion injury. The high uptake of [^{11}C]PJ 34 was distal to the site of the coronary artery ligation (arrow) and is consistent with PARP-1 mediated necrosis. This is in contrast to uniform uptake of the metabolic radiotracer, [^{11}C]acetate, in normal heart.

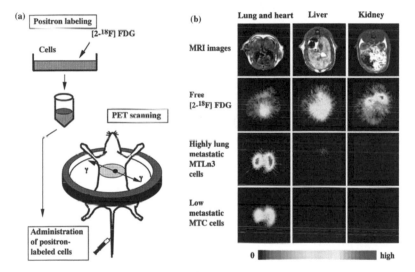

Figure 14.2 Experimental scheme of PET analysis for studying cell trafficking and accumulation of lung metastatic cells having differential metastatic potential in lungs. (a) First, cells are incubated with [2-^{18}F]FDG for 15–30 min at 37°C. Cells are washed to remove any free [2-^{18}F]FDG and are then injected into appropriate animals. PET imaging was started immediately after injection and performed for 60–120 min. Tissue radioactivity in the form of coincidence gamma photons was measured and converted to Bq/cm^3 of tissue volume by calibration. (b) Trafficking of [2-^{18}F]FDG-labeled highly lung metastatic MTLn3 cells and low metastatic MTC cells during the first 10 min after iv administration, as imaged by PET [reprinted with permission from Ref. (11)]. Images are in the coronal plane with a slice size of 3 mm. Scaling was corrected to be comparable in each organ. For reference to the PET images, magnetic resonance (MR) images of lungs, heart, liver, and kidneys are presented in the top panel. Lower three panels show PET images of free [2-^{18}F]FDG (upper), [2-^{18}F]FDG-labeled MTLn3 cells (middle), and [2-^{18}F]FDG-labeled MTC cells (lower).

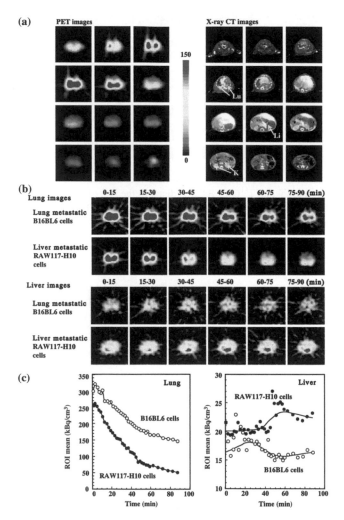

Figure 14.3 *In vivo* trafficking of lung metastatic B16BL6 melanoma cells and liver metastatic RAW117-H10 cells as determined by PET. (a) [2-¹⁸F]FDG-labeled B16BL6 cells were injected via the tail vein of a C57BL/6 mouse. Biodistribution during 30 min after administration of the cells was imaged by PET, and corresponding X-ray CT images are shown with a slice aperture of 3.25 mm [reprinted with permission from Ref. (28)]. Twelve slices from the head (upper left) to the tail (lower right) are shown. Scaling was corrected to be comparable between all images. Li, liver; Lu, lung; and K, kidney. (b) PET analysis of [2-¹⁸F]FDG-labeled B16BL6 and RAW117-H10 cells was performed over 90 min, and 15 min frames show cell accumulation in lungs and liver [reprinted with permission from Ref. (13)]. (c) Time–activity curves of ¹⁸F in lungs and liver after injection of [2-¹⁸F]FDG-labeled B16BL6 and RAW117-H10 cells were obtained from mean pixel radioactivity in the region-of-interest (ROI) of the PET images, where the injected dose was calibrated as 740 kBq.

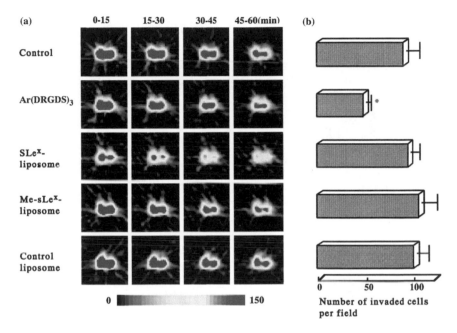

Figure 14.4 Effect of sLe^x-liposome or RGD-related peptide on the trafficking and invasion activity of B16BL6 melanoma cells. (a) C57BL6 mice were injected with [2-^{18}F]FDG-labeled B16BL6 cells (5 × 10^5 cells) with or without sLex-liposome, Me-sLex-liposome, empty liposome (3 nmol as egg yolk phosphatidylcholine), or Ar(DRGDS)$_3$. PET imaging of the lungs was started immediately after tumor cell injection and performed over 90 min and divided into every 15 min frames [reprinted with permission from Ref. (19)]. (b) B16BL6 cells (2 × 10^5 cells/well) were seeded with or without sLex-liposome, Me-sLex-liposome, empty liposome, or Ar(DRGDS)$_3$ into the upper compartment of a Transwell cell-culture chamber, the filters of which had been precoated with fibronectin on their lower surfaces and with Matrigel on their upper surfaces. After a 4 h incubation, cells per field which had invaded to the lower surfaces were counted [reprinted with permission from Ref. (13)]. *$P < 0.001$ vs. control.

(a)

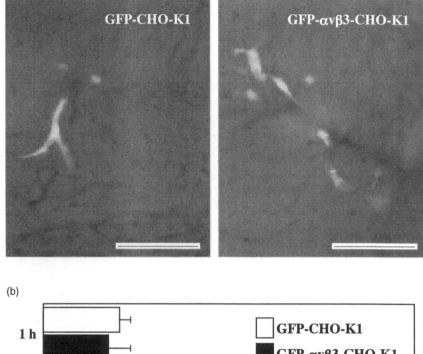

(b)

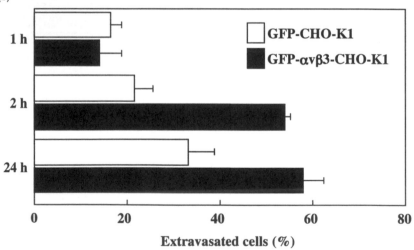

Extravasated cells (%)

Figure 14.5 IVM observation of GFP-CHO-K1 and GFP-αvβ3-CHO-K1 cells in liver after portal vein injection. (a) Invasion of GFP-CHO-K1 (left) and GFP-αvβ3-CHO-K1 (right) cells; 1×10^6 cells were injected into Balb/c nu/nu mice via a portal vein. At 24 h after the injection, liver was examined under a fluorescence microscope [reprinted with permission from Ref. (22)]. Bars represent 100 μm. (b) IVM analysis was performed as described in (a), at 1, 2, and 24 h after the injection of GFP-expressing CHO-K1 cells; the number of fluorescent cells sequestered in blood vessels or extravasated into surrounding tissue were counted under a fluorescence microscope. The data indicate the percentage of cells that had invaded into tissue vs. total cells counted.

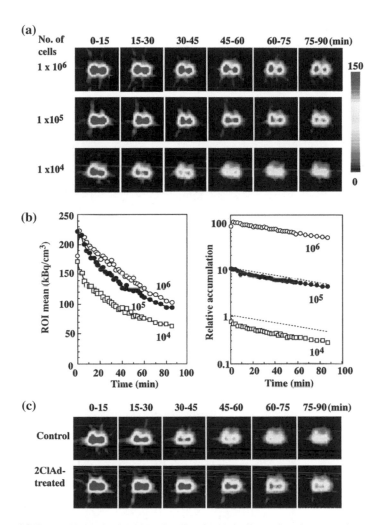

Figure 14.7 Trafficking of B16BL6 cells after injection of various numbers of cells. (a) [2-^{18}F]FDG-labeled B16BL6 cells (1 × 10^6 cells including [2-^{18}F]FDG-labeled 1 × 10^4 cells, 1 × 10^5 cells including [2-^{18}F]FDG-labeled 1 × 10^4 cells, and [2-^{18}F]FDG-labeled 1 × 10^4 cells) were injected into C57BL6 mice via the tail vein. PET imaging was started immediately after injection of the cells and was performed for 90 min in 15 min frames. The accumulation of B16BL6 cells in the lungs is shown [reprinted with permission from Ref. (28)]. (b) Time–activity curves of ^{18}F accumulation in the lungs were determined by analysis of the PET images (left panel). Relative cell accumulation is shown in the right panel where the highest accumulation after injection of 1 × 10^6 cells is 100. Dashed line shows 1/10 and 1/100 amount of the relative accumulation of cells after injection of 1 × 10^6 cells. (c) Mice were intraperitoneally pre-treated with 25 mg/kg of 2ClAd or PBS. Two days later, the mice were injected with [2-^{18}F]FDG-labeled B16BL6 cells (1 × 10^4 cells) via the tail vein. PET imaging, representing the accumulation of B16BL6 cells in the lungs, was performed as just described.

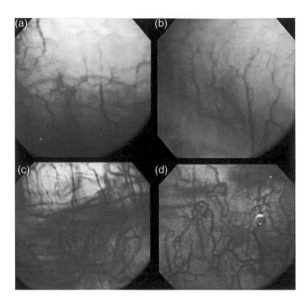

Figure 15.1 Side view and high-magnification bronchovideoscopic images of lower trachea of control subject (a), subject with COPD (b), steroid-naïve patient with newly diagnosed, stable asthma (c), and patient who has had stable asthma for >5 years, treated with inhaled corticosteroids (d). Fine vessel networks are prominently increased in the patients with asthma when compared with the control subject and the patient with COPD [From Tanaka et al. (12), by permission].

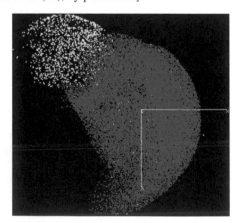

Figure 15.7 Fluorescent microspheres (15 μm) were injected into the jugular vein (grey) and left ventricle (white) 14 days after LPAL in mice. After histologic sectioning of the lungs and three-dimensional reconstruction of fluorescent images, the composite image shows that only spheres injected into the jugular vein appeared in the right lung and only spheres injected into the left side of the heart appeared in the upper left lung. In this experiment, no spheres were seen in the lower left lung (Image done in collaboration with Susan Bernard and Robb Glenny at the University of Washington).

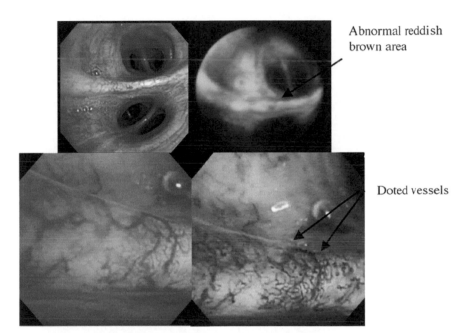

Abnormal reddish
brown area

Doted vessels

Figure 15.9 High-magnification bronchovideoscopy combined with NBI of the bronchial mucosa at sites of abnormal fluorescence. Shown are four different bronchoscopic findings (white light bronchoscopy, fluorescence bronchoscopy, high-magnification bronchovideoscopy, and high-magnification bronchovideoscopy with NBI) at the right basal bronchus of a patient with sputum cytologic findings suggestive of malignancy. Redness and swelling at the bifurcation were observed under white light examination, and an abnormal reddish-brown area was identified by fluorescence examination. Increased vessel growth and complex networks of tortuous vessels were observed at sites of abnormal fluorescence by high-magnification bronchovideoscopy with conventional RGB broadband filter. In the NBI images, the vessels were seen to be clearly dotted among the complex networks of tortuous vessels. The pathologic diagnosis, as determined by biopsy, was angiogenic squamous dysplasia [From Shibuya et al. (30), by permission].

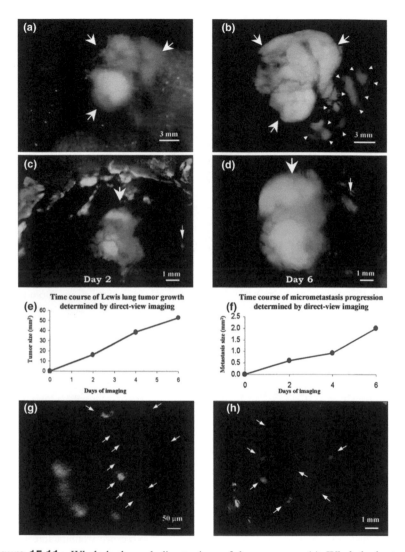

Figure 15.11 Whole-body and direct view of lung cancer. (a) Whole-body trans-cutaneous image of orthotopically growing Lewis lung tumor (arrows) in an intact live mouse on day 14 after surgical orthotopic implantation (SOI) (Bar = 3 mm). (b) Direct view of orthotopically growing Lewis lung tumor through skin-flap window also imaged in a (arrows). The primary tumor (large arrows) and invading tumor cells (small arrows) are visible. Vessels can also be visualized in the primary tumor (Bar = 3 mm). (c) Direct view of microfoci (arrows) on the ipsilateral lung on day 5 after SOI (Bar = 1 mm). (d) Same as c, day 9 after SOI (Bar = 1 mm). (e) Growth curve of large tumor determined by direct-view images (c and d, indicated by thick arrows). (f) Growth curve of microfocal tumor determined by direct-view images (c and d, indicated by fine arrows). (g) Two three-cell microfoci in the ipsilateral lung on day 5 after SOI visualized by direct-view imaging (Bar = 50 μm). (h) Micrometastases (arrows) in the contralateral lung on day 7 after SOI visualized by direct-view imaging (Bar = 1 mm) [From Yang et al. (33), by permission].

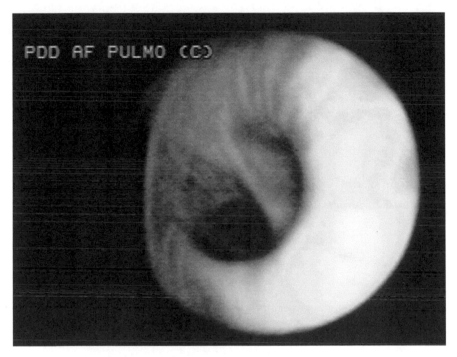

Figure 16.1 Normal airway with normal AF.

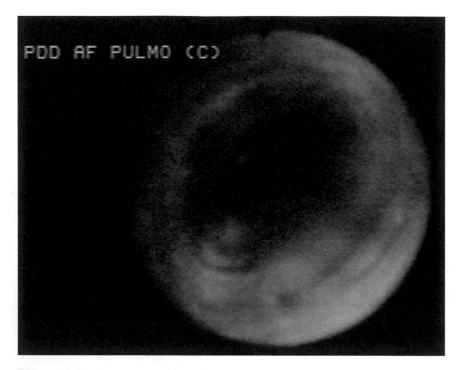

Figure 16.2 Abnormal AF due to airway neoplasia.

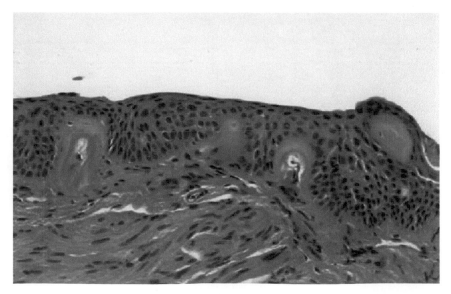

Figure 16.4 Histology section demonstrating ASD (courtesy of Dr. T. Fujisawa).

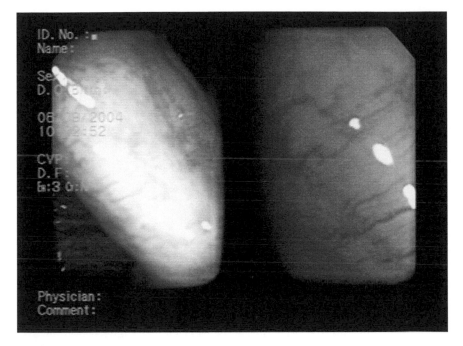

Figure 16.5 HMB image of ASD in an airway.

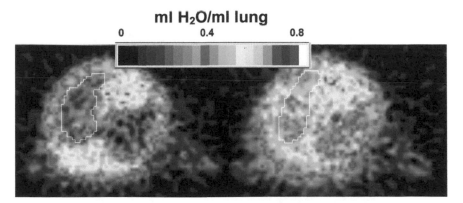

Figure 17.4 Lung water images from a normal rat (left) and a rat treated with OA (right) obtained by using a Concorde R4 microPET scanner after tail vein injection of $\sim$10 mCi of $[^{15}O]H_2O$. Images were referenced to a region over the heart, assumed to have a tissue water concentration of 0.84 mL/mL tissue. Note the increase in signal in the OA-treated rat, indicative of increased pulmonary edema as a result of the lung injury.

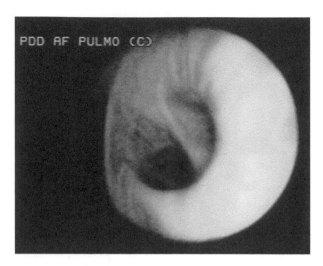

Figure 16.1   (**See color insert**) Normal airway with normal AF.

no photosensitizing agent is necessary to observe this effect (Fig. 16.1). As the airway becomes affected by dyplasia, metaplasia, and angiogenesis, the green fluorescence is lost and is replaced by a reddish-brown fluorescence (Fig. 16.2). This change in fluorescence occurs owing to progressive dysplastic airway mucosal cells crowding and replacing airway chromophores (5). Thus, the cellular and molecular changes occurring in the airway wall are detected by abnormal fluorescence to light of a given wavelength.

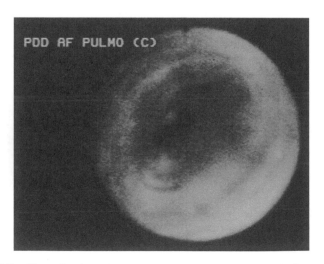

Figure 16.2   (**See color insert**) Abnormal AF due to airway neoplasia.

There is currently only one commercially available fluorescence broncho-scopy unit in the United States: the D-Light system (Karl Storz Endoscopy, Tuttlingen, Germany) (Fig. 16.3). The D-Light system employs a 300 W Xenon lamp to provide both white light (WL) and AF modes that are selected by use of a foot pedal. The light employed for fluorescence is of the range of 380–460 nm and detection is facilitated by a long-pass filter incorporated in the scope to block excitation light. The result is that crisp, clear images of the airway are provided, allowing for the endoscopist to rapidly switch between WL and AF modes.

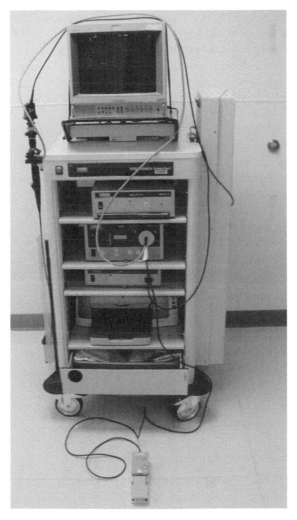

Figure 16.3 Storz D-Light system.

AF bronchoscopy has shown promise in the clinical setting to help guide interventions. To understand the utility of this technology, it will be helpful to review a study done by Sato et al. (6) reported in 1998. These investigators studied 180 patients with cancer positive sputum cytology. They conducted an average of three prolonged WL bronchoscopy sessions with brushings of all segments and subsegments. These sessions lasted an average of 45 min each. In total, 200 lesions were discovered, 175 of which were located in the main airways or segmental bronchi, within easy reach of the bronchoscope. The average delay in diagnosis was ~29 months. The same year that Sato's group published their findings, Lam et al. (5) published their study of the laser induced flourescence emission (LIFE)-lung system that resulted in its approval for clinical use by the FDA. These investigators studied 173 patients with suspected lung cancer in WL and AF modes and a total of 700 biopsies were taken. The detection of lesions of moderate dysplasia, severe dysplasia, and CIS was greatly facilitated by the AF mode. In fact, AF combined with WL bronchoscopy was roughly six times more sensitive when compared with WL bronchoscopy alone for the detection of these lesions. However, the false positive rate for the AF mode was 34% when compared with 10% for the WL mode alone. Any minor trauma that occurs during bronchoscopy, such as that due to patient coughing or liberal suctioning, may lead to mucosal injury and false positive findings during AF bronchoscopy. Therefore, the endoscopist must be careful to use adequate topical anesthetic, conscious sedation when needed, and avoid unnecessary suctioning in order to conduct an optimal exam.

Ernst et al. examined 300 patients with known or suspected lung cancer using the D-Light system in this largest study to date (7). Under the AF mode, the sensitivity of detecting premalignant lesions was 61.2% when compared with 10.6% under the WL mode. The specificity of the AF mode was 75.3% when compared with 94.6% for the WL mode. These findings are similar to the findings of other groups working with AF technology.

Thus, AF bronchoscopy has been shown to be a very useful screening tool with high sensitivity and acceptable specificity. Companies in the industry are all working to further advance this technology in order to improve upon the specificity in screening. It should be noted that AF bronchoscopy is best at detecting central airway tumors such as squamous cell carcinoma, and thus has a limited role in peripheral tumors such as adenocarcinoma. Now that physicians are equipped with this screening technology, studies are being designed to determine whether screening with AF technology will reduce cancer-related mortality.

B. High-Magnification Bronchovideoscopy

It is well known that a wide variety of malignancies in various organ systems recruit rich networks of vasculature, a process called neoangiogenesis, presumably to promote rapid growth of the cancer cells. In Chapter 15, a detailed discussion of neoangiogenesis is given. This process has been well described in the airway wall and has been termed angiogenic squamous dysplasia (Fig. 16.4). On histologic examination, plump capillary loops are seen penetrating into dysplastic bronchial epithelium. Many investigators feel that this is an early step in the development of dysplasia and that ASD may be a risk factor for development of CIS and carcinoma, but this remains to be determined.

Hoping to take advantage of the process of neoangiogenesis, Fujisawa et al. developed a high-magnification bronchovideoscope (HMB) with a 6 mm outer diameter capable of examining vessels in the bronchial submucosa at magnifications of up to 100× (8) (Fig. 16.5). These investigators initially studied 31 patients with sputum cytology positive for or suspicious of malignancy. All patients underwent WL and AF bronchoscopy before being examined by HMB. Abnormal areas, as assessed by AF, and adjacent normal areas were examined with the HMB system and biopsies were taken from 16 normal areas and 43 abnormal areas. An analysis of the histology of the lesions was done and compared to HMB observations. HMB was found to have a sensitivity of 71.4% and a specificity of 90.9% for detecting bronchial dysplasia. Neoangiogenesis was confirmed to be present in the malignant lesions as well.

C. Narrow-Band Imaging

Another promising technique is narrow-band imaging (NBI), a technology in which a narrow-banding filter is placed in a conventional videobronchoscope. The principal effect of this filter is to generate blue light in a narrower wavelength range of 400–430 nm when compared with 400–550 nm for a conventional system. This allows for better imaging of blood vessels, as the absorption wavelength of hemoglobin is 410 nm. NBI has allowed investigators to see changes in airway vasculature that has correlated with the presence of ASD (8). Preliminary results are very encouraging and bronchoscope manufacturers

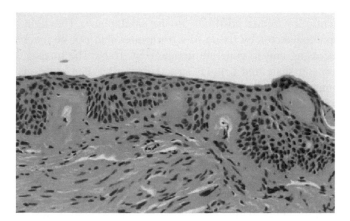

Figure 16.4 **(See color insert)** Histology section demonstrating ASD (courtesy of Dr. T. Fujisawa).

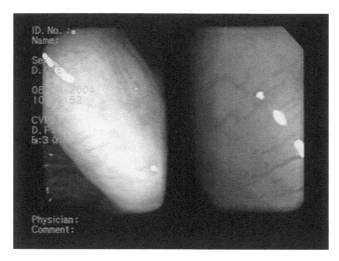

Figure 16.5   (See color insert) HMB image of ASD in an airway.

are working to further develop this technology. NBI may eventually allow physicians to detect ASD and other lesions in the airway without the need to take tissue biopsies.

D.   Optical Coherence Tomography

Optical coherence tomography (OCT) is a technology in which infrared light in the range of 800–1300 nm is employed in living tissue to generate high-resolution cross-sectional images. The technology works by scanning tissue with a beam of infrared light and then measuring the backscattered and reflected light at varying depths. The high velocity of light allows for taking several measurements at various positions in the axial plane. The light is reflected back to a photodetector by tissue microstructures that can be mapped out via a central processing unit to generate images (Fig. 16.6). The images depict tissue on a micrometer scale and cellular structures can be seen in astounding detail. OCT can image structures from 2 to 20 mm in depth depending on the properties of the tissue being imaged.

Spiteri and coworkers (9) reported their experience in comparing OCT images and histopathological sections in pig lungs. OCT images and corresponding histopathological sections were taken of the upper and lower airways of fresh pig lungs *ex vivo*. Data were analyzed and demonstrated excellent ability of OCT to image the trachea, main bronchus, and segmental bronchi. Penetration was up to 2 mm and resolution was clear to produce "living biopsies" of the epithelium, subepithelial tissues, and cartilage. These are also referred to as "optical biopsies" as cellular structures and components can be easily identified.

Fujimoto and coworkers (10) conducted a study of OCT imaging in rat organs, including lung, to determine if OCT images could guide laser ablation

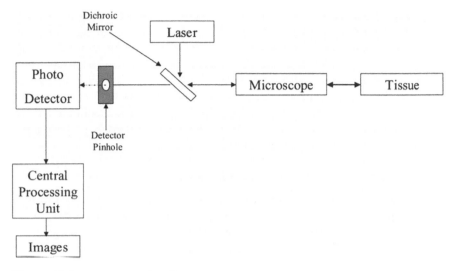

Figure 16.6 Schematic of an OCT system.

of tissue. Fresh rat brain, liver, lung, and kidney were collected and analyzed with OCT before and during argon laser treatment of the tissue. OCT images were compared with histological sections and were shown to correlate well with laser ablation of organ tissue (Fig. 16.7). These investigators proposed that

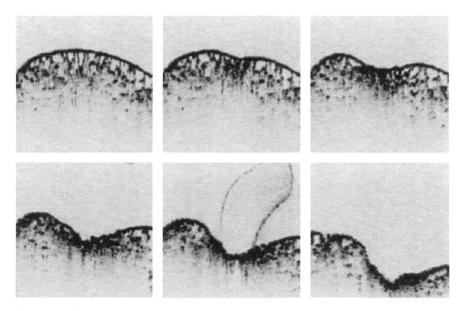

Figure 16.7 OCT images of lung after laser ablation (courtesy of Dr. S. Bopart).

real-time OCT may be used to guide laser surgery and allow surgeons to accurately achieve desired tissue effects. OCT continues to be studied further and its role in detection of airway neoplasia and endoscopic treatment of airway pathology is yet to be determined. The advantages of this technique include the ability to obtain cellular structure in great detail, a lack of crush artifact or biopsy artifact, and the ability to biopsy multiple sites without trauma. OCT is a very promising technology and has a wide range of potential applications in the airways, including the study of asthma, tracheobronchomalacia, relapsing polychondritis, and malignant and premalignant diseases.

E. Laser Scanning Confocal Microscopy

Laser scanning confocal microscopy (LSCM) is a technique that permits high-resolution two and three dimensional images of living tissue to be produced in a matter of seconds. The focal plane may be adjusted in 0.1 μm increments by many systems. LSCM utilizes properties of tissue–laser interaction discussed previously. Laser light is employed to scan tissue resulting in the usual absorption, reflection, and backscatter. The fluorescence produced from absorption is separated from most of the reflected light and backscatter by a small pinhole, known as a confocal aperature, placed in front of a photodetector. A central processing unit then constructs two dimensional images from the data collected by a photodetector (Fig. 16.8). A series of two dimensional images in a given area taken at varying depths can be employed to construct three dimensional images employing multimedia software. As the reflected light and backscatter are largely eliminated, the images are crisp and detailed down to the micron range.

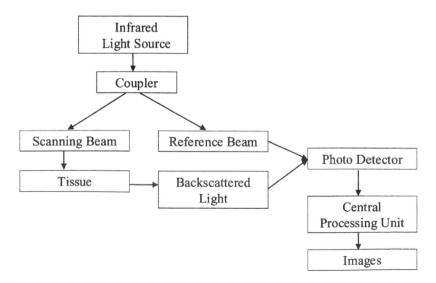

Figure 16.8   Schematic of an LSCM system.

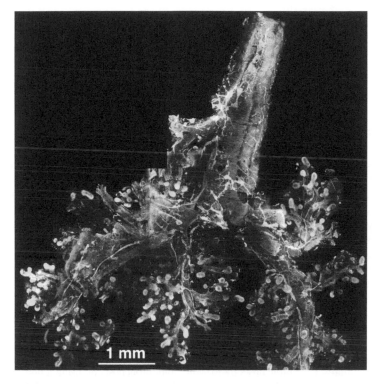

Figure 16.9 LSCM image of a fetal pig lung demonstrating neural ganglia outside the airways (courtesy of Dr. M. Sparrow).

Weichselbaum and Sparrow (11) have studied the development of neural tissue in pig lungs, and much of their work has involved LSCM. In one study, these investigators employed LSCM and immunohistochemistry techniques to study the development of ganglia in fetal and postnatal pigs. The images they obtained were striking, with montages of three dimensional images of nerves and smooth muscle allowing for an excellent view of neural tissue growth along bronchi (Fig. 16.9). MacAulay et al. (12) have hypothesized that LSCM may have some applicability in screening for lung cancer. Although this technology has previously been available to analyze specimens only *ex vivo*, these investigators are currently developing an LSCM device for *in vivo* applications.

IV. Conclusions

In the past 15 years, molecular imaging of the airways has evolved from science fiction to science. The possibility of employing optical modalities to take real-time histology-quality "living biopsies" of lung tissue is before us. These technologies are developing rapidly to help physicians in the fight against lung cancer and other diseases affecting the central airways such as relapsing polychondritis and tracheobronchomalacia. We predict that, in the next 5 years, these modalities will be employed in clinical trials proving their utility in diagnostics and in assisting with therapeutic airway interventions.

References

1. Jemal A, Tiwari R, Murray T, Ghafoor A, Samuels A, Ward E, Feuer E, Thun M. Cancer statistics 2004. CA Cancer J Clin 2004; 54:8–29.
2. Becker H. History of the rigid bronchoscope. In: Bollinger CT, Mathur PN, eds. Interventional Bronchoscopy. Vol. 30. Basel: Karger, 2000:2–15.
3. Auerbach O, Stout A, Hammond E et al. Changes in bronchial epithelium in relation to sex, age, residence, smoking, and pneumonia. N Engl J Med 1962; 267:111–119.
4. Auerbach O, Stout A, Hammond E et al. Bronchial epithelium in former smokers. N Engl J Med 1962; 267:119–125.
5. Lam S, Kennedy T, Unger M et al. Localization of bronchial intraepithelial neoplastic lesions by fluorescence bronchoscopy. CHEST 1998; 113:696–702.
6. Sato M, Saito Y, Usuda K, Takahashi S, Sagawa M, Fujimura S. Occult lung cancer beyond bronchoscopic visibilityin sputum cytology positive patients. Lung Cancer 1998; 20:17–24.
7. Beamis J, Ernst A, Simoff M, Yung R, Mathur P. A multicenter study comparing autoflourescence bronchoscopy to white light bronchoscopy using a non-laser light stimulation system. CHEST 2004; 125:148S–149S.
8. Shibuya K, Hoshino H, Chiyo M, Yasufuku K, Iizasa T, Saitoh Y, Baba M, Hiroshima K, Ohwada H, Fujisawa T. Subepithelial vascular patterns in bronchial dysplasisa using a high magnification bronchovideoscope. Thorax 2002; 57:902–907.
9. Yang Y, Whiteman S, Gey van Pittius D, He Y, Wang R, Spiteri M. Use of optical coherence tomography in delineating airways microstructure: comparison of OCT images to histopathological sections. Phys Med Biol 2004; 49:1247–1255.
10. Boppart S, Herrmann J, Pitris C, Stamper D, Brezinski M, Fujimoto J. High resolution optical coherence tomography guided laser ablation of surgical tissue. J Surg Res 1999; 82:275–284.
11. Weichselbaum M, Sparrow M. A confocal microscopic study of the formation of ganglia in the airways of fetal pig lung. Am J Respir Cell Mol Biol 1999; 21:601–620.
12. MacAuley C, Guillaud M, LeRiche J et al. 2D and 3D quantitative microscopy for preinvasive lung cancer. Lung Cancer 2000; 29(suppl. 1):252.

17

Functional Imaging of Rodent Lungs

DELPHINE L. CHEN and DANIEL P. SCHUSTER

Washington University School of Medicine,
St. Louis, Missouri, USA

I. Introduction

Every day, clinicians use imaging to diagnose disease and to assist in therapeutic decision-making. The value of anatomic imaging of lung structure with X-ray computed tomography (CT) is well known to every clinician. Advances in molecular imaging that may eventually be used to guide gene therapy or to evaluate biologic processes *in vivo* at the cellular and even subcellular levels hold great promise. Recent improvements in instrumentation are making it possible to combine different types of measurements into single multimodality imaging sessions (see Chapter 7).

Clinically, functional imaging (by, e.g., echocardiography or ventilation–perfusion scanning) provides useful information distinct from that obtained with either anatomic or molecular imaging. Because both anatomic and molecular imaging can now be extended to small animals such as rodents, it is important to develop and use functional imaging methods to complement other imaging techniques. In this chapter, we review some current methods for functional imaging of the lungs in small animals.

II. Definitions

Standard definitions for the terms *anatomic, functional*, and *molecular* imaging have yet to be developed. Generally, anatomic imaging techniques are used to display structure (e.g., airway diameter) or make measurements related to structure [e.g., lung volumes such as functional residual capacity (FRC)]. Molecular imaging, on the other hand, includes *in vivo* methods that are used to detect the presence or activity of specific molecular targets in tissues of interest (e.g., the expression of transgenes). Both anatomic and molecular imaging employ methods that depend primarily on static images, that is, images obtained at a single point in time.

In contrast, functional imaging methods almost always depend on obtaining repeated data over time to measure biologic processes such as ventilation, perfusion, or pulmonary artery (PA) pressures. Although anatomic imaging involves very long time constants—changes, if any, in the structure or process being imaged occur over a period of hours, days, or even years—changes mapped by functional imaging usually occur over seconds to hours.

Obviously, how a particular method is used can result in overlap among these different classifications. For example, measurements of FRC with X-ray CT provide not only anatomic information about lung volumes but also important information that can affect lung function. Likewise, measurements of [^{18}F]fluorodeoxyglucose uptake with positron emission tomography (PET) can be viewed as both "functional" (rates of tissue glucose utilization) and "molecular" (related to hexokinase or glucose transporter gene expression).

A. Lung Density

Clinical CT scanners have been used to evaluate lung density changes in rat models of radiation-induced lung injury (1–3). Because the resolution of most clinical scanners is ~0.5 mm, it is not possible, especially with breathing rodents, to obtain detailed anatomic images of the lungs in mice, whose whole-lung dimensions are on the order of millimeters (4). However, this resolution is adequate for assessing regional and overall density changes in rat lungs.

An example of how CT imaging can be used to monitor experimentally induced changes in lung density is provided in a study by Wiegman et al. (2). They evaluated the susceptibility of different areas of rat lungs to radiation injury by using a Philips Tomoscan SR 7000 high resolution scanner. In four groups of rats, 50% of the total lung volume at the apex, base, lateral, or mediastinal portions was irradiated. In another two groups, 50% of the total lung volume on either the right or left side was irradiated. For all irradiation treatments, a single dose of 18 cGy was used, and then animals were evaluated with CT scans at 4, 16, 26, and 52 weeks after irradiation. The dose from the CT scan itself, which was <1 cGy per session, was neglected. Average lung density over both lungs as well as regional lung density was determined from regions of interest (ROIs) placed over the first three slices ventral to the trachea, evaluating a total volume of 150 mm^3 in each region. CT numbers, expressed as Hounsfield units (HU), were used to obtain frequency distributions of density and to calculate average distributions within the ROIs and for the entire lung volume, where the numbers ranged from +1000 HU for bone to −1000 HU for air. Water was set to 0 HU. Rats that received mediastinal irradiation displayed the most significant increase in regional lung density by 16 and 26 weeks after irradiation (Fig. 17.1), and the density distribution also showed a significant shift toward higher-density numbers (Fig. 17.2), indicating that the lung tissue closest to the mediastinum is more susceptible to lung injury. Those rats that had radiation exposure on the left lung also showed a tendency

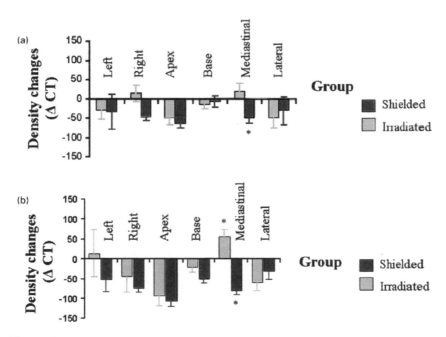

Figure 17.1 Density changes (in HU) in rat lungs, as measured by CT, (a) 16 and (b) 26 weeks after irradiation of 50% total lung volume in areas as indicated in charts. Only rats that had 50% of mediastinal lung volume irradiated had density changes that were significantly different. [Reprinted from Wiegman et al. (2) with permission from Elsevier.]

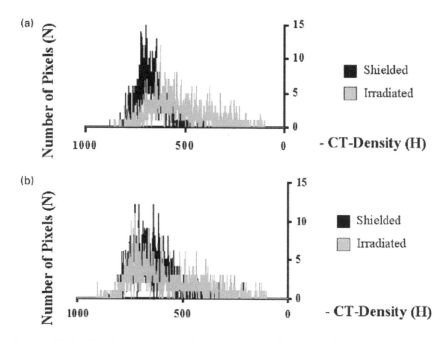

Figure 17.2 Density histograms of rat lungs exposed to irradiation of the (a) mediastinal or (b) left 50% of total lung volume. Note the shift in the peak of the irradiated pixels in the mediastinal group, indicating higher HU and thus more fibrosis as a result of the irradiation. [Reprinted from Wiegman et al. (2) with permission from Elsevier.]

toward an increase in density; however, all other groups showed a decrease in density over time, an indication of recovery from the radiation exposure (2).

The display of regional changes in lung density in small animals is markedly improved with the introduction of microCT scanners, given the higher spatial resolution available with these types of scanners (see Section II.B). We have recently generated images of oleic acid (OA)-induced lung injury in mice (Fig. 17.3) using an Imtek micro-CAT II scanner. OA is known to cause heterogeneous lung injury and noncardiogenic pulmonary edema that mimics the acute respiratory distress syndrome in humans. Figure 17.3 shows a clear increase in the lung density as a result of OA-induced lung injury. Thus, microCT may allow detection and quantification of acute changes in lung density that may be due to increases in lung water or atelectasis (5).

B. Lung Volumes

Lung volumes in rats and mice can also be measured by using clinical CT scanners (1,2,6). Mitzner et al. (6) used a Siemens Somatom IV scanner to calculate *in vivo* lung volumes in mice with a window level of -450 HU and a window width of 1350 HU, settings that have been shown to be accurate in obtaining

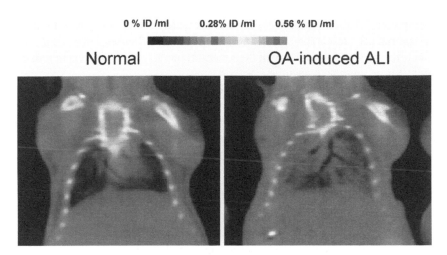

0 % ID /ml   0.28% ID /ml   0.56 % ID /ml

Normal   OA-induced ALI

Figure 17.3 Coronal images of a normal mouse and a mouse with OA-induced lung injury obtained with an Imtek microCAT II scanner. Note the overall increase in lung density in the OA-treated mouse. The trachea and major bronchi are also visible (reconstructed at a resolution of 200 μm).

measurements of airways approaching 1 mm in size. NIH Image software was used to convert HU to a percentage of air. Air percentage and the threshold area of each slice were used to calculate the volume of air in all the slices showing lung. Calibration of the measurement technique with known volumes of instilled air in dead mice showed a coefficient of variation of 10% in the measurement. For *in vivo* imaging, two different strains, C3H/HeJ and A/J, were followed up from ages 4 to 12 weeks with serial CT measurement of lung volumes, which Mitzner et al. (6) denoted as the FRC. All mice were anesthetized and breathing throughout the 15 s image acquisition. In their repeat measurements of FRC in the living mice, done 10 min apart, they saw variations of up to 21% of baseline, and in seven out of eight animals, the repeated measurement was <10% of baseline. Mitzner et al. (6) attributed this high degree of reproducibility in the measurement to the fact that the motion of the mouse diaphragm is on the order of the resolution of the CT scanner. However, they did notice significant variability, up to 25%, in measurements for each mouse over time, which was most likely due to a combination of technical and physiologic variables.

With the development of microCT scanners, the estimation of lung volumes by CT should be far more accurate because the voxel size of these scanners can be 2000× smaller than that of clinical CT scanners (4). However, because of the high doses of radiation involved in obtaining high-resolution images, radiation dose becomes a limiting factor for repeating studies. It is estimated that the life of a mouse is shortened by 7.2% per Gy of radiation exposure, and residual effects from sublethal radiation doses can accumulate (7). In developing experiments in which microCT is used for repeated measurements, researchers will need to balance obtaining the appropriate resolution needed for accuracy in their measurements with the effects of radiation exposure on animals over time.

Magnetic resonance imaging (MRI) with hyperpolarized (HP) gases can also be used to estimate ventilation volumes in small animals (8). The signal intensity generated by the HP gases in the peripheral airspaces should correlate to the ventilating volume in the ROI. This technique and its applications in ventilation assessments are discussed in more detail in Section II. D.

C. Lung Water and Blood Volume Measurements

Lung water can be estimated by changes in lung density by CT or by measurements of water density by MRI (9–11). However, lung water measurements obtained by these methods are limited in that there is no way to distinguish changes in extravascular lung water from changes in intravascular (blood) volume. With PET imaging, it is possible to determine not only the total lung water concentration by using oxygen 15-labeled water ($[^{15}O]H_2O$) but also the extravascular lung water component, because blood volume can be measured independently by using ^{15}O-labeled carbon monoxide ($[^{15}O]CO$) (12).

The resolution of currently available microPET scanners may still limit the ability to obtain these types of measurements in small animals, particularly in mice. The problem lies in the positron range of the tracer, $[^{15}O]H_2O$. For example, fluorine-18, one of the most commonly used radionuclides for clinical PET imaging, has a maximum positron range of 1.8 mm, with an average range of 0.35 mm in water, compared with a maximum range of 7.0 mm and an average range of 2 mm for ^{15}O (13). Given that the average chest diameter of a mouse is 20–25 mm, the resolution may not be adequate to provide accurate measurements of lung water in mice. Additionally, because PET imaging is done on actively breathing animals, partial volume effects caused by motion of the diaphragm, chest wall, and heart result in further blurring of the signal at the edges of the lungs, making it difficult to identify ROIs that do not include these surrounding structures in small animals. With rats, whose chest diameters are significantly larger, the resolution of current microPET scanners should be adequate for making such measurements. In addition, the development of multimodality imaging with microCT should help to prevent this problem.

We recently performed PET imaging in an OA injury model in rats using $[^{15}O]H_2O$ to determine total lung water accumulation that is characteristic of this model (Fig. 17.4). Images were obtained with a 5 min scan, beginning 4 min after tail vein injection of ∼10 mCi of $[^{15}O]H_2O$. Radioactivity measurements were decay-corrected to the time of tracer injection. Lung water concentration is calculated as the activity during the equilibrium $[^{15}O]H_2O$ scan in any lung ROI divided by the activity over the heart, with the assumption that the water content of blood or cardiac tissue is ∼0.84 mL H_2O/mL of tissue (12).

ml H₂O/ml lung

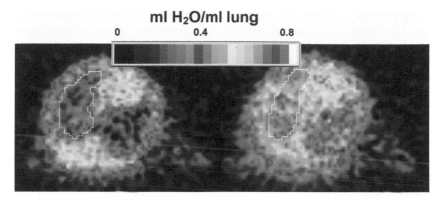

Figure 17.4 (See color insert) Lung water images from a normal rat (left) and a rat treated with OA (right) obtained by using a Concorde R4 microPET scanner after tail vein injection of ~10 mCi of $[^{15}O]H_2O$. Images were referenced to a region over the heart, assumed to have a tissue water concentration of 0.84 mL/mL tissue. Note the increase in signal in the OA-treated rat, indicative of increased pulmonary edema as a result of the lung injury.

The lung water concentration increased from 0.48 to 0.76 mL H_2O/mL lung, a 57% increase compared with baseline before injury. This increase in lung water concentration matched a comparable increase in postmortem lung weight, compared with normal rat lung weights in our laboratory. Further validation experiments are necessary to determine the accuracy of these measurements.

PET with $[^{15}O]CO$ can be used to measure pulmonary blood volume (14). However, this technique has not yet been developed for use in small animals.

D. Lung Ventilation and Perfusion

Recent advances in MRI with HP gases have allowed investigators to measure ventilation in rodents. With the development of new techniques for synchronizing magnetic resonance (MR) scan acquisition with ventilation, detailed maps of the lungs can now be created with high resolution (15). One of the challenges in using HP gases for pulmonary imaging is that these gases do not naturally maintain a polarized state for long. Thus, any polarized gas that is subjected to a magnetic field with a direction that is significantly different from the direction of the gas polarization will rapidly depolarize the gas and render it unusable for further study. In the lungs, this phenomenon results in loss of the MR signal before the HP gas has a chance to reach the periphery. To use HP gases to monitor ventilation throughout the lungs, investigators must manipulate MR data acquisition protocols to preserve signal intensity long enough to allow the gas to reach the periphery of the lungs while the gas is still in a state of hyperpolarization. Chen et al. (8) recently described such a technique with radial acquisition cine pulse sequence in conjunction with a skipping scheme in the applied radiofrequency pulse sequences. This technique requires imaging over multiple breaths of HP gases to generate the final images. By using this dynamic scanning technique, Chen et al. (8) were able to generate images showing clearly the peripheral lung as well as the major airways (Fig. 17.5). In addition, airflow in the major airways could be measured by normalizing the MR signal intensity in an ROI placed over an airway to the diameter of the airway. Because the right side of the lung receives 10% to 20% more of the total volume of gas in a single breath compared with the left side and because the diameter of the airways on the right was 21% to 47% larger than that of the airways on the left (depending on position), they predicted that the airflow in the left airways would actually be faster than that observed on the right. They found that the measured signal intensity in their selected ROIs, when normalized for airway diameter, was in agreement with these predictions. Regional ventilation could also be calculated, as it would be proportional to the signal intensity in the periphery of the lung as long as care was taken to preserve the polarization of the gas in the area of interest (8).

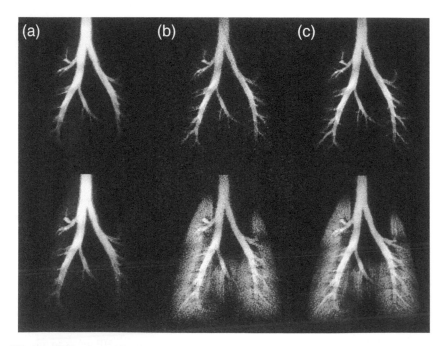

Figure 17.5   Lung images in normal rats obtained by using HP helium 3 gas. (a) Images were obtained by using a flip angle of 24° and skip factor of 1. (b) Images obtained by using a flip angle of 6° and skip factor of 1. (c) Images obtained with a flip angle of 12° and skip factor of 2. Note that by skipping every other frame, a higher flip angle can be used while maintaining gas polarization at the periphery of the lungs. [Reprinted from Chen et al. (8) by permission of Wiley-Liss, Inc., a subsidiary of John Wiley & Sons, Inc., copyright 2003.]

Dupuich et al. (16) used a single-breath technique with a different image acquisition and data processing protocol, which they called *sliding pulmonary imaging for respiratory overview*, a combination of a radial acquisition protocol with a sliding window method, to assess ventilation in rats (16). When this technique was used, pixel-by-pixel parametric maps of gas arrival time, filling time-constant values, average inflation rate, and gas volume values during a single breath of HP helium-3 (^{3}He) gas were generated. These values were then used to calculate overall gas flow rates and lung volumes in comparison with the actual gas flow delivery rate and the actual injected volume of gas. Dupuich et al. (16) found that the error rates in their calculated gas flow values ranged from 3% to 8%, whereas the error rates in estimating lung volumes ranged from 4.7% to 11.1%. Because they did not use slice selection in their data acquisition protocol, they noted that the values generated for the parametric maps of gas volume and average inflation rate values were a function of the thickness of the lung tissue. They hypothesized that using slice selection would improve the accuracy of their measurements (16).

Ventilation–perfusion studies are also now possible in rats. HP ^{3}He has been used in conjunction with gadolinium diethylene triamine pentaacetic acid or superparamagnetic iron oxide nanoparticles as intravenous contrast agents to obtain ventilation–perfusion images in rats (15,17,18). One advantage of using superparamagnetic iron oxide nanoparticles as a perfusion contrast agent is that they induce local magnetic field inhomogeneities in the lung after injection, which in turn causes a decrease in the signal from the HP ^{3}He present in the lung that is predictable and quantifiable (15) (Fig. 17.6). Hence, relative pulmonary blood volume can be calculated from these signal changes, as well as ventilation parameters.

Although ventilation–perfusion measurements have been obtained with PET and CT in large animal models (19,20), these techniques have not yet been translated into small animal models.

E. PA Pressures and Right Ventricular Function

Echocardiography, CT, and MRI are now being used to assess pulmonary arterial pressures and right ventricular function in rat models of disease. Although echocardiography has been used extensively in clinical practice, technical limitations have prevented its use in small animal models of disease until recently. We have recently used transthoracic echocardiography (TTE) to evaluate right ventricle (RV) changes in a rat model of pulmonary hypertension using a Siemens Acuson C256 ultrasound system equipped with 13 MHz and 8 MHz transducers (21). RV chamber size was determined by tracing the endocardial border of the RV on end-diastolic image frames. RV wall thickness was measured by using two-dimensional guided M-mode images of the inferior portion of the RV free wall. Doppler echocardiography was also used to noninvasively estimate systolic PA pressure by two methods. Images obtained by this protocol are shown in Fig. 17.7.

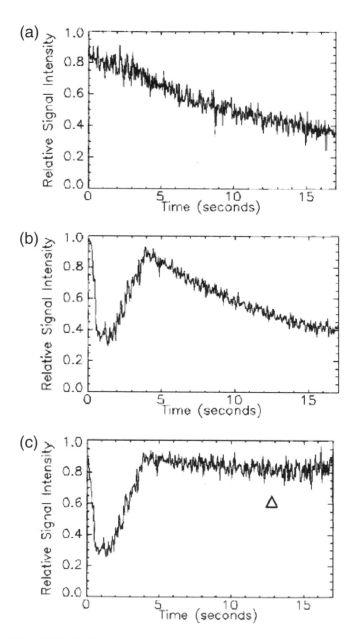

Figure 17.6 NMR helium 3 signal intensity over time. (a) Normal decay of signal intensity of ^{3}He. (b) Drop in ^{3}He signal intensity caused by first pass of ferromagnetic contrast agent. (c) Signal intensity of ^{3}He after correction for radiofrequency pulse effects (triangle shows slight drop, presumably caused by second pass of contrast agent). [Reprinted from Viallon et al. (15) by permission of Wiley-Liss, Inc., a subsidiary of John Wiley & Sons, Inc., copyright 2000.]

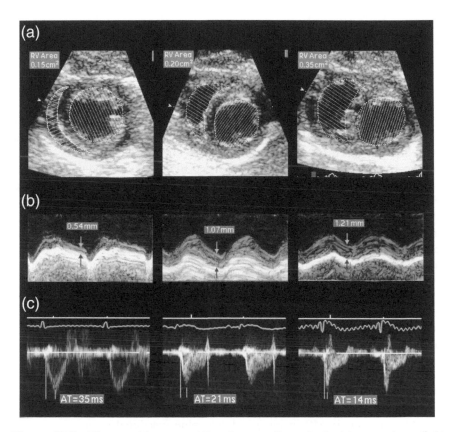

Figure 17.7 Ultrasound images and Doppler recordings obtained in normal rats (left) and rats with mild (center) and severe (right) pulmonary hypertension. (a) End-diastolic images of the right (crescent region) and left (round region) along the short-axis view. (b) M-mode images of the inferior portion of the right ventricular free wall. (c) Pulse-wave Doppler recordings of pulmonary outflow velocity. [Parts (a) and (b) reprinted from Schuster et al. (21) with permission.]

Jones et al. (22) also used TTE to follow the development of pulmonary hypertension in rats over a 6 week period. With TTE, they measured PA flow, PA flow acceleration time (PAAT), RV wall thickness, RV end-diastolic dimension, and tricuspid regurgitation velocity, which could then be used to derive the PA systolic pressure (PASP) (23). They also made direct measurements of PASP by means of direct cannulation of the PA. They found that TTE was capable of quantifying PA flow in all animals and that PAAT, over the range of 20–33 ms, could be used to predict the measured PASP; outside this range, PAAT failed to change as PASP changed. They also found that TTE could accurately quantify tricuspid regurgitation velocity only when significant tricuspid regurgitation was present (velocity >3 m/s) or when PASP was

>65 mm Hg and that using the gradient across the RV and right atrium to predict PASP systematically underestimated the PASP. RV free-wall thickening by TTE proved to be a consistent feature in the development of pulmonary hypertension (22), in agreement with our observations.

Scherrer-Crosbie et al. (24) published results of a study in which they used transesophageal echocardiography (TEE) in mice. Using a 3.5 F/30 MHz intravascular ultrasound probe, they performed TEE after intubation by tracheostomy in mice and compared RV wall thickness, volume, and mass measurements with those obtained by *ex vivo* casts and dissection of the RV. They obtained good correlations between TEE measurements of RV volume and those obtained by echocardiography of RV casts ($r = 0.88$). Although TEE measurements of RV free-wall mass and total RV mass were also correlated with true RV free wall and total weight ($r = 0.81$ and 0.77, respectively), there was a consistent underestimation by TEE, which they attributed to tracing errors because the epicardium near the pulmonary outflow tract and the apex was difficult to visualize. TEE and RV wall thickness measured by MRI were also comparable (0.41 ± 0.11 mm vs. 0.46 ± 0.10 mm) (24).

MRI has also been used to assess right ventricular function and PA pressures (25,26). The RV has been difficult to assess functionally because its morphology does not lend itself to modeling on the basis of typical geometric assumptions (i.e., its shape and motion cannot be represented by a simple ellipsoid, crescent, or other standard definable shape) (26). However, because of the high resolution of MRI and its ability to capture images over frames on the order of milliseconds, it is possible to visualize the walls of the right side of the heart very clearly (as a result of the intrinsic contrast between blood and myocardial tissue in MR images) and determine functional parameters such as ejection fraction, PA pressure, and PAAT by using manually placed ROIs (26).

Wiesmann et al. (26) used MRI to study changes in right ventricular function in a mouse model of myocardial infarction-induced heart failure. An electrocardiography-triggered fast gradient echo cine sequence (FLASH) was used to acquire 12 cine frames within each cardiac cycle with a temporal resolution of 8.6 ms. An example of the images obtained is shown in Fig. 17.8. The contrast seen between the myocardial tissue and blood pool is a result of inherent characteristics of these tissues when they are visualized with MRI. Normal mice were compared with mice in which ligation of the left anterior descending coronary artery had been performed (heart failure group). Wiesman et al. (26) found that intra- and interobserver variabilities in right ventricular volume measurements (7.9% and 7.7%, respectively, for RV stroke volume measurements) were lower than that seen in the study by Scherrer-Crosbie et al. (24) described previously, in which TEE was used (10.3% $\pm$ 13.6% and 13.5% $\pm$ 20.0%, respectively, for RV stroke volume). *In vivo* MR measurements of RV mass (26.8 $\pm$ 1.8 mg) were comparable to *ex vivo* RV wet weights (23.1 $\pm$ 1.4 mg). In the mice in the heart failure group, RV stroke volume and ejection fraction were decreased as determined by MR measurements, and RV diastolic wall thickening, indicating RV hypertrophy, was present (26).

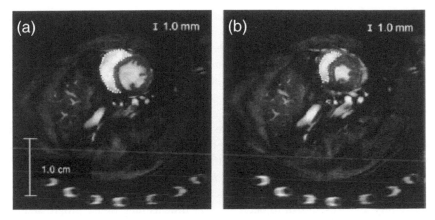

Figure 17.8 Images of normal mouse ventricles, short-axis view, obtained by MRI. The contrast between the blood pool and myocardial tissue is characteristic of these tissues when imaged using MRI. (a) Midventricular view at end diastole. (b) Same view at end systole. [Reprinted with permission from Wiesmann et al. (26).]

At this time, no reports are available regarding the use of CT for *in vivo* measurements of the pulmonary vasculature. Intravascular contrast is required to distinguish the vessels from surrounding soft tissue, and considerable effort is being devoted to developing this application of microCT. However, Karau et al. (27) used microfocal X-ray CT imaging specifically to assess the distensibility of pulmonary arteries in intact excised rat lungs filled with perfluorooctyl bromide to improve X-ray absorbance. From the CT measurements, they estimated the airway diameter at different points along the pulmonary vascular tree over a range of arterial pressures. Images were obtained over a range of pressures (5.4–30 mm Hg), and the actual pressure within a given artery, relative to atmospheric pressure, was determined by the vertical distance of the artery from the pressure reference height and the density of the perfluorooctyl bromide. The range of arterial diameters was ∼106–1861 μm at the lowest pressure and ∼151–2743 μm at the highest pressure. From their data, they found that distensibility was independent of the airway diameter. As microCT develops, it may be possible to make these types of morphometric measurements *in vivo* in small animals.

F. Diffusion

MRI techniques can be used to measure properties related to gas diffusion capacity of the lung. By using HP ^{3}He, it is possible to calculate the apparent diffusion coefficient (ADC). The ADC gives a measure of how freely gas can diffuse within the airways of the lungs. (This is different from diffusion *across* the airways as, for instance, is done when CO diffusing capacity is measured.) As ^{3}He, with a diffusion length of 0.042 cm (28) in air, moves out to the lung periphery, where the average diameter of the alveoli is $\sim$0.025 cm at end-inspiration (29), its diffusion becomes more restricted. Hence, in the periphery, the measured diffusion coefficient of the gas (and thus the term ADC) is much smaller than that measured in larger airways. This property makes it possible to use the ADC as a surrogate measure of airway diameter—an example of functional imaging being used to measure a structural or anatomic property of the lungs.

A number of groups have used the diffusion properties of HP ^{3}He to calculate ADC in various rat models of lung disease. ADC increases in rat models of emphysema; because the alveolar destruction in this disease results in larger-sized alveolar sacs, diffusion is less restricted, and hence a larger ADC is measured (30,31). The ADC has also been measured in a rat model of radiation lung injury and was shown to decrease over time as lung injury progressed and fibrosis developed, corresponding with the associated decrease in alveolar space (32).

HP xenon-129 has also been used in a rat model of lipopolysaccharide (LPS)-induced lung inflammation to quantify changes in diffusion. As ^{129}Xe is soluble in the blood and tissues (33), Mansson et al. (34) developed a model for the diffusion of ^{129}Xe from the alveolar space into the lung tissue and intravascular spaces. From this model, they were able to calculate total diffusion length, capillary diffusion length, tissue thickness, and perfusion. Tissue thickness in controls (5.6 $\pm$ 0.6 μm) and LPS-treated rats (6.0 $\pm$ 0.8 μm) was in agreement with the 5–6 μm range measured by microscopic methods (35). Both total diffusion length (8.5 $\pm$ 0.5 μm in controls vs. 9.9 $\pm$ 0.6 μm in the LPS group) and capillary diffusion length (2.9 $\pm$ 0.4 μm in controls vs. 3.9 $\pm$ 1.0 μm in the LPS group) significantly increased as a result of the LPS-induced inflammation, which is consistent with the known edema, mucus production, and cellular recruitment that occur with LPS exposure in lungs (36) and with the known effect membrane thickness has on lung diffusion capacity (37).

Because the ADC in normal lungs is homogeneous, alterations in the distribution of the ADC may also be useful in detecting disease. Yablonskiy et al. (38) showed, in humans, that because diffusion is anisotropic (gas moves more freely along the direction of the airway at all levels of the pulmonary tree), directional measurements of diffusion (across the diameter of an airway) can be used to detect the presence of emphysema in humans. Such techniques should also be applicable in small animal models of lung disease.

III. Conclusion

As techniques for imaging in small animals are developed, more tools will be available for assessing *in vivo* lung function in mice and rats. This will be particularly useful because expression of various disease states can be studied by using genetically modified animals. Additionally, more studies can be performed in a shorter period, with less cost, using smaller animals. Multimodality imaging—the convergence of anatomic, functional, and molecular imaging methods in one session—will undoubtedly contribute a wealth of new information about the lungs in both healthy and diseased states.

References

1. Vujaskovic Z, Down JD, van t' Veld AA, Mooyaart EL, Meertens H, Piers DA, Szabo BG, Konings AW. Radiological and functional assessment of radiation-induced lung injury in the rat. Exp Lung Res 1998; 24(2):137–148.

2. Wiegman EM, Meertens H, Konings AW, Kampinga HH, Coppes RP. Loco-regional differences in pulmonary function and density after partial rat lung irradiation. Radiother Oncol 2003; 69(1):11–19.

3. Lehnert S, el-Khatib E. The use of CT densitometry in the assessment of radiation-induced damage to the rat lung: a comparison with other endpoints. Int J Radiat Oncol Biol Phys 1989; 16(1):117–124.

4. Corrigan NM, Chavez AE, Wisner ER, Boone JM. A multiple detector array helical x-ray microtomography system for specimen imaging. Med Phys 1999; 26(8):1708–1713.

5. Schuster DP, Marklin GF. Effect of changes in inflation and blood volume on regional lung density—a PET study: 2. J Comput Assist Tomogr 1986; 10(5):730–735.

6. Mitzner W, Brown R, Lee W. In vivo measurement of lung volumes in mice. Physiol Genomics 2001; 4(3):215–221.

7. Ford NL, Thornton MM, Holdsworth DW. Fundamental image quality limits for microcomputed tomography in small animals. Med Phys 2003; 30(11):2869–2877.

8. Chen BT, Brau AC, Johnson GA. Measurement of regional lung function in rats using hyperpolarized 3helium dynamic MRI. Magn Reson Med 2003; 49(1):78–88.

9. Cutillo AG, Goodrich KC, Ganesan K, Watanabe S, Ailion DC, Albertine KH, Morris AH, Durney CH. Lung water measurement by nuclear magnetic resonance: correlation with morphometry. J Appl Physiol 1995; 79(6):2163–2168.

10. Beckmann N, Tigani B, Ekatodramis D, Borer R, Mazzoni L, Fozard JR. Pulmonary edema induced by allergen challenge in the rat: noninvasive assessment by magnetic resonance imaging. Magn Reson Med 2001; 45(1):88–95.

11. Wegener T, Wegenius G, Hemmingsson A, Jung B, Saldeen T. Computed chest tomography in rats with pulmonary damage due to microembolism. Acta Radiol Diagn (Stockh) 1986; 27(6):723–728.

12. Schuster DP, Mintun MA, Green MA, Ter-Pogossian MM. Regional lung water and hematocrit determined by positron emission tomography. J Appl Physiol 1985; 59(3):860–868.

13. Laforest R, Rowland DJ, Welch MJ. MicroPET imaging with nonconventional isotopes. IEEE Trans Nucl Sci 2002; 49(5):2119–2126.

14. Schuster DP, Marklin GF, Mintun MA. Regional changes in extravascular lung water detected by positron emission tomography. J Appl Physiol 1986; 60(4):1170–1178.

15. Viallon M, Berthezene Y, Decorps M, Wiart M, Callot V, Bourgeois M, Humblot H, Briguet A, Cremillieux Y. Laser-polarized (3)He as a probe for dynamic regional

measurements of lung perfusion and ventilation using magnetic resonance imaging. Magn Reson Med 2000; 44(1):1–4.

16. Dupuich D, Berthezene Y, Clouet PL, Stupar V, Canet E, Cremillieux Y. Dynamic 3He imaging for quantification of regional lung ventilation parameters. Magn Reson Med 2003; 50(4):777–783.

17. Cremillieux Y, Berthezene Y, Humblot H, Viallon M, Canet E, Bourgeois M, Albert T, Heil W, Briguet A. A combined 1H perfusion/3He ventilation NMR study in rat lungs. Magn Reson Med 1999; 41(4):645–648.

18. Stupar V, Berthezene Y, Canet E, Tournier H, Dupuich D, Cremillieux Y. Helium3 polarization using spin exchange technique: application to simultaneous pulmonary ventilation/perfusion imaging in small animals. Invest Radiol 2003; 38(6):334–340.

19. Vidal Melo MF, Layfield D, Harris RS, O'Neill K, Musch G, Richter T, Winkler T, Fischman AJ, Venegas JG. Quantification of regional ventilation–perfusion ratios with PET. J Nucl Med 2003; 44(12):1982–1991.

20. Kreck TC, Krueger MA, Altemeier WA, Sinclair SE, Robertson HT, Shade ED, Hildebrandt J, Lamm WJ, Frazer DA, Polissar NL, Hlastala MP. Determination of regional ventilation and perfusion in the lung using xenon and computed tomography. J Appl Physiol 2001; 91(4):1741–1749.

21. Schuster DP, Kovacs A, Garbow J, Piwnica-Worms D. Recent advances in imaging the lungs of intact small animals. Am J Respir Cell Mol Biol 2004; 30(2):129–138.

22. Jones JE, Mendes L, Rudd MA, Russo G, Loscalzo J, Zhang YY. Serial noninvasive assessment of progressive pulmonary hypertension in a rat model. Am J Physiol Heart Circ Physiol 2002; 283(1):H364–H371.

23. Bossone E, Duong-Wagner TH, Paciocco G, Oral H, Ricciardi M, Bach DS, Rubenfire M, Armstrong WF. Echocardiographic features of primary pulmonary hypertension. J Am Soc Echocardiogr 1999; 12(8):655–662.

24. Scherrer-Crosbie M, Steudel W, Hunziker PR, Foster GP, Garrido L, Liel-Cohen N, Zapol WM, Picard MH. Determination of right ventricular structure and function in normoxic and hypoxic mice: a transesophageal echocardiographic study. Circulation 1998; 98(10):1015–1021.

25. Al-Shafei AI, Wise RG, Grace AA, Carpenter TA, Hall LD, Huang CL. MRI analysis of right ventricular function in normal and spontaneously hypertensive rats. Magn Reson Imaging 2001; 19(10):1297–1304.

26. Wiesmann F, Frydrychowicz A, Rautenberg J, Illinger R, Rommel E, Haase A, Neubauer S. Analysis of right ventricular function in healthy mice and a murine model of heart failure by in vivo MRI. Am J Physiol Heart Circ Physiol 2002; 283(3):H1065–H1071.

27. Karau KL, Johnson RH, Molthen RC, Dhyani AH, Haworth ST, Hanger CC, Roerig DL, Dawson CA. Microfocal X-ray CT imaging and pulmonary arterial distensibility in excised rat lungs. Am J Physiol Heart Circ Physiol 2001; 281(3):H1447–H1457.

28. Chen XJ, Moller HE, Chawla MS, Cofer GP, Driehuys B, Hedlund LW, Johnson GA. Spatially resolved measurements of hyperpolarized gas properties in the lung in vivo. Part I: diffusion coefficient. Magn Reson Med 1999; 42(4):721–728.

29. Schreider JP, Raabe OG. Structure of the human respiratory acinus. Am J Anat 1981; 162(3):221–232.

30. Peces-Barba G, Ruiz-Cabello J, Cremillieux Y, Rodriguez I, Dupuich D, Callot V, Ortega M, Rubio Arbo ML, Cortijo M, Gonzalez-Mangado N. Helium-3 MRI diffusion coefficient: correlation to morphometry in a model of mild emphysema. Eur Respir J 2003; 22(1):14–19.
31. Chen XJ, Hedlund LW, Moller HE, Chawla MS, Maronpot RR, Johnson GA. Detection of emphysema in rat lungs by using magnetic resonance measurements of 3He diffusion. Proc Natl Acad Sci USA 2000; 97(21):11478–11481.
32. Ward ER, Hedlund LW, Kurylo WC, Wheeler CT, Cofer GP, Dewhirst MW, Marks LB, Vujaskovic Z. Proton and hyperpolarized helium magnetic resonance imaging of radiation-induced lung injury in rats. Int J Radiat Oncol Biol Phys 2004; 58(5):1562–1569.
33. Wolber J, Cherubini A, Leach MO, Bifone A. Hyperpolarized 129Xe NMR as a probe for blood oxygenation. Magn Reson Med 2000; 43(4):491–496.
34. Mansson S, Wolber J, Driehuys B, Wollmer P, Golman K. Characterization of diffusing capacity and perfusion of the rat lung in a lipopolysaccaride disease model using hyperpolarized 129Xe. Magn Reson Med 2003; 50(6):1170–1179.
35. Tanaka R, Al-Jamal R, Ludwig MS. Maturational changes in extracellular matrix and lung tissue mechanics. J Appl Physiol 2001; 91(5):2314–2321.
36. Beckmann N, Tigani B, Sugar R, Jackson AD, Jones G, Mazzoni L, Fozard JR Noninvasive detection of endotoxin-induced mucus hypersecretion in rat lung by MRI. Am J Physiol Lung Cell Mol Physiol 2002; 283(1):L22–L30.
37. Roughton FJ, Forster RE. Relative importance of diffusion and chemical reaction rates in determining rate of exchange of gases in the human lung, with special reference to true diffusing capacity of pulmonary membrane and volume of blood in the lung capillaries. J Appl Physiol 1957; 11(2):290–302.
38. Yablonskiy DA, Sukstanskii AL, Leawoods JC, Gierada DS, Bretthorst GL, Lefrak SS, Cooper JD, Conradi MS. Quantitative in vivo assessment of lung microstructure at the alveolar level with hyperpolarized 3He diffusion MRI. Proc Natl Acad Sci USA 2002; 99(5):3111–3116.

18

Prospects for Molecular Imaging in Humans

JOHANNES CZERNIN

David Geffen School of Medicine at UCLA,
Los Angeles, California, USA

WOLFGANG WEBER

Technische Universitaet Muenchen,
Muenchen, Germany

I. Introduction

In 1906, Flexner and Jobling (1) established a tumor model by transplanting a spontaneously growing rat tumor into generations of rats. One of the tumor-bearing rats was shipped to Berlin where Warburg et al. (2) conducted their landmark studies on glucose metabolism of tumors, which revealed that the metabolism of tumors is predominantly one of anaerobic glycolysis. Thirty to forty years later, in the 1950s and 1960s, Sokoloff et al. (3) labeled deoxyglucose with carbon 14, and Reivich subsequently marked deoxyglucose with fluorine 18, thus providing radiolabeled analogs of glucose that could be used for tumor imaging. In the 1970s, Phelps et al. (5) built the first positron emission tomography (PET) scanner, enabling the translation of the fundamental discoveries by Warburg et al. (2) into the most innovative and exciting clinical imaging tool in oncology (6).

^{18}F-fluorodeoxyglucose PET (FDG-PET) and integrated PET/computed tomography (CT) are now used to diagnose, stage, and restage malignancies and to monitor treatment effects in patients with cancer. For most cancers, PET accomplishes these tasks with greater accuracy than conventional anatomic imaging. Nevertheless, limitations remain. Foremost among these is the nonspecific nature of FDG uptake in patients with cancer. As shown by Warburg et al. in 1924 (2), benign tumors can also exhibit increased rates of glucose metabolism and, hence, increased FDG uptake. Accumulation of FDG in white blood cells, macrophages, fibroblasts, and other cells can also result in increased FDG uptake because inflammatory cells require glucose as their energy substrate. Thus, FDG-PET imaging provides many but not all of the answers needed for comprehensive imaging in humans. Some cancers do not exhibit increased rates of glycolysis and are, therefore, not visible on FDG-PET images. For these, anatomic imaging remains the most important diagnostic tool. Despite these limitations, FDG will remain the most important molecular imaging probe in cancer diagnostics.

However, the field of molecular imaging is rapidly expanding. Its goal in humans is to provide an array of imaging probes and technologies that target specific molecular processes characteristic of individual cancers. This would not only allow for better diagnosis and staging but also for improved treatment monitoring. The advances in molecular imaging have been facilitated by discoveries in tumor biology as well as by advances in drug and technology development. Important new signal transduction pathways and their alterations have been discovered in recent years, leading to novel and exciting treatment strategies. The effects of such treatments can be evaluated with surrogate markers of disease and disease responses such as the glucose analog ^{18}FDG or the thymidine analog ^{18}F-fluorothymidine (FLT). Thus, molecular imaging benefits the drug evaluation process by providing a unique tool for measuring treatment responses *in vivo*. In addition, therapeutic drugs can be labeled with positron-emitting isotopes and might thus be useful for predicting their biodistribution, pharmacokinetics, and pharmacodynamics *in vivo*. Use of these approaches requires interdisciplinary collaboration among tumor biologists, experts in the field of molecular imaging, physicists, mathematicians, physicians, and leaders in the pharmaceutical industry. Together, this diverse group of scientists is shaping the field of molecular imaging.

This chapter briefly summarizes the currently available "micro" imaging assays and highlights from "bench to bedside" approaches that bring novel imaging probes into the clinical arena. It further describes how well-defined molecular targets can be used to develop targeted imaging probes that might be applicable to human diseases. Coverage of all imaging probes undergoing preclinical testing is beyond the scope of this review, which is aimed at demonstrating concepts rather than providing a comprehensive overview. The emphasis of this discussion is on those imaging probes that might be relevant for clinical use in patients with lung cancer. Some of the described probes are clinically established, whereas others are in the early stages of preclinical or clinical evaluation.

II. Molecular Imaging Assays

With the merger of PET and anatomic CT imaging into single PET/CT devices, the acceptance and visibility of molecular imaging has increased dramatically. More than 300 PET/CT scanners are now used clinically worldwide and PET/CT imaging is now the "state of the art" for diagnosing, staging, and restaging of cancer as well as for monitoring tumor responses to treatment.

At the same time, high-resolution molecular imaging devices designed for small animal research have been developed into valuable tools for drug evaluation and imaging probe design. These include micro-PET, micro-CT, and optical imaging devices.

The advantages of micro-PET over *in vitro* or *ex vivo* approaches can be summarized as follows: effects other than autoradiography treatment can be monitored longitudinally in small animals, obviating the need for killing large numbers of animals. With the use of appropriate tracer kinetic models, the observed processes can be quantified in dimensions such as milligrams per gram per minute (mL/g/min) for blood flow measurements or micromoles per gram per minute (μmol/g/min) for glucose metabolic rates. The strengths and limitations of molecular imaging techniques have been recently reviewed in great detail by Massoud and Gambhir (7). Micro-PET scanners now approach a spatial resolution of about 1 mm^3 (8,9). This excellent resolution permits the observation of the natural behavior of small tumors in small animals and monitoring of treatment effects *in vivo*. Because visualization of normal anatomic structures may be limited in micro-PET studies, micro-CT is frequently used to provide anatomic background information. Anatomic and molecular images can be fused by using specifically designed software that affords assignment of normal or abnormal molecular imaging findings to specific anatomic structures (10) (Fig. 18.1).

Another approach for visualizing tumors in small animals is optical imaging in which fluorescence or bioluminescence is used as a signal (11). For fluorescent imaging, light is shone on a living small animal, and in response

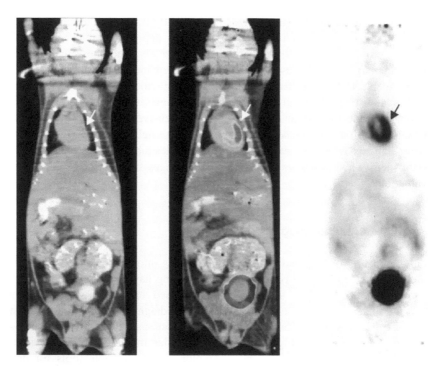

Figure 18.1 Mouse images obtained with micro-CT (left) and micro-PET (right). Images were fused to combine anatomic and molecular information (middle). Arrows point to normal cardiac anatomy (left) and physiologic myocardial glucose metabolic activity (middle and right).

to this, light of lower-energy wavelengths is emitted by a fluorescent molecule that is detected by a charged coupled device (CCD) camera. Most frequently, fluorescence imaging is used to detect cells that have been transfected with green fluorescent protein (GFP) from the jellyfish (*Aequorea victoria)* or similar fluorescent proteins. However, low-molecular-weight fluorescent dyes such as cy5 may also be coupled to peptides or proteins and used for fluorescence imaging (12). In bioluminescence imaging, light is emitted as a consequence of an intracellular enzymatic reaction. The most frequently used enzyme for bioluminescence is firefly luciferase, which oxidizes D-luciferin in the presence of adenosine triphosphate (ATP), resulting in the emission of yellow–green light (wavelength, 575 nm). For luciferase imaging, tumor cells must first be transfected with the luciferase gene. Luciferase-expressing cells can then be detected *in vivo* after injection of D-luciferin. Optical imaging has several advantages and shortcomings. One of the advantages is the ability to examine large numbers of small animals quickly and inexpensively. In addition, optical imaging is very sensitive, and just a few thousand cells transfected with GFP or luciferase can be detected by optical imaging. However, this is only the case when the cells are located near the body surface. Because of the limited penetration of light in tissue and the large amount of photon scattering, the sensitivity of optical imaging rapidly degrades for deeper-seated lesions. A specific limitation of fluorescence imaging is the autofluorescence of many tissues. Therefore, it can be difficult to differentiate between a specific signal originating from transfected cells and nonspecific autofluorescence. Because of limits to tissue penetration and the need to transfect cells, neither bioluminescence nor fluorescence imaging is likely to become a clinically applicable imaging technique for patients with lung cancer.

III. Imaging Targets, Probes, Processes, and Applications

A. Imaging Glycolytic Activity

Otto Warburg (13) studied the metabolism of tumor cells and found that their glycolytic rates were 124 times greater than those of blood. In frogs, carcinoma tissue produced 200 times as much lactic acid as a resting muscle and 8 times more lactic acid than a working muscle. He evaluated the contribution of oxidative and "cleavage" (i.e., anaerobic) metabolism to overall tumor metabolism and observed that, of 13 sugar molecules metabolized, only one was oxidized and the rest were "fermented." He thus proved that the metabolism of rat tumor cells is predominantly one of glycolysis. Increased rates of glycolysis are required to accommodate the high metabolic demands of rapidly proliferating tumor tissue. In addition, accelerated rates of the hexose monophosphate pathway provide the carbon backbone for DNA and RNA synthesis in growing tumors (14,15). Activity of glucose transporters and hexokinase is upregulated in tumor cells to facilitate glucose utilization. The glucose analog FDG follows the same cellular uptake mechanism as glucose; that is, it is taken up by cancer cells via facilitative glucose transporters and is subsequently phosphorylated by hexokinase to FDG-6-phosphate, which unlike glucose-6-phosphate, is not a substrate for glycolysis and thus remains trapped intracellularly (Fig. 18.2).

The molecular targets for FDG imaging, therefore, include glucose transporters and hexokinase. The whole-body distribution of FDG-6-phopshate provides unique information regarding the extent of cancer and its response to treatment. Anatomic imaging results in incorrect staging of cancer for many patients (16). For instance, the size of lymph nodes does not reliably predict the presence of cancer metastases (17). Dwamena et al. (18) conducted a meta-analysis to compare the performance of PET and CT for mediastinal lymph node staging in patients with lung cancer. This analysis included 514 patients with lung cancer evaluated with PET and 2226 patients with lung cancer evaluated with CT and revealed that the sensitivity (79% vs. 60%) and specificity (91% vs. 77%) were significantly higher for PET than for CT. In addition, as a

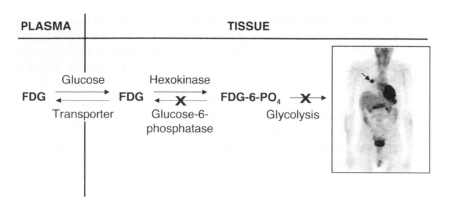

Figure 18.2 Kinetics of ^{18}F-FDG: FDG is taken up by tumor cells via glucose transporters that are overexpressed in cancer. Hexokinase phosphorylates FDG to FDG-6-phosphate, which is not a substrate for glycolysis and is essentially trapped in tumor cells. The arrow on the inserted FDG-PET image shows abnormal glycolytic activity corresponding to a newly diagnosed NSCLC. Note the normal myocardial and bladder activity.

whole-body technique, FDG-PET detects unexpected metastases in 10–16% of patients with lung cancer (19–21). Thus, PET is more accurate than CT for staging of lung cancer.

The superior accuracy of FDG-PET for staging of non-small-cell lung cancer (NSCLC) has also been shown to significantly improve disease management. In a multicenter study published by van Tinteren et al. (22), 188 patients with newly diagnosed NSCLC were randomly assigned to undergo either conventional CT-based staging or conventional staging and FDG-PET. The primary endpoint was the rate of futile thoracotomies. These were defined as tumor resections in patients with mediastinal lymph node involvement (tumor stage IIIA-N2 or IIIB), explorative thoracotomies of any kind, or tumor recurrence within 1 year after the thoracotomy. In patients whose cancer was staged by FDG-PET, the rate of noncurative thoracotomies was 51% lower than that in patients whose cancer was staged by conventional imaging techniques alone ($P = 0.003$). Thus, FDG-PET is one of the few imaging tests that has been found to significantly improve disease management in a randomized trial. A recent prospective study indicated additional diagnostic gains from using integrated PET/CT, whereby PET/CT provided additional "important" information over PET and CT alone in 41% of the patients (23). Thus, FDG-PET, and more recently, PET/CT are considered the "state of the art" for staging and restaging of lung cancer.

Compared with research on NSCLC, only few studies have addressed the use of FDG-PET in small cell lung cancer. This is mainly because most patients with small cell lung cancer present with metastatic disease at the time of diagnosis and are treated with systemic chemotherapy. Therefore, exact tumor staging is generally of less clinical importance than it is for patients with NSCLC. However, several studies have now indicated that small cell lung cancer is characterized by high FDG uptake, and FDG-PET may be used for initial tumor staging as well as for follow-up of treated patients (24,25).

In addition to detection and staging of lung cancer, FDG-PET may also be used to monitor chemotherapy and chemoradiotherapy. MacManus et al. (26) evaluated tumor response to radical (chemo)radiotherapy by CT and FDG-PET in a prospective study that included 73 patients. Tumor response as determined by FDG-PET was defined as normalization of all sites with abnormal FDG uptake (complete response) or a significant reduction in FDG uptake of all known lesions without the appearance of new lesions (partial response). Tumor response as determined by FDG-PET was a better predictor of patient survival than tumor response determined by CT, pretreatment stage, or patient performance status. Quantitative measurements of tumor metabolism by FDG-PET may even allow the prediction of tumor response during chemotherapy. In a study that included 57 patients with advanced NSCLC, the reduction of tumor FDG uptake was highly significantly correlated with best response to therapy. Failure to achieve a measurable reduction in tumor FDG uptake at this time point was associated with 96% risk of not achieving an objective response with the first-line chemotherapy regimen. In addition, nonresponders, as determined by FDG-PET, were characterized by a 3× shorter time to tumor progression and a 1.7× shorter overall survival (27). These data suggest that a metabolic response demonstrated by FDG-PET is an early predictor of the final outcome of therapy in patients with NSCLC. Using a metabolic response determined by FDG-PET as an endpoint may shorten the duration of phase II studies evaluating new cytotoxic drugs and may decrease the morbidity and costs of therapy in patients with nonresponding tumors.

B. Imaging Bone Metastases with ^{18}F-Fluoride

Bone metastases occur in nearly 50% of patients with lung cancer (28). Staging of lung cancer, therefore, routinely includes whole-body bone scintigraphy with technetium-labeled diphosphonates. ^{18}F-fluoride has been used as a bone-imaging agent for many decades. The kinetics of ^{18}F-fluoride are shown in Fig. 18.3. For many reasons, such as better spatial and contrast resolution, PET bone imaging is likely to be superior to conventional planar whole-body bone imaging. In several studies, conventional bone scintigraphy has been compared with ^{18}F-fluoride PET scintigraphy of the skeletal system, and results have confirmed the superiority of PET imaging.

In a prospective comparison of planar bone imaging, single photon emission computed tomography (SPECT) and ^{18}F-fluoride PET bone scintigraphy in 53 patients with newly diagnosed lung cancer (29), ^{18}F-fluoride had the greatest accuracy for the detection of bone metastases. The accuracy of ^{18}F-fluoride

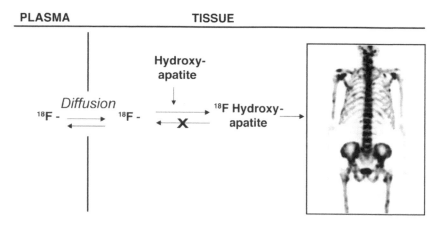

Figure 18.3 Kinetics of ^{18}F-fluoride. ^{18}F-fluoride diffuses into bone tissue and binds to hydroxy-apatite. The inserted PET image shows increased ^{18}F-fluoride accumulation in numerous bone metastases in this patient with prostate cancer.

imaging was significantly greater than that of the more frequently used planar bone imaging. Hetzel et al. (30) studied a total of 103 patients with lung cancer by using planar bone scintigraphy, SPECT, and ^{18}F-fluoride PET. PET had the lowest number of false-negative findings and a higher diagnostic accuracy than both conventional bone imaging techniques. More recently, Even-Sapir (31) reported an additional diagnostic advantage when ^{18}F-fluoride was used with combined PET/CT imaging. Addition of CT resulted in significantly improved specificity and diagnostic accuracy in 44 patients with cancer.

Hoegerle et al. (32) proposed an interesting comprehensive whole-body PET imaging approach, whereby FDG and ^{18}F-fluoride were administered in a single injection. This approach resulted in a sensitivity of 87% for the detection of bone metastases. Because of its superior diagnostic performance, ^{18}F-fluoride imaging will, in the near future, emerge as a commonly used bone survey for patients with cancer.

C. Imaging Amino Acid Metabolism

A large number of natural amino acids and amino acid analogs have been radiolabeled and evaluated for PET, and to a lesser degree for SPECT imaging of malignant tumors (Fig. 18.4). Radiolabeled amino acids show considerable differences with respect to ease of synthesis, biodistribution, and formation of radiolabeled metabolites that can confound image interpretation. For these reasons, in most of the clinical studies conducted so far, carbon 11-labeled methionine (Fig. 18.5), ^{11}C-tyrosine, or ^{18}F-labeled amino acid analogs such as fluoro-ethyltyrosine (FET) and fluoro-methyltyrosine (FMT) have been used.

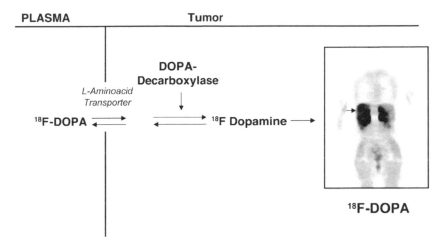

Figure 18.4 Kinetics of ^{18}F-DOPA. ^{18}F-DOPA is incorporated into tissue via the L amino acid transporter. In neuroendocrine tumors it is subsequently decarboxylated by DOPA-decarboxylase to ^{18}F-dopamine. The inserted image shows increased dopamine retention in liver metastases of a patient with carcinoid (arrow).

In addition, the amino acid analog alpha-iodo-methyl tyrosine (IMT) has been extensively used for SPECT imaging of brain tumors (33).

The main factor for the increased uptake of radiolabeled amino acids in malignant tumors appears to be the increased expression and activity of the so-called L-type amino acid transporter. This transport system mediates the movement of neutral amino acids across the cell membrane. It has long been characterized as a nonenergy-dependent bidirectional transport system, which

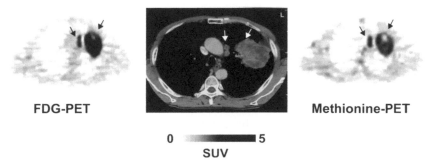

Figure 18.5 FDG (left) and ^{11}C-methionine (right) retention in NSCLC of the left upper lobe. The middle image represents the corresponding CT slice. FDG accumulation was more prominent (arrow), but the tumor was also clearly visible with methionine-PET (arrow). All three—FDG-PET, CT, and methionine PET-identified ipsilateral lymph node involvement (arrows). Both PET images are normalized to the same maximum SUV.

is specifically inhibited by the artificial amino acid BCH (2-aminobicyclo[2.2.1]-heptane-2-carboxylic acid). However, it was only in 1998 that the first L-type transporter molecule was identified (34,35). Currently, there are three known subtypes of the L-type carrier, designated *LAT1*, *LAT2*, and *LAT3* (36). The LAT1 subtype has been found to be overexpressed in several malignant tumors (37) and to transport IMT (38). The L-type carrier also accepts ^{18}F-fluorodopa ([18]FDOPA) as a substrate (39). [18]FDOPA was initially developed for imaging the cerebral dopaminergic system. In the brain [18]FDOPA undergoes decarboxylation to fluoro-dopamine, which is then stored intracellularly. However, [18]FDOPA has also been shown to accumulate in tumors without DOPA decarboxylase activity. In these tumors [18]FDOPA uptake is likely to reflect the increased activity of the L-type transporter and has been shown to be closely correlated to methionine uptake in a clinical study of brain tumors (40).

Since amino acid uptake of normal gray matter is much lower than glucose uptake, radiolabeled amino acids provide markedly better contrast for imaging of brain tumors. In addition, radiolabeled amino acids are efficiently transported across the blood-brain barrier and allow superior visualization of the local extension of brain tumors when compared with magnetic resonance imaging (MRI) or CT (41). Therefore, imaging of brain tumors has been the main clinical application of all amino acid tracers. Systematic comparative studies have shown little difference in the uptake of natural amino acids and amino acid analogs, which are not incorporated into proteins (42,43). In some animal models, uptake of radiolabeled amino acids in inflammatory processes has been shown to be lower with uptake of FDG (44,45). Therefore, PET with radiolabeled amino acids may be more specific than FDG-PET for tumor staging. However, in clinical studies this potential advantage has not been confirmed thus far. In patients with lung cancer, radiolabeled methionine and tyrosine are significantly accumulated by the primary tumors and metastases (46–49). The diagnostic accuracy of PET with methionine for mediastinal staging of NSCLC was comparable to that of FDG-PET in small series of patients (48). A disadvantage of the natural amino acids is their high uptake by the liver and pancreas, which limits their sensitivity for tumor detection in the upper abdomen. Overall, it is not expected that radiolabeled amino acids will replace FDG for staging of lung cancer.

In patients with lung cancer, the only important clinical application appears to be the evaluation of cerebral metastases, particularly after radiotherapy, when viable tumor tissue and reactive changes cannot be differentiated by CT or MRI.

D. Imaging Cell Membrane Synthesis

Choline, an amino alcohol, is the precursor of phospholipids, which are ubiquitous components of cell membranes. Choline can be labeled with [11]C (50) or [18]F (51,52) and is taken up by tumor cells via an active transport mechanism. It is subsequently trapped through phosphorylation by choline kinase to phosphorylcholine, which is incorporated into phospholipids, most notably, phosphatidylcholine (52) (Fig. 18.6). Several fluorinated choline analogs have been synthesized. All exhibit rapid blood clearance, allowing for early imaging after intravenous tracer injection (51). One potential advantage for imaging prostate cancer is that choline accumulates with some delay and only to a small degree in the urinary bladder. Thus, images can be obtained before the prostate bed is obscured by tracer accumulation in the urinary bladder. A disadvantage is that background activity in normal liver, spleen, and bowel, and to a certain degree, lung is fairly high so that primary or metastatic lesions in these organs would need to exhibit high tracer accumulation for detectability. In human plasma, ~85% and 48% of the administered ^{11}C-choline remains unmetabolized after 5–10 min, respectively, and ^{11}C-betaine is the major metabolite in human plasma (53).

Animal studies that describe the uptake of choline analogs in xenografts are sparse. One group reported that ^{11}C-choline accumulates in MCF-7 breast cancer xenografts (54). More information is available from clinical studies performed in patients with brain tumors, prostate cancer, and—to a lesser degree—lung cancer. The largest comparison between FDG and ^{11}C-choline PET to date included 100 patients who underwent restaging for prostate cancer. ^{11}C-choline findings were more frequently in agreement with conventional imaging findings than with findings from FDG-PET (55). PET with

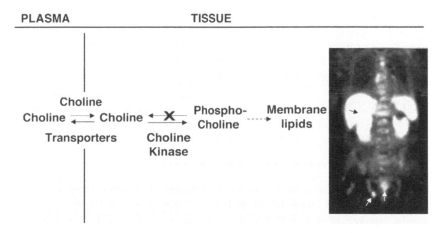

Figure 18.6 Kinetics of ^{18}F-choline. After transport into cells, choline is phosphorylated by choline kinase, and via intermediate steps, to phosphatidylcholine, a ubiquitous component of cell membrane lipids. Inserted image on the right demonstrates high physiologic hepatic tracer retention (arrow). Focally increased activity in the region of the bladder (arrow) is consistent with primary bladder carcinoma, since physiologic urine activity appears later during imaging. The focus of increased activity in the right lower pelvis corresponds to a bone metastasis (arrow).

[11]C-acetate (56), another tracer that has been used for prostate cancer imaging, and ^{18}F-choline PET appear to have a similar ability for imaging prostate cancer (57). ^{11}C-acetate also appears to be incorporated into phosphatidylcholine and neutral lipids.

[11]C-choline PET has also been used for imaging lung cancer. The cohort in Hara et al. (58) included 97 patients with lung cancer, 14 with pulmonary tuberculosis, and 5 with atypical mycobacterial infection. They reported concordantly high ^{11}C-choline and FDG uptake in patients with cancer and concordantly low uptake in those with atypical mycobacterial infection. A discordant uptake pattern with high FDG uptake but low choline uptake in patients with tuberculosis suggested that combined imaging with both probes might be useful for characterizing lung lesions as malignant with a high specificity.

However, some limitations of ^{11}C-choline imaging in patients with lung cancer were reported by Khan et al. (59). First, tumor to background ratios, semiquantitative measures of tracer uptake intensity, were more than twice as high for FDG than for ^{11}C-choline. ^{11}C-choline PET failed to reveal lymph node metastases in two patients. Finally, only tumors >2 cm were reliably detected with ^{11}C-choline PET. This was largely explained by relatively high ^{11}C-choline background activity in normal lung tissue. In a population of patients with lung cancer, Pieterman et al. (60) were able to clearly visualize all brain metastases with ^{11}C-choline, whereas FDG-PET failed to detect almost 90% of brain metastases. However, the detectability of intrapulmonary pleural metastases was lower with ^{11}C-choline than with FDG-PET (60). Using autoradiography, Wyss et al. (61) unequivocally demonstrated substantially increased ^{18}F-choline uptake in benign inflammatory tissue (abscess). This was subsequently confirmed for ^{11}C-choline in 10 patients with inflammatory joint disease (62). Thus, the question of whether choline analogs are more specific cancer imaging probes than FDG remains to be answered, and their clinical role needs to be defined. However, it is conceivable that dual isotope imaging with FDG and choline will increase the specificity of PET imaging for characterizing solitary pulmonary nodules and lymph nodes in patients with lung cancer.

E. Imaging Tumor Cell Proliferation

Abnormal cell proliferation is one of the hallmarks of cancer. Imaging of tumor cell proliferation or even DNA replication might, therefore, provide a more specific marker of tumor behavior and tumor responses to treatment than imaging of glycolysis. Several attempts have been made to synthesize radiolabeled analogs of nucleosides (63) for tumor imaging. These include ^{11}C-thymidine, ^{18}F-thymidine, iodo-deoxyuridine ([124]I-IudR, ^{125}I-IudR), [77]Br-deoxyuridine, [76]Br-uracil, 1-(2′-deoxy-2′-fluoro-beta-D-arabinofuranosyl)-(52) thymine ([11]CFMAU), and others.

Among these, FLT has been most widely studied in animal experiments and humans (64). Cellular uptake of FLT is determined by the activity of the thymidine salvage pathway. In this pathway extracellular thymidine is transported across the cell membrane by nucleoside transporters, phosphorylated three times to thymidine-triphosphate, and then incorporated into the DNA. FLT is transported across the cell membrane in a similar way as thymidine and phosphorylated by thymidine kinase 1 (TK1) to FLT-monophosphate (Fig. 18.7). However, during imaging, only minimal amounts of FLT are incorporated into the DNA. Nevertheless, FLT remains trapped intracellularly, since the polar FLT-monophosphate cannot cross the cell membrane. Although most FLT is not incorporated into DNA, it is still a marker of cellular proliferation because TK1 activity is generally closely regulated by the cell cycle and relevant TK1 activity is only observed during DNA synthesis (65). The correlation of TK1 activity, cellular FLT uptake, and tumor cell proliferation has been documented for various cell types (66,67).

Schwartz et al. (68) investigated the relationship between tumor cell proliferation and FLT uptake *in vitro*. Using various human and murine tumor cell lines, these authors demonstrated that for all tumors whose growth was strongly TK1 dependent, FLT phosphorylation, and hence, retention was high. Some tumors, however, exhibit growth activity that is not highly dependent on TK1 activity. For instance, KHTn and RIF1 tumor cell lines grew more independently of TK1 activity, and the overall correlation between tracer uptake and TK activity was poor. Thus, growth of some tumors might depend primarily on *de novo* nucleotide synthesis rather than on the salvage pathway (68). The biodistribution of FLT is species dependent. For instance, hepatic tracer accumulation was observed in humans but not in dogs, likely because of the lack of liver

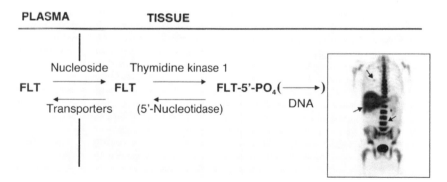

Figure 18.7 Kinetics of ^{18}F-FLT. After transport into cells via nucleoside transporters, FLT is phosphorylated by thymidine kinase 1 to FLT-5-phosphate, of which only a small portion is incorporated into DNA. Most of the FLT accumulates in small cytoplasmic molecules. The inserted image shows a patient with non-small cell lung cancer and mildly increased uptake in the primary lesion (upper arrow). Note the increased physiologic FLT activity in normal proliferating tissue such as bone marrow (lower arrow). Liver activity is high because of hepatic glucuronidation of FLT (arrow).

glucuronidase in the latter (64). However, the physiologically high uptake of tracer in tissues such as liver and bone marrow might limit the usefulness of FLT for cancer staging in humans (Fig. 18.8).

The ability of FLT-PET to detect malignant tumors in humans has now been confirmed by several studies. Furthermore, in several studies, investigators observed a correlation between tumor FLT uptake and cellular proliferation as determined by immunohistochemistry.

In contrast to observations in animal studies, FDG uptake in human lung cancer lesions is consistently two times higher than that of FLT (69,70). The sometimes low tumoral FLT uptake results in a small number of false-positive findings, and hence, a high specificity for malignancy. However, the sensitivity of FLT-PET might be too low for reliable lung cancer staging. Similarly, a study in patients with colorectal cancer (71) demonstrated relatively low FLT uptake values in primary tumors [standardized uptake value-(SUV): 2.1 $\pm$ 5.6] and extrahepatic metastases (2.2 $\pm$ 6.1). In this study, <30% of documented liver metastases were detected, and this was ascribed to high normal background activity in the liver.

Dittmann (69) used FLT to characterize thoracic lesions in 16 patients who were scheduled to undergo surgical resection, radiotherapy, or chemotherapy. The study group included patients with esophageal carcinoma, sarcoma, Hodgkin's disease, and NSCLC. Although uptake of FDG was consistently higher than that of FLT, the sensitivity for lesion detection was excellent for FLT, with a particular advantage for detecting brain metastases as a result of

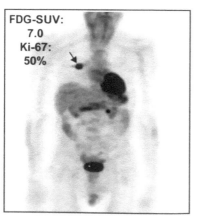
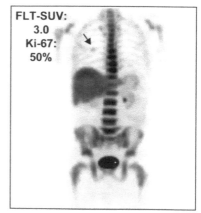

FDG-PET   **FLT-PET**

Figure 18.8 FDG and FLT study in a patient with NSCLC. The primary tumor was visible on both studies (arrows). However, FDG uptake was much more intense than FLT uptake despite a relatively high immunohistochemical index of tumor cell proliferation (Ki-67 index: 50%). SUV, an index of degree of tracer retention in tumor tissue, was markedly higher for FDG (7.0) than for FLT (3.0).

absent background FLT accumulation in this organ (69). However, no significant relationship between Ki-67 labeling index as a marker of tumor cell proliferation and FLT accumulation was observed. Another study (70) did show a close relationship between FLT uptake and the Ki-67 labeling index ($r = 0.92$; $P < 0.0001$) in a population of patients with lung cancer. These discrepant findings may be explained by differences in the studied tumor types, the proliferation of which is, to a varying degree, dependent on the thymidine salvage pathway.

In summary, FLT probes tumor cell proliferation *in vivo* and its uptake in tumors is TK1 dependent. It can be used to detect primary lung cancer and metastatic lesions in humans. However, most malignant lesions accumulate less FLT than FDG. Hence, the role of FLT for diagnosing and staging of cancer is evolving. A more important role of FLT-PET might be related to treatment monitoring, for which a more specific marker of tumor response than FDG would be desirable. One study in patients with breast cancer, which demonstrated a good predictive value of FLT-PET for treatment responses, supports this notion (72).

IV. Using Analogs of Therapeutic Drugs as Imaging Probes

Cyclo-oxygenase 2 (COX-2) has been proposed as a target for noninvasive imaging of inflammation and cancer. This is based on the notion that COX is the critical enzyme in prostaglandin synthesis. COX-2, a membrane-bound enzyme, has potent inflammatory effects but is also overexpressed in colon, breast, lung, and other cancers. COX-2 overexpression results in decreased apoptosis and increased cell migration and proliferation.

Radiolabeled COX-1 and COX-2 analogs have been recently synthesized (73). The first, ^{18}F-SC63217, has a low inhibitory concentration of 50% of enzyme activity of <10 nmol/L, and the latter has a less favorable one of <86 nmol/L. Both compounds were evaluated *in vitro*, and the cold, unlabeled analog (i.e., the parent drug) completely inhibited uptake of the radioactive analog in J774 cells for the COX-1 analog. Biodistribution studies revealed increased accumulation of the COX-1 analog in the small intestine, whereas uptake of the COX-2 analog was less prominent. Moreover, the COX-2 analog showed high nonspecific binding, which will limit the usefulness of this imaging probe *in vivo*. Another radiolabeled analog of a COX-2 inhibitor was synthesized at our institution by Satyamurthy and Barrio (unpublished data; Fig. 18.9). Biodistribution studies in mice revealed rapid defluorination and accumulation of the radioactive label in bone, which made it unfit for tumor imaging in this species. However, studies in vervet monkeys revealed much later and much less prominent defluorination, suggesting a potential role for imaging in humans. An imaging study recently completed in a healthy volunteer revealed a favorable biodistribution with low normal background activity in the abdomen and chest. Further, defluorination occurred late and only to a

PLASMA   **TISSUE**

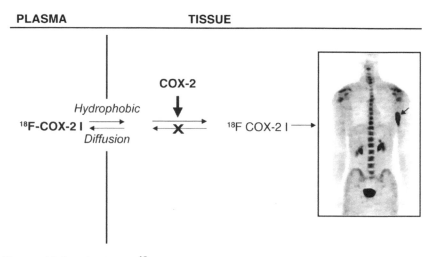

Figure 18.9 Kinetics of ^{18}F-COX-2 inhibitor. The imaging probe enters tissue via hydrophobic diffusion and binds to COX-2, which is overexpressed in cancer. The inserted image, obtained 25–50 min after tracer injection, demonstrates low liver and lung background activity but moderate tracer accumulation in the skeleton, which is explained by late defluorination of the compound. Focally increased tracer activity in the left axilla is due to tracer contamination (arrow).

moderate degree (Fig. 18. 9). The potential applications of this novel imaging probe are evident and include treatment monitoring of patients with inflammatory diseases, as well as patients with cancer.

V. Imaging Tyrosine Kinase Receptor Densities

Phosphorylation of proteins is an important signal transduction pathway by which extracellular signaling molecules regulate a number of critical cellular functions such as mitogenesis, protein translation, gene transcription, and cell cycle progression and differentiation (74). A large class of enzymes termed protein kinases (PKs) catalyzes protein phosphorylation reactions by transferring the γ-phosphate from ATP to the alcoholic group in serine and threonine or to the phenolic moiety of tyrosine. So far, more than 200 PKs have been identified and sequenced (75). An important subset of PKs is the protein tyrosine kinases (PTKs). A number of them are transmembrane glycoproteins with an extracellular ligand-binding domain and an intracellular tyrosine kinase regulatory domain (76). Such PTKs are also known as receptor tyrosine kinases (RTKs). Binding of specific peptide growth factor ligands to the extracellular receptor sites to activate the kinase domain of the RTKs is a necessary event in normal regulation of cell growth (76). However, under certain conditions, as a result of either mutation or overexpression, these RTKs can become deregulated and phosphorylate substrates inappropriately, leading to tumor formation and progression (77). The role of RTKs in tumor genesis is also supported by the fact that a number of proto-oncogenes encode for proteins having RTK activity (78). Thus, substantial efforts have been directed toward developing specific inhibitors of these enzymes as chemotherapeutic agents (79), the most prominent of which is the tyrosine kinase inhibitor STI 571 (Gleevec). This inhibitor of the constitutively activated tyrosine kinase BCR-ABL has successfully induced long-lasting remissions in patients with CML (80). In NSCLC, gefitinib (Iressa), a drug that targets the epidermal growth factor receptor (EGFR)—which is intimately involved in tumor proliferation, angiogenesis, metastatic spread, and invasiveness—has been introduced clinically. These and other small-molecule inhibitors exhibit high binding affinities for EGFR and result in growth arrest of tumor xenografts.

Several EGFR inhibitors are chemically based on a quinazoline structure. Radiolabeled quinazoline derivatives, which specifically and reversibly or irreversibly bind to EGFR and HER-2, have been synthesized at the University of California, Los Angeles (UCLA) and elsewhere. In a recent biodistribution study performed at UCLA, A-431 tumor cells overexpressing EGFR were implanted into the flanks of severe combined immunodeficient (SCID) mice. For the purpose of monitoring the biodistribution of the radiolabeled drug analog, dynamic micro-PET studies were performed over 3 h in A-431 tumor-bearing SCID mice. Tumors were visible on micro-PET images and exhibited a rim of mildly increased activity surrounding the center of the tumor. Pretreatment with a tyrosine kinase inhibitor resulted in accelerated washout kinetics of the imaging probe, suggesting that the imaging probe binds to EGFR *in vivo*. Several analogs of therapeutic tyrosine kinase inhibitors have been synthesized and are currently being evaluated in animal studies (Fig. 18.10).

Imaging of the expression of EGFR or other receptors of the ErbB family may allow selection of patients for treatment with ErbB antagonists and documentation of successful blockade of these receptors by therapeutic agents. Currently, only a subgroup of patients appears to benefit from treatment with ErbB antagonists and the molecular determinants for tumor response are unknown. Therefore, noninvasive imaging with ErbB receptor ligands could play an important role in treatment planning and monitoring.

VI. Imaging the Distribution of Radiolabeled Chemotherapeutic Agents

Several analogs of chemotherapeutic agents have been synthesized. These include paclitaxel, cyclophosphamide, 5-fluorouracil (5-FU), and others. The most widely studied labeled chemotherapeutic agent is 5-FU, a drug that has been used for cancer treatment for several decades. The drug inhibits DNA synthesis by inhibition of thymidylate synthase, which is in turn the key

PLASMA   **TISSUE**

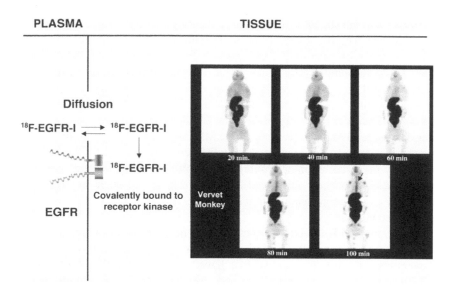

Figure 18.10   Kinetics of ^{18}F-EGFR-kinase inhibitors. The inhibitor enters the cell by diffusion and binds covalently to the intracellular kinase domain of the EGFR. The inserted images demonstrate the biodistribution of the labeled compound in a vervet monkey. At 20 min after injection, the tracer shows rapid biliary clearance into the bowel. At 80–100 min, tracer uptake in the skeleton consistent with defluorination is noted (arrow).

enzyme for *de novo* DNA synthesis (81). Radiolabeled analogs of 5-FU have been synthesized (82) and radiolabeled 5-FU has been used for cancer imaging in humans (83). Dimitrakopoulou et al. (84) reported an inverse relationship between degree of tumor tracer uptake and tumor growth rates, suggesting that treatment effectiveness could be predicted with ^{18}F-5-FU. More recently, Saleem et al. (81) demonstrated in humans with PET the effects of eniluracil, a drug that inhibits 5-FU degradation, on 5-FU pharmacokinetics in normal and abnormal tissue. Six patients with metastatic colorectal cancer were studied. Before eniluracil was added to 5-FU, the ^{18}F-5-FU accumulated more prominently in normal tissue than in abnormal tissue; in other words, tumors appeared as cold spots. After eniluracil administration, normal tissue uptake decreased and plasma levels of unmetabolized ^{18}F-5-FU increased, suggesting increased accumulation of the imaging compound in tumors.

VII.   Imaging of the $\alpha_v\beta_3$ Integrin

Binding and responsiveness of cells to the extracellular matrix is mainly mediated by integrins, a large family of cell adhesion molecules. Each integrin is composed of two noncovalently associated transmembrane glycoprotein subunits called *the α chain* and *the β chain*. So far, 18 α and 8 β chains have been identified, which form at least 24 receptors with different substrate specificities (85). One of the best characterized of these receptors is the $\alpha_v\beta_3$ integrin, which plays an important role in endothelial cell migration and survival during angiogenesis (86). In addition to activated endothelial cells, $\alpha_v\beta_3$ integrin is expressed by various tumor cells, such as malignant melanoma, in which it increases the metastatic potential (87).

The binding mechanisms of $\alpha_v\beta_3$ integrin to its ligands (e.g., vitronectin, fibronectin, fibrinogen, and osteopontin) have been extensively studied in recent years (88). It is now well established that $\alpha_v\beta_3$ binds to matrix proteins with an exposed RGD (arginine-glycine-aspartate) sequence (89). This binding motif is also used by several other integrin subtypes (e.g., $\alpha_v\beta_5$ and $\alpha iib\beta 3$) (88). However, the binding affinity of different integrins to an RGD sequence is critically influenced by its steric configuration as well as by the flanking amino acid residues (88). Intensive structure/activity investigations have resulted in the development of cyclic pentapeptides that specifically bind to $\alpha_v\beta_3$, but not to other related RGD-binding integrins. By radiolabeling these peptides with radioiodine, indium 111, technetium 99 m and ^{18}F, various imaging agents have been developed that specifically localize to tumors expressing $\alpha_v\beta_3$ (90). Recently, the $\alpha_v\beta_3$-ligand F-18-galacto-RGD (91) has also been shown to accumulate in human tumors expressing $\alpha_v\beta_3$ (Fig. 18.11). In clinical

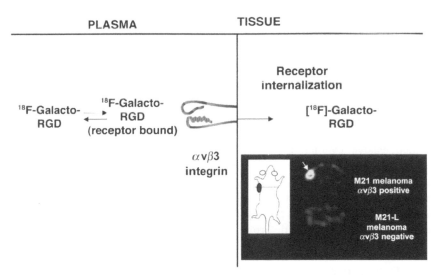

Figure 18.11 Kinetics of ^{18}F-galacto-RGD. The tracer binds to the extracellular portion of the $\alpha_v\beta_3$ integrin, which is subsequently internalized. The inserted images show PET studies of tumor-bearing mice. The $\alpha_v\beta_3$-positive M21 melanoma demonstrates intense tracer uptake, whereas the $\alpha_v\beta_3$-negative M21-L melanoma is not visualized in the PET study, confirming the receptor-specific tracer uptake.

studies, radiolabeled RGD peptides may be used to document $\alpha_v\beta_3$ expression of the tumors before the administration of therapeutic doses of $\alpha_v\beta_3$ antagonists, thus allowing appropriate selection of patients for clinical trials. Furthermore, radiolabeled RGD peptides may be used to assess the inhibition of the $\alpha_v\beta_3$ integrin by specific antagonists. Thus, imaging may be used to define the optimal dose and dose schedule for $\alpha_v\beta_3$ antagonists. Because expression of $\alpha_v\beta_3$ appears to be a general characteristic of activated endothelial cells, reduction of the uptake of radiolabeled RGD peptides may also be used as a marker for successful inhibition of angiogenesis by other therapeutic agents. Finally, $\alpha_v\beta_3$ expression has been reported to be an important factor in determining the invasiveness and metastatic potential of malignant tumors in experimental tumor models, as well as in clinical studies. Therefore, noninvasive imaging of $\alpha_v\beta_3$ expression may also provide a unique means of characterizing the biologic aggressiveness of a malignant tumor in an individual patient.

VIII. Summary

The traditional view of cancer as an anatomic disease is rapidly evolving into an understanding of cancer as a systemic molecular disease. More and more physicians now detect differences between anatomic masses by anatomic imaging and tumor viability by PET imaging of molecular processes.

The paradigm of pharmaceutical companies for evaluating the effects of novel drugs is also changing and is now departing from a simple anatomic concept. Tumor responses are being defined by molecular rather than anatomic changes, and molecular PET imaging provides the new means for these assessments.

Diverse disciplines such as tumor biology, physics, mathematics, pharmacology, drug development, medicine, and imaging have merged to create the new field of molecular imaging. PET imaging probes can now be used to monitor tumor-specific processes and their responses to therapeutic interventions. More comprehensive evaluations of patients with cancer are becoming possible, including whole-body surveys of glucose metabolism, bone matrix formation, amino acid metabolism, enzyme expression, tumor cell proliferation, and hormone receptor and tyrosine kinase receptor density. At the same time, micro-PET imaging assays greatly aid in the drug discovery process by allowing serial preclinical response determinations in small living animals.

References

1. Flexner S, Jobling S. Studies upon a transplantable rat tumour. New York: Monographs of the Rockefeller Institute for Medical Research, 1910.
2. Warburg O, Posener K, Negelein E VIII. The metabolism of cancer cells. Biochem Z 1924; 152:129–169.

3. Sokoloff L, Reivich M, Kennedy C, Des Rosiers MH, Patlak CS, Pettigrew KD, Sakurada O, Shinohara M. The [14C]deoxyglucose method for the measurement of local cerebral glucose utilization: theory, procedure, and normal values in the conscious and anesthetized albino rat. J Neurochem 1977; 28:897–916.
4. Reivich M, Kuhl D, Wolf A, Greenberg J, Phelps M, Ido T, Castella V, Fowler J, Gallagher B, Hoffman E, Alavi A, Sokoloff L. Measurement of local cerebral glucose metabolism in man with ^{18}F-fluoro-2-deoxyglucose. Acta Neurol Scand Suppl 1977; 64:190–191.
5. Phelps ME, Hoffman EJ, Mullani NA, Ter Pogossian MM. Application of annihilation coincidence detection to transaxial reconstruction tomography. J Nucl Med 1975; 16:210–224.
6. Phelps ME. Inaugural article: positron emission tomography provides molecular imaging of biological processes. Proc Natl Acad Sci USA 2000; 97:9226–9233.
7. Massoud TF, Gambhir SS. Molecular imaging in living subjects: seeing fundamental biological processes in a new light. Gene Dev 2003; 17:545–580.
8. Cherry SR, Gambhir SS. Use of positron emission tomography in animal research. Ilar J 2001; 42:219–232.
9. Chatziioannou A, Tai YC, Doshi N, Cherry SR. Detector development for microPET II: a 1 microl resolution PET scanner for small animal imaging. Phys Med Biol 2001; 46:2899–2910.
10. Townsend DW, Cherry SR. Combining anatomy and function: the path to true image fusion. Eur Radiol 2001; 11:1968–1974.
11. Weissleder R, Ntziachristos V. Shedding light onto live molecular targets. Nat Med 2003; 9:123–128.
12. Petrovsky A, Schellenberger E, Josephson L, Weissleder R, Bogdanov A Jr. Near-infrared fluorescent imaging of tumor apoptosis. Cancer Res 2003; 63:1936–1942.
13. Warburg O. Metabolism of tumors. In: Smith RR, ed. New York: Richard R. Smith, 1931:129–169.
14. Weber G. Enzymology of cancer cells (second of two parts). N Engl J Med 1977; 296:541–551.
15. Weber G. Enzymology of cancer cells (first of two parts). N Engl J Med 1977; 296:486–492.
16. Mountain CF. Value of the new TNM staging system for lung cancer [published erratum appears in Chest 1990; 97(3):768]. Chest 1989; 96:47s–49s.
17. McKenna RJ Jr, Libshitz HI, Mountain CE, McMurtrey MJ. Roentgenographic evaluation of mediastinal nodes for preoperative assessment in lung cancer. Chest 1985; 88:206–210.
18. Dwamena BA, Sonnad SS, Angobaldo JO, Wahl RL. Metastases from non-small cell lung cancer: mediastinal staging in the 1990s—meta-analytic comparison of PET and CT. Radiology 1999; 213:530–536.
19. Valk PE, Pounds TR, Hopkins DM, Haseman MK, Hofer GA, Greiss HB, Myers RW, Lutrin CL. Staging non-small cell lung cancer by whole-body positron emission tomographic imaging. Ann Thorac Surg 1995; 60:1573–1581; discussion 1581–1582.
20. Weder W, Schmid RA, Bruchhaus H, Hillinger S, von Schulthess GK, Steinert HC. Detection of extrathoracic metastases by positron emission tomography in lung cancer. Ann Thorac Surg 1998; 66:886–892; discussion 892–893.

21. Pieterman RM, van Putten JW, Meuzelaar JJ, Mooyaart EL, Vaalburg W, Koeter GH, Fidler V, Pruim J, Groen HJ. Preoperative staging of non-small-cell lung cancer with positron-emission tomography. N Engl J Med 2000; 343:254–261.

22. van Tinteren H, Hoekstra OS, Smit EF, van den Bergh JH, Schreurs AJ, Stallaert RA, van Velthoven PC, Comans EF, Diepenhorst FW, Verboom P, van Mourik JC, Postmus PE, Boers M, Teule GJ. Effectiveness of positron emission tomography in the preoperative assessment of patients with suspected non-small-cell lung cancer: the PLUS multicentre randomised trial. Lancet 2002; 359:1388–1393.

23. Lardinois D, Weder W, Hany TF, Kamel EM, Korom S, Seifert B, von Schulthess GK, Steinert HC. Staging of non-small-cell lung cancer with integrated positron-emission tomography and computed tomography. N Engl J Med 2003; 348:2500–2507.

24. Hauber HP, Bohuslavizki KH, Lund CH, Fritscher-Ravens A, Meyer A, Pforte A. Positron emission tomography in the staging of small-cell lung cancer: a preliminary study. Chest 2001; 119:950–954.

25. Pandit N, Gonen M, Krug L, Larson SM. Prognostic value of [(18)F]FDG-PET imaging in small cell lung cancer. Eur J Nucl Med Mol Imaging 2003; 30:78–84.

26. MacManus MP, Hicks RJ, Matthews JP, McKenzie A, Rischin D, Salminen EK, Ball DL. Positron emission tomography is superior to computed tomography scanning for response-assessment after radical radiotherapy or chemoradiotherapy in patients with non-small-cell lung cancer. J Clin Oncol 2003; 21:1285–1292.

27. Weber WA, Petersen V, Schmidt B, Tyndale-Hines L, Link T, Peschel C, Schwaiger M. Positron emission tomography in non-small-cell lung cancer: prediction of response to chemotherapy by quantitative assessment of glucose use. J Clin Oncol 2003; 21:2651–2657.

28. Toloza EM, Harpole L, McCrory DC. Noninvasive staging of non-small cell lung cancer: a review of the current evidence. Chest 2003; 123:137S–146S.

29. Schirrmeister H, Glatting G, Hetzel J, Nussle K, Arslandemir C, Buck AK, Dziuk K, Gabelmann A, Reske SN, Hetzel M. Prospective evaluation of the clinical value of planar bone scans, SPECT, and (18)F-labeled NaF PET in newly diagnosed lung cancer. J Nucl Med 2001; 42:1800–1804.

30. Hetzel M, Arslandemir C, Konig HH, Buck AK, Nussle K, Glatting G, Gabelmann A, Hetzel J, Hombach V, Schirrmeister H. F-18 NaF PET for detection of bone metastases in lung cancer: accuracy, cost-effectiveness, and impact on patient management. J Bone Miner Res 2003; 18:2206–2214.

31. Even-Sapir E, Metser U, Flusser G, Zuriel L, Kollender Y, Lerman H, Lievshitz G, Ron I, Mishani E. Assessment of malignant skeletal disease: initial experience with 18F-fluoride PET/CT and comparison between 18F-fluoride PET and 18F-fluoride PET/CT. J Nucl Med 2004; 45:272–278.

32. Hoegerle S, Juengling F, Otte A, Altehoefer C, Moser EA, Nitzsche EU. Combined FDG and [F-18]fluoride whole-body PET: a feasible two-in-one approach to cancer imaging? Radiology 1998; 209:253–258.

33. Jager PL, Vaalburg W, Pruim J, de Vries EG, Langen KJ, Piers DA. Radiolabeled amino acids: basic aspects and clinical applications in oncology. J Nucl Med 2001; 42:432–445.

34. Mastroberardino L, Spindler B, Pfeiffer R, Skelly PJ, Loffing J, Shoemaker CB, Verrey F. Amino-acid transport by heterodimers of 4F2hc/CD98 and members of a permease family. Nature 1998; 395:288–291.

35. Kanai Y, Segawa H, Miyamoto K, Uchino H, Takeda E, Endou H. Expression cloning and characterization of a transporter for large neutral amino acids activated by the heavy chain of 4F2 antigen (CD98). J Biol Chem 1998; 273:23629–23632.
36. Babu E, Kanai Y, Chairoungdua A, Kim do K, Iribe Y, Tangtrongsup S, Jutabha P, Li Y, Ahmed N, Sakamoto S, Anzai N, Nagamori S, Endou H. Identification of a novel system L amino acid transporter structurally distinct from heterodimeric amino acid transporters. J Biol Chem 2003; 278:43838–43845.
37. Yanagida O, Kanai Y, Chairoungdua A, Kim DK, Segawa H, Nii T, Cha SH, Matsuo H, Fukushima J, Fukasawa Y, Tani Y, Taketani Y, Uchino H, Kim JY, Inatomi J, Okayasu I, Miyamoto K, Takeda E, Goya T, Endou H. Human L-type amino acid transporter 1 (LAT1): characterization of function and expression in tumor cell lines. Biochim Biophys Acta 2001; 1514:291–302.
38. Shikano N, Kanai Y, Kawai K, Inatomi J, Kim do, K, Ishikawa N, Endou H. Isoform selectivity of 3-125I-iodo-alpha-methyl-L-tyrosine membrane transport in human L-type amino acid transporters. J Nucl Med 2003; 44:244–246.
39. Yee RE, Cheng DW, Huang SC, Namavari M, Satyamurthy N, Barrio JR. Blood-brain barrier and neuronal membrane transport of 6-[18F]fluoro-L-DOPA. Biochem Pharmacol 2001; 62:1409–1415.
40. Becherer A, Karanikas G, Szabo M, Zettinig G, Asenbaum S, Marosi C, Henk C, Wunderbaldinger P, Czech T, Wadsak W, Kletter K. Brain tumour imaging with PET: a comparison between [18F]fluorodopa and [11C]methionine. Eur J Nucl Med Mol Imaging 2003; 30:1561–1567.
41. Grosu A, Weber W, Feldmann HJ, Wuttke B, Bartenstein P, Gross MW, Lumenta C, Schwaiger M, Molls M. First experience with 1-123-alpha-methyl-tyrosine SPECT in the 3-D radiation treatment planning of brain gliomas. Int J Radiat Oncol Biol Phys 2000; 47:517–526.
42. Langen KJ, Clauss RP, Holschbach M, Muhlensiepen H, Kiwit JC, Zilles K, Coenen HH, Muller-Gartner HW. Comparison of iodotyrosines and methionine uptake in a rat glioma model. J Nucl Med 1998; 39:1596–1599.
43. Weber W, Wester H, Grosu A, Herz M, Dzewas B, Feldmann H, Molls M, Stoecklin G, Schwaiger M. O-(2-[18F]fluoroethyl)-L-tyrosine and L-[methyl-11C] methionine uptake in brain tumors: initial results of a comparative PET study. Eur J Nucl Med 2000; 27:542–549.
44. Rau F, Ziegler S, Weber W, Daum S, Herz M, Wester H, Schwaiger M, Senekowitsch-Schmidtke R. *In vivo* differentiation of tumor and inflammation by 18F-fluoroethyl--tyrosine PET with a small animal PET scanner. J Nucl Med 2001; 42:1070P.
45. Kubota R, Kubota K, Yamada S, Tada M, Ido T, Tamahashi N. Microautoradiographic study for the differentiation of intratumoral macrophages, granulation tissues and cancer cells by the dynamics of fluorine-18-fluorodeoxyglucose uptake. J Nucl Med 1994; 35:104–112.
46. Kubota K, Matsuzawa T, Fujiwara T, Abe Y, Ito M, Hatazawa J, Ido T, Ishiwata K, Watanuki S. Differential diagnosis of solitary pulmonary nodules with positron emission tomography using [11C]L-methionine. J Comput Assist Tomogr 1988; 12:794–796.
47. Nettelbladt OS, Sundin AE, Valind SO, Gustafsson GR, Lamberg K, Langstrom B, Bjornsson EH. Combined fluorine-18-FDG and carbon-11-methionine PET for diagnosis of tumors in lung and mediastinum. J Nucl Med 1998; 39:640–647.

48. Yasukawa T, Yoshikawa K, Aoyagi H, Yamamoto N, Tamura K, Suzuki K, Tsujii H, Murata H, Sasaki Y, Fujisawa T. Usefulness of PET with 11C-methionine for the detection of hilar and mediastinal lymph node metastasis in lung cancer. J Nucl Med 2000; 41:283–290.

49. Pieterman R, Willemsen A, Appel M, Pruim J, Koeter G, Vaalburg W, Groen H. Visualisation and assessment of the protein synthesis rate of lung cancer using carbon-11 tyrosine and positron emission tomography. Eur J Nucl Med Mol Imaging 2002; 29:243–247.

50. Hara T, Yuasa M. Automated synthesis of [11C]choline, a positron-emitting tracer for tumor imaging. Appl Radiat Isot 1999; 50:531–533.

51. DeGrado TR, Coleman RE, Wang S, Baldwin SW, Orr MD, Robertson CN, Polascik TJ, Price DT. Synthesis and evaluation of 18F-labeled choline as an oncologic tracer for positron emission tomography: initial findings in prostate cancer. Cancer Res 2001; 61:110–117.

52. Hara T, Kosaka N, Kishi H. Development of (18)F-fluoroethylcholine for cancer imaging with PET: synthesis, biochemistry, and prostate cancer imaging. J Nucl Med 2002; 43:187–199.

53. Roivainen A, Forsback S, Gronroos T, Lehikoinen P, Kahkonen M, Sutinen E, Minn H. Blood metabolism of [methyl-11C]choline: implications for *in vivo* imaging with positron emission tomography. Eur J Nucl Med 2000; 27:25–32.

54. Zheng QH, Stone KL, Mock BH, Miller KD, Fei X, Liu X, Wang JQ, Glick-Wilson BE, Sledge GW, Hutchins GD. [11C]Choline as a potential PET marker for imaging of breast cancer athymic mice. Nucl Med Biol 2002; 29:803–807.

55. Picchio M, Messa C, Landoni C, Gianolli L, Sironi S, Brioschi M, Matarrese M, Matei DV, De Cobelli F, Del Maschio A, Rocco F, Rigatti P, Fazio F. Value of [11C]choline-positron emission tomography for re-staging prostate cancer: a comparison with [18F]fluorodeoxyglucose-positron emission tomography. J Urol 2003; 169:1337–1340.

56. Seltzer MA, Barbaric Z, Belldegrun A, Naitoh J, Dorey F, Phelps ME, Gambhir SS, Hoh CK. Comparison of helical computerized tomography, positron emission tomography and monoclonal antibody scans for evaluation of lymph node metastases in patients with prostate specific antigen relapse after treatment for localized prostate cancer. J Urol 1999; 162:1322–1328.

57. Kotzerke J, Volkmer BG, Glatting G, van den Hoff J, Gschwend JE, Messer P, Reske SN, Neumaier B. Intraindividual comparison of [11C]acetate and [11C]choline PET for detection of metastases of prostate cancer. Nuklearmedizin 2003; 42:25–30.

58. Hara T, Kosaka N, Suzuki T, Kudo K, Niino H. Uptake rates of 18F-fluorodeoxyglucose and 11C-choline in lung cancer and pulmonary tuberculosis: a positron emission tomography study. Chest 2003; 124:893–901.

59. Khan N, Oriuchi N, Zhang H, Higuchi T, Tian M, Inoue T, Sato N, Endo K. A comparative study of 11C-choline PET and [18F]fluorodeoxyglucose PET in the evaluation of lung cancer. Nucl Med Commun 2003; 24:359–366.

60. Pieterman RM, Que TH, Elsinga PH, Pruim J, van Putten JW, Willemsen AT, Vaalburg W, Groen HJ. Comparison of (11)C-choline and (18)F-FDG PET in primary diagnosis and staging of patients with thoracic cancer. J Nucl Med 2002; 43:167–172.

61. Wyss MT, Weber B, Honer M, Spath N, Ametamey SM, Westera G, Bode B, Kaim AH, Buck A. 18F-choline in experimental soft tissue infection assessed with autoradiography and high-resolution PET. Eur J Nucl Med Mol Imaging 2004; 31:312–316.

62. Roivainen A, Parkkola R, Yli-Kerttula T, Lehikoinen P, Viljanen T, Mottonen T, Nuutila P, Minn H. Use of positron emission tomography with methyl-11C-choline and 2-18F-fluoro-2-deoxy-D-glucose in comparison with magnetic resonance imaging for the assessment of inflammatory proliferation of synovium. Arthritis Rheum 2003; 48:3077–3084.

63. Lu L, Samuelsson L, Bergstrom M, Sato K, Fasth KJ, Langstrom B. Rat studies comparing 11C-FMAU, 18F-FLT, and 76Br-BFU as proliferation markers. J Nucl Med 2002; 43:1688–1698.

64. Shields AF, Grierson JR, Dohmen BM, Machulla HJ, Stayanoff JC, Lawhorn-Crews JM, Obradovich JE, Muzik O, Mangner TJ. Imaging proliferation *in vivo* with [F-18]FLT and positron emission tomography. Nat Med 1998; 4:1334–1336.

65. Sherley JL, Kelly TJ. Regulation of human thymidine kinase during the cell cycle. J Biol Chem 1988; 263:8350–8358.

66. Rasey JS, Grierson JR, Wiens LW, Kolb PD, Schwartz JL. Validation of FLT uptake as a measure of thymidine kinase-1 activity in A549 carcinoma cells. J Nucl Med 2002; 43:1210–1217.

67. Waldherr C, Safaei A, Mellinghoff I, Tran C, Phelps M, Sawyers C, Czernin J. Micro-PET with 18F-FLT and 18F-FDG for monitoring targeted tumor therapy in SCIC mice. Society of Nuclear Medicine Annual Meeting, New Orleans, LA, June 2003.

68. Schwartz JL, Tamura Y, Jordan R, Grierson JR, Krohn KA. Monitoring tumor cell proliferation by targeting DNA synthetic processes with thymidine and thymidine analogs. J Nucl Med 2003; 44:2027–2032.

69. Dittmann H, Dohmen BM, Paulsen F, Eichhorn K, Eschmann SM, Horger M, Wehrmann M, Machulla HJ, Bares R. [18F]FLT PET for diagnosis and staging of thoracic tumours. Eur J Nucl Med Mol Imaging 2003; 30:1407–1412.

70. Buck AK, Halter G, Schirrmeister H, Kotzerke J, Wurziger I, Glatting G, Mattfeldt T, Neumaier B, Reske SN, Hetzel M. Imaging proliferation in lung tumors with PET: 18F-FLT versus 18F-FDG. J Nucl Med 2003; 44:1426–1431.

71. Visvikis D, Francis D, Mulligan R, Costa DC, Croasdale I, Luthra SK, Taylor I, Ell PJ. Comparison of methodologies for the *in vivo* assessment of (18)FLT utilisation in colorectal cancer. Eur J Nucl Med Mol Imaging 2003; 31:169–178.

72. Pio B, Park C, Pietras J, Satyamurthy N, Pegram M, Czernin J, Phelps M, Silverman D. Five minutes of imaging with [F-18]fluoro-L-thymidine predicts long-term post-therapy response in breast cancer patients, Society of Nuclear Medicine Annual Meeting, Philadelphia, PA, June 2004.

73. McCarthy TJ, Sheriff AU, Graneto MJ, Talley JJ, Welch MJ. Radiosynthesis, *in vitro* validation, and *in vivo* evaluation of 18F-labeled COX-1 and COX-2 inhibitors. J Nucl Med 2002; 43:117–124.

74. Schlessinger J. Cell signaling by receptor tyrosine kinases. Cell 2000; 103:211–225.

75. Manning G, Whyte DB, Martinez R, Hunter T, Sudarsanam S. The protein kinase complement of the human genome. Science 2002; 298:1912–1934.

76. Carpenter G. Receptors for epidermal growth factor and other polypeptide mitogens. Annu Rev Biochem 1987; 56:881–914.

77. Porter AC, Vaillancourt RR. Tyrosine kinase receptor-activated signal transduction pathways which lead to oncogenesis. Oncogene 1998; 17:1343–1352.

78. Heldin CH, Westermark B. Growth factors: mechanism of action and relation to oncogenes. Cell 1984; 37:9–20.

79. Levitt ML, Koty PP. Tyrosine kinase inhibitors in preclinical development. Invest New Drugs 1999; 17:213–226.

80. Druker BJ, Talpaz M, Resta DJ, Peng B, Buchdunger E, Ford JM, Lydon NB, Kantarjian H, Capdeville R, Ohno-Jones S, Sawyers CL. Efficacy and safety of a specific inhibitor of the BCR-ABL tyrosine kinase in chronic myeloid leukemia. N Engl J Med 2001; 344:1031–1037.

81. Saleem A, Yap J, Osman S, Brady F, Suttle B, Lucas SV, Jones T, Price PM, Aboagye EO. Modulation of fluorouracil tissue pharmacokinetics by eniluracil: in-vivo imaging of drug action. Lancet 2000; 355:2125–2131.

82. Shani J, Wolf W. A model for prediction of chemotherapy response to 5-fluorouracil based on the differential distribution of 5-[18F]fluorouracil in sensitive versus resistant lymphocytic leukemia in mice. Cancer Res 1977; 37:2306–2308.

83. Hohenberger P, Strauss LG, Lehner B, Frohmuller S, Dimitrakopoulou A, Schlag P. Perfusion of colorectal liver metastases and uptake of fluorouracil assessed by H2(15)O and [18F]uracil positron emission tomography (PET). Eur J Cancer 1993; 12:1682–1686.

84. Dimitrakopoulou A, Strauss LG, Clorius JH, Ostertag H, Schlag P, Heim M, Oberdorfer F, Helus F, Haberkorn U, van Kaick G. Studies with positron emission tomography after systemic administration of fluorine-18-uracil in patients with liver metastases from colorectal carcinoma. J Nucl Med 1993; 34:1075–1081.

85. van der Flier A, Sonnenberg A. Function and interactions of integrins. Cell Tissue Res 2001; 305:285–298.

86. Eliceiri BP, Cheresh DA. The role of alpha v integrins during angiogenesis: insights into potential mechanisms of action and clinical development. J Clin Invest 1999; 103:1227–1230.

87. Felding-Habermann B, Mueller BM, Romerdahl CA, Cheresh DA. Involvement of integrin alpha V gene expression in human melanoma tumorigenicity. J Clin Invest 1992; 89:2018–2022.

88. Plow EF, Haas TA, Zhang L, Loftus J, Smith JW. Ligand binding to integrins. J Biol Chem 2000; 275:21785–21788.

89. Xiong JP, Stehle T, Zhang R, Joachimiak A, Frech M, Goodman SL, Arnaout MA. Crystal structure of the extracellular segment of integrin alpha Vbeta3 in complex with an Arg-Gly-Asp ligand. Science 2002; 296:151–155.

90. Haubner RH, Wester HJ, Weber WA, Schwaiger M. Radiotracer-based strategies to image angiogenesis. Q J Nucl Med 2003; 47:189–199.

91. Haubner R, Wester H, Weber W, Ziegler S, Senekowitsch-Schmidtke R, Kessler H, Schwaiger M. Non-invasive imaging of avb3 integrin expression using a 18F-labeled RGD-containing glycopeptide and positron emission tomography. Cancer Res 2001; 61:1781–1785.

Index